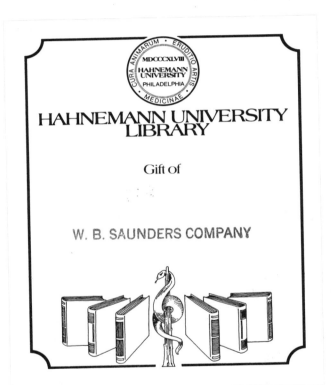

Surgical Obstetrics

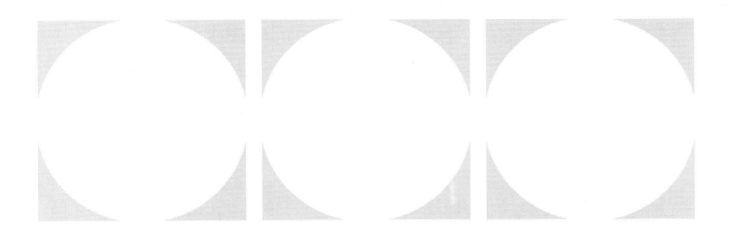

Illustrated by EUGENE NEW
Photography by RITA LETELLIER

WARREN C. PLAUCHÉ, M.D.
Associate Dean for Clinical Affairs
Professor, Department of Obstetrics and
Gynecology
Louisiana State University Medical Center
School of Medicine
New Orleans, Louisiana

JOHN C. MORRISON, M.D.
Professor of Obstetrics and Gynecology
Division of Maternal–Fetal Medicine
University of Mississippi Medical Center
Jackson, Mississippi

MARY JO O'SULLIVAN, M.D.
Professor and Director of Obstetrics
Perinatal Division
Department of Obstetrics and Gynecology
University of Miami School of Medicine
Miami, Florida

Surgical Obstetrics

W.B. SAUNDERS COMPANY
Harcourt Brace Jovanovich, Inc.

Philadelphia London Toronto Montreal Sydney Tokyo

W. B. SAUNDERS COMPANY
Harcourt Brace Jovanovich, Inc.

The Curtis Center
Independence Square West
Philadelphia, Pennsylvania 19106

Editor: W. B. Saunders Staff
Designer: Ellen Bodner-Zanolle
Production Manager: Linda R. Garber
Manuscript Editor: Karen Neff
Illustration Specialist: Lisa Lambert
Indexer: Nancy Weaver

Surgical Obstetrics   ISBN 0–7216–3049–9

Printed in Mexico.

Last digit is the print number: 9   8   7   6   5   4   3   2   1

The senior author dedicates this book to his teachers:

To Michael Newton, M.D. (deceased),
who taught the basics,

To Frank G. Gruich, M.D.,
who polished a very rough apprentice surgeon,

To Abe Mickal, M.D.,
who opened the door to academic medicine,

To a generation of obstetric residents
who inspired truth and strove for excellence.

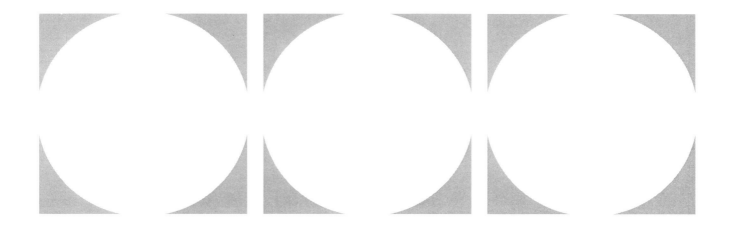

Contributors

ALFRED ABUHAMAD, M.D.
Fellow, Maternal-Fetal Medicine, University of Miami School of Medicine, Department of Obstetrics and Gynecology, Miami, Florida. Fellow, Maternal-Fetal Medicine, Jackson Memorial Hospital, Miami.
Operative Techniques for Cesarean Section

HAYWOOD L. BROWN, M.D.
Associate Professor, Maternal-Fetal Medicine, Indiana University School of Medicine, Department of Obstetrics and Gynecology, Indianapolis, Indiana. Director of Obstetric Services, Wishard Memorial Hospital, Indianapolis.
Pregnancy Termination; Puerperal Tubal Sterilization

ROBERT C. CEFALO, M.D., Ph.D.
Professor of Obstetrics and Gynecology and Assistant Dean, Office of Graduate Medical Education, University of North Carolina School of Medicine, Chapel Hill, North Carolina. Director of Maternal-Fetal Medicine, University of North Carolina Hospitals, Chapel Hill.
Anesthesia for Obstetrics

JANE CHUEH, M.D.
Assistant Professor, Obstetrics and Gynecology, University of California, San Francisco, California.
Fetal Invasive Procedures

BRYAN D. COWAN, M.D.
Associate Professor and Director, Division of Reproductive Endocrinology, Department of Obstetrics and Gynecology, University of Mississippi Medical Center, Jackson, Mississippi; Associate Professor of Obstetrics and Gynecology, University of Mississippi, Jackson. Staff Physician, Department of Obstetrics and Gynecology, Veterans Administration Medical Center, Jackson; Staff Physician, Department of Obstetrics and Gynecology, Mississippi Methodist Hospital and Rehabilitation Center, Inc., Jackson.
Management of Tubal Pregnancy

RANDALL C. FLOYD, M.D.
Fellow, Division of Maternal-Fetal Medicine, Department of Obstetrics and Gynecology, University of Mississippi Medical Center, Jackson, Mississippi.
Postpartum Hemorrhage

HARVEY A. GABERT, M.D.
Professor and Head, Division of Maternal-Fetal Medicine, Louisiana State University School of Medicine, New Orleans, Louisiana; Staff Physician, Southern Baptist Hospital and Charity Hospital, New Orleans.
Complications Common to Obstetric Operative Procedures

THOMAS J. GARITE, M.D.

Department of Obstetrics and Gynecology, University of California College of Medicine, Irvine, California.
Surgical Correction of Uterine Anomalies

RAYMOND F. GASSER, Ph.D.

Professor of Anatomy, Louisiana State University School of Medicine, New Orleans, Louisiana.
Surgical Obstetric Anatomy

LARRY C. GILSTRAP III, M.D.

Professor, Obstetrics and Gynecology and Director of Maternal-Fetal Medicine Fellowship and Clinical Genetics, University of Texas Southwestern Medical Center at Dallas, Dallas, Texas.
Placental Abnormalities: Previa, Abruption, and Accreta

MITCHELL S. GOLBUS, M.D.

Professor Department of Obstetrics and Gynecology, University of California, San Francisco, School of Medicine, San Francisco, California.
Fetal Invasive Procedures

VERDA J. HUNTER, M.D.

Assistant Professor of Gynecology and Obstetrics, Division of Gynecologic Oncology, University of Kansas College of Medicine, Kansas City, Kansas. Staff Physician, University of Kansas Medical Center, Kansas City; University of Missouri–Kansas City College of Medicine, Kansas City, Missouri.
Surgical Management of Trophoblastic Disease

DAVID N. JACKSON, M.D.

Department of Obstetrics and Gynecology, University of California College of Medicine, Irvine, California.
Surgical Correction of Uterine Anomalies

ROBERT JOHNSON, M.D.

Clinical Instructor, Department of Obstetrics and Gynecology, University of Miami School of Medicine, Miami, Florida. Jackson Memorial Hospital, Miami.
Vaginal Delivery of Twins

JAMES N. MARTIN Jr., M.D.

Professor and Director, Division of Maternal-Fetal Medicine, University of Mississippi School of Medicine, Jackson, Mississippi.
Nonobstetric Abdominal Surgery During Pregnancy

JOSEPH M. MILLER, Jr., M.D.

Professor of Obstetrics and Gynecology, Louisiana State University Medical Center, New Orleans, Louisiana. Medical Director of Obstetrics and Nurseries, Charity Hospital at New Orleans; Consultant Perinatologist, Southern Baptist Hospital, New Orleans.
Identification and Delivery of the Macrosomic Infant

JOHN C. MORRISON, M.D.

Professor of Obstetrics and Gynecology, Division of Maternal-Fetal Medicine, University of Mississippi Medical Center, Jackson, Mississippi.
Management of Tubal Pregnancy; Postpartum Hemorrhage

MARY JO O'SULLIVAN, M.D.

Professor and Director of Obstetrics, Perinatal Division, Department of Obstetrics and Gynecology, University of Miami School of Medicine, Miami, Florida.
Assisted Breech Extraction; Vaginal Delivery of Twins; Cesarean Section: History, Incidence, and Indications; Operative Techniques for Cesarean Section; Problems Encountered During Cesarean Delivery

JOSEPH G. PASTOREK II, M.D.

Associate Professor of Obstetrics and Gynecology; Chief, Section of Infectious Disease; Member, Section of Maternal-Fetal Medicine, Louisiana State University Medical Center, New Orleans, Louisiana.
Puerperal Tubal Sterilization

WARREN C. PLAUCHÉ, M.D.

Professor of Obstetrics and Gynecology and Executive Associate Dean for Clinical Affairs, Louisiana State University, School of Medicine, New Orleans, Louisiana. President of Staff, Charity Hospital, New Orleans.
Teaching Clinical Competence in Obstetric Surgery; Wound Management and Basic Surgical Principles; Extratubal Ectopic Gestation; Surgical Problems Involving the Pregnant Uterus: Uterine Inversion, Uterine Rupture, and Leiomyomas; Forceps Delivery; Vacuum Extraction; Operative Vaginal Delivery of Abnormal Vertex Presentations; Episiotomy and Repair; Obstetric Genital Trauma; Peripartal Hysterectomy

KAREN A. RAIMER, M.D.

Fellow, Maternal-Fetal Medicine, Department of Obstetrics and Gynecology, University of Miami/Jackson Memorial Hospital, Miami, Florida.
Cesarean Section: History, Incidence, and Indications

SUSAN M. RAMIN, M.D.

Assistant Professor of Obstetrics and Gynecology, University of Texas Southwestern Medical Center at Dallas, Dallas, Texas.
Placental Abnormalities: Previa, Abruption, and Accreta

STERLING E. SIGHTLER, M.D.

Staff Physician, Women's Hospital, Our Lady of the Lake Regional Medical Center, Baton Rouge General Medical Center, Medical Center of Baton Rouge, Baton Rouge, Louisiana.
Clinical Pelvimetry

FRED J. SPIELMAN, M.D.

Associate Professor of Anesthesiology and Obstetrics and Gynecology, University of North Carolina School of Medicine, Chapel Hill, North Carolina. Staff Anesthesiologist, University of North Carolina Hospitals, Chapel Hill.
Anesthesia for Obstetrics

DAVID L. WALTON, M.D.

Fellow, Maternal-Fetal Medicine, Department of Obstetrics and Gynecology, University of Miami School of Medicine, Miami, Florida.
Problems Encountered During Cesarean Delivery

JOHN C. WEED Jr., M.D.

Professor of Gynecology and Obstetrics and Director of the Division of Gynecologic Oncology, University of Kansas College of Medicine, Kansas City, Kansas. Staff Physician, University of Kansas Medical Center and University of Missouri–Kansas City College of Medicine, Kansas City, Missouri.
Surgical Management of Trophoblastic Disease

SALIH YASIN, M.D.

Assistant Professor of Clinical Obstetrics and Gynecology, Division of Maternal-Fetal Medicine, University of Miami School of Medicine, Miami, Florida. Attending Physician, Obstetrics and Gynecology, Medical Director/Postpartum Service at the University of Miami/Jackson Memorial Medical Center, Miami.
Assisted Breech Extraction; Problems Encountered During Cesarean Delivery

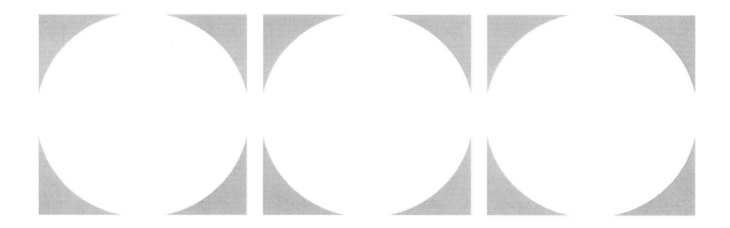

Acknowledgments

The authors wish to acknowledge the dedicated work of our photographer Rita Letellier and our graphic artist, Eugene New.

We gratefully acknowledge the help of our Editors at W.B. Saunders, Darlene Pedersen, Martin Wonsiewicz, and Joan Meyer, and the careful work of their designers, artists, copy editors, and printers.

Special thanks to our manuscript managers, Connie Rivette, Louise Baker, Donna Williams, and Liz Small.

We thank the contributors to this volume whose life's work shines upon these pages.

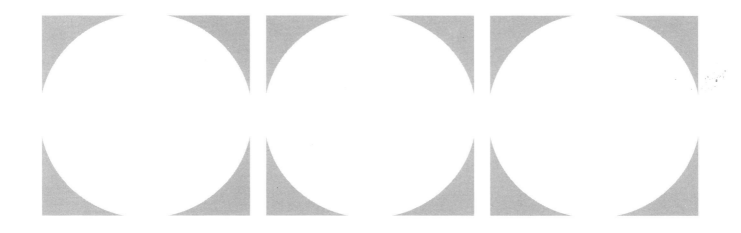

Preface

I HEAR, I FORGET
I SEE, I REMEMBER
I DO, I UNDERSTAND

Haida Tribal Proverb

Obstetric surgery has an illustrious history marked by long periods of slow, steady progress and times of pivotal change. We are entering an era of such change.

Obstetricians of the present replace many of the arts and skills of operative vaginal delivery with those of abdominal delivery. Training programs teach few transvaginal manipulations of the fetus and only the simplest of forceps maneuvers. Breech extraction and vaginal delivery of twins have all but disappeared from the training of a generation of obstetricians. These skills should not be lost.

This book describes many obstetric skills, old and new, in the terminology of modern obstetrics. A unique first chapter deals with methods of teaching obstetric surgical skills to trainees at all levels.

The number of cesarean births continues at an unprecedented rise. Pressure is building from colleagues and consumers to reduce the rate of cesarean delivery. This book reexamines the dictum, "Once a cesarean, always a cesarean" that governed the decisions of obstetricians for 50 years. A new slogan, "Vaginal birth after cesarean (VBAC)," competes to replace the old tenet. Such inclusive slogans necessitate the kind of comprehensive examination found in this book.

Vaginal births after cesareans only affect repeat cesarean deliveries. Reduction in primary cesarean births necessitates renewed interest in and acceptance of vaginal operative deliveries. Training in operative vaginal procedures is a prerequisite to safe reduction of abdominal delivery rates.

Those contemplating a renaissance in training in operative vaginal delivery will find help in several chapters. Clinical pelvimetry is reassessed as a useful prognostic tool. Basic anatomy and principles of anesthesiology are reviewed. Procedures are described for vaginal delivery of twins, breech extraction, and emergency operative vaginal deliveries. Forceps maneuvers and vacuum extraction are described in detail.

This book also describes procedures to manage obstetric emergencies such as postpartum hemorrhage, shoulder dystocia, uterine inversion, and uterine rupture. The obstetrician repeatedly exercises clinical judgment in every difficult case. *Surgical Obstetrics* emphasizes obstetric judgment and facilitates decision making.

Intrauterine fetal surgery, fetal blood sampling and direct transfusion, and chorionic villus sampling are among the newest obstetric surgical procedures. This book offers an introduction to these procedures, which define the leading edge of the specialty.

This book was written for obstetric students, residents, fellows, and their teachers. Together we advance surgical obstetrics.

WARREN C. PLAUCHÉ, M.D.

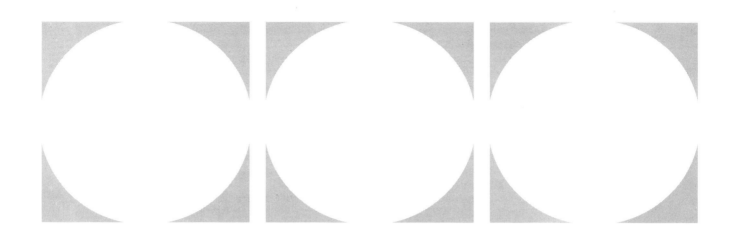

Contents

I

Surgical Principles

Teaching Clinical Competence in Obstetric Surgery

Warren C. Plauché

- DEFINITION OF CLINICAL COMPETENCE
- SURGICAL APPRENTICESHIP MODEL
- COMPONENTS OF CLINICAL COMPETENCE
- EVALUATION OF SURGICAL COMPETENCE
- GRANTING SURGICAL PRIVILEGES AND
  CREDENTIALING
- ROLE OF THE SURGICAL TEACHER

  Surgical Problem-Solving Skills
  Procedural Skills
- PATIENT-CENTERED SURGICAL TEACHING
- ALTERNATIVES TO PATIENT-CENTERED
  SURGICAL TEACHING
- CONCLUSIONS

DEFINITION OF CLINICAL COMPETENCE IN OBSTETRIC SURGERY

The word *clinical,* in *Webster's New Universal Unabridged Dictionary (2nd Edition. New York: Simon & Schuster, 1979.)* refers to ". . . medical practice based on actual treatment and observation of patients, as distinguished from experimental or laboratory study." The first definition of the word *competence* is "capacity equal to requirement." The root word is the Latin verb, competere, meaning "to strive together." These basic definitions can be combined to characterize the phrase *clinical competence* as "striving together to develop medical practice capacity equal to requirements."

Defining clinical competence is clearly not as simple as defining its component words. Senior,[1] in a conference sponsored by the National Board of Medical Examiners, stated that "the definition of competence has been an incomplete concept. . . . There are those who doubt whether competence really is a definable entity."

SURGICAL APPRENTICESHIP MODEL

Historical examples of evaluation and transference of surgical competence seem simple at first examination. An apprenticeship model has always dominated surgical training systems. Generations of surgeons acquired surgical competence by observing master surgeons and emulating their work under supervision.

Residency programs grew from early attempts by Osler and Halsted at Johns Hopkins to codify and focus medical and surgical apprenticeship training. The "house officer" was created so that trainees could observe the course of disease first-hand over extended periods of time. Surgical decisions and manual skills of trainees were examined by the observations of peers and supervisors during all levels of training.

A system developed that granted surgical privileges to trainees when their performance of surgical tasks was deemed adequate by peers and supervisors. Responsibility and privilege progressed at a rate commensurate with observed, demonstrated knowledge and skill. These principles still govern surgical competency evaluation in most current surgical programs. The ultimate responsibility for certification of clinical competency of residents and granting of surgical privileges in such a system rests with the attending surgical staff.

Regulating and supervising agencies and committees insist on clarification of the parameters of clinical competence that they are asked to certify. The evaluation of competence has become a national health management priority. Subjective traditional evaluation of competence is no longer accepted.

The traditional evaluation method of observed performance is being questioned on the grounds of subjectivity and lack of validity and reliability.[9, 10] Alternative evaluation systems suggest that competency is more accurately assessed by methods such as chart reviews and peer questionnaires. These studies include examination of elements of the system environment (equipment, consultants, nursing, support staff, and transport) as well as the skills of the physician.[11] Patient simulations, computerized management problems, and written tests examine clinical database acquisition and decision efficiency. Each approach contributes some information on specific elements of competency; none describes the complete, competent physician.

Evaluation specialists have attempted to apply the principles of educational evaluation and psychometrics to the task of improving competence evaluation. Educational and psychometric terminology, when applied to issues of medical competence, sometimes confuse rather than facilitate understanding by clinicians.

The following definition illustrates this terminology barrier: "A theory of clinical competence is defined as a measurement model containing one or more operationally defined constructs structurally inter-related to maximize the prediction or explanation of subsequent clinical performance."[2] Despite interpretation difficulties, educational and psychometric disciplines have important insights to offer physicians charged with the evaluation of medical and surgical competence. Competence evaluation couched in clinical terms facilitates both understanding and progress.

The American Board of Orthopedic Surgery was the first supervising agency of a clinical discipline to investigate the validity of its method of clinical competence evaluation. Levine and co-workers[3] found five resident clinical activities that best correlated with performance on subsequent orthopedic board certification examinations. The factors identified were general ability, general knowledge, inductive reasoning ability, performance on oral examinations, and decisiveness/efficiency.[3]

Subsequent studies in other clinical fields supported or negated the importance of one or more of these factors. Several theories of competence measurement emerged from these studies.

Ebel held that all tests measure only knowledge factors and that competence is just a form of special knowledge.[1] Senior[1] believed that knowledge factors correlated, albeit weakly, with general performance.[2] Maatsch proposed three active factors, knowledge, reasoning ability, and clinical performance.[4] Levine and McGuire insisted that all five factors cited by Levine's original proposal be considered in the evaluation of clinical competence.[3, 5]

Maatsch and Huang investigated the construct validity of these four competing theories of the components of clinical competence.[1] They concluded that "measurement of a general competence factor (in contrast to multiple specific ability or skill tests) is the most accurate method of predicting subsequent job performance." These investigators advised medical educators to "decompose the sophisticated, goal-oriented clinical interaction process into component tasks and skills in order to teach and evaluate mastery of those components in an orderly medical education curriculum."

The American Medical Association held a national conference on physician competence and its assessment in 1989. A number of complex and intricate methods of evaluation based on psychometric theory were presented. Petersdorf,[6] discussing the evaluation of clinical competence, questioned whether or not "we have become slaves to the psychometric gymnastics." He affirmed his belief in clinical skills assessment. He expressed concern that "we are applying standards which are psychometrically so strict that we cannot succeed."

Gonella,[7] in the same discussion, confirmed that "we have made our faculties so uneasy about the limitations of evaluation that they are tempted not to evaluate at all." Melnick[8] described an "undue awe of the number-crunching psychometricians by clinicians."

All of the above statements point to problems when we try to reduce the evaluation of clinical competence to an exercise "by the numbers."

Evaluating clinical competence is an important task for physicians. Resident credentialing issues are increasingly important to teaching hospitals. Liability issues bring pressure on hospitals to be certain that procedures are done or supervised by properly certified practitioners. Hospital and residency accreditation agencies encourage documentation of clinical competence and clear definition of privileges for both attending staff and residents. Training programs continue to search for accurate, objective ways to evaluate and document the attainment of clinical surgical competence.

THE COMPONENTS OF CLINICAL COMPETENCE

Tables 1–1, 1–2, and 1–3 outline some of the characteristics that describe clinical competence, as viewed by an obstetric surgeon. The obstetric surgeon must know how to, when to, and when not to operate. Most simply expressed, the obstetric surgeon must know what to do.

Ebel argued that "the knowledge of what to do is a major element in competence to do, and hence in performance."[1] His comment arose in discussions of the use and limitations of computer evaluation of clinical competence. The comment is even more to the point when directed at surgical skills.

Knowing what to do has many facets, as seen in Tables 1–1 to 1–3. Sufficient knowledge base, ability to gather data, and good problem-solving skills are necessary.

The knowledge base required in surgical disciplines begins with the basic sciences. Principles

Table 1–1. CHARACTERISTICS OF SURGICAL COMPETENCE

Knowing What Operation To Perform
Sufficient knowledge base
Background science—anatomy, physiology, pharmacology
Treatment alternatives
Data-gathering skills
Physical examination, laboratory, imaging, and ancillary services
Human interaction and communication
Problem-solving abilities
Application of history and examination of findings
Evaluation of laboratory and other data
Reasonable differential diagnostic choices
Reasonable treatment options and choices
Flexibility to change with new information and conditions
Resolution of complications and crises

Table 1–2. CHARACTERISTICS OF SURGICAL COMPETENCE

Knowing How To Do the Operation
Manual skills
Surgical skills appropriate to the task, alternative operations and complications
General support skills
Performance in crisis conditions

such as surgical anatomy, wound healing, fluid and electrolyte physiology, and drug effects and reactions are indispensible to the surgeon's armamentarium. One could make a long list of such knowledge requirements. Such a list for training in obstetrics and gynecology is contained in the educational objectives of the Council on Resident Education in Obstetrics and Gynecology (CREOG).[12]

The surgeon must be skilled at gathering information. He or she seeks all possible clues from the patient's history and supplements these with information obtained by physical examination, imaging, and laboratory testing. The surgeon must possess the ability to synthesize and interpret this information.

Once the case-specific information is gathered, collated, and processed, the surgeon must be able to formulate a plan to address the problem. The plan must include a reasonable differential diagnosis list and action items to establish working and definitive diagnoses. The surgeon must have the flexibility to change his or her plan with changing information and circumstances. He or she must be able to act reasonably in times of crisis.

Surgeons must possess the physical skills to perform the required operations. They must know their limitations and know when to seek consultation. All surgical activities require drive and energy that must be sustained under critical and changing circumstances.

The obstetric surgeon must know when obstetric problems necessitate operative intervention. This implies both recognition of conditions and choice of the correct moment to intervene in the course of a developing disorder. Knowing when not to operate is of equal importance.

Absolute personal and medical honesty, integrity, and ethical behavior are needed for proper implementation of these decisions. A very complex

Table 1–3. CHARACTERISTICS OF SURGICAL COMPETENCE

Knowing When To Operate
Knowledge of when to operate and when not to
Absolute clinical honesty
Ethical behavior
Resolve and motivation
Sensitivity to ethical, moral, and religious issues
Dependability and availability
Clinical flexibility when faced with situational changes

set of human activities emerges as one reviews the many elements of surgical competence.

EVALUATION OF CLINICAL COMPETENCE

The most difficult evaluations in medical education are the assessment of the student in clerkship and the evaluation of clinical competence of house officers. The number of factors involved in clinical competence and their interactions are complex and change continuously during training. The competence of house officers in training defies stipulation that is both completely accurate and completely current. This difficulty conflicts with the urgent requests of regulating agencies for minutely accurate delineation of surgical privileges for residents based on competency evaluation.

It is possible to recognize surgical competence. Such recognition depends on observation by qualified surgeons trained in the same discipline. Good obstetric surgeons can recognize the level of surgical skills of trainees and peers by direct observation of obstetric surgical procedures.

Close observation at the operating table yields a clear initial impression of the operator's skills. First impressions are modified by observed changes in the performance characteristics of the trainee over time. Such evaluation is admittedly subjective, complex, and difficult to describe. It is subject to human error and bias. Firsthand estimations of surgical skills by peers are our best, most valid, and most useful clinical evaluation tools.

Extremes of surgical competence or incompetence are the easiest traits to recognize. It is more difficult to stratify degrees of competence across the middle range. Perhaps this level of microdifferentiation is not necessary. We are usually asked simply to identify competence, not degrees of mastery.

All residents, beginning early in training, should operate with faculty members who specifically evaluate their surgical skills. These evaluations help assign appropriate surgical privileges at each level of training. Problems should be identified and specific skill remediation should be instituted if necessary. This process is continuous throughout the training experience.

The evaluation of surgical competence of house officers must include all the elements that define competence, not just manual skills or knowledge of certain operating procedures. Each training unit establishes a system of regular evaluation of each element of cumulative training experience. Training departments commonly develop evaluation instruments that list important characteristics and skills and provide rating scales for each. These

ratings can be tracked in simple computer databases.

Neither the American College of Obstetrics and Gynecology nor the Joint Commission on Accreditation of Hospitals dictates the exact method for delineation of hospital privileges.[14] Many hospitals use either a checklist of procedures or illnesses or a review of body systems by specialty. Pressure is building for hospitals to undertake comprehensive matching of current physician competence evaluation to the granting of privileges. The latter system, as described previously, is complex and difficult to implement. It offers a more precise delineation of privileges for trainees in surgical specialties.

Trainee evaluation instruments are both evaluation documents and feedback tools. Include items that assess a broad range of characteristics of quality professional work and conduct, not just procedural skills. Many evaluators include personality traits, work efficiency, communication skills, basic and current patient knowledge, problem-solving abilities, research aptitudes, teaching skills, and interaction with patients and co-workers. Provide space for the evaluator to record narrative comments and general impressions. These lines often hold the most telling evaluations and the most powerful feedback items for trainees.[13]

Summary assessment codes placed in the upper right-hand corner of the front page of each evaluation form facilitate rapid sorting and easy review of progress over time.

All supervising staff and senior residents complete evaluation instruments on each trainee near the end of each training rotation. Multiple evaluators ensure fairness and dilute interpersonal relationship bias. The program director reads all evaluations and collates the file of each trainee. These files accurately track the progress of the surgeon in training. Problems of trainees surface quickly, feedback to trainees is prompt and specific, and remediation needs are readily identified and tracked.

The phrase "quality assurance" has crept into the vocabulary of physicians and administrators. Compliance with quality assurance requirements falls to the officers of hospital staffs and the leaders of training programs. Effective evaluation systems are the strongest tools for assisting accurate assignment of privileges and credentials and the quality assurance efforts of training programs and hospitals.

The training department is the trusted grantor and arbiter of trainee credentials and privileges. Hospitals in which training experiences occur should look to the training departments for the most accurate resident evaluations and credentialing. Hospital accrediting agencies should validate and accept the credentialing decisions of accredited training departments.

Issues of confidentiality and limitation of access

to evaluation forms may arise. Trainees should have free access to their evaluations. These evaluations are very effective performance feedback instruments. The evaluation files should be confidential and not available to unauthorized personnel. The training director supervises their use. Evaluation files are available for use for trainee progress assessment within the department and for credentialing in the hospital.

Requests to certify the clinical surgical competence of ex-trainees arrive regularly from licensing boards, hospitals, and prospective partners. These requests are easy to answer when the evaluation files contain the observations of several training evaluators. Specific permission from the ex-trainee to release information should accompany all such requests.

GRANTING SURGICAL PRIVILEGES TO RESIDENTS

One of the most important uses of a resident evaluation system is the assignment of successive surgical privileges. Responsibility must not outstrip capability. Surgical responsibilities must be progressive in order to allow training to advance and to develop self-confidence in the resident. Training directors need to know the current level of competence of each trainee to properly assign privileges.

All elements of clinical and surgical competence are important in determining the level of privileges to be granted. In surgical specialties special attention is directed to procedural skills. Progressive acquisition of these surgical skills must be accurately tracked by the evaluation system.

All obstetric teaching programs keep statistics on the obstetric deliveries and operations performed by individual residents. Documented supervision of surgical experiences provides the data for a logical system for granting progressive surgical privileges. There is no substitute, in the assessment of operating skills, for direct observation by supervising surgeons.

Privileges are not granted simply for time in training or number of cases performed. Procedure-specific case lists only count experience events. This may suffice to document capability in simple procedures early in training. The sequences of decisions and skills required for advanced surgical operations call for direct, on-site evaluation.

Case lists and accumulated training time do not account for differences in entry skills and the variable progress rates of trainees. Written rotation exit evaluations by attending physicians and senior residents give clues to some facets of surgical competence. The knowledge base, problem-solving skills, and personal characteristics and motivation of individual residents are tracked by these documents.

Direct observations of performance are the most critical elements of evaluation for the appropriate assignment of specific advanced operating privileges.

If the operating privileges of a resident must be delayed for any reason, the program should offer supportive remediation opportunities. Specify remediation criteria and prescribe a range of programs and exercises suited to the needs of the trainee. When remediation goals are attained, confer the delayed privileges without prejudice. Frequent progress conferences with empathetic faculty during the remediation period help maintain the dignity and confidence of the trainee.

THE ROLE OF THE TEACHING SURGEON

Physicians have always been teachers. It is most fortunate for surgical novices that so many of our profession are willing to share their hard-won knowledge.

Residents in training begin their preparation for the operating room in the early years of medical school. Those who are best prepared come to postgraduate programs with a knowledge of surgical knot tying, skin preparation, draping, hand scrubbing, and other basic surgical skills. Many have sutured lacerations or surgical incisions. Despite all this experience, very few junior residents have thought through all aspects of complex surgical operations when they first acquire operating room responsibility.

Residents must know the function of all the instruments to be used in the proposed operation. They must be able to properly apply and remove each instrument. They must be able to choose the correct instrument for each surgical need.

Preliminary experiences with surgical tools can be gained in settings outside the operating theater. There comes a time when hands-on patient experience is the only way to advance the skills of trainees. This is the realm of the surgeon-teacher.

The surgeon-teacher imparts knowledge on several levels. The teacher describes his or her reasoning method for the choice and timing of operations. He or she discusses decision options for the preparation for and accomplishment of surgical procedures. These interactions teach surgical problem solving.

The surgical teacher demonstrates, observes, and critiques the many steps of operative procedures. This activity corresponds closely to the direct teaching of manual skills to an apprentice in industry.

The surgical teacher is a role model for the principles of medical ethics, clinical honesty, and effective interpersonal relationships. Exposition of the role of the obstetric surgeon is most effective during on-site responses to day-to-day surgical problems. The surgical trainee learns, by repeated observation of mature clinicians, to think and behave like an obstetric surgeon.

The surgical teacher instills in residents the ability and desire to share their knowledge and to teach their skills to junior residents, students, and colleagues. Residents and fellows are among our most important teachers. Teaching must be inculcated as an essential part of the resident's job. The attitude that teaching is an important function for all residents must be supported by faculty and heads of departments in tangible ways. Feedback on teaching skills is treated with the same seriousness in the evaluation process as feedback on surgical skills.

The surgical teacher who fulfills all of the activities above is in the best possible position to evaluate the progress of his or her trainees. His or her frequent updates on trainee performance in formal and informal evaluations provide the department with the highest quality information for performance tracking and credentialing.

The teaching and evaluation tasks outlined for the surgical teacher are difficult and time-consuming. Not all obstetric surgeons perform these functions happily or well. Teaching and evaluation processes are critical to the continuity of obstetric surgery.

Effective Teaching in the Operating Room

How can an obstetric resident or surgeon be most effective and efficient in his or her teaching role in the operating room? The operating room is an ideal teaching environment. The operating theater provides intense images on which the trainee can attach packets of new knowledge.[17] The attention of the trainees is riveted to the process. Motivation is high. Feedback is immediate and focused. Many of the requirements for effective teaching are provided by the environment.[9, 20] The surgeon provides knowledge, energy, and direction to the process.

Be certain that all members of the operating team know what operation is to be done, how, and why. A preoperative conference is an effective way to focus the attention of the operating team. The teaching surgeon, the residents, students, and other members of the surgical team should be present. Review the patient's history, physical examination and laboratory findings, and the indications for surgery. Discuss the choice of operation and its timing. Review surgical approaches and techniques. Point out options for solving anticipated problems. Review the choices of anesthetic methods and agents. Decide together the appropriate suture materials and instruments. Check the availability of support materials, such as blood products, special instruments, retractors, or packs.

Review the entire operative procedure with the team step by step. Diagram incisions and clamp placements on chalkboard or paper to enliven anatomic descriptions. Encourage and respond to questions from all members of the operating team.

Verbal description of thought processes helps trainees learn how surgeons resolve clinical problems. Verbalization during procedural demonstrations is an important part of the teaching process.[19] Reviewing the technique of the anticipated operation in detail makes for better coordination and assistance at all levels.

The surgeon must know the level of skill and experience of key members of his or her team. Ask at the preoperative conference about the experience of team members with the planned operation. Assign operating responsibilities based on this knowledge as well as that gained by direct observation.

During actual surgery, the bilateral symmetry of the human pelvic anatomy provides a superb opportunity to teach surgical skills. Demonstrate a portion of the operation on one side of the dissection, talking the team through each new step. Ask the trainee to repeat the procedure exactly as demonstrated on his or her side. Offer immediate and specific feedback to the trainee.[19, 20] Over time, a selection of acceptable alternative operative techniques can be introduced and demonstrated. Repeated practice by the trainee under varied conditions, with supervision and timely feedback, leads to mastery of the procedure.

The Resident as Surgical Teacher

The resident in training shares the obligation, the burden, and the pleasure of the surgical teaching role. At some time during training, residents teach junior obstetric residents, interns and residents from other services, students, and allied operating personnel.

Apter and colleagues[15] surveyed resident teaching activities at Northwestern University Medical School. They found that residents enjoyed teaching and considered it a critical component of their experience and education. Physicians in surgical specialties recognize that fellow residents immediately senior to them in training were often their most effective teachers. They hold these mentors in high esteem.

Stenchever and colleagues[16] determined by national survey that approximately 70% of clinical learning among medical students was provided by house officers. The exact quantity of teaching by residents varies among schools, but it is always an important component of both undergraduate and graduate teaching. Teaching is, therefore, one of the skills that resident physicians must acquire and is one of the resident's most important responsibilities.

Teaching skills do not come naturally to all prospective surgeons. They are seldom taught in schools of medicine. A surgical teacher must first be in firm possession of the broad content of his or her subject. A variety of teaching techniques, such as those described previously, can then be used to enhance the transfer of surgical knowledge and skills to students and junior residents.

Most activities are best performed when some reward is perceived. What is the resident's reward for teaching? Apter and colleagues[15] found that residents considered the major personal benefit of their teaching to be thorough learning of the subject matter. Seventy-four percent of residents in the survey believed that their teaching efforts were appreciated by their trainees. Appreciative trainees become the most enthusiastic and helpful members of ward and operating teams.

Plauché and Edwards[17] suggested that there are few stronger stimuli to learning and retention of learned material than the combination of intense images and emotional involvement that occurs at the surgical table. These dramatic graphic cases are stored in memory as energized, image-indexed packets on which subsequent related knowledge is appended.

Irby[18] described the knowledge base of physicians as constructed of thousands of such packets stored in memory and connected in complex networks of related information. The physician's collection of memory packets may be thought of as his or her "experience," dearly acquired over considerable time.

Rapid relational sorting and subconscious correlation of many networks of information allow the mature physician to almost magically produce instantaneous differential diagnoses and management plans. These begin to surface the moment elements of a new case are presented. Diagnoses are constantly and automatically sifted and updated as additional facts surface. This integration of stored experience and instantaneous correlation with current facts is referred to as "clinical judgment."

Consider this example of the power of imagery in surgical teaching. The chief resident says, "This patient goes to surgery tomorrow," without explanation. Junior members of the surgical team learn very little about the case. The chief resident could create an important teaching episode by explaining his or her thought processes. His or her explanation can be illustrated by demonstrations of physical findings augmented by drawings, pictures, or verbal images.

The chief resident might say, "This patient has an adnexal mass and is 20 weeks pregnant. We believe the mass to be a benign cystic teratoma because of the characteristic 'snowflake' ultrasound pattern." (The resident shows the ultrasound images or draws the pattern.)

"She is experiencing intermittent severe pain that leads me to believe the mass is twisting on its pedicle." (The chief resident gently demonstrates the patient's abdominal guarding.)

"We will remove the mass to avoid the acute episode that could occur if the pedicle twisted sufficiently to cause infarction of the mass. The mass appears benign, but we can never be certain, so we will approach it as though it could be malignant. The informed consent of the patient must include that possibility."

Junior members of this resident's team hear a respected physician's diagnostic thinking. They know the reasons for this physician's choice of therapy. The lessons in surgical management are emotionally charged and likely to be retained.

The active, striking images of the pregnant patient twisting uncomfortably in bed, the chief giving his or her opinion, and the appearance of the tumor at the surgical table provide the strongest possible stimuli to the student's memory system. It is likely that students and junior residents will forever carry this episode in their memory banks to be called up whenever the key word "teratoma" or the key phrase "abdominal pain in pregnancy" is encountered.

Teaching in the manner described takes considerable effort on the part of the resident. Energy and enthusiasm are often cited by students as among the most important traits of their best teachers.[17] Surgical teaching requires that the teacher hold the undivided attention of his or her learners. The teacher must project comprehensive knowledge and intense interest in the subject at hand. Nothing is more boring than a subject presented in a disinterested monologue. There is no substitute for animation and enthusiasm on the part of the teacher.

Good surgical teachers often combine detailed descriptions of their decision-making processes with related personal case anecdotes. This case material is laced with open questions directed toward the personal and intellectual interests of the learners.[19, 20]

Many residents are effective teachers by intuition. Those of us who are not innately skilled teachers can learn to verbalize our thought processes, to question skillfully, and to enrich the experience of our learners.[19] Surgical trainees who are taught in this manner move toward clinical maturity guided by clear examples of decision making by experienced surgeons.

Teaching Surgical Procedures

Surgical procedures are complex sequences of manual skills. They are taught somewhat differently from general medical material and decision-making processes. Anderson[21] and Fitts[22] described three stages in the learning of procedural skills (Fig. 1–1).

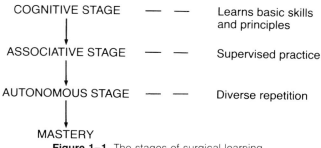

Figure 1–1. The stages of surgical learning.

The first stage, the "cognitive stage," is when the students learn the basic elements of the procedure. They learn how the skill is applied and the details of its performance (Fig. 1–2).

The second, the "associative stage," occurs during supervised practice of the procedure with appropriate feedback.

The third, the "autonomous stage," is attained through continued practice under diverse circumstances.[19, 22] In this phase, the procedure becomes an automatic routine that can be performed despite distractions to concentration.

"Mastery" is attained at the peak of this learning curve. Fitts[22] found that performance continued to improve when good outcomes resulted (Fig. 1–3).

The apprenticeship model for teaching manual skills has been carefully studied by the industrial sector. Complex procedures can usually be broken down into a series of simpler activities, which are more easily taught.[22]

Visual aids facilitate the demonstration of procedures and add active images to the learning process. One example is the use of blackboard or line drawings of the steps of a procedure while describing each step (Fig. 1–4). Another example is demonstration of procedures on structurally accurate anatomic models. The trainee becomes more comfortable with a procedure if he or she handles the real tools to be used.

After the teacher has described and illustrated the steps of a procedure, the student should repeat the steps in detail and receive immediate feedback.[19] Practice should be provided initially with verbal repetition, then with models when possible, and eventually with actual cases. These principles, developed in industry, apply nicely to the teaching of surgical operative skills.

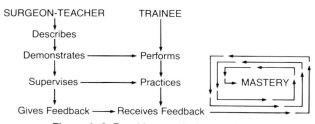

Figure 1–2. Teaching surgical procedures.

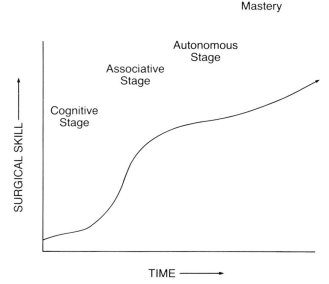

Figure 1–3. Surgical learning curve.

Critique of Surgical Skills

Surgeon-teachers must be able and willing to offer critique and feedback, both positive and negative, to their trainees. Without feedback, recurrent mistakes enter the trainees' knowledge base. Biehler[23] stated that feedback is one of the most important facilitators of the learning process. Ende[24] identified timeliness and specificity as the keys to effective feedback.

It is critical to give feedback to surgical trainees as close in time to the surgical event as possible.[24] The resident should never receive the first adverse criticism months after an occurrence as part of a probation hearing. He or she equally should not hear words of praise and encouragement only at the graduation party.

The surgeon-teacher reserves critical comments during the performance of intricate procedures. Critique at such times creates a counterproductive atmosphere of nervousness and anxiety. Immediately on finishing a case, the teacher should take the trainee aside for a private debriefing on the surgical events. Praise can be public, but adverse criticism should be private.

Feedback should always be procedure-specific and not personal.[21–24] Picture a surgical situation in which the surgeon-teacher makes the following comments to the trainee.

"You really messed up. You cut the damn ureter. You never get anything right."

Such an outburst would only gain the animosity of the trainee and teach him or her nothing. A more effective response might be:

"I think you should have handled the dissection of that right ureter differently. Here's how we approach the ureter to prevent injury in such a case. I'm sure you won't make that same mistake when we operate together again."

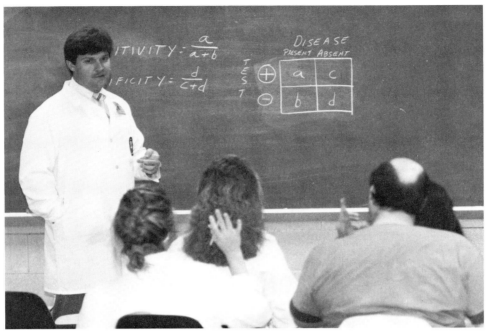

Figure 1—4. Small group teaching. Students have a visual image before them, which enables them to actively participate in analysis and resolution of the problem.

Corrective dialogue, however phrased, should express the specific technical error, offer suggestions for improvement, and indicate a measure of continued respect.

Edwards and colleagues[25] believed that the instructor should not blame a bad outcome on unfortunate circumstances but relate it to specific flaws in technique. Good outcomes should be related to excellence in technique, skill, and preparation, not attributed to luck or good fortune.

PATIENT-CENTERED SURGICAL TEACHING

The ideal surgical training environment offers progressive supervised practice involving human surgical patients. Today's medical realities have threatened this ideal because of inadequate numbers of teaching cases and insufficient supervision.

Training environments that chiefly utilize private patients face the problem of inadequate numbers and scope of surgical cases available to the resident for training. Private patients sometimes object to the participation of the resident in their examination and care. Gynecologic and obstetric patients can be particularly reluctant unless forewarned. An environment must be created in which the participation of trainees at all levels is the accepted norm.

The private practitioner is sometimes loathe to allow the resident to have direct surgical responsibility for his or her private patients. This is particularly true in the earlier years of residency training, just when the practice of surgical skills is most critical.

Supervision of individual procedures in the private environment is often very carefully done, and this resource deserves careful nurturing. Simply watching a master at work, however, is not an optimal or even adequate method by which to learn complex surgical procedures.

Experiences of high quality in the private environment often accrue only to residents who already display mastery of procedures. Privately controlled training environments must ensure careful attention to the preliminary steps in surgical teaching. Procedures must be demonstrated and progressive practice provided with appropriate feedback.

Training programs in public institutions face problems that are quite different from those in the private sector. Funding of public hospitals and training programs has diminished in many regions. The surgical faculties have increasingly turned to private practice or research grants for their basic support. There is danger that supervision of surgical trainees in public hospitals may diminish as the priorities of the faculty change.

Public hospitals are often overburdened with patients. Residency programs in these environments may be driven by the need to provide service rather than by educational needs. A balance must be found. Training departments must insist on protected study time and schedules that ensure adequate rest and relaxation time for trainees.

Public teaching hospitals usually provide a broad scope of surgical experiences. A problem of high priority in public programs is getting attending physicians to attend. Adequate faculty time must be devoted to teaching surgical principles, demonstrating techniques, and supervising resident practice in the operating room. To accomplish this goal, governments, medical schools, and public institutions must provide stable subsidies for teaching programs in public hospitals. Incentives must be sought to encourage medical school faculty to return to the public clinics, wards, and operating rooms.

Residents whose opportunities for surgical practice lack supervision and critique incorporate poor surgical habits into their arsenal of techniques. Techniques and procedures that are not ideal or standard enter the practice habits of these physicians. These flawed techniques become icons in memory because they were acquired during training, and they are very difficult to alter once they are fixed in place by repetition.

Some surgical teaching in programs based in public hospitals can be diverted successfully to the personal practices of faculty in private hospitals. Capable private practitioners who are interested in working with residents are major resources for these teaching programs.

Faculties must develop renewed dedication to the goal of teaching the next generation of obstetric surgeons. This goal must be promulgated by the highest administrative levels of our teaching institutions and filter through to every teaching staff member. It is difficult to imagine a goal of greater importance to a training program than dedication to the highest quality surgical teaching.

ALTERNATIVES TO PATIENT-CENTERED TEACHING

Advanced surgical procedures allow few alternatives to patient-centered teaching. Specially designed environments can be utilized for the early cognitive stages of learning procedural skills. Animal laboratories and procedural skills laboratories provide such opportunities.

The time-honored "dog lab" provides surgical opportunities for trainees using live animal models. Anesthetic and aseptic techniques duplicate those of the hospital operating room. Animal laboratories are surgical teaching environments of proven effectiveness.

The animal surgical laboratory, however, has been beset with problems and has largely fallen into disuse. Animal care facilities are very expensive to maintain and subject to complicated and frequently changing regulations. Animal rights activists have raised questions about the propriety and ethics of the use of animals for medical research and practice of surgical skills.

Heads of surgical departments have expressed concern that animal laboratory experience might supplant true clinical expertise. Residents might sense that the single performance in the laboratory of a difficult procedure such as ureteral transplantation gives them permission to perform the operation in humans. Practice with inanimate objects does not stimulate these feelings.

Procedural Skills Laboratories

Procedural skills laboratories historically began with knot-tying boards and anatomic mannequins. Many basic surgical skills can be taught in a coordinated laboratory setting. Examples of skills suited to this teaching style are suturing, knot tying, incisions, aspiration techniques, biopsy techniques, endoscopies, microsurgical techniques, diagnostic imaging, interpretation of laboratory data, endotracheal intubation, cardiopulmonary resuscitation, and the demonstration of normal anatomy and pathology. The procedural skills laboratory can be expanded to teach interviewing skills, physical examination, and problem solving. Computer support, video demonstrations, standardized patients, and supervised practice further extend the versatility of the procedural skills laboratory.

The procedural skills laboratory can become very sophisticated and bring together in one site the facilities necessary to teach basic surgical skills in all disciplines. Training at all levels, from introductory hand washing for medical students to microsurgical techniques for subspecialty fellows, can be provided.

The procedural skills laboratory avoids duplication of facilities across departments. Trained auxiliary personnel teach basic skills. Faculty teaching time is preserved for operating room supervision of residents and teaching advanced techniques.

The procedural skills laboratory allows direct observation and tracking of student-resident skill acquisition and provides many opportunities for direct feedback. Support and praise help build the trainee's confidence in his or her ability to work with living patients.

Once a trainee has acquired the necessary knowledge base and manual surgical skills, he or she is introduced into an operating team. He or she begins the "associative stage" of skill perfection first as an observer, then as an assistant, and eventually as a responsible surgeon.[20, 21] The associative and autonomous stages of incorporating a skill into the surgical repertory and working toward mastery necessitate patient-centered environments. Direct bedside and operating table teaching supervision and critique are irreplaceable elements of advanced surgical training.

CONCLUSIONS

Teaching surgical concepts and procedures to students and residents should be a major mission of medical school obstetric faculty. Residents must invest in their important role as surgical mentors of junior residents and students.

Individual faculty members add their authority to departmental surgical teaching goals by being role models of good teaching techniques. Timely, specific feedback and evaluation can be incorporated into everyday ward and operating room experiences. Teaching can be made part of the routine of surgical teams and can improve surgical teaching at all levels.

The surgical work of every resident should be carefully evaluated. The best evaluation systems go beyond simple counting of experiences and evaluate all parameters of surgical competence. Procedural skill evaluation and critique necessitate observation at the operating table by experienced surgical teachers. Direct faculty supervision prevents the acquisition and fixation of poor surgical habits.

A carefully designed evaluation system that incorporates the above principles makes easy the tasks of granting surgical privileges, certifying of physician competence, and preparing for program accreditation.

References

1. Senior JR: Toward the Measurement of Competence in Medicine. Philadelphia: National Board of Medical Examiners, 1976, p. 16.
2. Maatsch JL, Huang R: An evaluation of the construct validity of four alternative theories of clinical competence. Proc Annu Conf Res Med Educ 25:69, 1986.
3. Levine HG, McGuire CH, Nattress LW Jr: The validity of multiple-choice achievement tests as measures of competence in medicine. Am Ed Res J 7(1):69, 1970.
4. Maatsch JL: Predictive validity of medical specialty examinations. Final Report for the National Center for Health Services Research (Grant No. HS 02038-4), 1983.
5. Levine HG, McGuire CH: The validity and reliability of oral skills in assessing cognitive skills in medicine. J Ed Measurement, 7 (2):63, 1970.
6. Petersdorf RG: Discussion following: Evaluation of competence and skills. Proceedings of AMA conference, Physician Competence: Whose responsibility? Singer I (ed.): Medical Education Group of the AMA, 1989, p. 103.
7. Gonella JS: Discussion following: Evaluation of competence and skills. Proceedings of AMA conference, Physician Competence: Whose responsibility? Singer I (ed.): Medical Education Group of the AMA, 1989, p. 104.
8. Melnick DE: Discussion following: Evaluation of competence and skills. Proceedings of AMA conference, Physician Competence: Whose responsibility? Singer I (ed.): Medical Education Group of the AMA, 1989, p. 104.
9. Gonella JS: Competence assessment during medical school. Proceedings of AMA conference, Physician Competence: Whose responsibility? Singer I (ed.): Medical Education Group of the AMA, 1989, p. 55.
10. Barro AR: Survey of evaluation of approaches to physician performance measurement. J Med Educ (Suppl) 48:1053, 1973.
11. Gonella JS, Goran MJ, Williamson JW et al: Evaluation of patient care: An approach. JAMA 214:2040, 1970.
12. Educational Objectives for Residents in Obstetrics and Gynecology. Council on Residency Education in Obstetrics and Gynecology. 4th Edition. Unit five, pp. 45–47; Unit eleven, pp. 99–103.
13. Edwards JC, Plauché WC, Randall H et al: Guidelines for evaluating, referring and supporting students in the clinical years. Baton Rouge: LSU Press. 1987, p. 37.
14. Quality Assurance in Obstetrics and Gynecology. Washington, DC: The American College of Obstetricians and Gynecologists. 1989 Edition. 1989, p. 76.
15. Apter A, Metzger R, Glassroth J: Residents' perceptions of their role as teachers. J Med Ed 63:900, 1988.
16. Stenchever MA, Irby DM, O'Toole B: A national survey of undergraduate teaching in obstetrics and gynecology. J Med Ed 54:467, 1979.
17. Plauché WC, Edwards JC: Images and emotion in patient-centered clinical teaching. Perspect Biol Med 31:4, 1988.
18. Irby DM: Clinical teacher effectiveness in medicine. J Med Educ 53:808–815, 1978.
19. Edwards JC, Marier RL (eds.): Clinical Teaching for Medical Residents: Roles, Techniques and Programs. New York: Springer Publishing Company, 1988, pp. 72–74.
20. Edwards JC, Plauché WC, Marier RL: Handbook of Conferences on Teaching Skills for Residents. New Orleans: LSU School of Medicine, 1987.
21. Anderson JR: Cognitive Psychology and its Implications, 2nd Edition. New York: W.H. Freeman, 1985.
22. Fitts PM: Factors in complex skill training in training research and evaluation. In Glaser R (ed): Training Research and Education, New York: John Wiley and Sons, Inc., 1962.
23. Biehler RF: Psychology Applied to Teaching, 3rd Edition. New York: Houghton Mifflin Company, 1978.
24. Ende J: Feedback in clinical medical education. JAMA 250:777, 1983.
25. Edwards JC, Kissling GE, Brannan JR et al.: Study of teaching residents how to teach. J Med Ed 63:603–609, 1988.

2

Surgical Obstetric Anatomy

Raymond F. Gasser

- **NONGRAVID STATE**
  - Vulva
  - Perineum
  - Vagina
  - Anterior Abdominal Wall
  - Pelvis
  - Uterus
  - Pelvic Portion of the Ureter

  - Bladder and Urethra
  - Sigmoid Colon, Rectum, and Anal Canal
  - Posterior Abdominal Wall Structures
- **ANATOMIC CHANGES DURING PREGNANCY**
  - Gravid Uterus
  - Changes in Related Organs
  - Placenta

NONGRAVID STATE

Vulva

The female external genital organs, collectively referred to as the *vulva*, or the *pudendum*, lie in front of and below the pubic symphysis (Fig. 2–1). They consist of the *mons pubis*, the *labia majora*, the *labia minora*, the *clitoris*, and the *vestibule of the vagina*. Opening into the vestibule are the vagina, the urethra, and the ducts of the paraurethral and vestibular glands.

Mons Pubis

The mons pubis is a rounded, median elevation lying anterior to the pubic symphysis and pubic bones. It is covered with hair after puberty and elevated by a subcutaneous fat pad.

Labia Majora

A broad, longitudinal fold of skin called the labium majus is located on each side of the vulva. It is largely filled with subcutaneous fat and contains the fibrous termination of the round ligament of the uterus. The pudendal cleft is located between the folds in the midline. Anteriorly, the subcutaneous fat within the labium majus is continuous with that of the mons pubis. Posteriorly, it joins the ischiorectal fat. After puberty, the skin of the lateral surface of each labium majus is pigmented and covered with hair. It contains sweat and se-

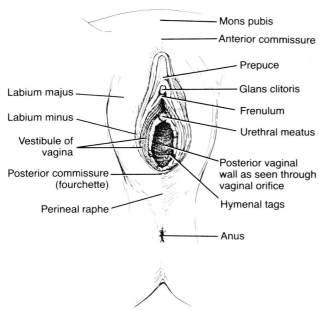

Mons pubis
Anterior commissure
Prepuce
Glans clitoris
Frenulum
Urethral meatus
Labium majus
Labium minus
Vestibule of vagina
Posterior commissure (fourchette)
Perineal raphe
Posterior vaginal wall as seen through vaginal orifice
Hymenal tags
Anus

Figure 2–1. The vulva, or pudendum.

baceous glands. The medial surface is smooth, hairless, and studded with sebaceous glands. The anterior junction of the labia majora is sometimes referred to as the *anterior commissure;* where the labia joins it posteriorly is the *fourchette,* or *posterior commissure.* The narrow space in front of the fourchette is called the *navicular fossa.*

LABIA MINORA

A fleshy, smaller fold of skin called the labium minus is located medial to the labium majus and is of variable size and shape. In contrast to the labium majus, it is hairless and contains no fat. Its lateral surface is in contact with the smooth, inner surface of the labia majora; its medial surface is in contact with the medial surface of its counterpart on the other side. The vaginal vestibule is between them and becomes apparent only when the labia minora are separated. Anteriorly, as the labium minorus approaches the clitoris, it divides into two small folds that fuse around the clitoris with its counterparts on the other side. The upper folds unite above the clitoris to form the *prepuce of the clitoris;* the lower folds join one another on the underside of the clitoris as the *frenulum of the clitoris.* A whitish, sebaceous material that is secreted by the glands in the skin of the two folds may collect around the glans clitoris.

CLITORIS

The clitoris lies between the anterior ends of the labia minora under cover of the prepuce. Like the penis, it is composed of erectile tissue and is capable of erection. The *body* of the clitoris consists of two corpora cavernosa that are enclosed in a

fibrous sheath. Each corpus cavernosum begins as a *crus,* which is attached to the medial edge of its respective ischiopubic ramus. The *suspensory ligament* attaches the clitoris to the pubic symphysis. The crura unite in the midline to form the body. At the free end of the body is a small elevation of erectile tissue called the *glans.* It plays an important role in the excitatory phase of the sexual response because of its rich supply of sensory nerve endings. An oval mass of erectile tissue, called the *bulb of the vestibule,* is located along the deep aspect of each labium minus next to the vaginal vestibule. Each bulb is attached to the inferior fascia of the urogenital diaphragm and is covered externally by the thin *bulbospongiosus (bulbocavernosus) muscle.* Anteriorly, the bulb tapers as it approaches the clitoris, ending in tiny vascular channels (called *pars intermedia*) that connect to the underside of the glans.

VESTIBULE OF THE VAGINA

Between the labia minora is the vestibule of the vagina, where the vagina opens as a vertical slit. The opening of the vagina (called the *vaginal orifice,* or the *introitus*) is rimmed with variably sized nodes of fibrous tissue known as *hymenal tags.* The vaginal orifice is sometimes partially or totally closed by a fold of mucous membrane, the *hymen.* If the hymen does not rupture by the time of puberty, it prevents the exit of menstrual fluids and must therefore be incised.

Immediately anterior to the vaginal orifice in the midline is the *urethral meatus.* The urethra opens there as a small, vertical slit about 2 cm below the glans clitoris. The margins of the meatus are usually raised, giving it a puckered appearance. On each side of the meatus are the minute openings of the *paraurethral glands* (of Skene). The small space in the vaginal vestibule that is posterior to the vaginal orifice is called the *vestibular fossa.* The duct of the *greater vestibular gland* (of Bartholin) opens there on each side. The gland is a small, lobulated, pea-sized body at the posterior edge of the bulb of the vestibule. It, along with the numerous *lesser vestibular glands,* which also open into the vaginal vestibule, secretes mucus that lubricates the region.

Perineum

The perineum is the diamond-shaped region at the most inferior part of the trunk between the thighs and the buttocks (Fig. 2–2). The urethra, the vagina, and the anal canal pass through it. The *pubic symphysis* bounds it anteriorly, the tip of the *coccyx* posteriorly, and the *ischial tuberosity* on each side laterally. Anterior to the ischial tuberosity, the lateral wall is bound by the medial surface of the *ischiopubic ramus;* posterior to the

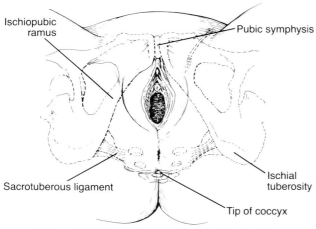

Figure 2–2. The perineum, with bony landmarks.

tuberosity, it is limited by the *sacrotuberous liga-ment*, which is overlapped by the *gluteus maximus muscle* (Fig. 2–3). This osseoligamentous, dia-mond-shaped frame also forms the *inferior pelvic aperture.* The deeper part of the lateral wall is bound by that part of the obturator internus mus-cle that extends below the attachment of the lev-ator ani muscle along with its fascial covering. The skin limits the perineum superficially (inferi-orly), and the pelvic diaphragm bounds it deeply (superiorly) (Fig. 2–4). For descriptive purposes, the perineum is divided into two triangular regions by an imaginary line connecting the two ischial tuberosities; anteriorly, the subdivision is called the *urogenital region* or *triangle,* and posteriorly it is called the *anal region* or *triangle.* Located in the center of the perineum between the anal canal and the lower vagina is a fibromuscular mass

called the *perineal body,* or *central tendon, of the perineum* (see Fig. 2–3). It contains smooth and skeletal muscle fibers bound together with collag-enous and elastic tissue and is the point of attach-ment of several sets of perineal muscles and fascial layers.

UROGENITAL REGION

In the urogenital region, a muscular shelf called the *urogenital diaphragm* stretches between the ischiopubic rami (see Figs. 2–3, 2–4). It is trav-ersed by the urethra and vagina and serves as a foundation for the attachment of the external gen-ital organs. The urogenital diaphragm is limited superficially (inferiorly) by a strong, whitish layer of collagen fibers called the *perineal membrane* (or the *inferior fascial layer of the urogenital dia-phragm*). The perineal membrane divides the uro-genital region into two thick anatomic layers of considerable clinical importance, the superficial and the deep perineal compartments or pouches.

Superficial Perineal Compartment. The su-perficial compartment (see Figs. 2–3 and 2–4) lies superficial to the perineal membrane and contains, on each side, the *greater vestibular gland*; the *crus of the clitoris,* with its overlying *ischiocavernous muscle*; the *bulb of the vestibule,* with its overlying *bulbospongiosus (bulbocavernous) muscle*; and the small *superficial transverse perineal muscle.* The ischiocavernous muscle covers the crus of the cli-toris and is important in the maintenance of cli-toral erection because it compresses the crus against the ischiopubic ramus, thereby retarding blood flow from the erectile tissue. The bulbospon-giosus muscle arises from the body of the clitoris

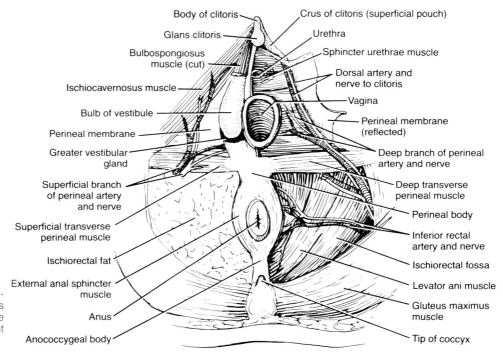

Figure 2–3. The perineum. Mus-cles, fascia, vessels, and nerves are shown. The left side of the drawing is superficial, the right side is deep.

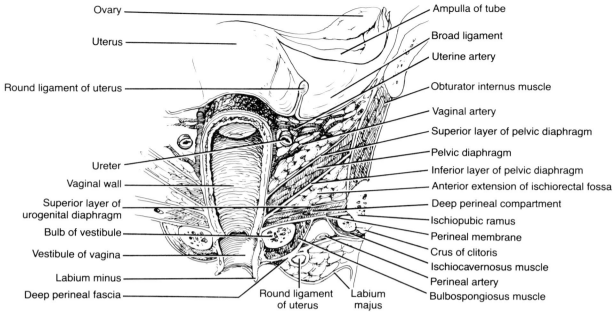

Ovary —————

Uterus —————

Round ligament of uterus —————

Ureter —————
Vaginal wall —————
Superior layer of —————
urogenital diaphragm
Bulb of vestibule —————
Vestibule of vagina —————
Labium minus —————
Deep perineal fascia —————

————— Ampulla of tube
————— Broad ligament
————— Uterine artery
————— Obturator internus muscle
————— Vaginal artery
————— Superior layer of pelvic diaphragm
————— Pelvic diaphragm
————— Inferior layer of pelvic diaphragm
————— Anterior extension of ischiorectal fossa
————— Deep perineal compartment
————— Ischiopubic ramus
————— Perineal membrane
————— Crus of clitoris
————— Ischiocavernosus muscle
————— Perineal artery
————— Bulbospongiosus muscle

Round ligament   Labium
of uterus   majus

Figure 2–4. Frontal view of vagina and nongravid uterus showing lateral relations.

and the adjacent pubic bone, then passes posteriorly around the lower part of the vagina, covering the bulb of the vestibule to insert in the perineal body. The muscle can act as a sphincter with its counterpart on the other side to constrict the lower part of the vagina. The poorly developed, insignificant, superficial transverse perineal muscle arises from the inner surface of the ischium near the tuberosity and courses transversely to insert in the perineal body. All of the muscles in the superficial compartment are covered by *deep perineal fascia* and are innervated by the *perineal branch of the pudendal nerve.*

Deep Perineal Compartment. The deep perineal compartment lies between the perineal membrane (inferior fascial layer of the urogenital diaphragm) and the relatively indistinct *superior fascial layer of the urogenital diaphragm* (see right sides of Figs. 2–3, 2–4). The urogenital diaphragm is composed of a sheet of muscle that is divided into two parts: anteriorly, the *sphincter muscle of the urethra*, and posteriorly, the *deep transverse perineal muscle.* The urethra and the vagina pass through the urogenital diaphragm. The muscle fibers in the urogenital diaphragm mainly course transversely from the ischiopubic ramus to join in the midline with their counterparts on the other side. Some of the fibers of the sphincter muscle of the urethra arch over the urethra, whereas others are arranged in a circular fashion around it. The muscle fibers of the sphincter of the urethra also course around the vagina and blend with its lower portion in the region where the urethra is embedded in its anterior wall. The muscle plays an important role in urinary continence because it constricts the urethra when the bladder is filled with urine; it can also cause interruption of the

urine stream. The deep transverse perineal muscle inserts into the perineal body behind the vagina. When it contracts bilaterally, it puts tension on the perineal body, thereby contributing to the support of the perineum and the three visceral structures passing through it. The *perineal branch of the pudendal nerve* innervates both muscles in the deep compartment.

The *dorsal nerve of the clitoris* and the accompanying internal pudendal vessels course anteriorly in the lateral part of the deep compartment close to the ischiopubic ramus, where they are susceptible to injury. Along the anterior margin of the urogenital diaphragm, the two fascial layers of the diaphragm fuse to form the *transverse perineal ligament.* Anterior to this fascial thickening is the *arcuate pubic ligament,* which lies along the inferior edge of the pubic symphysis. A small gap between the two ligaments transmits the *deep dorsal vein of the clitoris* from the perineal region into the pelvic cavity.

ANAL REGION

The anal region contains the *anus,* the *external anal sphincter muscle,* and the *ischiorectal fossa.* The anus is the opening of the anal canal at the surface of the perineum after the anal canal passes through the pelvic diaphragm. The skin around it is pigmented and contains sebaceous and sweat glands. The external anal sphincter is composed of voluntary, striated muscle fibers that surround the anal canal after it passes through the pelvic diaphragm. It has been described as consisting of subcutaneous, superficial, and deep parts. The subcutaneous part is the most superficial and circles the lowermost wall of the anal canal. The deep part of the sphincter is composed of circularly arranged fibers that fuse with the levator ani muscle. The intervening, superficial part is made up of muscle fibers that course mainly longitudinally along the sides of the anal canal and decussate in front of and behind the anus to insert in front into the perineal body and behind into an ill-defined fibrous mass called the *anococcygeal body*, or *anococcygeal ligament* (see Fig. 2–3). The anus presents externally as a longitudinal, slitlike opening rather than a circular one, probably because of the anteroposterior direction of many of the external anal sphincter muscle fibers.

The *ischiorectal fossa* is a wedge-shaped, fat-filled space that is limited superficially by the skin. The skin forms the base of the wedge. The vertical, lateral wall of the fossa is formed by the obturator internus muscle. The sloping superomedial wall is composed of the levator ani muscle (see Fig. 2–3). Ischiorectal fat allows for the distension of the rectum and anal canal during defecation. The fossa is traversed by fibrous strands but because the strands do not form well-defined compartments, abscesses in the fat can spread without generating pain from tension. The fossa and its contained fat extend anteriorly, deep (superior) to the urogenital diaphragm but below the levator ani muscle. The extension is called the anterior recess. Posteriorly, the fat in the fossa passes deep to the gluteus maximus muscle to the vicinity of the sacrotuberous ligament. Laterally, the fossa is limited by the ischium and the obturator fascia covering the lower part of the obturator internus muscle. Internal pudendal vessels and branches of the pudendal nerve course in the lateral wall of the fossa through a channel in the obturator fascia called the *pudendal canal* (of Alcock). Posteriorly, these vessels and the nerve give off their *inferior rectal* (hemorrhoidal) *branches*, which run across the fossa to supply the external anal sphincter and the skin and fascia around the anus. Other cutaneous nerves that run through the fossa are the *perforating branch of the second and third sacral nerves* and the *perineal branch of the fourth sacral nerve*.

BLOOD VESSELS OF THE PERINEUM

The *internal pudendal artery* is the principal artery to the perineum (see Fig. 2–3). It arises from the internal iliac artery in the pelvic cavity, leaving the cavity by coursing out the lower part of the greater sciatic (ischiatic) foramen. It passes around the ischial spine and enters the pudendal canal in the lateral wall of the ischiorectal fossa by traversing the lesser sciatic foramen. The first branch is the *inferior rectal artery*, which crosses the ischiorectal fossa to supply the skin and muscles around the anus. A *perineal branch* supplies the structures in the superficial perineal compartment and continues as *posterior labial branches* to

the labia majus and minus. As the internal pudendal artery enters the deep perineal compartment, it gives branches to the bulb of the vestibule, the greater vestibular gland, and the urethra. It terminates by dividing into *deep and dorsal arteries to the clitoris* near the pubic symphysis.

The *superficial external pudendal artery* arises from the medial side of the femoral artery and sends anterior labial branches to the anterior part of the labium majus. It courses medially in front of the terminal part of the round ligament of the uterus. The *deep external pudendal artery* also arises from the femoral artery, but at a deeper and more distal site. It courses medially and pierces the fascia lata at the medial side of the thigh, to be distributed to the lateral part of the labium majus. Its branches anastomose with the anterior and posterior labial arteries.

The veins draining the perineum are mainly tributaries of the internal iliac vein. For the most part, they accompany the arteries. The *deep dorsal vein of the clitoris* is an exception because it drains blood from the erectile tissue of the clitoris through a gap below the pubic symphysis to the venous plexus around the neck of the bladder. *External pudendal veins* help drain the labium majus by coursing laterally to empty into the great saphenous vein.

LYMPHATIC DRAINAGE OF THE PERINEUM

The lymph from most perineal structures drains to the *superficial inguinal lymph nodes*, with some also passing to the *deep inguinal nodes* (see Fig. 2–9). Enlargement of the superficial nodes may be the first sign of an infection or neoplasm in the superficial tissues of the perineum. Some lymphatics from the clitoris accompany the deep dorsal vein inside the pelvic cavity to drain to the *internal iliac nodes*. Lymphatics from deep perineal structures, including the membranous urethra, follow the internal pudendal vessels to the internal iliac nodes.

PERINEAL INNERVATION

The *pudendal nerve* is the principal nerve to the perineum (see Fig. 2–3). It is a branch of the sacral plexus and is formed by the ventral rami of S–2, S–3, and S–4. It leaves the pelvic cavity through the greater sciatic foramen in company with the internal pudendal vessels. After passing behind the ischial spine, it reaches the lateral wall of the ischiorectal fossa by coursing through the lesser sciatic foramen. The nerve divides into three branches near the ischial spine: (1) the *inferior rectal nerve*, which crosses through the fat in the ischiorectal fossa to innervate the skin around the anus, the external anal sphincter muscle, and the lining of the anal canal below the pectinate line; (2) the *perineal nerve*, which breaks up into two superficial cutaneous branches to the posterior part of the labium majus and lower vagina and a deep muscular branch that supplies all of the muscles in the superficial and deep perineal compartments, part of the external anal sphincter and levator ani muscles, and the bulb of the vestibule; and (3) the *dorsal nerve of the clitoris*, which continues forward in the urogenital diaphragm near the ischiopubic ramus, passing through the perineal membrane to the dorsum of the clitoris, where it terminates in the glans.

The areas of skin at the periphery of the perineum are innervated by various other cutaneous nerves. The mons pubis and the anterior part of the labia are supplied by the genitofemoral nerve and the anterior labial branches of the ilioinguinal nerve (L–1). Skin over the lateral part of the ischiorectal fossa is innervated by the perineal branch of the posterior femoral cutaneous nerve.

The visceral motor (parasympathetic) nerve fibers required for clitoral erection are derived from the pelvic splanchnic nerves. They reach the clitoris by passing through the urogenital diaphragm with the urethra and may be damaged in pelvic fractures.

Vagina

The vagina (sheath) extends from its vestibule to the uterus, passing superiorly with a posterior inclination through the urogenital and pelvic diaphragms (Fig. 2–5; see Fig. 2–4). It is approximately 10 cm in length and is located mainly in the pelvic cavity, where it terminates by fusing around the cervix of the uterus. It is very distensible and serves as the female organ of copulation as well as the lower end of the birth canal. The anterior and posterior walls are usually in contact with each other in the lower part, having the shape of an *H* on transverse section. The upper end is sometimes called the *vaginal vault* because the lumen forms recesses, or *fornices*, around the vaginal part of the cervix. Because the vagina forms an angle of about 90 degrees with the uterus, the posterior wall is considerably longer than the anterior wall and the posterior fornix is deeper than the anterior and lateral fornices. The lateral wall of the vagina is attached to the cardinal ligament and to the pelvic diaphragm. The wall is made up mainly of smooth muscle and dense connective tissue with many elastic fibers. The outer layer is largely connective tissue, containing the vaginal arteries, nerves, and a plexus of veins. The mucosa is thrown into small transverse folds called *rugae*, and an anterior and a posterior longitudinal fold called a *vaginal column*. The stratified squamous epithelium at the surface undergoes cyclic changes that correlate with the ovarian cycle.

RELATIONSHIPS

The anterior wall of the vagina lies adjacent to the urethra and the base of the bladder, with the terminal part of the urethra embedded in its most inferior portion (see Figs. 2–4 and 2–5). The thin layer of connective tissue that separates the anterior wall from the bladder is called the *vesicovaginal septum*. Anteriorly, the vagina is indirectly connected to the back of the pubic bone through fascial thickenings at the base of the bladder known as *pubovesical ligaments*. Posteriorly, the lowest part of the wall is separated from the anal canal by the perineal body. The middle portion lies adjacent to the ampulla of the rectum, and the uppermost segment lies adjacent to the rectouterine pouch (of Douglas) of the peritoneal cavity, from which it is separated by only a thin layer of peritoneum. The greater vestibular gland, bulb of the vestibule, and bulbospongiosus muscle lie lateral to the lowest portion of the vagina. More superiorly, the pubococcygeus portion of the levator ani muscle courses lateral to the vagina and, with its counterpart on the other side, acts as a sphincter. The ureter, uterine vessels, and nerves lie very close to the lateral wall, superiorly.

BLOOD SUPPLY, LYMPHATICS, AND NERVES

The lower part of the vagina is supplied by the internal pudendal artery, and the middle portion receives blood from the inferior vesical and middle rectal branches of the internal iliac artery (Fig. 2–6). However, its chief blood supply is through vaginal branches of the uterine artery, which form single longitudinal channels anteriorly and posteriorly (called *azygos arteries*) that anastomose with the arteries supplying the middle and lower portions of the vagina. Vaginal veins drain into the venous plexus, which is located in its outer wall. The plexus mainly drains superiorly to the uterine venous plexus, then laterally to the internal iliac veins.

Lymph from the lower part of the vagina near the vestibule drains to the superficial inguinal lymph nodes. The middle part drains mainly to the internal iliac nodes, whereas the upper part drains to these as well as to the external iliac nodes.

The pudendal nerve innervates the lower part of the vagina and arises from spinal cord segments S–2, S–3, and S–4, to which vaginal pain sensations are conducted. Most of the vaginal nerves are derived from the uterovaginal portion of the hypogastric plexus, located retroperitoneally on the front of the fifth lumbar vertebra. Sympathetic, parasympathetic, and visceral sensory fibers pass through the plexus to supply the superior part of the vagina. Little is known about the function of the visceral motor nerves. The visceral sensory fibers appear to be stimulated mainly by tension in the vaginal wall rather than by lacerations.

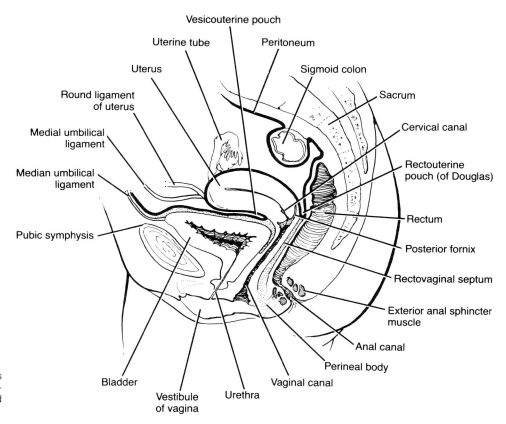

Vesicouterine pouch

Uterine tube

Peritoneum

Uterus

Sigmoid colon

Round ligament
of uterus

Sacrum

Medial umbilical
ligament

Cervical canal

Median umbilical
ligament

Rectouterine
pouch (of Douglas)

Pubic symphysis

Rectum

Posterior fornix

Rectovaginal septum

Exterior anal sphincter
muscle

Anal canal

Perineal body

Bladder

Vaginal canal

Vestibule
of vagina

Urethra

Figure 2–5. Sagittal view of pelvis showing anterior and posterior relations of vagina and nongravid uterus.

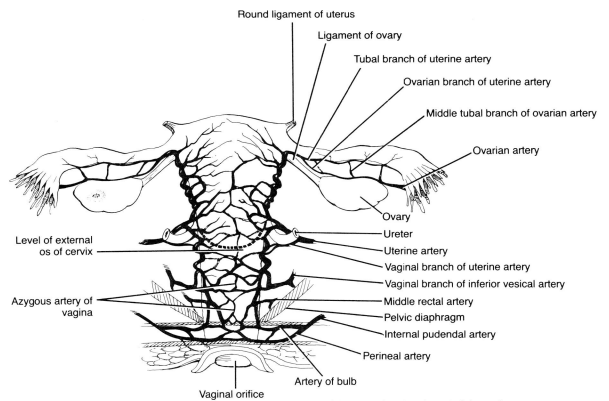

Round ligament of uterus

Ligament of ovary

Tubal branch of uterine artery

Ovarian branch of uterine artery

Middle tubal branch of ovarian artery

Ovarian artery

Ovary

Level of external
os of cervix

Ureter

Uterine artery

Vaginal branch of uterine artery

Vaginal branch of inferior vesical artery

Azygous artery of
vagina

Middle rectal artery

Pelvic diaphragm

Internal pudendal artery

Perineal artery

Vaginal orifice

Artery of bulb

Figure 2–6. Frontal view of vagina and nongravid uterus showing the arterial supply.

Anterior Abdominal Wall

BOUNDARIES AND LANDMARKS

In the midline, the anterior abdominal wall is bound above by the *xiphisternal junction* and below by the *pubic symphysis*. The convexly arching lower costal cartilages join together to form a rim (the *costal margin*) that limits the upper part of the wall laterally. Inferiorly, the lateral part of the anterior wall extends, medially to laterally, from the *pubic crest*, the *inguinal ligament* (of Poupart), and the *iliac crest* (Fig. 2–7). There are no bony structures laterally, the wall being limited above by the tenth rib and below by the iliac crest. Other bony landmarks include the *xiphoid process* in the midline above, the *pubic tubercle* (at the lateral end of the pubic crest) and the *anterior superior iliac spine* (at the anterior end of the iliac crest) below. Inferiorly, the pubic bone and the pubic symphysis separate the anterior wall from the vulva; the inguinal ligament that courses from the pubic tubercle to the anterior superior iliac spine separates the inferior part of the wall from the anterior thigh.

Several soft tissue landmarks can be seen, but their degree of visibility is largely dependent on the amount of fat in the subcutaneous tissue, age, muscular status, parity, and period of gestation. The *umbilicus* is most obvious and lies in the midline. Its vertebral level varies, but it is consistently innervated by the T–10 spinal cord segment. The aponeuroses of the lateral abdominal wall muscles join in the midline with their counterpart on the other side to form the *linea alba*. The linea alba runs from the xiphoid process to the pubic symphysis and is usually the strongest part of the aponeurotic portion of the abdominal wall. It may be represented on the surface in lean, muscular patients as a vertical, midline depression. In such patients, a slightly curved, vertical depression can be seen on each side that corresponds to the lateral border of the rectus abdominis muscle (called the *linea semilunaris*).

SKIN AND SUBCUTANEOUS LAYER

In the healthy state, the skin of the anterior wall is smooth and very elastic. It is usually attached to the deeper tissues in the midline. The cleavage lines of the skin (called Langer lines) are shown in Figure 2–7. Above the umbilicus, they mainly run transversely; below the umbilicus, they slant more inferiorly as the midline is approached. The cleavage lines in the groin generally parallel the inguinal ligament; those slightly below the ligament spiral inferiorly around the medial aspect of the upper thigh. Retraction of skin incisions is minimal when cuts are made parallel to the lines and maximal when made at right angles to the lines. Although the importance of the scar in abdominal surgery is often greatly overshadowed by more major issues, incisions parallel to the lines tend to result in finer, more linear scars than those made at right angles (see Chapter 3). Microscopic examination of the tissues shows that the direction of the cleavage lines is parallel to the direction of the majority of underlying connective tissue fibers. Variations in the direction of the lines seem to be influenced more by body shape than by age.

The subcutaneous layer of the wall is composed of a variable amount of fat and connective tissue and contains the cutaneous blood vessels, lymphatics, and nerves (Figs. 2–8 and 2–9). In obese patients, the outer portion of the subcutaneous

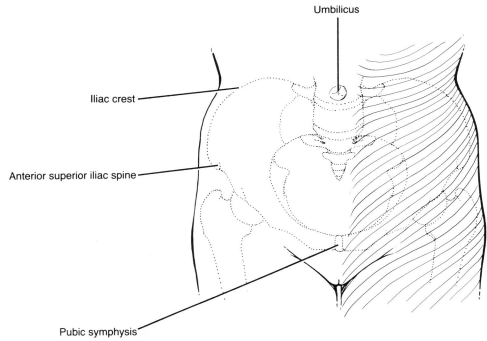

Umbilicus

Iliac crest

Anterior superior iliac spine

Pubic symphysis

Figure 2–7. Langer cleavage lines in the anterior abdominal wall.

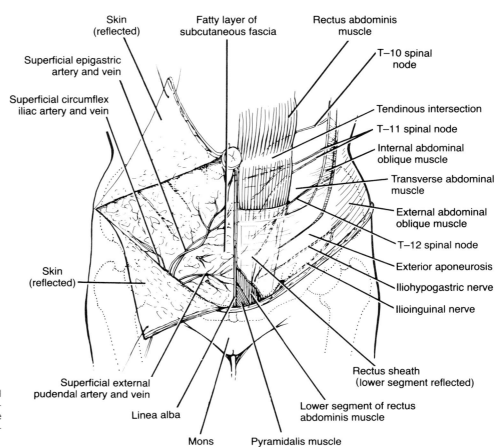

Skin (reflected)
Fatty layer of subcutaneous fascia
Rectus abdominis muscle
Superficial epigastric artery and vein
T–10 spinal node
Superficial circumflex iliac artery and vein
Tendinous intersection
T–11 spinal node
Internal abdominal oblique muscle
Transverse abdominal muscle
External abdominal oblique muscle
Skin (reflected)
T–12 spinal node
Exterior aponeurosis
Iliohypogastric nerve
Ilioinguinal nerve
Rectus sheath (lower segment reflected)
Superficial external pudendal artery and vein
Linea alba
Lower segment of rectus abdominis muscle
Mons
Pyramidalis muscle

Figure 2–8. Anterior abdominal wall. Muscles, fascial layers, vessels, and nerves are shown. The left side of the drawing is superficial, the right side is deep.

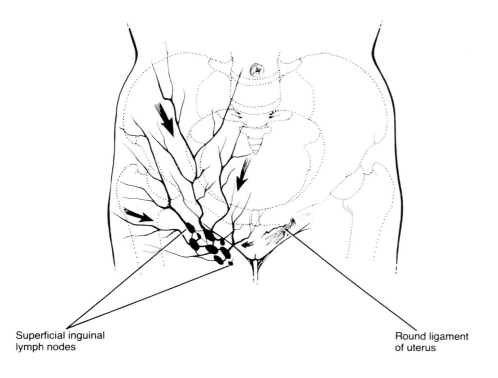

Superficial inguinal lymph nodes
Round ligament of uterus

Figure 2–9. Infraumbilicial part of the anterior abdominal wall showing the course of the round ligament and lymph drainage.

layer (superficial part) in the lower abdominal region has a more fatty texture than the deeper portions, where there may be a concentration of overlapping, fibrous sheets, or lamellae. Fat may collect deep to the fibrous sheet as well. In thin patients, it may be impossible to identify distinct fatty and fibrous portions. The superficial fatty layer continues inferiorly over the pubic bone, where it forms a pad in the midline that produces the mons pubis of the vulva. More laterally, it is continuous with the fatty layer in the labium majus. A vertically coursing, fibrous band of variable extent often is present in the midline just above the symphysis pubis. The band is adherent to the linea alba and is the equivalent of the fundiform ligament of the penis. The subcutaneous layer is only loosely attached to the deep fascia over the external abdominal aponeurosis and rectus sheath on each side of the midline. The loose attachment can become a fascial cleft that may extend into the urogenital part of the perineum.

Arteries in the subcutaneous layer freely anastomose with each other and arise from various sources. Below the umbilicus, most of the skin is supplied by three small branches that ascend from the femoral artery and pass superficial to the inguinal ligament (see Fig. 2–8). They are, from medial to lateral: the *superficial external pudendal artery*, which courses medially, superficial to the round ligament of the uterus, to supply the lower part of the wall and the anterior part of the perineum; the *superficial epigastric artery*, which runs obliquely toward the umbilicus; and the *superficial circumflex iliac artery*, which courses laterally just above the iliac crest.

The subcutaneous veins accompany the arteries but are more numerous and form extensive anastomoses. Below the umbilicus, they mainly drain inferiorly, passing superficial to the inguinal ligament to empty into the terminal part of the great saphenous vein in the upper thigh (see Fig. 2–8). Above the umbilicus, the subcutaneous veins drain superiorly and laterally to the axillary vein or its tributaries.

The subcutaneous lymph vessels mainly follow the course of the veins (Fig. 2–9). A horizontal line at the level of the umbilicus represents the peak of a watershed: below the umbilicus, the lymph travels inferiorly and laterally to the *superficial inguinal nodes* located just below the inguinal ligament; above the umbilicus, it mainly travels superiorly and laterally to the *axillary lymph nodes*.

The skin of the anterior wall is innervated by cutaneous branches of the lower six thoracic and the first lumbar spinal nerves (T–7 to T–12 and L–1). The dermatomes are arranged in serial bands from superior to inferior. The seventh thoracic nerve innervates the skin over the xiphoid process; the tenth thoracic nerve courses to the umbilicus; the subcostal nerve (T–12) supplies the suprapubic skin; and the iliohypogastric nerve (L–1) innervates the skin over the groin. The intervening areas are innervated by the intervening spinal nerves. The lower intercostal nerves maintain their downward and medial slope into the abdominal wall after they leave their intercostal spaces. Cutaneous branches enter the subcutaneous layer on each side in two vertical rows—a small, anterior series that pierces the anterior rectus sheath a short distance from the midline and a larger, lateral series near the midaxillary line. Most of the skin of the anterior wall is supplied by the anterior branches of the lateral series of cutaneous nerves.

MUSCLES AND RECTUS SHEATH

There are five pairs of muscles in the wall that support and protect the abdominal viscera in front and laterally (see Fig. 2–8). They attach above and laterally to the sternum and lower ribs and below to the pelvic bone. The three lateral muscles superimpose as sheets, one on the other. From superficial to deep, they are the *external oblique,* the *internal oblique,* and the *transverse muscles.* The *rectus* and *pyramidalis muscles* constitute the medial group and lie adjacent to the linea alba enclosed in the *rectus sheath.* The rectus sheath is formed by the fusion of the aponeuroses of the three lateral muscles as they course to the midline. The collagen fibers in the fused aponeuroses decussate in the linea alba with their counterpart on the other side, thereby forming a very strong union in the midline.

The external oblique muscle arises from the outer surface of the lower eight ribs. Its fibers course in a manner similar to putting a hand in a pocket, downward and forward. The posterior fibers insert directly on the outer lip of the iliac crest. The remaining fibers give rise to a broad aponeurosis soon after they curve around the side of the abdomen. The aponeurosis passes in front of the rectus muscle to insert in the linea alba. It attaches above to the sternum and below to the anterior superior iliac spine, pubic tubercle, and pubic symphysis. The lower edge of the aponeurosis is thick and folded back on itself, forming the inguinal ligament (of Poupart) in the groin region. The ligament courses between the anterior superior iliac spine and the pubic tubercle and is bound down to the deep fascia of the thigh (fascia lata femoris). The *superficial inguinal ring* is a small opening in the external aponeurosis located about 2.5 cm above and lateral to the pubic tubercle (see Fig. 2–9). The superficial ring lies just above the inguinal ligament. The round ligament of the uterus courses through the ring, then runs inferiorly to attach to the subcutaneous tissue in the labium majus. Accompanying the round ligament through the ring are a variable amount of fat, the genital branch of the genitofemoral nerve, and the artery of the round ligament. The cutaneous portion of the ilioinguinal nerve commonly pierces the external aponeurosis just above the superficial ring.

The internal oblique muscle lies beneath the external oblique muscle. Most of its fibers run at right angles to those of the external oblique muscle. Such an arrangement provides maximal strength to the wall. The internal oblique muscle arises from the lateral half of the inguinal ligament, the iliac crest, and the lumbodorsal fascia. The posterior fibers course upward and forward to insert into the lower ribs and their costal cartilages. The anterior fibers course medially and give rise to an aponeurosis that separates at the lateral border of the rectus muscle into anterior and posterior lamellae. The anterior lamella joins the aponeurosis of the external oblique muscle to form the *anterior rectus sheath* in front of the rectus and pyramidalis muscles. The posterior lamella joins the aponeurosis of the deeper transverse muscle in the upper three fourths of the anterior wall to form the *posterior rectus sheath*. The posterior sheath passes deep to the rectus muscle to attach in the midline to the linea alba. Midway between the umbilicus and the symphysis pubis, the entire internal oblique aponeurosis joins with the external oblique and transversus aponeuroses, and together they form the anterior rectus sheath, which passes in front of the most inferior segment of the rectus muscle and the pyramidalis muscle. The posterior sheath therefore ends about midway between the umbilicus and the pubic symphysis, causing the deep side of the rectus muscle to be bare of the posterior sheath below this point. The lower border of the posterior sheath is referred to as the *arcuate* or *semicircular line*.

The transverse muscle is the deepest of the three lateral muscles. Like the internal oblique muscle, its fibers also originate from the inguinal ligament, iliac crest, and lumbodorsal fascia. The transverse muscle has an additional origin from the inner surface of the lower six costal cartilages. Its fibers mainly run transversely toward the midline. At the lateral border of the rectus muscle, it gives rise to an aponeurosis that helps to form the posterior rectus sheath in the upper three fourths of the wall and the anterior rectus sheath in the lower one fourth. The muscle fibers in the inferior part of the muscle join with similar fibers in the internal oblique muscle and together arch medially and inferiorly over the inguinal canal as the *falx inguinalis*. The most medial part of the falx inguinalis gives rise to the *conjoined tendon* that inserts on the pecten of the pubis. The conjoined tendon lies behind the superficial inguinal ring, giving strength to this area of weakness. Medially, it is continuous with the lower part of the anterior rectus sheath.

The rectus muscle arises above from the xiphoid process of the sternum and the anterior surface of the costal cartilages of the fifth through the seventh ribs. It courses inferiorly as a flat, straplike muscle to insert on the front of the pubic bone and the pubic symphysis (see Fig. 2–8). It is broad and thin above but narrows and thickens as it courses inferiorly. The rectus muscle is enclosed by the rectus sheath except posteriorly in its lower one fourth. It is attached anteriorly to the rectus sheath above the umbilicus at three transverse bands called *tendinous intersections*.

When present, the small pyramidalis muscle is located deep to the lowest part of the anterior rectus sheath in front of the rectus muscle (see Fig. 2–8). It arises from the pubic crest and courses superiorly and medially to insert in the linea alba.

BLOOD VESSELS OF THE ABDOMINAL WALL

Branches of the *lower five intercostal arteries* and the *subcostal artery* accompany their respective nerves to help supply the deep part of the anterior wall. They enter the lateral aspect of the rectus sheath, where they anastomose with the *superior* and *inferior epigastric arteries*. The superior epigastric artery is the inferior continuation of the internal thoracic (mammary) artery. It courses inferiorly behind the seventh costal cartilage, where it enters the rectus sheath. As it continues inferiorly, it becomes buried in the rectus muscle. The larger inferior epigastric artery takes origin from the external iliac artery at the level where the latter passes behind the middle of the inguinal ligament. It courses medially and upward between the transversalis fascia and the peritoneum, passing near the medial edge of the deep inguinal ring (Fig. 2–10). The inferior epigastric artery pierces the transversalis fascia as it approaches the rectus muscle, then enters the rectus sheath by coursing in front of the arcuate line. It ascends in the posterior part of the rectus muscle and, about half the time, anastomoses with the superior epigastric artery, forming a vertically coursing arterial channel within the rectus sheath. The lower, lateral part of the wall is supplied by the *deep circumflex iliac artery* that arises from the external iliac artery and ascends between the internal oblique and transverse muscles.

The veins draining the deep part of the anterior wall generally accompany the arteries. Above the umbilicus, they course upward to the internal thoracic (mammary) vein and laterally to the lower intercostal veins; below the umbilicus, the inferior epigastric vein drains into the external iliac vein.

MOTOR NERVES IN THE ANTERIOR ABDOMINAL WALL AND THEIR JEOPARDY IN SURGICAL INCISIONS

The *lower six thoracic nerves* (T–7 to T–12) supply the principal motor innervation to the anterior wall muscles (see Fig. 2–8). The seventh

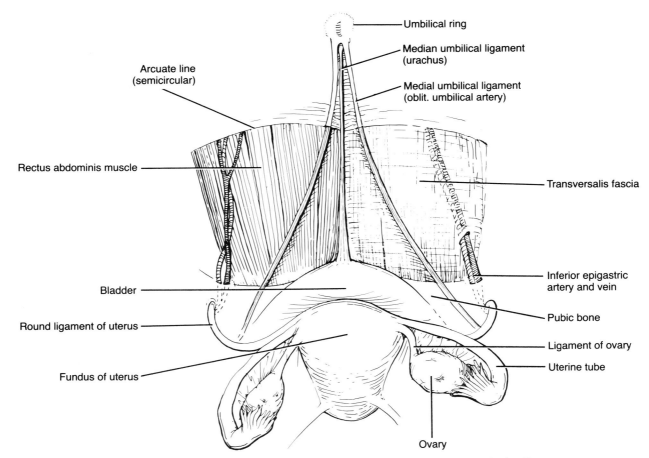

Figure 2–10. Posterior view of the infraumbilical part of the anterior abdominal wall.

through the eleventh intercostal nerves and the subcostal nerve enter the wall at the costal margin and spiral forward and inferiorly between the internal oblique and transverse muscles. They give off important motor branches to these two muscles and to the more superficial external oblique muscle. The thoracic nerves continue medially, where they enter the lateral border of the rectus sheath to innervate the rectus muscle. They terminate as anterior cutaneous nerves after piercing the anterior rectus sheath. Motor innervation to the infraumbilical portion of the wall, including the lower part of the rectus muscle, is supplied by the tenth, eleventh, and twelfth thoracic nerves. The pyramidalis muscle just above the pubic symphysis usually is supplied by the subcostal nerve (T–12). The iliohypogastric and ilioinguinal nerves often arise in common from the first lumbar nerve (L–1), which enters the lateral part of the anterior wall just below the subcostal nerve. The two branches arise close to the iliac crest, but usually neither enters the rectus sheath. The ilioinguinal branch innervates the lower part of the internal oblique muscle, then courses through the inguinal canal to become cutaneous by passing out the superficial ring. The iliohypogastric branch is

mainly a cutaneous nerve to the lower, lateral part of the wall.

Because the motor nerves to the rectus muscle enter along its lateral border, this muscle cannot be easily freed and retracted medially without injuring its nerve supply. However, it is safe to retract the muscle laterally. The commonly used *median vertical incision* has the advantage of not cutting through any motor nerves or muscle fibers. The linea alba is cut in this incision, and the medial margins of the rectus and pyramidalis muscles are retracted laterally. In the *paramedian vertical incision*, the anterior rectus sheath, rather than the linea alba, is cut. The rectus muscle is then retracted medially or laterally. However, medial retractions jeopardize its nerve supply. In muscle-splitting incisions, the rectus muscle is separated vertically along its length. Such incisions may denervate that part of the rectus muscle on the medial side of the wound. Deep to the rectus muscle, the transversalis fascia is encountered immediately if the incision is below the arcuate line, where the posterior rectus sheath is absent.

Transverse incisions are made in a curved manner and cut through the anterior rectus sheath on both sides. No motor nerves are in jeopardy when the rectus muscles are retracted laterally. Detachment of the rectus and pyramidalis muscles from their insertion on the pubis causes little nerve damage as long as the detachment is below the entrance of the subcostal nerve (T–12). Some denervation is produced when the rectus muscle is cut transversely above its pubic attachment. The closer the cut is made to the entrance of a motor nerve, the more nerve fibers are interrupted, since the nerves course vertically after their entrance into the muscle. The *oblique incision* is often made in the lower lateral part of the anterior wall. It is usually a muscle-splitting incision that divides the three lateral muscles in the direction of their fleshy and tendinous fibers. Oblique incisions near the anterior superior iliac spine can injure the ilioinguinal nerve and possibly denervate the lower part of the internal oblique muscle (falx inguinalis). Oblique incisions at higher levels jeopardize the lower thoracic nerves as they course to the rectus muscle between the internal oblique and transverse muscles. Transecting them denervates a segment of the rectus muscle.

TRANSVERSALIS FASCIA, EXTRAPERITONEAL TISSUE, AND PERITONEUM

The *transversalis fascia* is subserous fascia located on the deep side of the transverse muscle. It is usually thicker and stronger than the deep fascia between the muscles in the wall. It is the anterior part of the endoabdominal fascial layer that lines the abdominal cavity. In the midline, deep to the linea alba, it is continuous with that on the other side. Above the arcuate line, the transversalis fascia lies adjacent to the deep surface of the posterior rectus sheath. Below the arcuate line in the lower one fourth of the wall, it lies adjacent to the rectus muscle itself, where the posterior rectus sheath is absent (see Fig. 2–10). The transversalis fascia attaches inferiorly to the posterior surface of the pubis, but more laterally it helps form the femoral sheath around the femoral artery and vein and blends with the iliopsoas fascia.

The transversalis fascia is separated from the peritoneum by loose *extraperitoneal* (preperitoneal) *tissue* that contains a variable quantity of fat. In the lower part of the wall, remnants of fetal structures course superiorly through this layer to the deep side of the umbilicus (see Fig. 2–10). In or near the midline is the single *median* (middle) *umbilical ligament,* the remains of the fetal urachus, which connects to the apex of the bladder. It is often hypertrophied during pregnancy and may be sectioned during bladder mobilization. Located farther laterally on either side is the *medial* (formerly called lateral) *umbilical ligament.* It is the remnant of the distal part of the umbilical artery that carries blood to the placenta during fetal life. This ligament also has been called the obliterated umbilical or hypogastric artery. It is surgically

important that the extraperitoneal tissue in the lower abdominal wall is continuous below with the retropubic or prevesical space (of Retzius), allowing for easy anterior mobilization of the bladder.

The *peritoneum* is the deepest layer of the anterior wall and is the serous membrane lining the peritoneal cavity. In the lower part of the wall, it continues laterally on the deep side of the inguinal canal and reflects superiorly to line part of the iliac fossa. Inferiorly, the peritoneum on the wall (parietal layer) becomes visceral by continuing onto the superior surface of the bladder, then lining the vesicouterine pouch to reach the anterior aspect of the uterus (see Fig. 2–5). This part of the peritoneum is mobilized in an extraperitoneal cesarean section by the development of a space from the suprapubic approach.

Pelvis

The pelvis (basin) consists of the *pelvic* (innominate or coxal) bone on each side anteriorly and laterally and the *sacrum* and *coccyx* in the midline posteriorly. The two pelvic bones articulate in the midline anteriorly at a fibrocartilaginous joint, the *pubic symphysis.* Limited movement takes place at the pubic symphysis, and it is thought that there is some softening of the fibrocartilage near term, allowing some separation of the pubic bones during parturition. Posteriorly, the pelvic bone articulates with the sacrum at the *sacroiliac joint.* This joint is partly cartilaginous and partly synovial in type, permitting some limited movement.

The pelvis is divided into a *true (minor)* and a *false (major)* pelvis. The boundary between the false (a part of the abdomen) and the true pelvis is the *superior pelvic aperture,* or pelvic inlet. The superior pelvic aperture is bounded on each side by the *linea terminalis,* in the front by the upper edge of the pubic symphysis, and in the back by the sacral promontory. The linea terminalis is a line on the bony pelvis that runs through the pecten of the pubis and the arcuate line of the ilium. Although the superior pelvic aperture opens freely above into the abdominal cavity, the *inferior pelvic aperture,* or pelvic outlet, is closed by muscles that form most of the rounded bottom of the basin and surround the viscera that open to the outside through it.

Two muscles form the floor of the pelvis, and together they constitute the *pelvic diaphragm.* They are the *coccygeus,* a simple muscle between the coccyx and the ischial spine, and the complex *levator ani,* which passes from one side of the pelvis to the other and from the pubis anteriorly to the coccyx posteriorly (see Fig. 2–3). The levator ani portion of the pelvic diaphragm attaches to pelvic viscera and is considered important in support of the uterus and in voluntary control of the bladder and rectum (see Fig. 2–4). Two muscles, the obturator internus and the piriformis, line the posterior and lateral walls of the pelvis. They are considered muscles of the lower extremity and are not part of the pelvic diaphragm.

The muscles lining the pelvis and forming the pelvic floor are covered by the endoabdominal fascial layer, which continues downward into the pelvis from the abdominal cavity. Various parts of the fascia have received special names. Pelvic fasciae can be divided into two portions: the *parietal fascia,* which covers the walls of the pelvis, and the *visceral fascia,* which is associated with the pelvic viscera. Parietal fascia may be subdivided into the *obturator fascia* over the obturator internus muscle and the *superior fascia of the pelvic diaphragm,* which covers the muscles of the diaphragm (see Fig. 2–4). The pelvic visceral fascia has been described in many different ways, but a generally valid concept is that it forms thin sheaths around the various viscera and blends with the fascia on the pelvic diaphragm. Nerves and vessels coursing along the posterolateral wall of the pelvis are surrounded by neurovascular sheaths that are attached to the parietal pelvic fascia and course medially to supply pelvic viscera.

Uterus

SIZE AND POSITION OF THE NONGRAVID UTERUS

The nongravid uterus is located in or near the midline of the pelvis between the bladder and small intestine in front and the rectum and sigmoid colon behind (see Fig. 2–5). It has an inverted pear shape, with thick, muscular walls and a triangle-shaped lumen that is narrow in the sagittal plane but broad in the frontal plane. The three major subdivisions of the uterus are the upper, triangular portion, called the *body;* a lower, tubular portion, called the *cervix;* and a short, intervening, constricted portion called the *isthmus.* The domed portion of the body above the entrance of the uterine tubes is the *fundus.* The vaginal wall attaches to the cervix obliquely, being higher posteriorly than anteriorly. The line of attachment divides the cervix into vaginal and supravaginal segments. In the nongravid state, the convex fundus is directed anteriorly, with the body forming nearly a 90-degree angle with the vagina (anteverted), and bent slightly inferiorly (anteflexed). The anterior surface of the body is flat and lies adjacent to the superior surface of the bladder. The posterior surface is convex and faces superiorly and posteriorly near the sigmoid colon and rectum.

The cervix is directed downward and backward, in contact with the posterior wall of the vagina. Its opening, or *external os,* lies in or near a plane at the level of the ischial spines and the upper end of the pubic symphysis. The ureter courses imme-diately lateral to the cervix, making it very susceptible to injury at this point (Fig. 2–11*B;* see Figs. 2–4, 2–6).

The peritoneum covers the body of the uterus, including the fundus portion (see Figs. 2–4, 2–5). Anteriorly, at the level of the isthmus, the peritoneum is reflected onto the upper surface of the bladder, forming the shallow *vesicouterine pouch.* Posteriorly, the peritoneum extends farther inferiorly, covering the isthmus, the supravaginal cervix, and the posterior fornix of the vagina before reflexing onto the anterior surface of the rectum, forming the deep *rectouterine pouch* (of Douglas).

The dimensions of the nongravid uterus vary considerably, and the uterus is usually slightly larger when it has accommodated a previous pregnancy. The body of the uterus averages approximately 5 cm in length. The isthmus and the cervix together measure approximately 2.5 cm long and 2 cm in diameter. The size of the cervix in relation to the body of the uterus varies with age and parity. In a young child, the cervix is twice the size of the uterine body, about equal to that in a nulliparous woman, and about one third the size of the uterine body in a multiparous woman.

The wall of the uterus is made up of a thin outer covering of peritoneum *(serosa),* a thick intermediate layer of variable proportions of smooth muscle and connective tissue *(myometrium),* and an inner mucosal layer *(endometrium).* The body of the uterus contains the most muscle fibers, with the amount diminishing inferiorly as the cervix is approached. The cervix is made up of only about 10% muscle, with the balance being mainly connective tissue. As a result of its development from the fused portion of the paramesonephric (müllerian, or female) ducts, the muscle fiber arrangement in the uterine wall is complex. The *outer layer* of the myometrium contains mostly vertical fibers that course laterally in the upper part of the body to become continuous with the external longitudinal muscle layer of the uterine tubes. The *middle layer* constitutes the bulk of the uterine wall and is made up of an interlacing network of spiraling muscle fibers that are continuous with the inner circular muscle layer of each tube. Bundles of smooth muscle fibers in the supportive ligaments interlace and blend with this layer. The *inner layer* consists of circularly arranged fibers that may have a sphincter-like function at the isthmus and at the orifices of the tubes. Two muscle fascicles in the lateral wall run from the cervix to the fundus and may play a role in the coordination of muscle contraction.

The uterine cavity in the nongravid state is little more than a slit when viewed laterally, with close anterior and posterior walls (see Fig. 2–5). The cavity has the shape of an inverted triangle when viewed from the front, with a *base* superiorly, where it is continuous on each side with the lumen of the uterine tube, and an *apex* inferiorly, where

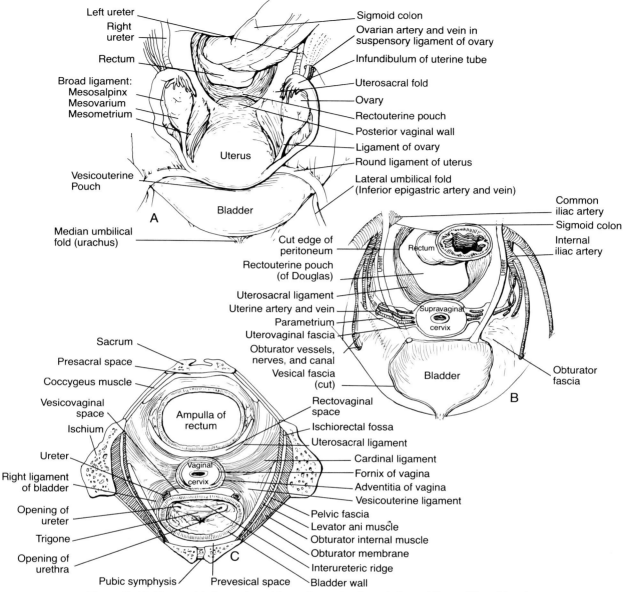

Figure 2–11. Nongravid uterus viewed from above showing relations at three different levels.

it is continuous with the canal coursing through the isthmus and the cervix (see Fig. 2–14, nongravid). The canal of the isthmus is constricted and may be 6 to 10 mm in length. Where its upper end widens into the uterine cavity, the canal is called the *anatomic internal os*. Where the lower end of the isthmic canal widens into the cervical canal, the canal of the isthmus is known as the *histologic internal os* because it is the level where an abrupt microscopic change occurs in the mucosa. The cervical canal is slightly expanded in its middle and opens into the vagina at the external os.

ADNEXA OF THE NONGRAVID UTERUS
Uterine Tube

Extending laterally from each side of the body of the uterus is a long, narrow, trumpet-shaped uterine tube (fallopian tube, salpinx, or oviduct) (see Figs. 2–4 and 2–11A). It occupies the upper border of the broad ligament and arches laterally over the upper pole of the ovary, then downward over the posterior part of the medial surface of the ovary. The lumen, or canal, of the tube runs from the superior angle of the uterine cavity to the ovary, gradually increasing in diameter as it courses laterally. In the nongravid state, the tube is approximately 10 cm long when straightened. Four different segments can be distinguished. The *intramural portion* is within the wall of the uterus that communicates with the uterine cavity. Its lumen has the smallest diameter (a millimeter or less). The narrow segment extending laterally from the lateral margin of the uterus is called the *isthmus*. At its lateral extent, the tube enlarges and becomes somewhat tortuous, forming the *am-*

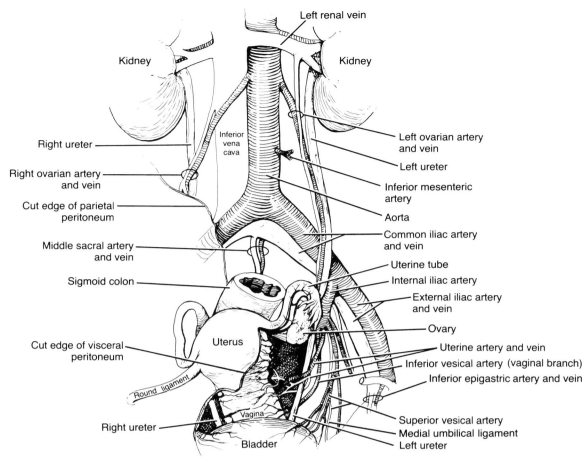

Figure 2–12. Posterior abdominal and pelvic walls showing relationships to the nongravid uterus.

pulla. The tube terminates near the ovary as the funnel-shaped *infundibulum.* Finger-like *fimbriae* extend from the periphery of the infundibulum surrounding the *abdominal ostium.* One or more fimbriae are in contact with the ovary *(ovarian fimbria).* The wall of the tube is made up of three layers: an outer layer composed mainly of the peritoneum *(serosa),* an intermediate smooth muscle layer *(myosalpinx),* and an inner mucosal lining *(endosalpinx).* The mucosal lining is arranged in longitudinal folds that extend into the lumen. The folds are highly branched in the ampullary segment.

Ovary

The oval or almond-shaped ovary is the female gonad (see Fig. 2–11A). It is located medial to the curved portion of the uterine tube and is somewhat flattened, measuring approximately 2 cm wide, 4 cm long, and 1 cm thick. It usually has a grayish-pink coloration and a puckered, uneven surface. The long axis of the ovary is almost vertical, the upper pole being located close to the uterine tube, with the lower pole nearer the uterus. The surfaces face medially and laterally. The posterior border is free; the anterior border is attached to the broad ligament by a short, two-layered fold of peritoneum

called the *mesovarium.* Vessels and nerves course through the mesovarium to reach the ovarian *hilum.* In nulliparous women, the ovary usually lies in the upper part of the pelvic cavity in a shallow depression on the lateral wall between the diverging external and internal iliac vessels *(ovarian fossa).* In multiparous women, it may lie anywhere on the lateral pelvic wall or even extend into the rectouterine pouch. The ovary becomes displaced during the first pregnancy and usually never returns to its original position. In nulliparous women, the upper pole usually lies near the external iliac vein. Attached to the upper pole is a vascular fold of peritoneum, the *suspensory ligament of the ovary* (infundibulopelvic), that contains the ovarian vessels and nerves (Fig. 2–12; see Figs. 2–4, 2–6, 2–11A). The lower pole is attached to the uterus by a round, fibromuscular cord called the *ligament of the ovary.* This ligament joins the lateral margin of the uterus in the angle where the tube joins the body of the uterus.

Uterine Ligaments

The *broad ligament of the uterus* is a double fold of peritoneum or mesentery that extends laterally from the uterus on each side (see Figs. 2–4, 2–11). The peritoneum on the anterior and posterior surfaces of the uterus continues laterally as the anterior and posterior layers of the broad ligament. The two layers join superiorly, where they enclose the uterine tube at the upper border of the broad ligament. A double layer of peritoneum, the *mesovarium,* extends posteriorly from the posterior surface of the broad ligament to the ovary. That part of the broad ligament above the origin of the mesovarium is called the *mesosalpinx* because it contains the uterine tube in its free border. That part below the origin of the mesovarium is called the *mesometrium.* The suspensory ligament of the ovary and its contained vessels and nerves are continuous with the lateral part of the broad ligament. The ligament of the ovary lies within the free borders of the mesovarium as the former courses to the lateral side of the uterus. The base of the broad ligament (mesometrial portion) encloses the uterine vessels and nerves.

The subserous connective tissue of the uterus continues laterally into the broad ligament as the *parametrium.* It contains some smooth muscle fibers and anchors the broad ligament to the lateral pelvic wall. The parametrium is scant medially near the uterus and superiorly near the tube where the two peritoneal layers of the ligament are close. The parametrial tissue is more abundant laterally and inferiorly where the broad ligament thickens. The connective tissue in the base of the ligament is continuous with the connective tissue of the pelvic floor (superior fascia of the pelvic diaphragm). Its densest portion is named the *cardinal ligament* (transverse cervical or Mackenrodt); it attaches medially to the upper vaginal wall and supravaginal portion of the cervix and laterally to the parietal fascia on the lateral pelvic wall (see Fig. 2–11*C*). Another fascial thickening, known as the *uterosacral ligament,* is continuous with the posterior aspect of the cardinal ligament. It attaches to the supravaginal cervix, then passes posterolaterally around the lateral side of the rectum to become continuous with the fascia covering the front of the second and third sacral vertebrae. The peritoneum covering the ligament is named the *uterosacral fold* and forms the lateral boundary of the rectouterine pouch. On occasion, there is a thickened band of fascia coursing between the supravaginal cervix and the posterior surface of the bladder called the *vesicouterine* (anterior) *ligament.* Its peritoneal covering forms the *vesicouterine fold.* Often the cardinal and uterosacral ligaments are not distinct anatomic ligaments but mainly neurovascular sheaths or fascial condensations. However, they have long been regarded as clinically important supports of the uterus.

The *round ligament of the uterus* is attached to the lateral side of the uterus in front of the attachment of the ligament of the ovary (see Fig. 2–11*A*). It courses laterally through the broad ligament to reach the lateral pelvic wall, where it ascends over the external iliac vessels to enter the deep inguinal ring lateral to the inferior epigastric vessels (see Fig. 2–10). It passes through the inguinal canal and anchors in the tissue of the labium majus (see Fig. 2–9). The round ligament of the uterus is 3 to 5 mm in diameter and is composed of smooth muscle fibers and connective tissue. It and the ligament of the ovary are remnants of the gubernaculum of the ovary, found in late embryos.

UTERINE BLOOD VESSELS, LYMPHATICS, AND NERVES

Arteries

Knowledge of the origin, course, and branching pattern of the arteries that supply the uterus is very important in controlling bleeding during surgery. The main blood supply to the uterus is the *uterine artery,* which arises in a variable manner from the anterior division of the internal iliac (hypogastric) artery (see Figs. 2–4, 2–6, 2–11*B*, 2–12). Nearly half of the time, the uterine artery arises independently from the internal iliac artery. At other times, it may originate from the umbilical, internal pudendal, inferior vesical, or vaginal branches, or from a stem in common with one or more of these branches. A double uterine artery has been observed. The *ovarian artery* assists in supplying the uterus through its large anastomosis with the uterine artery in the broad ligament (see Fig. 2–6).

The uterine artery courses downward from its origin in the lateral pelvic wall, then forward and medially, passing above and in front of the ureter, to which it may send a branch. It turns sharply medially in the base of the broad ligament, running toward the cervix. The parametrium binds the artery to the accompanying veins, nerves, ureter, and cardinal ligament. As the uterine artery approaches the cervix, it supplies the latter with several tortuous, penetrating branches. The arrangement of the cervical branches allows for rapid cervical expansion without interruption of the blood supply. The uterine artery then divides into one large, very tortuous ascending branch and one or more smaller descending branches that supply the upper vagina and adjacent part of the bladder (see Fig. 2–6). The ascending main branch courses superiorly along the lateral margin of the uterus, sending arcuate branches to the uterine body. The *arcuate arteries* circle the uterus beneath the serosa. At intervals, they give off *radial branches,* which penetrate the interlacing muscle fibers of the myometrium by passing directly inward. When the interlacing muscle fibers contract after delivery, they function as ligatures by constricting the radial branches. The arcuate arteries quickly diminish in size as they course toward the midline. Because of this, there tends to be less bleeding with midline incisions of the uterus than with lateral ones. When the ascending branch of the uterine artery reaches the uterine tube, it turns laterally in the upper part of the uterine tube, dividing into *tubal* and *ovarian branches* (see Fig. 2–6). The tubal branch runs laterally in the mesosalpinx close to the uterine tube, which it supplies through a series of branches. The ovarian branch courses into the mesovarium, where it has a large anastomosis with the ovarian artery that arises from the aorta. The anastomotic channel supplies the ovary and sends a series of tubal branches through the mesosalpinx that anastomose with the tubal branch of the uterine artery.

Veins

The venous plexus that drains the uterus passes inferiorly, whereas the one draining the vagina passes superiorly. Both plexuses are continuous with a plexiform arrangement of uterine veins that surround the uterine artery lateral to the cervix. As the veins approach the lateral pelvic wall, they usually join to form two trunks that empty into the internal iliac vein. Although the major portion of blood from the uterus drains inferiorly by way of the uterine veins, some drains superiorly through the suspensory ligament of the ovary as the *ovarian*, or *pampiniform plexus*. On the right side, the ovarian venous plexus, in company with the ovarian artery, crosses the ureter obliquely and empties into the inferior vena cava (see Fig. 2–12). On the left side, the ovarian plexus does not cross the left ureter and drains into the left renal vein.

Lymphatics

Lymph channels are very numerous in the walls of the entire genital tract. Intramural plexuses drain the endometrium and myometrium into a subserosal plexus, which is drained by efferent vessels. Lymph from the lower uterus drains mainly to the sacral, external iliac, and common iliac nodes, some also emptying into the lower lumbar nodes along the abdominal aorta and the superficial inguinal nodes. Most of the lymph from the upper uterus passes laterally in the broad ligament, where it joins with that from the uterine tube and ovary. It then leaves the pelvis by coursing superiorly through the suspensory ligament of the ovary in company with the ovarian vessels. It travels on the posterior body wall, draining into nodes along the lower part of the abdominal aorta.

Nerves

Nerves to the uterus course through the pelvic plexus and consist primarily of afferent and sympathetic fibers, with few parasympathetic fibers. Uterine and vaginal fibers course medially together around the uterine vessels in the upper part of the cardinal ligament. Most of the nerves accompany the branches of the uterine artery, with the cervix receiving more fibers than the body of the uterus. Afferent pain fibers from the body appear to travel through the hypogastric plexus and lumbar sympathetic chain to enter the spinal cord through the T–11 and T–12 spinal nerves. Uterine pain has been relieved by blocks of the first three lumbar sympathetic ganglia. Sectioning the hypogastric plexus makes biopsy of the fundus painless. Pain from the cervix and upper vagina passes through the pelvic plexus to enter the spinal cord through sacral spinal nerves S–2, S–3, and S–4. Preganglionic sympathetic fibers to the uterus course from the aortic plexus, through the hypogastric plexus just inferior to the sacral promontory, and to the pelvic plexus, where they synapse in small ganglia within the plexus.

Pelvic Portion of the Ureter

This segment of the ureter is most susceptible to injury during surgery, its ligation being the most common accident. The ureter enters the pelvic cavity by crossing either the common iliac artery or the external iliac artery (see Fig. 2–12). The attachment of the sigmoid mesocolon to the posterior wall lies between the left ureter and the midline. In the pelvis, the ureter on both sides passes medial to the internal iliac and obturator vessels. It takes a curved course medially on the upper part of the pelvic wall, where it runs just posterior to the ovary beneath the peritoneum (see Fig. 2–11A). The ureter passes close to the suspensory ligament of the ovary, where it is in jeopardy when the ovarian vessels within the ligament are clamped.

The course of the ureter toward the cervix often can be seen without dissection through the transparent peritoneum and the posterior layer of the broad ligament when the uterus is elevated anteriorly by traction. As the ureter courses near the uterosacral fold, it passes deeper into the connective tissue of the uterosacral and cardinal ligaments at the base of the broad ligament of the uterus. It then runs obliquely medially, behind and under the uterine artery (see Figs. 2–4, 2–6, 2–11B, 2–12).

The ureter, uterine artery, and nerves are enclosed in a common connective tissue sheath for 1 to 2.5 cm of their length. At this point, the ureter usually lies 1.5 to 2 cm lateral to the cervix. The distance from the cervix varies from 1 to 4 cm, and at this point the ureter is most susceptible to injury. Following the cord-like medial umbilical ligament (obliterated hypogastric or umbilical artery) to its origin in the lateral pelvic wall can help locate the distal part of the ureter.

After the ureter leaves the base of the broad ligament, it inclines medially and downward in front of the upper vaginal wall to terminate in the bladder. This segment of the ureter is easy to palpate. Dissection of the bladder off the anterior surface of the supravaginal cervix displaces the ureters downward and laterally. At the posterior wall of the bladder, the ureters are approximately 5 cm apart, but the slit-like openings inside the bladder are only half this distance apart because of their very oblique downward and medial course through the thick wall of the empty bladder. The oblique course of the ureter through the bladder wall is thought to be important in preventing reflux of urine from the bladder into the ureter.

The main arterial supply to the pelvic portion of the ureter arises close to the pelvic brim from the common, external, or internal iliac arteries rather than from higher levels that descend with it. Because the branches reach the ureter from its lateral side, the pelvic ureter should be exposed from its medial side. The lowest segment of the ureter near the bladder usually receives a branch from the uterine and the inferior vesical arteries. The anastomoses of arteries in the wall of the pelvic ureter are not always adequate, so that interruption of one of the supplying vessels can cause damage.

Nerves to the pelvic portion of the ureter are sparse and arise from the hypogastric and pelvic plexuses. Although ureteric peristalsis is independent of an extrinsic nerve supply, the lower part of the ureter receives both sympathetic and parasympathetic nerve fibers.

Bladder and Urethra

The hollow, muscular *bladder* is lined with a mucous membrane and covered superiorly with peritoneum (see Fig. 2–5). Its shape and relations depend on its state of distension. When empty, the bladder has a pyramid shape, with an *apex* pointed forward and upward, a *base* (fundus) pointed backward and downward, and one *superior* and two *lateral* surfaces. The superior surface is flat or concave and in contact with the anterior surface of the nongravid uterus.

As the bladder fills, the superior surface becomes convex and comes into contact with the small intestine. The lateral surfaces are separated from the symphysis pubis and the pubic bones by loose connective tissue, forming a potential space called the *prevesical,* or *retropubic,* space (of Retzius) that allows for easy surgical separation of the bladder from the pubis. The potential space may contain large amounts of fat and extends around the sides of the bladder and upward through the extraperitoneal tissue to the umbilicus. The two lateral surfaces meet the base at the *neck* of the bladder, which lies adjacent to the superior fascial layer of the urogenital diaphragm. The neck of the bladder is continuous inferiorly with the *urethra.* Superi-

orly, the *median umbilical ligament* attaches to the apex.

Below the vesicouterine pouch, the base of the bladder lies adjacent to the cervix and anterior vaginal wall, being separated from them by a layer of connective tissue called the *vesicovaginal septum.* The septum contains the vesical venous plexus (also called the pudendal or Santorini plexus), which drains the posterior surface of the bladder, the cervix, and the upper vagina. These veins are encountered during total hysterectomy and during a low cesarean section. Because the connective tissue lateral to the bladder surrounds the vessels and nerves to the bladder and the terminal part of the ureter, it is sometimes called the *lateral* (true) *ligament of the bladder* (see Fig. 2–11C). It blends laterally with the fascia on the pelvic surface of the levator ani muscle which, when thickened, forms the vesicouterine ligament that laterally bounds the shallow vesicouterine pouch.

Because the mucosa lining the bladder is only loosely attached to the muscular layer, it is folded when the bladder is empty. In an empty bladder, the lining is smooth only in a triangular area at the bladder base called the *trigone.* The lateral angles of the trigone are formed by the ureteral orifices, with the urethral opening in the midline forming the anterior angle. Underlying muscle fibers raise the mucosa between the ureteral orifices into an *interureteric ridge.*

The *urethra* is a short tube in the female, extending approximately 3 cm from the bladder neck to its orifice *(meatus)* in the vestibule of the vagina (see Fig. 2–1). It begins at the bladder neck at the level of the middle of the pubic symphysis, where it is surrounded by dense fascia and the vesical venous plexus. After a short downward and forward course, it terminates posterior to the lower edge of the pubic symphysis. The upper half of the urethra is close to the anterior vaginal wall and is separated from it by dense connective tissue and blood vessels. Its lower half is actually embedded in the anterior wall of the vagina. The vesicovaginal septum separating the bladder and vagina does not extend inferiorly to separate the urethra and vagina. As the urethra pierces the urogenital diaphragm, it is surrounded by the sphincter muscle of the urethra. Because the urethral mucosa is arranged into longitudinal folds, it is relatively easy to dilate.

The arteries supplying the bladder are variable in number, origin, and branching pattern. One to four *superior vesical arteries* supply the apex and superior and lateral surfaces. They usually arise from the proximal, patent segment of the umbilical artery, but about 10% of the time they arise from the uterine artery. The *inferior vesical artery* is usually a single branch of the internal iliac artery; it supplies the base and neck of the bladder and the upper part of the urethra and vagina. Anastomoses have not been found in the bladder wall. Most of the bladder wall drains into the *vesical venous plexus* around the bladder neck. This venous plexus receives the deep dorsal vein of the clitoris anteriorly and communicates with the vaginal plexus posteriorly. It drains laterally through three channels into the internal iliac vein. Lymphatics from the bladder course laterally to the *external* and *internal iliac nodes*.

Nerves to the bladder course through the hypogastric plexus, the sacral sympathetic trunk, and the pelvic splanchnic nerves, all of which unite in the pelvic plexus. The vesical nerve plexus is an anteroinferior extension of the pelvic plexus that runs medially to the bladder. Cholinergic (parasympathetic) fibers have been observed in the bladder neck and proximal urethra. There are few adrenergic (sympathetic) fibers in these two regions, but they are abundant in the trigone area.

Sigmoid Colon, Rectum, and Anal Canal

The *sigmoid colon* is the continuation of the descending colon and because of its location in the pelvic cavity is sometimes referred to as the pelvic colon. It begins in the left iliac fossa near the pelvic brim and ends in front of the third sacral vertebra by becoming the rectum (see Fig. 2–11*A*). The S-shaped sigmoid colon enters the true pelvis by passing over the medial border of the left greater psoas muscle, crosses the midline in front of the sacrum, then swings back to the left and inferiorly to become the rectum in the posterior part of the lower pelvic cavity. The uterus, uterine tubes, and ovaries are located anteriorly and inferiorly. Structures that cross the left part of the pelvic brim pass posterior to the sigmoid colon. The most significant are the left common iliac vessels, the left ureter, and the left ovarian vessels (see Fig. 2–12). The sacral promontory and first three sacral vertebrae are posterior to the sigmoid colon as it crosses the midline. This segment of the colon is covered completely with peritoneum and is suspended throughout its length by a mesentery, the *sigmoid mesocolon*. Because of its peritoneal outer surface, the sigmoid colon sometimes is used to cover the operative site during pelvic surgery to prevent adhesions to the adjacent small intestine.

The *rectum* begins in the midline at the level of the third sacral vertebra, where the sigmoid colon loses its mesentery. It is approximately 10 cm in length and follows the concave surface of the lower sacrum and coccyx as it courses inferiorly and forward (see Fig. 2–5). Below the coccyx it turns sharply backward to become the anal canal. The superior one third of the rectum is covered with peritoneum on its front and sides. Only the front of the middle one third is covered with peritoneum,

which reflects anteriorly onto the posterior fornix of the vagina and supravaginal cervix, forming the floor of the rectouterine pouch. The lowest one third of the rectum has no peritoneal covering and may be dilated to form the *ampulla* (see Fig. 2–11*C*). The lower sacrum, coccyx, and anococcygeal raphe are posterior relations. Laterally, from above downward, are the sigmoid colon in the pararectal fossa, the sacral plexus of nerves, and the piriformis, coccygeus, and levator ani muscles.

The upper part of the rectum is usually separated anteriorly from the cervix and posterior fornix of the vagina by coils of small intestine that fill the rectouterine pouch. The posterior vaginal wall lies anterior to the lower part of the rectum and is separated from it by a thin layer of fascia named the *rectovaginal septum*. The rectum and vagina can be separated surgically by developing a space in the septum.

The anal canal is the terminal segment of the large intestine. It begins at the lower flexure of the rectum as the intestine passes through the pelvic diaphragm between the pubococcygeus portions of the levator ani muscles (see Figs. 2–3, 2–5). The canal is about 3 cm in length and extends in a posteroinferior direction to end in the perineum as the *anus*. The levator ani muscle separates it from the ischiorectal fat. An involuntary *internal anal sphincter* surrounds its upper part, and a voluntary *external anal sphincter* surrounds its lower part. A large venous plexus lies just deep to the surface lining of the canal. It can drain superiorly into the hepatic portal system by way of the superior rectal (hemorrhoidal) vein or inferiorly into the inferior vena caval system of veins by way of the middle and inferior rectal veins.

Posterior Abdominal Wall Structures

The *abdominal aorta* courses inferiorly in the midline, anterior to the upper four lumbar vertebrae and to the left of the inferior vena cava (see Fig. 2–12). It ends in front of the fourth lumbar vertebra by dividing into left and right common iliac arteries. The latter course inferior and laterally, to terminate in front of the sacroiliac joint by dividing into external and internal iliac branches. The abdominal aorta supplies the gastrointestinal tract, pancreas, liver, suprarenal glands, kidneys, ovaries, and posterior body wall.

The *inferior vena cava* begins at the union of the common iliac veins in front of the fifth lumbar vertebra. It ascends to the right of the abdominal aorta (see Fig. 2–12) but has fewer visceral tributaries than the aorta has branches because the gastrointestinal tract and pancreas drain into the liver by way of the hepatic portal vein. The remaining branches of the abdominal aorta have corresponding veins that drain into the inferior vena cava. An important difference in the tributary pattern is the drainage of the suprarenal gland and ovary on the left side. The veins from these two viscera drain first into the left renal vein rather than directly into the inferior vena cava. The left renal vein crosses the midline in front of the aorta to terminate in the inferior vena cava.

Each bean-shaped *kidney* lies retroperitoneally, adjacent to the superior part of the posterior body wall and lateral to the vertebral column and greater psoas muscle. The renal artery and vein, together with the renal pelvis, course through a vertical cleft in the medial margin of the kidney called the *renal hilum*. Both hila are at the level of the first lumbar vertebra, with the right one being slightly lower than the left because the large liver is directly above the right kidney. The renal veins leave the kidneys anterior to the renal arteries which, in turn, are anterior to the renal pelvis.

The thick, muscular, walled *ureter* is the inferior continuation of the renal pelvis. It runs retroperitoneally on the posterior body wall for about 12 to 15 cm before coursing over the pelvic brim to enter the pelvic cavity. It may exhibit considerable variation in diameter and descends slightly medially on the greater psoas muscle. On the right side, the ovarian vessels cross anterior to the ureter in an oblique manner, whereas the vessels on the left side stay medial to the ureter. Anteriorly, the left ureter is protected more than the right one because it is crossed by the root of the sigmoid mesocolon and the left colic vessels.

ANATOMIC CHANGES DURING PREGNANCY

Gravid Uterus

Size and Position

Uterine enlargement during pregnancy is not symmetric; it is sometimes most marked in the body below the tubes and at other times in the fundus above the tubes. Variations in the site of enlargement are probably influenced greatly by the location of the implantation site.

First Trimester. The original pear shape is maintained during the first few weeks of pregnancy. The uterus triples in size by the end of the second month and changes from a flat, pear shape to a rounded form (Fig. 2–13). The rapid increase in size and weight during the second month may result in the uterus's being in exaggerated positions of anteflexion, retroflexion, or retroversion. The fundus usually can be palpated above the pubic symphysis by the end of the first trimester.

Second Trimester. The uterus usually retains its rounded shape throughout the second trimester.

It expands superiorly out of the pelvic cavity, into the abdominal cavity, and through the superior pelvic aperture. Midway through pregnancy (fifth month), the fundus is at the level of the umbilicus, making contact with the anterior abdominal wall by displacing the intestines and greater omentum superiorly and laterally.

Third Trimester. At the beginning of the third trimester, the uterus assumes an ovoid shape as the vertical dimensions increase more rapidly than either the transverse or anteroposterior dimensions. The gravid uterus is quite mobile and tends to rotate, usually to the right, with the left side moving anteriorly and toward the midline. Rotation to the right is thought to be caused by pressure from the sigmoid colon, which lies on the left posterior side of the pelvic cavity. Rotation to the left may occur when there is a pelvic or lower abdominal mass on the right side. In the erect position, the greatly enlarged uterus gets considerable support from the abdominal wall, which stretches as it enlarges. When the mother is in the supine position, the heavy uterus places backward pressure on the aorta and the inferior vena cava (see Fig. 2–12). By 8 months' gestation, the fundus extends superiorly to the level of the xiphoid process. During the last month of pregnancy, the presenting part of the fetus descends into the pelvis (this process is called *lightening*), thereby causing the fundus to recede slightly inferiorly.

Myometrium

Uterine enlargement during pregnancy is accompanied by stretching and marked hypertrophy of the myometrium. The body of the uterus weighs approximately 70 g in the nongravid state and increases to over 1000 g at term. Mitotic figures are rarely observed in the muscle layer during pregnancy, suggesting that the smooth muscles undergo hypertrophy rather than hyperplasia. New muscle cells that do form probably originate in the media of growing myometrial arteries and veins. Hypertrophy of the myometrium begins during the first few weeks but occurs mainly during the third month. Muscle fascicles in the lower portion of the uterus overlap one another like shingles on a roof. Increases in the fibrous and elastic tissue accompany the hypertrophy. The increased uterine size during the second and third trimesters is caused mainly by the pressure of the expanding conceptus. The myometrium of the body is 2 to 3 cm thick in early pregnancy but thins to 1 to 2 cm thick in late pregnancy. Uterine wall thinning may be exaggerated in multigravid women, during multiple pregnancy, and in hydramnios.

During labor, the musculature in the wall of the isthmus must dilate rather than contract. The isthmic musculature is poorly defined in the early weeks of pregnancy, when the area feels softer

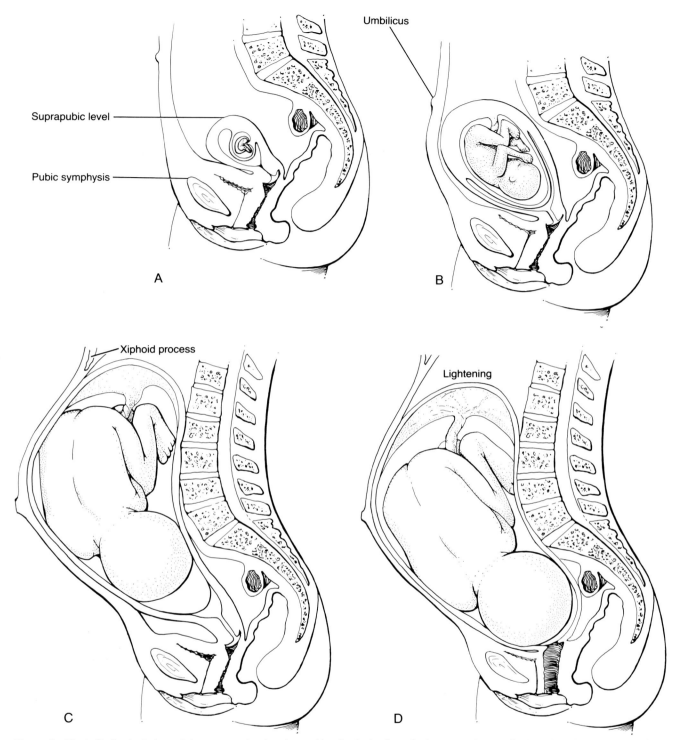

Figure 2–13. *A–D,* Sagittal view of the uterus showing its position in *A,* the first, *B,* the second, and *C,* the third trimesters, and *D,* at term.

than either the body or the cervix. After the second month, musculature in the isthmus hypertrophies like that in the body and makes up the major portion of the *lower uterine segment* (Fig. 2–14). The isthmic canal triples in length to approximately 3 cm. During the second trimester, the isthmus becomes incorporated into the uterus and the isthmic canal becomes part of the uterine cavity. The junction between the body and the isthmus is no longer visible externally, since their walls are approximately the same thickness. This condition lasts until the middle of the third trimester, when a transverse linear depression appears in the junction region. The musculature above the

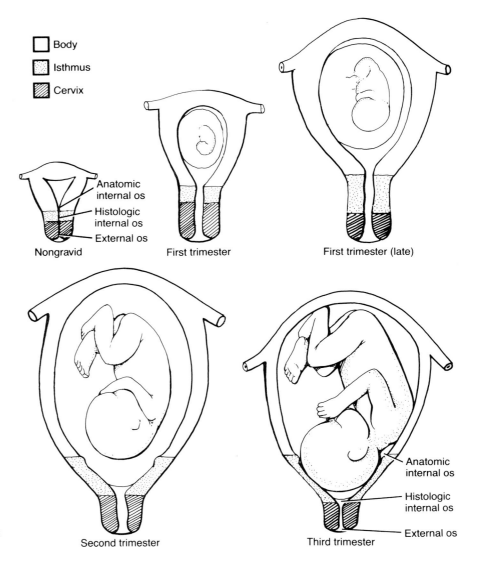

Body
Isthmus
Cervix

Anatomic internal os
Histologic internal os
External os
Nongravid

First trimester

First trimester (late)

Second trimester

Third trimester

Anatomic internal os
Histologic internal os
External os

Figure 2–14. Frontal view of the uterus showing the location and extent of the three parts of the uterine wall at different periods of gestation.

depression is thicker than that below. The depression is located just below the vesicouterine pouch, corresponding to the level of the anatomic internal os. It is sometimes called the "physiologic contraction ring," which moves to a higher level during labor. After delivery, the ring becomes a marked constriction area between the body of the uterus and the cervix.

CERVIX

The cervix changes remarkably during pregnancy and labor. Two of the earliest signs of pregnancy are cervical softening and cyanosis caused by edema and increased vascularity. Shortly after conception, the glands lining the cervical canal secrete a very thick mucus, forming a plug that seals off the uterine cavity during gestation. The glands usually make up only a fraction of the cervical mass in the nonpregnant state, but during pregnancy they undergo consid-

erable proliferation so that by term they make up about half the mass. The muscle content of the cervix does not change appreciably.

During labor, the cervix dilates after softening as a result of dissociation of the collagen fibers within it. During the second and early third trimesters, an incompetent cervix may dilate painlessly, causing premature rupture of the membranes and the delivery of a previable fetus. Previous cervical trauma appears to change the muscle to collagen ratio, resulting in an increase of muscle fibers.

UTERINE CAVITY

The uterine cavity in the gravid condition enlarges as the myometrium hypertrophies. Its rate of enlargement is greater initially than the growth rate of the conceptus. During the early part of the second trimester (fourth month), the cavity is completely filled by the rapidly expanding conceptus and remains obliterated until delivery.

ADNEXA, BLOOD VESSELS, AND NERVES

As pregnancy progresses, the adnexal structures move superiorly (see Fig. 2–16). An adnexal mass may present in the upper abdominal quadrant during the last trimester. The *uterine tubes* in the upper border of the *broad ligament* stretch with the ligament as tension is exerted on them by the rising, gravid uterus. The tubes become hyperemic but undergo little hypertrophy during pregnancy. The *ovary* enlarges during the first month of pregnancy when the *corpus luteum* reaches its maximal diameter of 2 to 2.5 cm. Regressive changes appear in the corpus luteum within 2 to 3 weeks after implantation. After the second month, the ovary becomes smaller and its surface often is covered by patches of the reddish decidual reaction taking place in the underlying stroma. Parts of the corpus luteum persist until the middle of pregnancy. The corpus luteum eventually involutes and becomes the *corpus albicans*. As the gravid uterus rises, the *round ligament of the uterus* increases substantially in length and diameter (see Fig. 2–16).

Both the uterine and ovarian arteries undergo marked enlargement during pregnancy. The tortuous arrangement of the ascending branch of the uterine artery and its broad anastomosis with the ovarian artery allow the arterial channels to elongate and accommodate the enlarging uterus. The more linear descending branches can be felt along the lateral side of the cervix at vaginal examination as a result of their increased size. A vast ipsilateral and contralateral arterial anastomotic network forms throughout the uterus. The arcuate arteries in and around the implantation site increase in size and degree of branching.

The veins surrounding the uterus, including those at the base of the bladder, within the broad ligament, and around the cervix and upper vagina, become greatly enlarged during pregnancy. The ovarian veins on both sides enlarge to enormous size and are possible sites for thrombus formation. They may be injured by external trauma and sometimes rupture spontaneously. The diameter of the ovarian vascular pedicle nearly triples during pregnancy. Dissection during cesarean section is performed near the midline to avoid excessive bleeding from the dilated venous plexus. The veins in the broad ligament appear medusa-like and can be a centimeter or more in diameter. Because the ovarian and uterine veins are devoid of valves, constant venous pressure within the uterine wall probably results from their dilation and contraction. Hypervascularity of the uterine wall may occur in 20% of pregnancies and likely results from the dilation of myometrial veins. There may be excessive bleeding during surgery on the anterior uterine wall because of hypervascularity.

The nerve supply to the uterus hypertrophies during pregnancy, and the pelvic plexus increases in size. The function of the motor nerves to the uterus is poorly understood. Motor nerves are not essential to normal activity at parturititon.

Changes in Related Organs

BLADDER AND URETER

As the gravid uterus enlarges, it compresses the superior surface of the bladder from above (Fig. 2–15; see Fig. 2–13). After the fourth month of gestation, the bladder become hyperemic, the trigone region elevates, and the interureteric ridge thickens. The trigone region progressively deepens and widens until term. Toward the end of pregnancy, the base of the bladder is moved superiorly out of the pelvis by the enlarging uterus to a position in the lower abdomen. The pressure of the

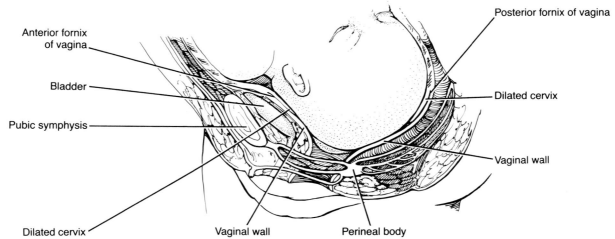

Figure 2–15. Sagittal view showing anatomic relations of the lower uterine segment to other pelvic structures and to the fetal head during labor with a partially dilated cervix.

presenting part near term may impair drainage of blood and lymph from the base of the bladder, causing the area to swell and become traumatized. During prolonged parturition, the anterior vaginal wall is stretched so severely that it is sometimes the site of vesicovaginal fistulas. An extraperitoneal cesarean section that is performed through the upper part of the prevesical or retropubic space necessitates the mobilization of the peritoneum over the bladder if the peritoneal cavity is to be avoided (see Figs. 2–5, 2–15).

It is unclear whether or not reflux, which may occur with chronic bladder distension, causes hydroureter, which often accompanies pregnancy. The connective tissue sheaths that enclose the lower third of the ureter, uterine vessels, and nerves hypertrophy during pregnancy. This condition, together with the accompanying massive enlargement of the uterine vessels, favors urinary stasis and dilation of the upper portion of the ureter. Another mechanism may also be a factor: when the expanding uterus rises completely out of the pelvis during the fourth month, it may possibly compress the ureter at the pelvic brim, resulting in hydroureter. The right ureter above the brim usually dilates more than its counterpart on the left. One possible explanation for this is the oblique path the right ovarian vessels take across the right ureter. The right ovarian vessels become greatly enlarged during pregnancy, possibly putting pressure on the right ureter. The enlarging uterus frequently causes lateral displacement and elongation of both the abdominal and pelvic portions of the ureter. Because a connective tissue sheath encloses and binds the ureter and the uterine vessels to the lateral side of the cervix (see Figs. 2–4, 2–6, 2–11B, 2–12), when the latter dilates during delivery, the distal ureter must necessarily move to a more lateral position.

ANAL CANAL AND ANUS

Anorectal varicosities or hemorrhoids frequently occur during pregnancy. They arise from the venous plexus, located just beneath the surface lining of the anal canal. The upper part of the plexus drains by way of the superior rectal vein into the hepatic portal system. The lower part drains into the inferior vena cava through the lower and middle rectal and iliac veins. There are no valves in the portal system of veins; the anal venous plexus, therefore, is affected particularly by the increasing venous pressure resulting from the enlarging uterus.

POSITION OF ABDOMINAL VISCERA

Abdominal viscera that have a mesentery can be pushed away from their normal anatomic location by the expanding uterus. The position of such viscera is said to be intraperitoneal, and several of them are relocated during pregnancy.

By the end of the first trimester, the uterus rises out of the true pelvis. During the second trimester, it makes contact with the anterior body wall. The jejunum and ilium of the small intestine are pushed superiorly and laterally, ultimately reaching the vicinity of the liver near term (Fig. 2–16). The enlarging uterus also distorts the anatomic location of the cecum and appendix, displacing them progressively laterally and superiorly (Fig. 2–17). At the middle of the second trimester, the appendix is at the level of the iliac crest, and by the middle of the third trimester, it is located just below the subcostal margin. The ascending and descending colons are displaced laterally, and the transverse colon with the attached greater omentum is pushed superiorly. The sigmoid colon is displaced superiorly and may be compressed against the pelvic brim by the gravid uterus. The pressure and mechanical tension produced by the expanding uterus, together with the decreased intestinal motility that accompanies pregnancy, can precipitate intestinal obstruction (see Chapter 14).

VISCERA ON THE POSTERIOR ABDOMINAL WALL

The additional weight of the enlarged uterus can project posteriorly and narrow the lumen of several structures located there, namely, the abdominal aorta and some of its branches, the inferior vena cava and some of its tributaries, and the abdominal portion of the ureter (see Fig. 2–12). Many complications affecting the kidney result from compression of its vessels or drainage system. By 16 weeks' gestation, the uterus reaches the lumbar region and begins to exert pressure on the lower posterior structures when the mother is in the supine position. As pregnancy advances, more superior structures can become affected. Pressure is greatest on the second through the fourth lumbar vertebrae because they are most prominent. Their prominence is accentuated by the progressive lordosis that compensates for the anterior position of the enlarging uterus. These vertebrae act as a fulcrum for the left displacement of the aorta. In addition to displacement, the pressure exerted by the uterus also can compress the aorta and common iliac arteries, producing a blood pressure drop distal to the point of compression.

Both the inferior vena cava and the common iliac veins may be compressed in late pregnancy. Occlusion of the inferior vena cava can occur when the mother is in the supine position; the common iliac veins may become blocked when she is in the sitting or standing position. Such conditions produce edema and varicose veins in the lower extremities. Responses vary, depending on the duration of the blockage and the extent of the collateral circulation, by which blood is returned

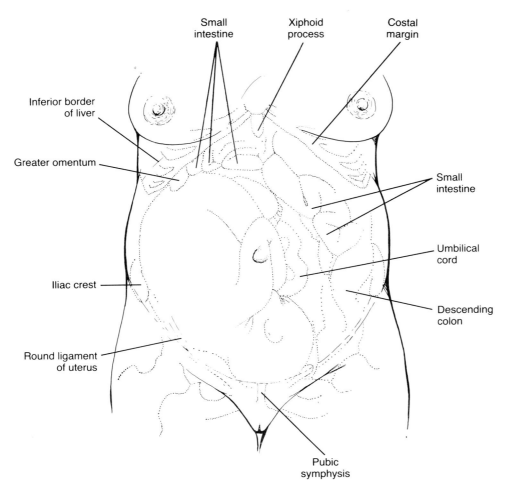

Small intestine

Xiphoid process

Costal margin

Inferior border of liver

Greater omentum

Small intestine

Umbilical cord

Iliac crest

Descending colon

Round ligament of uterus

Pubic symphysis

Figure 2–16. Anterior view of the uterus showing the position of abdominal and pelvic organs near term.

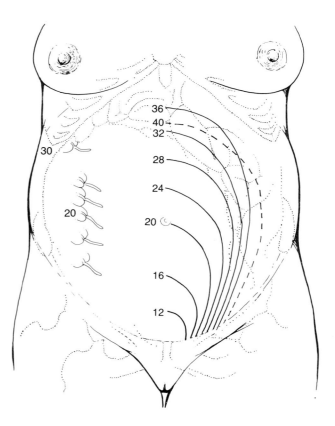

36
40
32
30
28
24
20
20
16
12

Figure 2–17. Anterior view of the abdominal wall showing the superior extent of the uterus at different stages of gestation and the position of the cecum-appendix.

to the heart. In prolonged blockage, the anterior wall veins become enlarged. In the second half of pregnancy, venous return to the heart is increased when the mother moves from lying on her back to lying on her side, relieving part of the venous compression.

The abdominal portion of the ureter often elongates and dilates during pregnancy, producing hydroureter. There is controversy over whether the dilation is hormonally or mechanically caused. The fact that posture affects the left ureter only supports the mechanical cause. The condition can arise by the end of the first trimester and persist until the sixteenth postpartum week.

ANTERIOR ABDOMINAL WALL

Many changes in the soft tissue landmarks of the anterior abdominal wall can be observed during pregnancy. The umbilicus and linea alba may be accentuated because of the distension of the wall by the enlarged uterus. The tension exerted on the wall may widen the linea alba, thereby separating the rectus abdominis muscles, resulting in a condition known as *diastasis recti.* In severe cases, the wall over the uterus may be little more than skin, a thin layer of fascia and peritoneum. Abdominal contents can protrude through a weakened umbilicus, causing a *hernia.*

A brown-blackish pigment frequently is deposited in the midline skin, forming a *linea nigra.* About half of all pregnant women develop reddish, slightly depressed, mainly vertical streaks (called *striae gravidarum*) in the abdominal skin in the later months of pregnancy. Multiparous patients often show glistening, silvery, vertical lines that are scars left from previous striae. If the deeper, main venous drainage of the lower extremity becomes obstructed, the subcutaneous venous anastomoses in the anterior wall may dilate to assist venous return to the heart. A large, vertically coursing venous channel called the *thoracoepigastric* vein may form that acts as a bypass connecting the great saphenous vein in the thigh with the axillary vein in the shoulder.

Placenta

The *fetal part* of the placenta develops from the *trophoblasts* that form the outer layer of the blastocyst. The *maternal part* arises from the endometrium deep to the implantation site which, after having undergone the decidual reaction, is known as the *decidua basalis.* Finger-like chorionic villi, which form from the trophoblasts, contain capillary channels of the fetus that are supplied by branches of the *two umbilical arteries* and drained by tributaries of the *single umbilical vein.* The three umbilical vessels course through the umbilical cord and connect the blood vessels inside the body of the fetus to those in the placenta.

Intervillous spaces contain maternal blood and are supplied by endometrial spiral arteries and drained by endometrial veins. As pregnancy progresses, the villi associated with the decidua basalis rapidly increase in number, branch profusely, and enlarge. Simultaneously, the blood-filled intervillous spaces enlarge at the expense of the decidua basalis.

The final shape of the placenta is determined by the form of the persistent area of villi. Usually this is circular, giving the placenta a discoid shape (Fig. 2–18). When villi persist elsewhere, several variations in placental shape occur, e.g., accessory placenta, diffuse placenta, horseshoe placenta, and bi-discoidal placenta. There are innumerable variations in size and shape, but most of them are of little functional significance.

As the villi invade the decidua basalis, they leave behind several wedge-shaped areas of decidual tissue called *placenta septae.* The septae divide the fetal part of the placenta into 10 to 38 irregular convex areas, composed of lobes called *cotyledons,* which are apparent only on the maternal surface. Each cotyledon consists of two or more main stem villi and their many branches. The fetal surface of the placenta does not show the cotyledon structure but instead is smooth and composed of an outer layer of *amnion,* which overlies a layer of connective tissue called the *chorionic plate.* A number of large chorionic arteries and veins that supply and drain the chorionic villi can be seen deep to the surface layer converging toward the umbilical cord. The attachment of the umbilical cord is usually slightly eccentric, but occasionally it is marginal (this is called *battledore placenta*); rarely, the insertion is into the thin chorionic membrane outside the placenta *(velamentous placenta)* (see Fig. 2–18).

The placenta enlarges as the fetus continues to grow and the uterus enlarges (Fig. 2–19). Its increase in surface area roughly parallels that of the expanding uterus. Throughout pregnancy it fairly consistently covers approximately 25 to 30% of the internal surface of the uterus. The increase in placental thickness results from the branching and enlargement of the existing villi rather than increased penetration into the uterine wall. Such thickening is largely complete by the middle of gestation. At full term, the placenta has a diameter of 15 to 25 cm, is approximately 3 cm thick, and weighs 500 to 600 g (approximately one sixth the weight of the term fetus).

The position of the placenta on the wall of the uterine cavity is determined largely by the site of implantation that occurs near the end of the first week after fertilization. The blastocyst usually implants in the upper part of the uterus, slightly more frequently on the posterior than on the anterior and fundal walls (Fig. 2–20). Rare implantations in the lower uterine segment near the internal os of the cervix result in *placenta previa.*

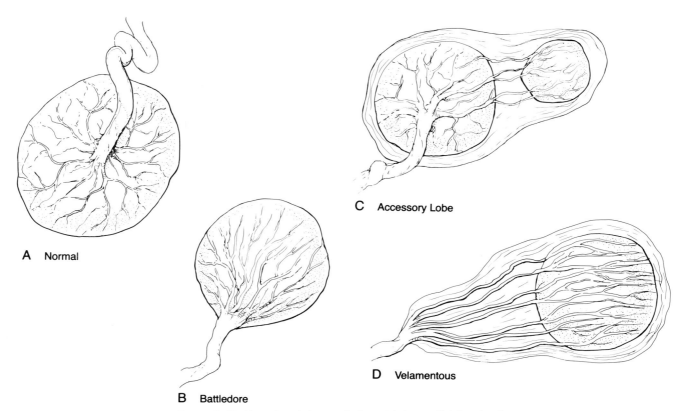

A   Normal

B   Battledore

C   Accessory Lobe

D   Velamentous

Figure 2–18. Normal and abnormal placental shapes (fetal surface).

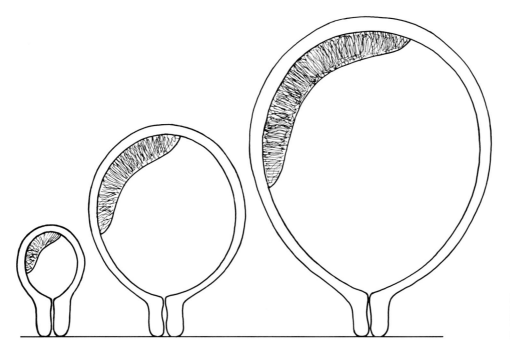

Figure 2–19. Normal placental position on the uterine wall in the first, second, and third trimesters *(left to right).*

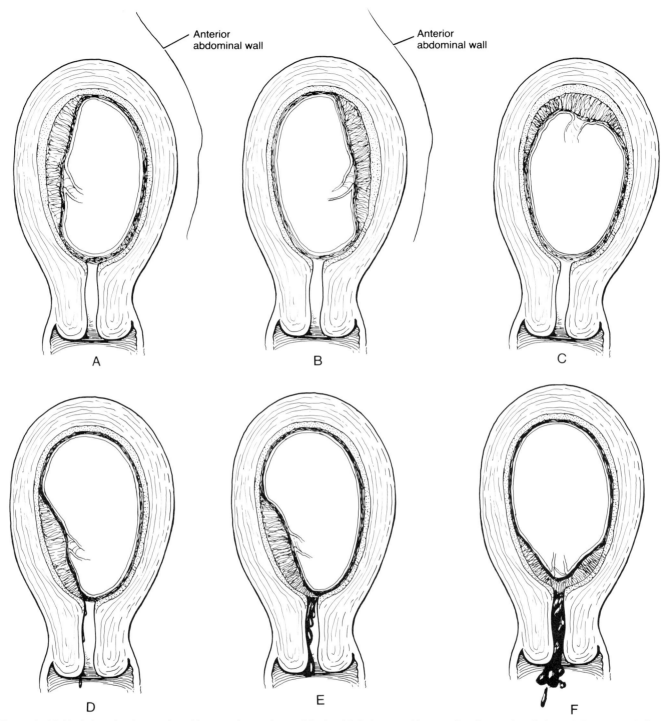

Figure 2–20. Variations in placental positions on the uterine wall in the third trimester (*A*, posterior, *B*, anterior, *C*, fundal, *D*, marginal, *E*, partial, and *F*, total placenta previa).

The placenta that develops from such implantation encroaches on or covers the cervical canal. *Total* placenta previa completely covers the cervical os, *partial* placenta previa partially covers the os, and *marginal* placenta previa is low on the uterine wall but does not actually extend over the os. Placenta previa may cause severe bleeding during pregnancy or at the time of delivery (see Chapter 12). Implantation below the internal os of the cervix (called a *cervical pregnancy*) is very rare and inevitably leads to spontaneous abortion and severe maternal hemorrhage (see Chapter 9).

Abnormal adherence of part or all of the placenta to the uterine wall with partial or complete absence of the decidua basalis is called *placenta accreta*. Premature detachment of a normally implanted placenta in the latter half of pregnancy is called *abruptio placentae*.

3

Wound Management and Basic Surgical Principles

Warren C. Plauché

WOUND HEALING

The ability of the human body to heal itself after illness or injury is one of the wonders of physiology. Ellis[1] said, "Every operation is an experiment in wound healing." Wound healing is truly the basis of all surgery, for without assurance of this process, even the most aggressive surgeon would not dare to remove or repair any physical defect. Despite the importance of the healing process, "wound healing is the Cinderella of clinical and experimental surgical research."[1] In other words, the subject of wound healing comes late to the research

"ball," a stepsister who has until now received little attention.

Many of the principles of wound healing that deal with tensile strength of wounds, contraction of scars, and placement of incisions were developed over a century ago. Modern cell biology investigations clarify the physiologic and biochemical mechanisms that control wound healing events. A new scientific floor exists beneath surgical tenets empirically developed through observation of outcomes. Future progress in wound healing will come from investigators of the new biology. This chapter reviews principles of wound management and dis-

45

Table 3–1. PHASES OF WOUND HEALING

Substrate phase—inflammation
Proliferative phase—granulation tissue
Remodeling phase—matrix, collagen, contraction

coveries about wound healing that apply to the work of the obstetric surgeon.

How do wounds heal? Any wound, regardless of site or cause, goes through a prescribed process of restructuring of the defect. The healing of the skin best describes the continuum of the healing process. Investigators in the field of dermatology have performed much of the recent work on the cell biology of cutaneous healing. A 1986 prize paper by Kanzler and colleagues[2] reviewed the phases of healing of the skin in great detail. There are many lessons for the obstetric surgeon contained in these studies.

Cutaneous wound healing occurs in three phases (Table 3–1). This artificial division into phases oversimplifies a continuous process (Fig. 3–1). The first substrate phase, also called the inflammatory or exudative phase, occurs from shortly after the wound event through the third or fourth day. This phase initiates all the biochemical events that are necessary to begin the repair. Injured cells release thromboplastin, which activates the coagulation cascade. Small-vessel hemostasis derives from blood coagulation, vasoconstriction, and platelet aggregation.

Platelets activate on exposure to mature collagen in the wound. Fibronectin facilitates the attachment of platelets to collagen fibrils. Activated platelets elongate, and their internal organelles release thromboxane A_2, adenosine diphosphate, and other substances. The platelets and collagen coagulum plug open vessels and begin the formation of a healing matrix in the wound. Activated platelets also release proteolytic enzymes that attract leukocytes to the wound site. Other plasma proteins activate plasminogen and bradykinin, which increase the permeability of blood vessels to proteins and leukocytes.[4]

Neutrophils first appear in the wound just 6 hours after the traumatic event. They rapidly increase in number and decline after 2 to 3 days if there is no infection.

Lymphocytes build slowly to a maximum concentration on the sixth day after injury. Lymphocytes produce macrophage activation factor (MAF) and interleukin-1 and -2.[4] These substances induce the proliferation of thymocytes. The further synthesis of lymphokines causes proliferation of granulocytes and fibroblasts.[4]

Macrophages appear early and accumulate in the wound matrix for 4 to 5 days, then decline in numbers. Macrophages derive from monocytes and are critical to wound healing. Macrophages survive in the low-oxygen tensions at the avascular center of the wound clot. Once activated, macrophages begin to débride the wound with a variety of enzymatic proteases and with phagocytosis. Macrophages also actively manage wound collagen[5] and degrade collagen denatured by the wound event. After the first week, macrophages foster new collagen synthesis. Macrophages also stimulate the growth of new blood vessels into the wound space.[6]

Epidermal growth factor in wound serum stimulates collagen synthesis by fibroblasts.[3] Fibrin monomers polymerize to form an early fibrin scaffold, which adds to hemostatic security. This fibrin scaffold lends transient stability to the wound and forms a framework for migration of repair fibroblasts and new epithelial cells covering the wound.

Fibroblasts and endothelial cells produce fibronectin very early in the healing process. This sticky-surfaced active protein coats cell surfaces. Fibronectin enhances platelet adhesion and facilitates mononuclear cell phagocytosis. Fibronectin

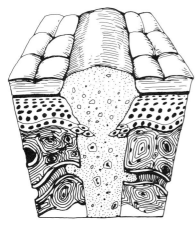
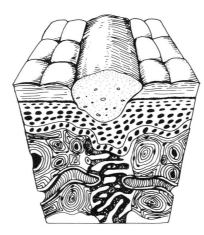
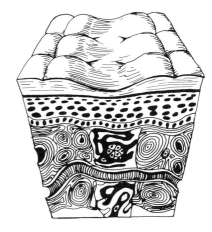

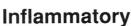
Inflammatory   **Proliferative**   **Remodeling**

Figure 3–1. The phases of wound healing. *Left,* inflammatory or substrate phase—days 1 through 4. *Center,* proliferative or granulation tissue phase—days 4 through 14. *Right,* remodeling or collagen contraction phase—day 14—6 to 12 months.

forms cross links that help new cells adhere to underlying tissues.[7] Healing fibroblasts and new epithelial cells migrate along fibronectin-coated fibrin scaffolding.[8] Later in the healing process, fibronectin hastens the process of remodeling of the wound by promoting phagocytosis of denatured collagen by macrophages.[7]

These early processes prepare the wound for active repair events. The proliferative or granulation tissue phase of wound healing begins about the third or fourth wound day and lasts 10 to 14 days. Proliferation actually begins during the latter part of the initial substrate or inflammatory phase. Fibroblasts enter the wound, proliferate, and produce immature new collagen. New blood vessels grow into this matrix to form classic granulation tissue. Re-epithelialization begins at the edges of the wound while granulation tissue is forming.

Epithelial cells slowly migrate from the edges of the wound to cover the defect. The "free edge" phenomenon also stimulates regeneration of epithelium. Cells without neighbors respond by proliferation and migration. Epithelial cells can move only over other living cells. In a properly moist environment, they move at a rate that is proportional to the amount of available oxygen.[8]

Epithelial growth factor binds to receptors on the surface of growing cells and activates enzymes that provide increased nutrient transport and protein synthesis. Fibronectin facilitates this growth and migration of epithelial cells, fibroblasts, and endothelial vascular cells.

Winter[9] characterized the movement of healing epithelial cells as a "leap frog" phenomenon. Each cell moves no more than two or three cell lengths. The cell then stops and becomes a basal cell over which the following line of cells migrates. This process continues along all wound edges. A sheet of epithelium several cells thick gradually advances to close the wound. A crust on the wound or a foreign object in the wound causes advancing cells to burrow beneath or around the obstruction to maintain the moist conditions necessary for further growth.[10]

The principle of contact inhibition comes into play when sheets of migrating cells from each side of a wound meet. Cells stop advancing, form new intercellular attachments, and resume their normal morphology and function.

The growth of new blood vessels in the wound depends on gradients of oxygen tension. Low oxygen levels allow only host monocytes and the cells of capillary buds to function and proliferate. Growth factors that increase vessel growth are released under low oxygen conditions. Capillaries grow and eventually branch. They join other capillaries and blood flow begins.[11] Oxygen tension rises when blood begins to flow once again in the new vessels. Oxygen inhibits growth factors and slows the growth of new vasculature.

Fibroblasts lay down immature collagen most efficiently in a slightly acidic environment with reducing qualities and high oxygen tension. Immature new collagen reaches its maximum production rate between 5 and 7 days after the wound event. Half of the new scar is made of this soft, jelly-like immature collagen. Other components include fibronectin, fibrin, glycosaminoglycans, and proteoglycans. The glycans control hydration of the wound matrix.

Large amounts of collagen are laid down during days 14 to 21. The remodeling phase begins as the proliferation of granulation tissue and new epithelium slows. The wound matrix is continuously altered over a period of months. The quantity of fibronectin in the wound diminishes. The character of wound collagen changes to firm, mature collagen.[12] The wound gains strength as larger collagen bundles form and linkages between bundles increase.[12] The tightly wound triple helix formation of mature collagen maximizes the tensile strength of the wound.

Wound contraction begins soon after granulation tissue is formed. Contraction occurs when activated fibroblasts differentiate into myofibroblasts and acquire motility and the ability to contract, much like smooth muscle cells.[13] High concentrations of actomyosin in granulation tissue confirm its contractile capacity.[13]

By the third week after injury, an epithelial wound reaches 20% of its final strength.[14] It will eventually reach approximately 70% of the strength of intact skin in 6 to 12 months.[15]

Wounds Other Than Epithelial Wounds

We have discussed the healing of epithelial wounds. Basic physiologic processes are similar for most wounds. The obstetric surgeon profits from examining studies of the healing properties of certain specific surgical wounds.

The early studies of Howes and colleagues,[14] in 1929, created the lasting impression that laparotomy wounds reached their peak of tensile strength at 14 days. More recent studies indicate that such wounds may steadily gain in strength for up to 42 days.[15] Such studies promoted the development of absorbable sutures that hold their strength in tissues longer than traditional catgut.

What of genital tract wounds? Good studies are few. Schlaff and co-workers[16] used paired rat uterine horns as a model for the healing of uterine muscle. They found that uterine wound–bursting strength peaked at 14 days and then exhibited a paradoxical decrease in strength. Added estrogen did not affect this phenomenon in the rat uterine horn. Increased progesterone levels adversely affect wound healing in other models.[17]

Dunihoo and co-workers[18] described the healing

of wounds in rabbit uterine horns. Matched incisions repaired by continuous and interrupted closure and by inverting and everting suturing methods were examined. Healing was incomplete in the animals sacrificed at 12 to 15 days. Healing was complete at 28 to 32 days. Scar strength was excellent with all methods. The uterine muscle burst under tension before scar separation occurred. There was no difference between suturing methods in quality of healing or strength of scar.[18]

Factors That Alter Wound Healing

The obstetric surgeon must know how wounds heal and how to assist their normal healing. He or she must also know those factors that impede wound healing. Reed and Clark,[19] in 1985, outlined numerous factors that may delay the healing of cutaneous wounds. They organized the principal causes of failure to heal into local factors, systemic factors, and exogenous factors (Table 3–2). The most important of these factors are examined in this chapter in detail.

Wound Infection

Infection is the most important and most common preventable cause of improper wound healing. All wounds, traumatic or surgical, receive some degree of bacterial inoculum with the first break in the integrity of the skin. Leukocytes promptly destroy most bacterial contaminants, provided they are present in sufficient numbers with their lytic and phagocytotic mechanisms intact.

Foreign bodies in the wound contribute huge bacterial inoculums. Necrotic tissues, wound hematomas, and seromas encourage growth of bacteria. Bacteria in a wound consume the oxygen

Table 3–2. FACTORS THAT DELAY WOUND HEALING*

Local factors
Infection
Foreign body in wound
Hypoxia
Desiccation
Seromas and hematomas
Friction and motion of wound
Systemic factors
Nutrition
Aging
Coagulation disorders
Vascular diseases
Chronic systemic diseases
Exogenous factors
Glucocorticoids
Antineoplastic drugs
Anticoagulants
Wound dressings
Wound care

*Modified from Reed BR, Clark RAF: Cutaneous tissue repair: Practical implications of current knowledge. II. J Acad Dermatol 13:919, 1985.

and nutrients necessary for healing tissues. Bacterial metabolism produces an intensely acidic environment that breaks down cells and digests matrix necessary for early wound healing. Bacterial endotoxins and exotoxins directly damage healing tissues.

Bacterial antigens attract leukocytes to the wound site. This might seem to be favorable for early healing, but the low oxygen tensions and acidic environment of an infected wound reduce the capability of leukocytes to perform phagocytosis and débridement. They prolong the inflammatory component of wound healing and slow the normal healing process.

Deficiencies in host defense mechanisms impede the destruction of bacteria in a wound.[19] Complement may be deficient from hereditary or autoimmune disease processes, such as lupus erythematosus or rheumatoid arthritis.

Several conditions produce deficiencies in the chemotactic mechanisms of leukocytes. A common cause of poor chemotaxis is diabetes mellitus.

Immunodeficiency states, sickle cell disease, and diabetes mellitus reduce the ability of leukocytes to opsonize and destroy the cell wall of bacteria. Chronic disease states, such as diabetes mellitus, chronic granulomatous diseases, leukemias, and certain enzyme deficiencies inhibit the ability of neutrophils to ingest bacteria.[19] The diabetic, who figures so prominently in obstetric high-risk populations, emerges as particularly susceptible to wound infections.

The surgeon must minimize the number of bacteria that remain in the wound after surgery. Precautions begin before the operation starts. Preoperative cleansing of the patient's skin and the hands of the surgical team is still important, even in this day of potent antimicrobial drugs.

Shaving the operative site, especially hours before surgery, increases contamination of the wound with skin bacteria. Clipping long hair usually suffices. If you must shave the skin, do so immediately before the operation.[20]

Polk and colleagues,[21] from the Centers for Disease Control, published guidelines for review of surgical wound infections that outline an accepted antiseptic regimen for preparation for surgery.

A 5-minute scrub with one of the iodophors, chlorhexidine or hexachlorophene, sufficiently cleans the hands of those participating in the first operation of the day. A 2- or 3-minute scrub will do for later cases. The skin of each patient receives a detergent scrub, followed by an application of chlorhexidine, iodophor, or iodine tincture.[21]

Wound Oxygenation

Ischemic wounds do not heal well.[19] Low oxygen tension exists in wounds with inadequate vascular supply, necrotic tissue, hematomas, foreign bodies, or excessive bacterial inoculum. These factors inhibit normal healing and favor the growth of anaerobic and facultative anaerobic organisms. Many of these organisms are intensely pathogenic and produce devastating endotoxins and exotoxins.

Foreign bodies in wounds reduce oxygen tensions to very low levels.[22] Excessive carbonization from use of the electrocautery has the same effect. All traumatic wounds must be carefully cleansed and débrided. Tightly drawn sutures and excessive edema contribute to wound hypoxia.[19]

Several factors alter wound oxygenation. Low levels of oxygen in the inspired anesthetic mixture during surgery increase wound ischemia. General and local anesthetic agents that cause vasoconstriction decrease oxygenation at the wound site. Avoid intense vasoconstrictor drugs, such as epinephrine and ergot alkaloids, when possible. Avoid the vasoconstriction caused by the patient's smoking in the perioperative period.

Winter[23] showed that epithelialization occurs most rapidly over the moist surface of clean granulation tissue. Drying out of wounds and the formation of crusts and eschars do not favor rapid wound healing. New epithelium has to burrow under eschar and around foreign material to heal. The prevention of desiccation of open wounds speeds healing. These findings changed the way surgeons cared for wounds and led to the development of occlusive dressing techniques.[24]

Nutrition

There are many nutritional substances that either are essential to wound healing or favor its processes (Table 3–3). Protein and calorie intake are critical because all healing tissues need essential amino acids and energy for the synthesis of new tissue proteins.

Levenson and Seifter[25] documented inhibition of all phases of wound healing by severe protein restriction. Antibody responses, early phagocytosis, matrix formation, and later fibroplasia are particularly sensitive to protein deprivation. Young[26] reported that human surgical patients with severe protein-calorie malnutrition experience delayed wound healing, decreased immunocompetence, and increased wound infection rates. They experienced longer hospital stays and higher rates of morbidity and mortality.

Table 3–3. NUTRITIONAL NEEDS IN HUMAN WOUND HEALING

Calories	Vitamin K
Protein	Zinc
Essential amino acids	Vitamin E*
Vitamin A	Vitamin B*
Vitamin C	

*Not proven required in the healing of wounds in humans; significant in the healing of wounds in animals.

The synthesis of compounds related to the formation of dermal elements of the skin necessitates vitamin A. Vitamin A affects adhesion of cells and the formation of keratin and collagen.[19] Animals with vitamin A deficiency display wounds that are slow to epithelialize and that frequently become infected. Low collagen content of wounds results in weaker tensile strength of the healed scar.

Vitamin B restriction in experimental animals causes deficient collagen deposition and weakened wound strength. Vitamin B deficiency in humans is rare and produces no known wound-healing problems.

Proper collagen synthesis necessitates vitamin C.[25] Without vitamin C, collagen fails to form its strong triple helix and remains in an unstable state subject to degradation. Beisel and colleagues[27] found that vitamin C deficiency inhibited fibroblast migration and neutrophil phagocytosis early in the healing process.

Vitamin E reduces the number of toxic free radicals arising from metabolic processes. The rapid events of early wound healing involve intense endogenous and exogenous metabolism. The exact role of vitamin E and free radicals is not clear. Runders and co-workers[28] showed that vitamin E improved cell-mediated immunity and wound healing in burn wounds in mice.

Vitamin K is essential to coagulation pathway factors VII, IX, and X. These factors and other specific coagulation proteins form the initial microvascular plugs in surgical wounds. Vitamin K helps prevent intraoperative and postoperative hematomas.

Zinc appears to be important to the integrity and function of cell membranes.[24] The association of zinc with many enzymatic processes gives it a critical role in cell growth and duplication and the synthesis of proteins and collagen.[29] Senapati and Thompson[30] found that zinc levels increased by 50% in tissues from healing wounds.

Aging and Chronic Disease

The older the patient, the more likely that wound healing is delayed or deficient. Goodson and Hunt[31] described reduction in cell replication and metabolism, wound contraction, and remodeling capability as aging progresses. The aged do not clear denatured collagen or synthesize new collagen rapidly. Wounds revascularize slowly in aged patients.[32]

Aged surgical patients, however, heal better than one would expect from this litany of physiologic deficiencies. Hosking and colleagues[33] reported the results of 795 operations at the Mayo Clinic on patients aged 90 and above. Overall serious morbidity within 48 hours after surgery was 9.4%, and the mortality rate was 1.6%. Emergency procedures carried a particularly high risk of early morbidity and mortality in these patients.

Wound-healing problems compound when poor nutrition is added to aging factors. Chronic diseases also complicate the healing process. Vascular diseases reduce blood flow to the wound site and reduce available oxygen. Venous stasis commonly interferes with wound healing in the extremities. Hosking and colleagues[33] found that early postoperative morbidity and mortality in elderly patients related directly to their physical status classification as defined by the American Society of Anesthesiologists.

Diabetes mellitus adversely affects several wound-healing processes. Chronic autoimmune diseases plague aged populations. Obstetric patients only occasionally suffer from degenerative or chronic diseases.

Physical Factors

Motion of wound edges slows healing or may make healing impossible, as with nonunion of osseous fractures. The constant motion of uterine contractions threatens the proper healing of cesarean incisions. Cesarean incisions usually heal firmly despite the progesterone-laden post-delivery environment and grinding motion. Some cesarean incisions heal poorly. Thin, pale, transverse scars are often seen at the time of repeat cesarean deliveries. Classic cesarean scars often show healing of only a portion of a full-thickness myometrial wound, leaving a deep, V-shaped defect.

Complete early dehiscences of cesarean scars occur particularly when severe endomyometritis complicates the post-cesarean course. The uterine wound dehiscence site adheres to the anterior abdominal wall, surrounded by adherent loops of bowel and omentum. Little or no myometrium remains between the abdominal wall and the endometrial cavity. Re-entry into such an environment risks injury to bowel, bladder, or other adhered organs.

Drug Effects

Several groups of drugs adversely affect wound healing. The most widely studied of these drugs are anti-inflammatory corticosteroids, antineoplastic agents, and antibiotics.

Glucocorticoids reduce fibroblast proliferation and leukocyte infiltration in the earliest phases of wound healing. They suppress the normal inflammatory process. Leukocytes that appear in the wound do not effectively kill bacteria or clear wound detritus.[34] Glucocorticoids reduce collagen synthesis, weakening the wound matrix. Steroid inhibition of prostinoid vasodilators reduces wound oxygenation. The reduced rate of cell differentiation slows epithelial coverage of the wound.[35]

Pollack,[36] in 1982, summarized the effects of antineoplastic drugs on wound healing. The lack of prospective controlled studies restricts firm conclusions about these powerful inhibitors of cell growth. Animal studies were often contradictory, depending on the aspect of healing studied. Anecdotal reports indicate that, in the few patients who require antineoplastic medications during pregnancy, wound healing appears to be acceptable.

Certain antibiotics have adverse effects on wound healing. Scher and co-workers[37] found that a 7-day course of cefazolin or cefonicid significantly reduced mean wound-breaking strength after midline celiotomy in rats. Antibiotic regimens shorter than 3 days showed no such effect. Borden and co-workers[38] found that metronidazole had a similar, though transient, effect.

Prophylactic antibiotic regimens do not appear to affect wound healing in the human patient. Adverse effects of antibiotics on human wound healing are not of sufficient import to preclude their indicated use in surgical patients.

PRINCIPLES OF OPERATIVE CARE

Preoperative Considerations

Preoperative management of the obstetric surgical patient begins long before the operation. The obstetric surgeon establishes an atmosphere of respect and trust with all of his or her patients and a sense of cooperative decision-making. The physician repeatedly shows his or her concern for the welfare of the mother and her baby. Rapport begins at the first prenatal visit and expands with every effort of the physician on the patient's behalf.

Education in prenatal nutrition, hygiene, and the physiology of pregnancy and labor is particularly effective in cementing physician-patient relationships. The physician gains the further confidence of the patient in the prenatal period by effective teaching and feedback. The patient is then prepared and capable of handling her part in making difficult decisions about operative procedures.

Informed Consent

The essence of preoperative care lies in the informed consent issue. Inform the patient in the broadest possible meaning of this term. Educate her about her condition, its potential complications, and options for solution of the problems at hand. Tell her the surgical complications possible with each option, including the option of no treatment. Explanations must be in language the patient understands, translated if necessary. Offer to answer any questions in a way that invites questions.

There is a fine line between telling the patient everything she needs to know to make informed decisions and frightening the patient with morbid details of rare potential problems. We must hope our legal requirements do not extend that far.

The patient who trusts the physician's ability to decide in concert with her own thinking, ethics system, and religious beliefs may release much of the decision-making to the physician. Without such knowledge and trust, the physician may have to offer full grim disclosure for all procedures to enable the patient and her family to participate in decisions with full knowledge of options and complications.

The medicolegal system is evolving in the direction of full disclosure, regardless of the effect this has on the patient. Legal advisors suggest that full disclosure is the best way to protect the physician in the event of rare surgical complications. Patient advocates claim the right to fully informed participation by patients in medical decisions about themselves. The phrase, "If I had known about that complication, I never would have had the operation," echoes in courtrooms across the land.

Some physicians deal with the issues of full disclosure, medical malpractice, and patient consumerism by taking themselves completely out of the decision loop. This places the entire burden of decision on the patient, with the physician only playing the role of information resource. Is this the best way to make critical medical decisions?

All medical decisions are, at last case, made by our patients. They decide whether to take our advice, do our exercises, abstain from harmful habits, and accept our proposals for cure. Most sick patients long to be told by someone they trust what to do to get better. Should the physician abrogate his or her responsibility as medical decision-maker? The decision-making process should involve us with our patients and be in concert with their wishes. Openly discuss options, using all avenues of consultative opinion in complex cases. A set of final decision options that include his or her own recommendations should be offered by the physician.

Patients expect knowledgeable advice and understandable explanations. Sick, troubled people want the educated opinion of a physician who holds as his or her guiding principle that which is best for the patient. Armed with the carefully considered opinions of one or more such trusted physicians, the patient makes her own choices. These choices will likely be very personal. They are sometimes unrealistic and seem illogical and difficult to understand. Physicians must become dedicated masters of education who carefully help their patients make standard and realistic therapeutic choices.

Other aspects of the preoperative care of the obstetric patient begin early in the prenatal care process. The well-nourished patient who has adequate iron stores is at much lower risk than the malnourished, anemic patient. Prenatal screening brings to light concurrent illnesses that may require treatment in order to prevent complications and minimize surgical risk. Careful monitoring of the mother and fetus may give early warning of developing problems and reduce the number of decisions to be made in a crisis.

The preoperative preparation of patients immediately before obstetric surgery increases the patient's safety during the anesthetic and surgical events. Review the patient's medical history and perform a general physical examination. Establish intravenous access lines according to need. Anticipate the need for blood and blood fractions. Unless an emergency exists, perform basic blood and urine tests with particular emphasis on electrolytes, hemoglobin and hematocrit levels, and coagulation parameters. Assess any concurrent medical disorders discovered in the history and examination.

A Foley catheter keeps the patient's bladder empty. Meticulous catheter insertion technique and early removal of indwelling catheters minimize postoperative urinary tract infections. Many surgeons prefer to empty the rectum with an enema or suppository before elective abdominal surgery, but this is certainly not mandatory. Remove abdominal or pubic hair by clipping shortly before surgery. A general body shower using bacteriostatic soaps the night and morning before elective surgery helps to reduce the number of skin pathogens. Skin preparation on the operating table was described earlier in this chapter.

Reduce the pH of gastric contents with liquid nonparticulate antacids to minimize the potential effect of any aspiration of gastric contents during anesthesia. Preoperative atropine-like medications help reduce bronchial secretions. Minimize preoperative narcotics, sedatives, or tranquilizer medications to avoid excessive sedative load on the newborn.

Sutures and Knots

SUTURE MATERIALS

There always has been controversy about the most appropriate suture materials and wound closures. Layer closure with either continuous or interrupted sutures works well in uncomplicated cases with no healing problems. Continuous unlocked suture closures of wound layers speeds the operation. If the suture breaks at any point along its length, the entire suture line opens. Continuous locked suture lines address this problem in part but may compromise the microcirculation at the wound edges. Interrupted suture lines are stable and provide suture-free gaps for rapid neovascularization. Mass closure methods improve the outcomes in problem wounds, such as secondary closures after wound dehiscence (Fig. 3–2).

The suture material chosen for each surgical task is partly a matter of personal choice. Many surgeons prefer inert, nonreactive nylon (Ethilon), dacron (Mersilene), or polypropylene (Prolene) nonabsorbable suture material for their strength and permanence. Other surgeons prefer absorbable suture.

Chromicized catgut is a long-time favorite absorbable suture. Surgical knots set and hold easily with chromic gut.

Synthetic absorbable sutures derived from polyglycolic acid (Dexon and Dexon S) or polyglactin (Vicryl and Tevdek), simple or braided, have become very popular. They possess strength in small calibers.[39] They are relatively inert in tissues. This allows protracted holding times followed by eventual resorption. These polyglycolic-polyglactin sutures hold their strength in tissues at least twice as long as catgut.[39] However, they are more difficult to tie securely and require multiple throws that create bulky knots.

The first throw of surgical knots with synthetic sutures is difficult to stabilize and tends to loosen unless held under tension. Practice with synthetic sutures produces satisfactory, stable knots.

A survey of the membership of the Society of Gynecologic Surgeons in 1987 revealed a wide variety of sutures chosen for gynecologic laparotomy. The sutures most often chosen were varieties of polyglycolic-polyglactin sutures.[40] Chromicized catgut led a similar survey conducted 10 years previously. Cotton, silk, and metal sutures were rarely used by those surveyed.

SURGICAL KNOTS

Choose the type of knot according to the type of suture material used and the purpose of the tie.

Monofilament nylon and similar sutures necessitate multiple throws of slip knots, similar to a fisherman's leader line. These knots form bulky masses of suture material in the tissue. Although these suture materials do not excite much local tissue response, the hard, bulky knots may be noticeable and uncomfortable if placed near the skin surface. In continuous monofilament closures, the first and last knots must be absolutely secure. The entire length of the suture line separates if either end unties.

Polyglycolic-polyglactin sutures require a tight first slip knot and four or five additional throws for knot security. They, too, produce bulky knots. The braided versions of these sutures seem to be less dependent on many throws for safety.

A single square knot secures catgut suture in all its variations. Most surgeons tie a third insurance throw. Catgut in tissues absorbs water,

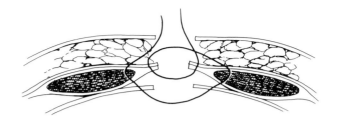
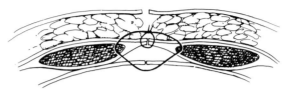

Figure 3–2. Mass abdominal closure: the Smead-Jones stitch.

swells, and becomes soft. If the ends of the suture beyond the knot are shorter than a centimeter, the knot may untie. Catgut rapidly loses strength in the presence of tissue fluids. It holds effectively for only 6 to 7 days.

Older materials, such as cotton and silk, are also securely tied with a single square knot. These materials are not hygroscopic, so the suture ends can be quite short. Natural-fiber sutures invoke intense inflammatory tissue responses. Synthetic, inert materials have essentially replaced natural fibers.

Circumstances affect how the surgeon ties his or her knots. The knot should draw the suture very tightly around vascular pedicles. Sutures should only loosely approximate the tissue layers in wound closure. The most common cause of wound dehiscence other than wound infection is necrosis of the fascia as a result of sutures too tightly drawn. Sutures do not generally tear through the fascia in dehiscence cases. The real problems are fascial ischemic necrosis or infection.

The square knot is the classic surgical knot taught in most surgical disciplines. The first throw of a square knot may loosen in the process of manipulating the suture to form the second throw. This is particularly likely if the encircled tissues are bulky or under tension. Avoid slippage of the first throw of the square knot by keeping tension on one arm of the suture or by using the surgeon's knot. The surgeon's knot ensures stability of the first throw by passing the suture around itself twice. This maneuver stabilizes a tie under tension, but adds bulk to the knot.

There can be advantages to other types of knots. Do not disparage the granny knot or the slip knot. There are many circumstances, particularly deep in the pelvis, where the ability to apply the first throw and add a second throw that can tighten the first is a major advantage.

INCISIONS

Abdominal Incisions. Most of the abdominal incisions associated with obstetric surgery are variations of the lower abdominal vertical or transverse incision. Special circumstances may occasionally dictate other abdominal incisions, but every obstetric surgeon must master the variants of low abdominal vertical and transverse incisions.

Lower Abdominal Vertical Incisions. The types of lower abdominal vertical incisions most often utilized in obstetric surgery are infraumbilical midline incisions and paramedian incisions (Fig. 3–3).

Midline incisions are quick, easy, and versatile. They allow good exposure of the pelvic organs and the pregnant uterus. Extension of the incision cephalad around the umbilicus allows the operator to obtain more room if procedures necessitate additional exposure.

Midline incisions are prone to postoperative hernia formation.[41] Blood supply to the midline is relatively poor. The oblique and transverse muscles of the abdominal wall constantly pull at the wound during healing. Vertical incisions are subject to disrupting stresses when the patient flexes the trunk, unlike transverse incisions, which simply fold together with this movement. Choose a paramedian or transverse incision if there is concern about the patient's wound-healing abilities.

Perform the midline incision by incising the skin in the midline of the lower abdomen from the top of the mons veneris to just below the umbilicus. The incision may curve around the umbilicus if necessary. This causes difficulty in cosmetic repair if the lateral jog is extensive or angular. Continue the incision with a scalpel through the subcutaneous fat to the white, opaque rectus fascia. Maintain meticulous hemostasis by clamping and ligating or cauterizing skin and subcutaneous tissue bleeding points.

Incise the fascia along the full length of the incision, beginning at midincision with the scalpel and continuing first caudad, then cephalad, with Mayo or similar heavy scissors. Separate the rectus muscles in the midline by sharp dissection and retraction. Be careful not to injure the perforator branches of the inferior epigastric vessels on the underside of the rectus muscles. Accidental disruption of these vessels may be missed at the time of the incision, only to appear later as a subfascial hematoma.

The thin, glistening, translucent sheet of peritoneum is the last structure between the operator and the peritoneal cavity. The posterior rectus fascial sheath accompanies the peritoneum above the semilunar line in the upper third of this incision.

Grasp and elevate the peritoneum at approximately the junction between the upper and middle thirds of the incision with a pair of hemostats placed a fingerbreadth apart. Take care not to injure the bowel, bladder, or other organs on entry into the peritoneal cavity. Alternately remove and replace the hemostats to be certain that the bowel has not been grasped. Palpate the peritoneum between the instruments. It should feel like a thin, slippery, double sheet, with no intervening tissue.

Incise the peritoneum with scalpel or fine scissors between the hemostats. Introduce a finger into the opening to confirm the absence of bowel or adhesions in the line of the incision. Complete the peritoneal incision with a Metzenbaum or other fine scissors, first cephalad, then caudad.

Check for the presence of an umbilical hernia. Extend the caudal end of the incision to the reflection of peritoneum over the bladder. The appearance of blood vessels coursing with the peritoneum often provides a warning that the bladder is near. Transillumination of the peritoneum during the dissection ensures the safety of the bladder.

The paramedian incision resembles the midline incision, except that it lies a centimeter or two lateral to the midline, left or right. Paramedian

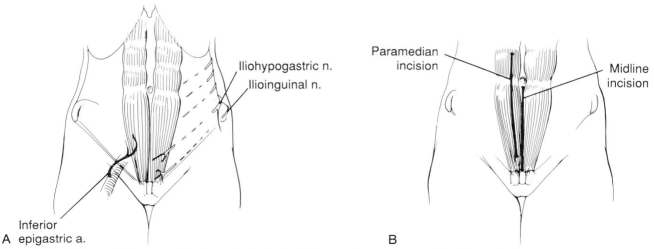

Figure 3–3. *A,* Anatomic features of the lower abdominal wall that may be encountered in either vertical or transverse incisions. *B,* Vertical abdominal incisions: right paramedian and low midline.

incisions may be extended cephalad without curving awkwardly around the umbilicus.

Paramedian incisions traverse the individual anterior and posterior rectus fascial sheaths rather than the central linea alba. Retract the rectus muscles laterally before making a vertical incision in the peritoneum. If the rectus muscles themselves are cut, the incision becomes a trans-rectus muscle–splitting incision. Advocates of paramedian incisions believe that the two fascial layers and the interposed rectus muscle lend strength and blood supply to the repair, which reduces postoperative hernias and wound dehiscence.

The lateral paramedian incision lies near the lateral margin of the rectus muscle, as does the right pararectus Battle incision. The lateral paramedian incision has not found wide favor in the United States, possibly because of cosmetic reasons. This incision has some use in appendectomies. It offers increased exposure over the gridiron muscle–splitting incisions that divide the muscles of the abdominal wall in the direction of each muscle.

Donaldson and colleagues,[41] in England, examined the incidence of wound complications in 850 lateral paramedian and midline incisions in general surgical patients. Their paired prospective series showed a 3.6% incidence of wound problems in lower midline incisions, compared with 0% complications in the lateral paramedian incisions.

The gridiron (Rocky-Davis) incision allows proper exposure only if the disorder is correctly diagnosed as appendicitis and the appendix cooperates by being in a classic position. Pregnancy displaces the appendix upward in 60% of cases, and the appendix lies behind the cecum in many of the remaining 40%. Adnexal disease mimics appendicitis and is not easily managed through the gridiron incision. The gridiron incision defies extension sufficient for major explorations.

Closure of the Vertical Abdomninal Incision. Before closing any abdominal incision, remove all instruments, packs, and sponges from the abdomen. Double check the sponge and instrument count with the circulating nurse. All surgical pedicles receive a final check for security of sutures and hemostasis. Clean up all secretions, blood, and other contaminants to prepare the wound for closure.

Close the peritoneal incision with a simple running suture of small-gauge catgut or polyglycolic-polyglactin suture (00 or 000). Lively discussion continues about the closing of the peritoneal layer, particularly the pelvic parietal peritoneum. Surgeons formerly believed that careful, almost watertight peritoneal closure gave best results. There is less emphasis now on such a meticulous peritoneal closure. Mass closure techniques have become very popular. Open spaces in the peritoneal closure heal rapidly, with few adhesions. Many surgeons

maintain that merit remains in neat anatomic reapproximation of each incised tissue layer.

Next, close the fascia with interrupted 0 or 00 sutures. Current practice favors inert, long-lasting polyglycolic-polyglactin suture material. Continuous suture technique is as reliable in uncomplicated, clean cases as is the interrupted method. It is certainly much faster. Whatever the choice, loose approximation of the wound maintains the microcirculation for proper healing.

Mass combined closure, such as the Smead-Jones suture technique (see Fig. 3–2), provides very effective secondary wound closures. It offers preventive insurance when the surgeon recognizes a special risk of poor wound healing.

After secure closure of the fascia, check hemostasis in the subcutaneous tissues. The subcutaneous fat rarely requires sutures. Suturing the fascial layer of Scarpa relieves tension on the overlying skin closure and stabilizes the wound line during early healing.

Personal choice largely governs skin closure methods. Interrupted vertical mattress sutures were formerly the most popular closure of the skin and immediate subcutaneous tissues. Many services now utilize skin staples to rapidly close the dermis and epidermis. Early staple removal (3 to 5 days) gives pleasing cosmetic results.

Techniques for managing wound dehiscences and other wound complications are described later in this chapter.

Transverse Abdominal Incisions. Transverse low abdominal incisions are popular incisions for both gynecologic and obstetric abdominal procedures. There is undeniable cosmetic advantage in the "bikini" incision. The fortunate surgeon who places his or her incision in just the proper wrinkle and sees healing proceed without incident anticipates an almost invisible scar. There are less ephemeral advantages to transverse incisions. Wound dehiscence, evisceration, and incisional hernias rarely occur with transverse incisions.[41]

The most common transverse incision in obstetrics and gynecology is the Pfannenstiel incision.[42] The Pfannenstiel elliptical transverse incision technique took the transverse skin incision recommended by Kustner and added a transverse incision of the fascia. Two complaints about the Pfannenstiel incision are the time required to accomplish it in an emergency and adequacy of exposure.

Concerns about adequacy of exposure brought modifications of the operation that transect the rectus muscle or its tendinous attachment to the pubic bone. Mackenrodt[43] originally recommended a transverse rectus muscle-splitting technique for radical pelvic surgery. Dividing the rectus abdominis muscle produces sufficient operating space for all but the most unusual upper abdominal procedures. Transection of the rectus muscle belly describes the Maylard incision. Transection of the tendons of the rectus muscle near their insertion on the pubic bone characterizes the Cherney incision (see Fig. 3–7).

The Pfannenstiel incision utilizes a transverse skin incision, a transverse fascial incision, and a vertical peritoneal incision. The anterior superior iliac spines on each side and the upper mons veneris about two fingerbreadths above the symphysis define the placement of the skin incision. The skin incision is a segment of a theoretical ellipse drawn through these points. This places the incision along one of the Langer skin tension lines and assures optimum cosmesis.

The length of the incision varies according to the anticipated needs of the operation. Incision length shortens as the operator gains experience. Length of the incision is not a critical factor, because wounds heal from side to side, not end to end.

When cosmesis is the pervading wish of the patient, choose the smallest skin incision consistent with adequate surgical exposure. A fold in the skin just above the mons veneris is an excellent guide for placement of the transverse incision. The crease helps to hide the resulting scar. Incisions placed too caudad traverse the fatty tissue of the mons. This adds unnecessary depth to the dissection and restricts operating space. Incisions are sometimes intentionally placed more cephalad to gain operating space. High transverse incisions may heal with less satisfying cosmetic appearance.

This author performs the Pfannenstiel incision, operating from the left side of the patient. A scalpel makes a single sweep that incises all layers of the skin and some of the superficial subcutaneous tissue along the previously chosen course. This incision lies on the underside of the curve of the abdomen. Keep the knife at right angles to the plane of the skin along the length of the incision to avoid beveling the skin (Fig. 3–4).

The ileohypogastric nerve or ileoinguinal nerve,

depending on the level of incision, lies near the lateral ends of this incision. These nerves are sensory to the mons and portions of the upper thighs and low lateral abdomen. Retract rather than cut these nerves whenever possible.

The inferior epigastric artery and vein pass through the subcutaneous tissues near the lateral extent of the Pfannenstiel incision. Try to identify and isolate the inferior epigastric vessels on each side by dissection with a hemostat. Plunge the hemostat into the subcutaneous tissue near the lateral extent of the incision. Open the hemostat to reveal any vessels and nerves traversing the area. Repeat this until you find the inferior epigastric vessels. Isolate and doubly clamp the vascular bundle on each side. Cut the vessels between clamps and replace each clamp with a catgut free tie (000 or 0000).

Incise the subcutaneous fat with a scalpel or scissors until the fascial layer is visible along most of the length of the incision. An assistant retracts the skin upward and cephalad in the corners of the incision with a Parker or similar retractor. Clamp all bleeding points and control them with fine catgut ties or cauterization.

Begin the semielliptic transverse incision in the fascial layer by incising with a scalpel all layers of fascia for a short distance across each side of the linea alba (Fig. 3–5).

An assistant grasps the upper and lower edges of the opened fascia on one side of the midline with Allis or Ochsner clamps and elevates the fascia. Grasp the edge of the fascia with toothed forceps and free the fascia from underlying muscle layers. Direct the curve of the Mayo scissors upward during this dissection to avoid damage to underlying structures. Track the scissors directly beneath the fascia, tenting it along the anticipated course of the incision. Withdraw the opened scissors to extend the dissection. Thrust, open, and withdraw the scissors to the lateral extent of the

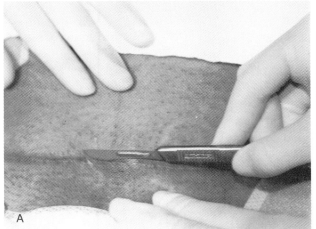

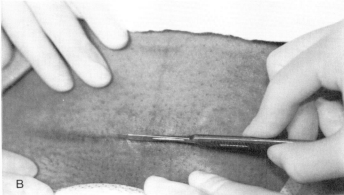

Figure 3–4. *A,* Incorrect scalpel angle for skin incision (beveled). *B,* Correct angle of scalpel blade for skin incision (courtesy Mohammed Bey, M.D.).

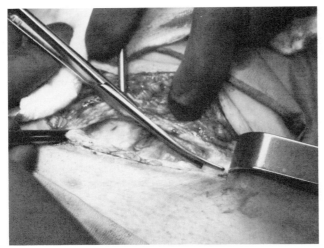

Figure 3–5. Transverse incision in the lower abdominal wall. Curved Mayo scissors incise the fascia on each side of the midline.

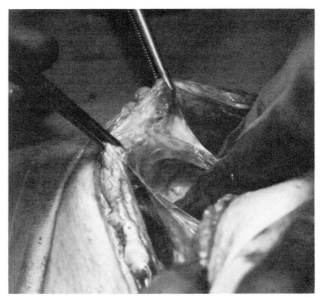

Figure 3–6. Transverse incision. Dissecting beneath the fascia on each side of the linea alba.

incision. The assistant once again retracts the skin and subcutaneous tissue upward and laterally during this procedure.

A firm push of slightly open scissors cleanly incises the rectus fascia and the fascia of the oblique and transverse muscles of the abdominal wall to the lateral extent of the skin incision. Ligate any perforating branches of the inferior epigastric vessels encountered near the lateral reaches of this incision. Incise the fascia on the other side of the linea alba in similar fashion.

The fascia remains firmly attached along the linea alba. Isolate the linea alba along the course of the anticipated vertical peritoneal incision.

Grasp the fascia on each side of the midline with Allis or Ochsner clamps and firmly elevate it upward (Fig. 3–6). Dissect a tunnel with your fingers on each side of the linea alba caudad between the fascia and the underlying rectus and pyramidal muscles. This isolates the linea alba to a point near its attachment on the pubic bone. Incise the isolated linea alba with Mayo scissors, curvature turned upward, near its fascial attachment along the length of the dissection.

Pfannenstiel operation continues on opposite page

Increasing Exposure for Complex Surgery

One may obtain additional operating space by transecting the rectus abdominis muscles (Maylard incision) or the tendinous insertion of the rectus muscles on the pubic bones (Cherney incision) (Fig. 3–7). Incise the peritoneum transversely to achieve maximum exposure. Operations like the cesarean delivery rarely require these special incisions, which facilitate removal of large tumors or other major procedures.

The Maylard incision begins by carefully passing a Kelly or other long curved clamp beneath the middle of the exposed length of rectus muscle.[42] Open the clamp slightly and divide the muscle, a small portion at a time, with a scalpel or cauterizing knife. Control all bleeding points and vessels encountered by ligature or cautery. The severed muscle retracts both caudad and cephalad.

Muscle tissue does not hold sutures well. Sutures that incorporate the posterior rectus sheath help approximate the ends of the rectus muscles at the time of incision closure. Some surgeons do not reapproximate the ends of the muscles during closure. The muscle heals within its sheath of fascia and still provides good abdominal support.

The author prefers the Cherney incision when additional room is needed in a low transverse incision.[43] Division of the stout fibromuscular rectus tendons is easier and faster than division of the rectus muscle, and the risk of bleeding is lessened. At closure, tendon ends are easily reapproximated to bring the rectus back into proper anatomic position.

Perform the Cherney modification of the transverse incision by first passing a finger or a long Kelly clamp beneath the rectus tendons near their insertions on the pubic bones. Do not dissect deeply because of the plexus of veins that overlie the anterior bladder wall. Open the guiding instrument and divide the rectus tendons with a scalpel. The recti retract cephalad. Open the peritoneum carefully in the midline and incise it transversely along the entire width of the incision.

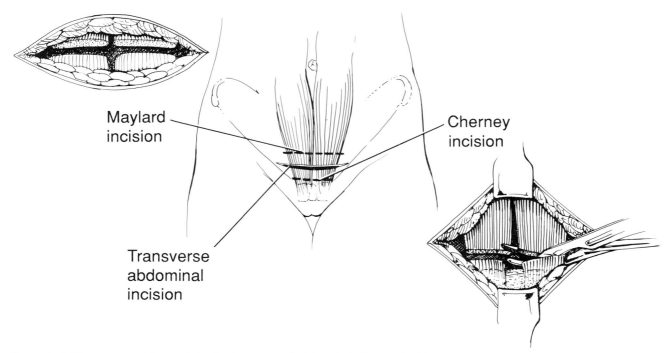

Figure 3–7. Three types of lower abdominal transverse incision. *Left,* Maylard incision divides to the bellies of the rectus muscles. *Center,* The three incision sites. The central Pfannenstiel incision retracts the rectus muscles without incision. *Right,* Cherney incision divides the tendons of the rectus muscles near their insertion on the pubic bone.

The standard Pfannenstiel operation (continued).
Switch the fascial clamps to the cephalad side of the incision and dissect the linea alba cephalad. Try for 3 or 4 inches of dissection length. Small arteries and veins perforate the fascia to supply the rectus muscles near the upper extent of this dissection. Avoid or clamp and ligate these if necessary. Incise the isolated linea alba with scissors under direct vision cephalad to the topmost extent of the dissection.

Separate the rectus and pyramidalis muscles in the midline to approach the peritoneum. Do not allow the fingers or instruments to dig beneath the undersurface of the recti. Large perforating vessels are easily damaged, and resulting hematomas beneath the rectus muscles are not easily recognized or controlled.

Identify the peritoneum in the upper third of the dissection and open it vertically, as described for the vertical abdominal incision. Continue with the chosen operation.

Closure of low abdominal transverse incisions begins with reapproximation of the peritoneal incision with a continuous suture of fine catgut or polyglycolic-polyglactin suture (00 or 000). Check the security of previous subfascial and subcutaneous vascular ties. Reapproximate the fascial layer with interrupted or continuous sutures of polyglycolic-polyglactin suture (0 or 00).

It is often difficult to draw the fascial edges together without tension at the time of closure. Flex the patient's trunk by manipulating the position of the operating table. The author first places a single figure 8 suture to approximate the midline of the fascial incision. This relieves tension along the remainder of the suture line and facilitates knot tying. The author uses a continuous 00 polyglactin suture, beginning at the lateral angle of the incision, for each half of the remaining fascial closure.

The weakest portion of transverse incisional repair is at the lateral ends of the wound, where the incision nears the inguinal canal. Carefully approximate all fascial layers at the lateral corners of the wound to prevent incisional herniation in this region.

Invert the large knot at each end of the closure beneath the fascia to prevent painful subcutaneous granulomas. The angle stitch begins beneath the fascia and then passes the needle upward through one leaf of fascia and down through the opposite leaf. Tie the knot beneath the fascia.

Next, approximate the fascia of Scarpa with continuous 000 absorbable suture. Many obstetric surgeons omit this step. We use it to relieve tension on the skin edges, hoping for a better cosmetic result.

Close the skin with subcuticular continuous suture, staples, or simple taping of the skin edges. Transverse incisions fall naturally together, and the skin edges need only be stabilized for a few days.

Subcuticular fine monofilament continuous suture placed in the dermis without knots makes a fine skin closure. Simply pull the suture out on the fourth or fifth day after surgery.

Place skin staples about a centimeter apart. Tent the skin upward before placing each staple to avoid inverting the skin edges. Remove staples after 3 to 5 days to avoid a visible line of puncture marks. Tape the skin edges with strips of sterile paper tape to sustain support of the incision line for a few additional days.

Steri-Strip taping of the skin edges as the original skin closure provides excellent approximation of the skin edges. Strength of closure is not needed, only accurate, tension-free approximation. The patient removes the tape in a bath or shower 5 to 7 days after surgery.

Instruct the patient to report any wound drainage, redness, or pain. Examine the wound at the time of discharge from the hospital and whenever a patient calls with a wound complaint. The next routine inspection of the wound occurs at postoperative examination 4 to 6 weeks after surgery. The scar initially is raised and pink. Wounds remodel toward their ultimate cosmetic appearance over 6 to 12 months.

WOUND DRESSINGS

Medicaments from honey to iodine have been applied to wounds for centuries to affect their healing. The intention was to suppress infection, but many of these potions suppress healing processes.[44, 46]

Magnetic and electrical fields and even ionic air have been tingled and wafted over wounds in efforts to enhance wound healing. These treatments do not have wide acceptance or use. The conclusion permitted by modern cell biology studies is that a wound heals most reliably when it is undisturbed in a warm, moist environment free of bacterial infection.

Wounds with dry, thick eschars heal more slowly than wounds that are kept moist. Pollack[3] strongly advocated semiocclusive dressings and a moist environment for the fastest, most secure healing. This concept is now incorporated in daily wound management.

Some of the first moisture-retaining surgical dressings were spray films or common adhesive polyvinyl plastic food wraps.[47] Thick laminates containing hydrophilic compounds attract liquid wound drainage and effectively cover large, weeping wound surfaces.

Surgeons question, without satisfactory scientific conclusion, whether dressings that adhere to the surface of the wound are preferable to those that adhere only to the wound edges. Adherence of a dressing to the wound prevents maceration and discourages the invasion of bacteria.[48] Adherent dressings efficiently débride large, granulating wound surfaces but disturb broad areas of delicate new epithelium.

Nonadherent dressings improve the environment for new epithelium. These products are taped to normal skin at the wound edges and do not stick to the wound surface.

The newer dressings are complex, flexible, adherent laminates of nylon and silicone. These dressings are especially useful on angular surfaces with large areas bare of epithelium. They hold to the wound surface by hydrophilic bonding to tissue fibrin.[47] Allergic responses may occur to almost any dressing adhesive. Dressings that adhere to the wound bed by hydrophilic bonding seldom cause allergic tissue reactions.

Gallico[49] developed an autologous skin graft-dressing from cultured epidermal cells obtained by skin biopsy specimens from patients. In a few days, the cells multiply rapidly in culture to cover an area many times the size of the biopsy specimen. The specimen is returned to the patient as a thin film of cells in much the same process as any skin graft. This very expensive process is rarely needed in obstetric surgery.

The clean incisions characteristic of obstetric operations usually necessitate only a simple dressing or no dressing at all. A nonadhesive strip and gauze covering held with tape suffices. We use a prepackaged sterile occlusive dressing for routine operations.

WOUND DRAINS

Draining a wound by placing an inert wick into the wound space to conduct away blood, serum, pus, or other ordure has a long and noble surgical history. Clean surgical wounds with good hemostasis do not need drains. Wound drainage is indicated for obviously infected wounds, certain patients at risk for poor healing, or coagulopathy that makes absolute hemostasis impossible. Drain the abdomen or deep pelvis when there is gross infection or hematoma. Drain the spaces near repairs of injuries to the bladder, ureter, or bowel.

There are valid reasons to avoid wound drainage when possible. Drains are foreign bodies that reduce oxygen tension in wounds and impair healing. Drains allow entrance of bacteria into the depths of the wound.

Drains are brought out through stab wounds separate from the surgical incision. The drain should exit in a somewhat dependent position if gravity drainage is expected. Gravity drains do not effectively drain the deep pelvis if they exit through the anterior abdominal wall. They are more effective when brought out through the vagina. Gravity drains are not completely satisfactory even when dependent drainage is possible.

Suction drainage systems are much more efficient than gravity systems. A good suction drainage system consists of a length of thin, flat, flexible tubing of an inert and nonadherent substance. It has multiple perforations to collect fluid along its entire length. Position these drains in the depths of the wound and connect them to a length of plastic tubing that attaches to a suction device, such as a plastic squeeze bottle.

The gentle, constant suction created by these devices ensures removal of any liquid material that accumulates in the wound. Wound edges remain apposed except at the actual drain site. Suction drainage systems effectively drain the deep pelvis through the anterior abdominal wall. Suction drainage makes the material drained from the wound readily visible, measurable, and disposable without mess.

Wound drains tend to retract into the wound as the patient moves about. Drain retraction is a particular problem with Penrose rubber drains. Some surgeons rely on a large safety pin placed through the drain near its exit to prevent retraction. Others suture such drains to the skin at the drain site. Suction drainage systems have a flared area in the suction tubing that prevents retraction into the wound. Suture fixation is unnecessary.

Remove drains from the wound as soon as drainage is minimal. Ten ml or less drainage in 12 hours is a good general rule. Gravity systems necessitate frequent changes of bulky dressings that are uncomfortable for the postoperative patient. Suction drainage systems necessitate frequent evacuation of the squeeze bottle and reestablishment of suction.

It is rarely necessary to leave drains in the subcutaneous space longer than 48 hours. Do not remove drains, however, as long as a large amount of drainage is coming from the wound.

Remove drains by simply pulling them out. The process is almost painless if the patient is distracted at the moment the drain is pulled. Cover the small stab wound at the site of exit of the drain with a simple adhesive dressing.

Delayed Wound Closures

Scott and colleagues[50] stated that delayed primary closure of skin and subcutaneous fat in contaminated laparotomy incisions virtually eliminates the risk of wound abscess in clinical practice. Delayed closure of the skin and subcutaneous layers may be better than wound drainage when obvious infection or wound dehiscence is present.

The skin and subcutaneous space remain open in delayed closures. Place nonabsorbable sutures an inch apart through skin and subcutaneous fat and leave them untied. If the wound is free of infection 4 to 5 days after surgery, gently tie these sutures to complete the delayed closure. This causes only minimal discomfort to the patient.

Scott and colleagues[50] found the tensile strength of secondary closures weaker at 5 days but stronger at all other times of testing than matched, closed wounds. Incisional hernias were rare in wounds managed with secondary closure. Incisional hernias develop most frequently in wounds that are complicated by hematomas or infection.[1]

Wound Seromas and Hematomas

Wound seromas are collections of sterile tissue fluids in the subcutaneous or subfascial wound spaces. A small quantity of tissue fluids is normal in healing wounds. A large collection of fluids separates the wound edges and lowers oxygen tension in the wound. The seroma is an ideal culture medium for any bacterial inoculum.

Wound seromas are frequent in transverse incisions. Some physicians drain the subcutaneous space in every transverse incision to prevent this wound complication. Hilton[53] polled the members of the Royal College of Obstetricians and Gynaecologists in 1988 regarding their wound drainage practices. This group drained the subcutaneous space in 4% of routine clean cases. They drained the subfascial space in 20% of cases. Complicated cases resulted in more frequent use of drains. Forty-six percent of potentially infected wounds were drained. Active suction drains were favored by 83% of respondents.

Extensive use of electrocautery and electrodesiccation increases the amount of tissue fluid that pours into the wound. Suture closure of the subcutaneous tissues does not prevent seromas.

Treat wound seromas by simple drainage. Because the wound is not infected, there is minimal delay in primary healing.

Hematomas form in wounds when severed subcutaneous or subfascial blood vessels are not adequately controlled. Meticulous hemostasis prevents wound hematomas. Subrectus hematomas in vertical abdominal incisions often result from torn perforator vessels beneath the rectus muscles. The operator may tear these vessels by hooking his or her fingers beneath the rectus muscles when separating them. Bleeding is often not immediately recognized. Pressure from the retractors during operation may interrupt bleeding temporarily. It often resumes, but remains hidden during closure. These subrectus hematomas can be large enough to cause severe anemia and vasomotor instability.

Subfascial and subcutaneous hematomas are the most common in obstetric surgery. These hematomas may become infected and develop into wound abscesses.

The treatment of wound hematomas is surgical drainage. Antibiotics are added if infection is suspected. Expand the blood volume with crystalloids and blood components if the patient becomes unstable.

Wound Infections: Cellulitis and Abscesses

Wound infections occur when the bacterial growth in the wound overwhelms defense mecha-

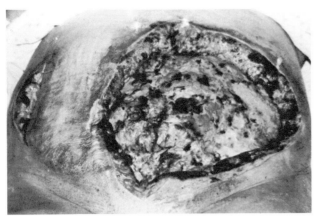

Figure 3–8. Necrotizing fasciitis following a low abdominal vertical incision, after débridement. (Photo courtesy G. Sotrel, M.D. Reprinted with permission of the American College of Obstetricians and Gynecologists. Obstet Gynecol 62:675, 1983.)

nisms. All wounds have some bacterial inoculum. The number of bacteria increases with inadequate skin preparation, when the skin is shaved hours before surgery, or when the operation involves pelvic infections.

Bacteria invade abdominal wounds from glands and crevices in the skin. The longer the procedure, the more the inoculum. Bacteria invade the uterine cavity during obstetric labor. The lower uterine segment, the site of cesarean incisions, is heavily inoculated with vaginal flora. Peripartal hysterectomy incisions enter the bacteria-laden vagina. Each of these circumstances increases the number of bacteria in obstetric surgical wounds.

Wound infections usually begin with cellulitis. The wound becomes red, hot, and tender, and the patient has a fever. Bactericidal antibiotics may arrest the process at this stage, provided there is no seroma or hematoma that requires surgical drainage.

Abscess formation proceeds from uncontrolled cellulitis. The wound becomes increasingly tender and swollen. The patient develops a spiking fever pattern. Other signs of systemic sepsis may or may not be present. The wound may open spontaneously and drain purulent material.

Wound abscesses must be surgically drained by being opened completely and by evacuation of the contents of the abscess. All pockets of pus must be opened and evacuated. Remove any foreign bodies. Débride necrotic tissues. Begin broad-spectrum antibiotics and adjust these according to reports of cultures obtained from the abscess cavity. Pack the wound cavity open with sterile surgical gauze. Change these wound dressings at least daily. Cleanse and débride the abscess cavity as necessary at each dressing change.

Complete wound healing by secondary intention may take 6 weeks or more. It is sometimes possible to speed healing by secondary closure when all wound edges are covered with clean granulation

tissue. Be very patient and do not close the wound prematurely.

Necrotizing fasciitis is feared by all surgeons. Wound infection by synergistic bacteria results in rapid liquefaction necrosis of fascia, subcutaneous tissue, and skin. The process quickly spreads to involve large areas of the abdominal wall (Fig. 3–8).

Management requires courageous débridement of all affected tissues back to clean, viable tissue. This often leaves large defects in the abdominal wall, but it is the only choice.

Multiple wound cultures, particularly of débrided tissues, yield knowledge of the panel of bacteria causing the problem. Order specific antibiotics, but remember that antibiotics do not solve the problem of necrotizing fasciitis without extended débridement.

Wound Dehiscence

Wound dehiscence is heralded by the unexpected painless drainage of serosanguineous fluid from a wound that was previously thought to be healing well. The patient usually calls the attendant because of suddenly soaked dressings or clothing. Examination reveals the drainage coming from an opening in the skin along the incision closure line. Dehiscence often occurs on the fifth to seventh day after surgery. Current trends toward short hospital stays preclude diagnosis of wound dehiscence while the patient is still in the hospital in many cases.

Sudden drainage of serosanguineous fluid from the wound could herald a wound seroma or a complete wound dehiscence. Seromas are usually subcutaneous, whereas wound dehiscence extends through the fascial layer and beyond.

Probe the wound under aseptic conditions with a sterile instrument. If the fascia feels intact and the instrument does not penetrate the fascia, the drainage is probably from a wound seroma. Manage as described earlier in this chapter.

True wound dehiscence allows the wound probe to drop through the fascial layer into the peritoneal cavity. Cover the wound and take the patient promptly to the operating room. Open the wound completely under appropriate anesthesia by blunt separation with the fingers and sharp dissection as necessary. Culture the wound site. Remove the bulk of previous wound suture material and any other foreign bodies. Explore the previous operative site, the pelvis, and the entire abdomen. Free any adhered loops of bowel or other adhesions. Drain and culture any hematomas or abscess sites. Irrigate the abdomen and wound with large quantities of saline. Begin secondary wound closure, as described subsequently.

SECONDARY CLOSURE OF WOUND DEHISCENCES

Mass closure techniques are excellent for primary laparotomy closure and approach standard practice for secondary closure of wound dehiscences. Mass closures, such as the Smead-Jones suture method, help reduce the incidence of wound dehiscence.[1] The chance of late herniation at the operative site is also reduced by these techniques.

Mass closures place sutures broadly through all support layers of the abdominal wall. They provide loose apposition of wound edges without strangulation of blood supply.[51] Less suture material clutters the wound, and the microcirculation near the wound site remains intact.

Mass closure techniques originated with the "retention sutures" of generations of surgeons. In the past, when a wound was thought to be likely to heal poorly in oncology patients, diabetic patients, or malnourished patients, retention sutures were placed. Standard layer closure was supported by large-caliber interrupted nonabsorbable sutures that encompassed all wound layers. These sutures were tied over plastic or rubber "booties" or gauze pads. These sutures relieved tension on the primary suture lines. Retention sutures were the surgeon's insurance against wound dehiscence and were often left in place 10 to 14 days or longer. Retention sutures have been replaced by current mass closure techniques.

The Smead-Jones mass closure is illustrated in Figure 3–2. There are many technical variations of this closure. Each suture incorporates the anterior rectus fascia, the rectus muscle, the posterior rectus fascia, and the peritoneum. The suture begins an inch or more back from the wound edge and pierces, from outside in, the anterior rectus fascia, the rectus muscle, the posterior rectus fascia, and the peritoneum on one side of the wound. The peritoneum must be traversed 1 cm from the wound edge, leaving a minimum of suture material within the peritoneal cavity. This prevents the accidental entrapment of the bowel, which could occur with a large loop of intraperitoneal suture.

The Smead-Jones suture continues on the other side of the wound. It passes first through the peritoneum from within, near the peritoneal edge. The needle then passes from below through the posterior rectus fascia, the rectus muscle, and the anterior rectus fascia an inch or more lateral to the wound edge. The suture next passes through the conjoined fascia from above near the edge on the original side and from below on the opposite side. The mnemonic far-far-near-near gets you through the steps.

Draw the suture just tight enough to approximate the tissues and tie it securely. Sutures are placed at intervals of 1.5 to 2 cm. The Smead-Jones closure approximates all the deep layers of the wound and provides a smooth, tension-free peritoneal and fascial closure.

Gallup and colleagues[52] reported excellent results in 1989 with primary mass closure of midline incisions in 210 gynecologic patients, using continuous monofilament suture. Although 60% of these patients were operated on for gynecologic cancers, only 3.4% experienced wound complications. There were no eviscerations and only one incisional hernia.

POSTOPERATIVE CARE AND COMPLICATIONS

Just as preoperative care begins in the prenatal period, postoperative care begins during the operation. Intravenous fluids infused during surgery ensure proper hydration of the patient. Oxytocics reduce blood loss from the postpartum uterus. Gentle handling of tissues and prevention of wound contamination prepare for rapid primary wound healing. Intraoperative blood loss should be estimated as an early guide to the possible need for transfusion. This estimate should be modified with postoperative determinations of the hematocrit value, vital signs, and continued estimates of blood loss.

In the recovery area, carefully monitor the airway until the patient is fully awake. Monitor vital signs, intravenous intake, and urine output. Give particular attention to the tone of the uterus and lochia flow in postcesarean patients.

Administer oxytocics and gently massage the uterus to prevent postpartum hemorrhage. Early postpartum hemorrhage usually occurs in the first hour or so after delivery. Make attendants aware of how exquisitely tender the uterus and abdominal wall are after cesarean delivery. Slow infusion of dilute oxytocin, 10–20 IU/L of intravenous fluids, for the first 12 hours after delivery ensures contraction of the uterus.

The patient should be attended constantly for the first few hours after obstetric surgery. Write orders for monitoring vital signs, drain flow, urinary output, and intravenous fluids for the first 12 to 24 hours. Tailor analgesic agents to patient need.

Patients transfer to a floor unit in a few hours, subject to the availability of continued close observation on the ward. Attendants must know what complications to look for and how to notify the surgeon immediately if an unforeseen event occurs. Remain available or supply appropriate coverage for emergencies.

Early ambulation is one of the most important principles of postoperative care. The patient exercises her legs in bed as soon as she is alert and gets up to walk by the first day after surgery. Early ambulation reduces phlebothrombosis and pulmonary embolism. Patients regain strength and confidence most rapidly when walking begins early in convalescence. This takes some persuading at first, but is well worth the effort.

Early ambulation also combats postoperative atelectasis. Low abdominal incisions reduce the splinting of diaphragmatic breathing. Encourage deep breathing and coughing in all surgical patients to clear any tracheobronchial secretions.

Positive-pressure breathing is the key to the management of focal atelectasis. Pulmonary therapists can assist with difficult cases. Mechanical positive pressure assists inflation of the alveoli and delivers aerosolized surfactant medications. Patients without complications benefit from any routine that encourages them to breathe deeply and exhale against mild resistance.

Care of the bladder and bowel in the postoperative period is very important. Most surgeons develop their own routine management designed to prevent paralytic ileus and stimulate normal bowel and bladder function.

Indwelling bladder catheters can usually be removed soon after operation unless there has been surgery on the bladder or ureters, or vulvar problems that make voiding difficult. Keep fluid intake sufficient to maintain copious urine output.

"Gas pains" cause the most bitter patient complaints after the first postoperative day. The surgeon welcomes these signs of return of bowel motility. Paralytic ileus is the most common postoperative gastrointestinal problem of the obstetric surgeon. Early ambulation encourages prompt return of bowel function. One may encourage a recalcitrant bowel with sublingual, oral, or even parenteral neostigmine (Prostigmin, ICN Pharmaceuticals, Inc., Costa Mesa, Calif.) analogues, but these are rarely necessary. The first passage of flatus by the patient marks the return of physiologic bowel function after abdominal surgery.

Ileus that lasts more than a few days may signal intestinal obstruction, peritonitis, or other intra-abdominal complications. The patient's abdomen becomes distended and uncomfortable. She tolerates oral feeding poorly and may vomit. Bowel sounds are sluggish or absent. Completely re-evaluate the patient with appropriate imaging and consultation if the patient has not passed flatus by the third postoperative day.

Progressive diet management begins with discontinuance of intravenous fluids after the first postoperative day. Progress to oral feedings of clear liquids, then semisolid, then soft foods, and finally a regular diet as bowel function returns. Some surgeons prefer to withhold all oral feeding except clear liquids until flatus is passed by the patient. Shorter hospital stays have encouraged earlier introduction of solid foods into the postoperative diet. Early feeding, carefully monitored, causes few complications and no apparent increase in the incidence of postoperative ileus.

Take special care to balance the calorie intake and insulin needs of diabetic patients. Recall the effects of diet change, the metabolic alterations of surgical stress, and the dramatic drop in insulin requirements after obstetric delivery.

The wound necessitates no care other than inspection until sutures or staples are removed on the fourth or fifth day after the procedure. The trend is toward earlier suture or staple removal. Support the skin incision with adhesive strips after suture or staple removal if necessary. The patient removes these easily several days later while bathing or showering at home.

SUMMARY

This chapter has discussed many aspects of the surgical wound. All obstetric surgeons must choose incision sites and produce and close wounds in the abdominal wall, perineum, and genital tract. Knowledge of the healing process allows the surgeon to enhance healing factors, such as nutrition, and reduce factors that delay healing, such as foreign bodies or infections.

Knowledge of wound-closure options, varied suture materials, drains, and dressings allows the surgeon to facilitate natural healing processes. Choose each technique to suit the needs of the individual patient and surgical procedure.

Obstetric surgeons are most fortunate that the physiologic processes of wound healing are so constantly reliable. Surgeons repeatedly enter the sanctum of the coelomic and uterine cavities with complete confidence that healing will take place.

In the rare instance when primary healing does not occur, the obstetric surgeon must recognize and manage wound complications. Humility comes with the realization that it is the surgeon who cuts and sews, but it is the body that heals.

References

1. Ellis H: What's new in wound healing. Aust NZ J Surg 57:341, 1987.
2. Kanzler MH, Gorsulowsky DC, Swanson NA: Basic mechanisms in the healing cutaneous wound. J Dermatol Surg Oncol 12:11, 1986.
3. Pollack SV: Wound healing 1985: An update. J Dermatol Surg Oncol 11:3, 1985.
4. Gillis S: Interleukin biochemistry and biology: Summary and introduction. Fed Proc 42:2635, 1983.
5. Leibovich SJ, Ross R: A macrophage-dependent factor that stimulates the proliferation of fibroblasts in vitro. Am J Pathol 84:501, 1976.
6. Thakral KK, Goodson WH III, Hunt TK: Stimulation of wound blood vessel growth by wound macrophages. J Surg Res 26:430, 1979.
7. Grinnell F: Fibronectin and wound healing. Am J Dermatopathol 4:181, 1982.
8. Clark RAF: Fibronectin in the skin. J Invest Dermatol 81:475, 1983.
9. Winter GD: Epidermal regeneration studied in the domes-

tic pig. In Maibach HI, Rovee DT (eds.): Epidermal Wound Healing. Chicago: Year Book Medical Publishers, Inc., 1972.

10. Krawczyk W: Pattern of epidermal cell migration during wound healing. J Cell Biol 49:247, 1971.
11. Folkman J: Angiogenesis: Initiation and control. Ann NY Acad Sci 401:212, 1982.
12. Clark RAF: Cutaneous tissue repair: Basic biologic considerations. I. J Am Acad Dermatology 13:701, 1985.
13. Majino G, Gabbiani G, Hirschel BJ, et al.: Contraction of granulation tissue in vitro: Similarity to smooth muscle. Science 173:548, 1971.
14. Howes EL, Sooy WJ, Harvey SC: The healing of wounds as determined by their tensile strength. JAMA 92:42, 1929.
15. Levenson SM, Geever EG, Crawley LV, et al.: The healing of rat skin wounds. Ann Surg 161:293, 1965.
16. Schlaff WD, Gittlesohn AM, Cooley BC, et al.: A rat uterine horn model of genital tract wound healing. Fertil Steril 48:866, 1987.
17. Nyman S, Lindhe J, Zederfeldt B: Impaired wound healing in progesterone treated rabbits. Acta Chir Scand 139:415, 1973.
18. Dunihoo DR, Otterson WN, Mailhes JB, et al.: An evaluation of uterine scar integrity after cesarean section in rabbits. Obstet Gynecol 73:390, 1989.
19. Reed BR, Clark RAF: Cutaneous tissue repair: Practical implications of current knowledge. II. J Am Acad Dermatol 13:919, 1985.
20. Alexander JW, Fischer JE, Boyajian M, et al.: The influence of hair removal on wound infection. Arch Surg 118:347, 1983.
21. Polk HL, Simpson CJ, Simmons BP, Alexander JW: Guidelines for review of surgical wound infection. Arch Surg 118:1213, 1983.
22. Hohn DC: Host resistance to infections: Established and emerging concepts. In Hunt TK (ed.): Wound Healing and Wound Infection. New York: Appleton-Century-Crofts, 1980, pp. 264–279.
23. Winter GD: Formation of the scab and the rate of epithelialization of superficial wounds in the skin of the young domestic pig. Nature 193:293, 1962.
24. Rovee DT, Kirrowaky CA, Labrin J, Downes AM: Effect of local wound environment on epidermal wound healing. In Maibach H, Rovee DT (eds.): Epidermal wound healing. Chicago: Year Book Medical Publishers, Inc., 1972, pp. 159–181.
25. Levenson SM, Seifter E: Dysnutrition, wound healing, and resistance to infection. Clin Plast Surg 4:384, 1977.
26. Young ME: Malnutrition and wound healing. Heart Lung 17:60, 1988.
27. Beisel WR, Edelman R, Nauss K, et al.: Single nutrient effects on immunologic function. JAMA 245:53, 1981.
28. Rundus C, Peterson VM, Zapata-Sirvent R, et al.: Vitamin E improves cell mediated immunity in the burned mouse: A preliminary study. Burns 11:11, 1984.
29. Neldner K: The biochemistry and physiology of zinc metabolism. In Goldsmith L (ed.): Biochemistry and physiology of the skin. New York: Oxford University Press, 1983, pp. 1082–1095.
30. Senapati A, Thompson RPH: Zinc deficiency and the prolonged accumulation of zinc in wounds. Br J Surg 72:583, 1985.
31. Goodson WH, Hunt TK: Wound healing and aging. J Invest Dermatol 73:88, 1979.
32. Yamaura H, Matsuzawa T: Decrease in capillary growth during aging. Exp Gerontol 15:145, 1980.
33. Hosking MP, Warner MA, Lobdell CM et al.: Outcomes of surgery in patients 90 years of age and older. JAMA 261:1909, 1989.
34. Fauci AS, Dale DC, Balow JE: Glucocorticoid therapy: Mechanisms of action and clinical considerations. Ann Intern Med 84:304, 1976.
35. Edwards JC, Dunphy JE: Wound healing. II. Injury and abnormal repair. N Engl J Med 259:275, 1958.
36. Pollack SV: Systemic medications and wound healing. Int J Dermatol 21:489, 1982.
37. Scher KS, Scott-Conner CE, Montany PE: Effect of cephalosporins on fascial healing after celiotomy. Am J Surg 155:361, 1988.
38. Borden EB, Sammartano RJ, Dembe C, et al.: The effect of metronidazole on wound healing in rats. Surgery 97:331, 1985.
39. Howes E: Strength studies of polyglycolic acid versus catgut sutures of the same size. Surg Gynecol Obstet 137:15, 1973.
40. Ling F: Personal communication, September, 1989
41. Donaldson BR, Hegarty JH, Brennan TG, et al.: The lateral paramedian incision: experience with 850 cases. Br J Surg 69:630, 1982.
42. Pfannenstiel HJ: Uber die Vorteile des suprasymphysaren Fascienquerschnitts fur die gynakologischen Koliotomien, zugleich ein Beitrag zu der Indikationsstellung der Operationswege. Samml Klin Vortr NF 268; Gynak 97, Feb 1900.
43. Mackenrodt A: Die Radikaloperation des Gebarmutterscheidendrebses mit Austraumung des Beckens. Verh Dtsh Gynakol 9:139, 1901.
44. Maylard AE: Direction of abdominal incisions. Br Med J 2:895, 1907.
45. Cherney LS: A modified transverse incision for low abdominal operations. Surg Gynecol Obstet 72:92, 1940.
46. Kozol RA, Gilles C, Elgebaly SA: Effects of sodium hypochlorite (Dakin's solution) on cells of the wound module. Arch Surg 123:420, 1988.
47. Wheelan RG: The newer surgical dressings and wound healing. Advanced Dermatol Surg 5:393, 1987.
48. Noe J, Kalish S: The problem of adherence in dressed wounds. Surg Gynecol Obstet 147:185, 1978.
49. Gallico GG, O'Conner NE, Compton CC, et al.: Permanent coverage of large burn wounds with autologous cultured epithelium. N Engl J Med 311:448, 1984.
50. Scott PG, Chambers M, Johnson BW, et al.: Experimental wound healing: Increased breaking strength and collagen synthetic activity in abdominal fascial wounds healing with secondary closure of the skin. Br J Surg 72:777, 1985.
51. Baggish M, Lee W: Prevention of abdominal wound disruption utilizing the Smead-Jones closure technique. Obstet Gynecol 46:530, 1975.
52. Gallup DG, Talledo OE, King LA: Primary mass closure of midline incisions with a continuous running monofilament suture in gynecologic patients. Obstet Gynecol 73:675, 1989.
53. Hilton P: Surgical wound drainage: A survey of practices among gynecologists in the British Isles. Br J Obstet Gynecol 95(10):1063, 1988.

4

Complications Common to Obstetric Operative Procedures

Harvey A. Gabert

Obstetric operative procedures may involve the abdomen, vulva, vagina, cervix, uterus, bladder, and ureter. Complications related to operative procedures may follow a spontaneous, forceps, or cesarean birth. The advancements in tech-nique, suture, fluid care, infection prevention, and treatment of shock have reduced maternal mortality and morbidity markedly over the last 4 to 5 decades. Prenatal care has identified and thereby reduced the complications related to high-risk

65

pregnancy. The newer, more effective antimicrobial drugs have played a great part in reducing intrapartum and postpartum infections. These drugs are now widely used in a prophylactic fashion as well as for definitive therapeutic treatment.

Attention directed toward euglycemic blood glucose control in diabetes mellitus, use of antihypertensives, immunization, and advanced treatment for other diseases has been instrumental in lowering maternal and fetal mortality and morbidity. Other dramatic changes have come about because of intensive care equipment and knowledge.

It is always important to realize that obstetric management includes both mother and fetus. In preoperative care, one must, therefore, always bear in mind that drugs or decreased maternal oxygen may affect the fetus and the newborn. Abdominal procedures during pregnancy must prevent undue manipulations to avoid premature labor or other trauma to the uterus. The obstetrician must choose the proper time, appropriate procedure, safest anesthetic, and supporting measures to prevent the morbidity and mortality of the mother. These measures safeguard the fetus and the newborn.

In deciding on the procedure, advantages and disadvantages of abdominal versus vaginal approach must be understood. The procedure should then proceed with high regard for tissue, avoidance of trauma, and good general surgical technique.

PREOPERATIVE EVALUATION

Appropriate physical examination should include the breasts, the abdomen, the pelvis, the lungs, and the cardiovascular system. In addition, an appropriate consent form spelling out possible complications must be obtained. The preoperative status of the patient needs to be assessed as to nutrition, anemia, shock, electrolyte balance, and infection. Laboratory tests should include a complete blood count and clotting status. A platelet count, including partial thromboplastin time and prothrombin time, is essential. Other hematologic tests needed may be a determination of bleeding time, the von Willebrand factor, and fibrinogen and fibrin split products. The Rh type and blood group should be ascertained. Type and screen are sufficient in uncomplicated procedures. Typed and crossmatched blood should be available if the patient is actively bleeding, has lost a good amount of blood, is in shock, or if excessive blood loss is anticipated during the surgical procedure (Table 4–1). This would include complications of placenta previa, abruptio placentae, large, bleeding lacerations, hematomas, and patients with a positive antibody screen. The last should be typed and crossmatched prospectively.

If infection is present, appropriate bacteriologic testing of the infected areas is needed. Urinalysis, urine cultures, and indicated blood cultures should

Table 4–1. BLOOD COMPONENT USES

1. One unit of whole blood equals 450 ml of blood + 63 ml of anticoagulant and preservative. This equals 1 unit packed red blood cells (PRBCs) + 1 unit platelets + 1 unit plasma.

2. One unit of PRBCs (265 ml of red blood cells), hematocrit 80%, contains most of the white blood cells from the whole blood and raises a 70-kg patient's hematocrit by 3%.

3. One unit platelet (60 ml of platelet-rich plasma), 5.5×10^{10} platelet, contains white cells, mostly lymphocytes, and raises a 70-kg patient's platelet count by 5000 to 7000.

4. One unit of plasma (170 to 220 ml of plasma), usually fresh frozen and thawed at 37° C—contains all coagulation factors—plasma can be kept liquid at 4° C, but loses factors V and VIII. Fresh frozen plasma can be thawed at 4° C to form cryoprecipitate, a high concentrate of factor VIII, von Willebrand factor, fibrinogen, factor XIII, and fibronectin.

5. To replace oxygen-carrying capacity, use PRBCs.

6. To treat bleeding tendencies resulting from platelet deficiencies, use platelets.

7. To treat bleeding tendencies resulting from coagulation factor deficiencies, use fresh frozen plasma or more highly concentrated products for specific deficiency.

8. For von Willebrand disease, hemophilia A, and disseminated intravascular coagulation, use cryoprecipitate.

be obtained. A urinary catheter should be inserted prior to surgery to ensure that adequate urine volume and concentration are maintained.

Preoperative abdominal radiographic films may be needed if perforation of the bowel or bladder is suspected. In addition, special studies, such as ultrasonography, may help to delineate the problem and its location if it is intra-abdominal.

If shock is present, appropriate blood and fluid replacement must be instituted to stabilize the patient prior to starting surgery. While waiting for blood, crystalloid or colloid solution at a rate of 3 ml for every milliliter of blood loss should be used. However, if bleeding is massive from a ruptured liver or spleen, immediate surgery may be needed to save the patient's life.

Blood Transfusion

There are adequate data to support storage of a patient's blood to be used in a later transfusion.[1] This avoids isoimmunization, transfusion reactions, and blood-borne infections. Information is also accumulating that pregnant women can, without jeopardy to the pregnancy, store their own blood.[1, 2]

The other methods of transfusion are from donors, either as whole blood or blood components (Table 4–2). Recent interest has turned toward recovery of lost blood at surgery with immediate replacement. This necessitates a specific piece of equipment, known as a cell-plasma saver, which is a source of volume and red blood cell mass. The most frequent complications during any of the transfusion methods are hyperkalemia, hemolysis,

Table 4–2. COMPONENT BLOOD PRODUCTS

Product	Content	Indications	Volume	Shelf Life
Whole blood	Red blood cells Leukocytes Platelets Plasma	Acute blood loss Neonatal exchange Transfusion	500 ml	35 days in CPDA-1* at 1–6° C
Red blood cells	Red blood cells Leukocytes Plasma	Anemia	200–300 ml	35 days in CPDA-1 at 1–6° C
Red blood cells, frozen-thawed	Red blood cells Few leukocytes Platelets Plasma	Anemia Prevents reactions to white blood cells, platelets, plasma proteins Storage of rare blood	170–190 ml	Frozen—3 yr Thawed—24 hr
Red blood cells, reduced leukocytes	Red blood cells Few leukocytes Some plasma	Prevents febrile white blood cell antibodies Anemia	200–250 ml	35 days in CPDA-1 at 1–6° C
Platelet concentrate	Platelets Few leukocytes Some plasma	Bleeding resulting from low platelet count or poor function	20–50 ml	72 hr
Leukocyte concentrate	Leukocytes, platelets, and few red blood cells	Serious infections in leukopenic patients	50–300 ml	24 hr
Fresh-frozen plasma	Clotting factors No platelets	Clotting disorders	10–25 ml	Frozen—1 yr Thawed—6 hr
Cryoprecipitated AHF (antihemophilic factor)	Factor VIII Factor XII Fibrogen von Willebrand factor Fibronectin	Deficiencies in factor VIII and factor XIII von Willebrand factor	Lyophilized powder	Frozen—1 yr Thawed—6 hr
Purified AHF concentrate	Factor VIII	Factor VIII deficiency	20 ml sterile water Lyophilized powder	Determined by manufacturer
Autoplex	Activated procoagulants	Inhibitor to factor VIII	20–40 ml sterile water Lyophilized powder	2 yr
Factor IX	Factors II, VII, IX, X	Factors II, VII, IX, X deficiency	20–40 ml sterile water Lyophilized powder	Determined by manufacturer
Albumin	5% Albumin or 25% albumin	Plasma volume expansion	5% 50–100 ml	3 yr
Plasma protein fraction	Albumin Alpha and beta globulins	Plasma volume expansion	5% 250–500 ml	3 yr
Rh (D) Immune globulin	Gamma globulin anti-D from immunized donors	Sensitization in Rh (D)–negative patients	1–2 ml	3 yr
Immune serum	Gamma globulin	Hypogamma-globulinemia or disease prophylaxis	2 ml 10 ml	3 yr

*CPDA-1—citrate-phosphate-dextrose-adenine.

febrile allergic reactions, and transfusion reaction (Tables 4–3, 4–4).

Blood transfusion is indicated in patients with severe anemia and blood loss. The total blood volume in a nonpregnant female varies from 64 to 80 ml/kg. A 70-kg woman would have a blood volume of 4500 to 5600 ml. During pregnancy, an increase in plasma volume and red blood cell mass occurs. The volume expansion can be increased by 50% over that of the nonpregnant state. The usual average plasma volume increase is about 1300 ml, whereas the red blood cell mass increases by 250 to 450 ml.[3, 4]

The average blood loss in a noncomplicated vaginal delivery approaches 500 ml, whereas the average at cesarean delivery is 1000 ml.[4] This is extremely important information because we do not have a rapid blood loss assessment laboratory test. In other words, replacement is based on the estimation of blood loss. It is said that the amount of blood lost is usually twice as much as the surgeon estimates and half as much as the patient or anesthetist thinks the patient lost. Blood loss can also be assessed on the basis of a blood pressure drop and an increased heart rate. Pregnant females can tolerate a low hematocrit if the blood

Table 4–3. STEPS FOR THE TREATMENT OF A
HEMOLYTIC TRANSFUSION REACTION

1. STOP THE TRANSFUSION.

2. Maintain the urine output at a minimum of 75 to 100 ml/hr by generously administering fluids intravenously and possibly mannitol, 12.5 to 50 g, over a 5- to 15-minute period. If intravenously administered fluids and mannitol are ineffective, then administer furosemide, 20 to 40 mg, intravenously.

3. Alkalinize the urine; because bicarbonate is preferentially excreted in the urine, only 40 to 70 mEq/70 kg of sodium bicarbonate is usually required to raise the urine pH to 8; repeat urine pH determination indicates the need for additional bicarbonate.

4. Assay urine and plasma hemoglobin concentrations.

5. Determine platelet count, partial thromboplastin time, and serum fibrinogen level.

6. Return unused blood to blood bank for repeat crossmatch.

7. Send patient's blood sample to blood bank for antibody screen and direct antiglobulin test.

8. Prevent hypotension to ensure adequate renal blood flow.

Table 4–4. COMPLICATIONS IN PACKED RED BLOOD CELL
(PRBC) TRANSFUSION

PRBC Complications
1. Depleted 2,3-diphosphoglycerate in stored PRBCs results in decreased oxygen capacity.
2. Citrate buffers in PRBCs may result in hypocalcemia and hyperkalemia.
3. Dilution of circulating clotting factors and platelets may occur.
4. Transfusion reaction.

Prevention of Coagulopathy
1. If > 10 U PRBCs are transfused, 1 U fresh frozen plasma/ 5 U PRBCs should be given.
2. If > 10 U PRBCs are transfused, 5 U of platelets should be given when platelet count decreases to 100,000 k or less.

volume is maintained. There is no evidence that routine blood replacement benefits pregnant women with a low hematocrit. It is extremely important to prevent blood transfusion if possible. In spite of excellent screening methods, risk of hepatitis B and C is as high as 1 in 100 and risk of human immunodeficiency virus is 1 in 46,000 to 1 in 1,000,000.

Anesthesia

It is important to have a large-bore intracatheter placed so that appropriate fluids and blood can be administered. Stabilization is needed prior to any surgical procedure and includes oxygenation, restoration of circulatory volume, and appropriate drug administration. Oxygen should be given at a rate of 6 to 7 L per minute by mask or, if needed, by intubation.

The vascular volume should be maintained by a crystalloid fluid, such as 0.9% sodium chloride or Ringer's lactate solution. Albumin or a 5% or 6% betastarch solution can be used if acute hypovole-

mia is present. These solutions maintain colloid oncotic pressure for about 24 hours. To have a similar effect with crystalloid fluid, a large-volume infusion is needed, which often markedly lowers colloid oncotic pressure and may result in movement of fluid from the vascular to the extravascular compartment. This can cause acute peripheral and pulmonary edema. If shock is present and large volumes of fluid infusion are anticipated, a Swan-Ganz catheter to monitor pulmonary capillary wedge pressure should be placed prior to surgery (Figs. 4–1, 4–2, and 4–3). This prevents inadvertent production of pulmonary edema.

In the presence of active bleeding and shock, either fresh whole blood or appropriate component therapy may be needed (see Table 4–2). Vasopressor drugs should be used only as a last resort.

The choice of anesthesia is important in either a pregnant or a postpartum patient. In the presence of a compromised intravascular volume, epidural or spinal anesthesia is contraindicated. A progressive motor block may further compromise the intravascular volume by a decrease in peripheral resistance, with a resultant decrease in the afterload volume accompanied by hypotension. Under these circumstances, appropriate fluid replacement may be impossible and may result in irreversible shock.

The best anesthesia to manage a complication in obstetrics is general anesthesia with intubation. This allows for good control over the mother and avoids aspiration. Regardless of the type of anesthesia used, safety to the mother and fetus must

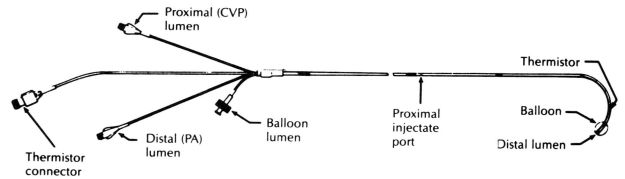

Figure 4–1. Schematic pulmonary artery catheter. CVP—central venous pressure; PA—pulmonary artery.

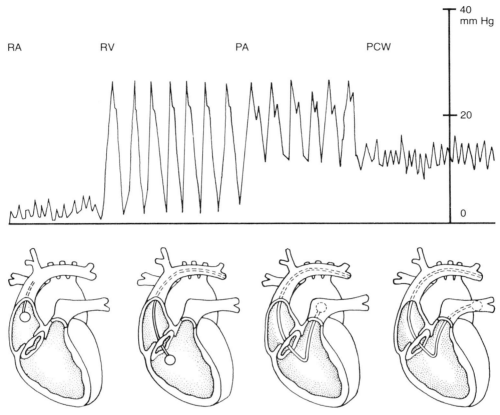

Figure 4–2. Pulmonary artery catheter pressure waves related to position.

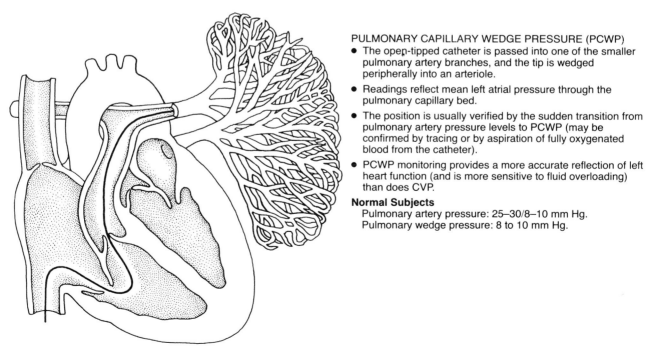

PULMONARY CAPILLARY WEDGE PRESSURE (PCWP)
- The open-tipped catheter is passed into one of the smaller pulmonary artery branches, and the tip is wedged peripherally into an arteriole.
- Readings reflect mean left atrial pressure through the pulmonary capillary bed.
- The position is usually verified by the sudden transition from pulmonary artery pressure levels to PCWP (may be confirmed by tracing or by aspiration of fully oxygenated blood from the catheter).
- PCWP monitoring provides a more accurate reflection of left heart function (and is more sensitive to fluid overloading) than does CVP.

Normal Subjects
Pulmonary artery pressure: 25–30/8–10 mm Hg.
Pulmonary wedge pressure: 8 to 10 mm Hg.

Figure 4–3. Pulmonary artery pressure catheter in schematic position.

be considered. Most complications occur after delivery, allowing more intensive anesthesia management of the mother.

Preoperative Preparation

A urinary catheter can be inserted and the preoperative site shaved and scrubbed after the start of anesthesia unless an acute emergency exists. The use of clippers for removal of pubic and perineal hair is more desirable than shaving because it tends to decrease the risk of lacerating the skin with a resulting skin infection.

There are numerous scrubs used to cleanse the surgical area, and most are effective. The use of alcohol or other degreaser followed by 10% iodine in alcohol decreases the necessity for prolonged scrubbing. The abdomen and vulva can be prepared in this manner, whereas povidone-iodine solution should be used for vaginal procedures.

ROUTINE CARE AFTER CESAREAN DELIVERY AND COMMON COMPLICATIONS

Vital Signs

Recovery from any procedure that necessitates anesthesia must include monitoring of all vital signs every 15 minutes until the patient has recovered from the anesthetic effects. In addition, bleeding from the vagina and the incision must be recorded along with uterine consistency and urine output. Complications, such as bleeding, shock, infection, urinary problems, and bowel problems, may occur after cesarean or other surgical procedures and often may result in excessive morbidity.[5] These complications can cause prolonged hospitalization and expense.

Fluid and Electrolytes

Fluid and electrolytes must be monitored closely because pregnancy often involves movement of water out of the vascular system into intracellular and extracellular compartments, especially if pre-eclampsia is present. A solution of 5% dextrose in water should be used only if there is no hypovolemia and cardiovascular stability is expected, because it diffuses into all spaces containing water to balance osmolality. If hypovolemia is present, normal saline or a crystalline solution should be used. If the colloid pressure is low, the use of albumin decreases the loss of water into the interstitial spaces.

Adequate urine output, at least 50 ml per hour, is a good sign of adequate blood volume. If oliguria is present, it may be the first sign of hypovolemia. It is important to check urine osmolarity because failure to concentrate is an early sign of acute renal failure.

The use of a central venous pressure monitor line, in the presence of severe hypovolemia, may prevent fluid overload and subsequent pulmonary edema. If severe pre-eclampsia or shock is present, the use of a pulmonary artery catheter allows more accurate monitoring (see Figs. 4–1, 4–2, and 4–3).[6] Direct arterial monitoring may be needed occasionally. This type of monitoring in the absence of obtainable cuff pressure allows blood pressure monitoring and access to blood sampling for blood gas determination (Fig. 4–4).

Analgesia

Analgesia must be used in adequate dosage to decrease the frequency of injections. The comfort of the patient is required, but respiratory depression must be avoided. Adequate dosages of the many pain killers available prevent swings in blood levels and keep the patient the most comfortable.

The use of intrathecal and epidural agents, such as morphine sulfate (Duramorph) and fentanyl, has had mixed reports. If used judiciously, opiates have been effective for over 24 hours, obviating the need for respiratory depressant agents.[7] The use of continuous fentanyl is showing promising results, with a decrease in the complications, such as itching and nausea, that some patients complain of when opiates are used.

Ambulation

The patient should have recovered from the initial reaction of the operation before ambulation is begun. The baby can nurse when the mother is able to. If prolonged bed rest is needed, leg movement is important to decrease the possibility of thrombophlebitis. Most patients tolerate early ambulation and appear to recover quickly.

SPECIFIC COMPLICATIONS
Anesthesia

Postoperative anesthesia complications are responsible for 10 to 15% of all maternal deaths. The most common cause is aspiration of gastric contents. Aspiration can be prevented in most cases by appropriate endotracheal intubation. The severity of this syndrome is related to either obstruction of the airway or burn of the bronchial tree by the acidic gastric contents. Pulmonary edema and hypovolemia can occur quickly and result in hypoxemia, hypotension, and shock. Treatment needs to be aggressive and may include intubation, suction, and positive-pressure ventilation and oxygen.

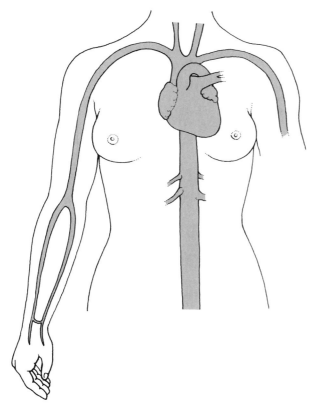

- Important when stroke volume is low and Korotkoff sounds are markedly reduced or cuff pressure is unobtainable (systolic pressure <55 mm Hg)

- *Note:* In 5 to 10% of patients with unobtainable cuff pressure, the intra-arterial pressure is normal or high

- An intra-arterial line in shock provides access to blood samples for serial blood gas determinations

- Provides precise beat-to-beat pressure assessment

Figure 4–4. Schematic direct arterial monitoring.

Positive end-expiratory pressure is excellent for pulmonary edema. Bronchoscopy is usually required when obstruction is present. The use of steroids is debatable, and their use does not appear to affect the outcome.[8, 10]

Problems such as uterine relaxation and liver damage have been reported with halothane exposure; the last is usually secondary to repeated use. Supportive therapy, such as good nutrition and correction of coagulation problems, allows the liver to recover.

Spinal anesthesia can result in headache because of leakage of spinal fluid. This occurs if a large-bore needle is used. Treatment includes strict bed rest, hydration, and sedation. If the headache continues, placement of a blood patch by injection of 10 ml of the patient's blood over the rent in the dura results in a high rate of success.

Bladder dysfunction after spinal anesthesia can result in overdistension. An indwelling catheter, to allow the bladder to regain its tone, usually corrects this problem. Sometimes prolonged use of the catheter is needed, and the patient should be given a prophylactic antibiotic, such as nitrofurantoin.

The subarachnoid space can be infected, and infection is usually blood-borne rather than from direct contamination. The infection may take the form of meningitis or abscess. Lumbar puncture is indicated, and broad-spectrum antibiotics should be started. If an abscess is suspected, a computed tomographic scan should be performed. An epidural abscess can cause paralysis and may require decompression.

Respiratory

Respiratory complications are common after abdominal procedures, especially if general anesthesia was used. Postoperative pain results in shallow breathing and produces a decrease in functional volume.[8, 9] Because of this, the initial effect tends to be atelectasis. Lower abdominal incisions and transverse incisions appear to be less of a problem because deeper respirations can usually be taken by the patient. It is important to use some type of apparatus, such as blow bottles, to aid in normal lung expansion and expiration.

Atelectasis tends to occur early but improves rapidly with good lung expansion. If it does not resolve, pneumonia follows, usually 4 to 10 days after surgery. This needs to be treated aggressively with antibiotics. In addition, incentive spirometry, intermittent positive-pressure breathing, and continuous positive airway pressure may be needed. Patients rarely need intubation or positive end-expiratory pressure ventilation unless some type of chronic or other restrictive respiratory lung disease is present.

Adult respiratory distress syndrome may result if shock, sepsis, or trauma occurs. These problems are usually secondary to marked hypovolemia and infection in obstetric patients.[7] Symptoms are severe and consist of tachypnea, dyspnea, and bronchoconstriction. If the condition continues for more than 5 days, the usual result is tissue destruction, with pulmonary fibrosis and eventual death. It is important to monitor these patients intensively as to respiratory and cardiac status and fluid and electrolyte balance.

Bowel

Postoperative nausea is usually short-lived and depends on the type of anesthetic used.[5] Once flatus has been passed and a bowel movement has occurred, normal function has returned. There is debate as to whether clear oral liquids should be withheld until bowel sounds are present; however, most patients can easily tolerate fluids after nausea has subsided. Once a patient claims to be hungry, bowel problems rarely are noted. The diet can usually be advanced within 24 hours in most cases. If bowel surgery or upper organ surgery was performed, a nasogastric tube should be inserted, and a long tube if appropriate.[10]

The most common bowel postoperative problem is adynamic ileus. This complication is related to peritoneal irritation, bowel manipulation, intra-abdominal sepsis, bleeding into the lumen or wall of the intestinal tract, or metabolic derangements, such as ketoacidosis and electrolyte imbalance. When additional surgery, such as bowel resection, liver repair, or spleen removal, was encountered at the original operation, ileus is very common. Some pain medications, such as codeine, can also contribute to a sluggish bowel. The small bowel usually returns to normal function within 12 hours, whereas the stomach and sigmoid colon are last to resume peristalsis, at times taking up to 3 to 5 days.

Post-cesarean ileus can cause nausea and vomiting, abdominal pain and distension, absent or minimal bowel sounds, and absence of passage of flatus. These signs, together with distended loops of bowel on abdominal radiograph, make the diagnosis. Ileus may require nasogastric suction and delay of oral food intake but tends to resolve in 24 to 48 hours with conservative treatment.

The usual cause of initial abdominal distension is probably swallowed gas. The high nitrogen content found in the bowel gas supports this contention.

By decreasing bowel manipulation, by minimal use of packing, and by early resumption of a general diet, adynamic ileus can be sharply reduced. In addition, good surgical technique and avoidance of peritoneal contamination result in a low incidence of ileus.

Potassium deficiency is a major cause of adynamic ileus and is usually accompanied by hypochloremic alkalosis. This problem is seen 3 to 6 days after surgery and results from excessive electrolyte loss from vomiting, gastric suction, or urine. An electrocardiogram confirms hypokalemia in most cases. The situation is corrected by appropriate potassium chloride replacement. The addition of 40 mEq of potassium chloride to each 1000 ml of solution is needed and should be given over a 6-hour time period.

Continued nausea, vomiting, and distension are usually related to a decrease in bowel activity. Withholding oral intake usually corrects the problem; if not, a Levin nasogastric and occasionally a Cantor or Miller-Abbott long tube may be needed for decompression.[10] Suction should be continuous. Balanced intravenous fluids, in volume of 2500 ml per 24 hours, are needed for baseline replacement. Gastric suction should be replaced on a volume-for-volume basis.

Progressive distension and lack of bowel sounds indicate obstruction and may necessitate abdominal exploration. Radiologic examination and aggressive fluid and electrolyte replacement are mandatory. Mechanical bowel obstruction may be caused by adhesions, torsion, vascular accidents, and inclusion of the bowel during closure of the abdominal incision. In these situations, surgical correction is needed. Presurgical decompression may be needed, depending on the site of obstruction. A long tube, such as a Cantor tube, can relieve the obstruction. Surgical decompression may necessitate lysis of adhesions and resection of devitalized bowel. Appropriate care after obstruction is relieved includes suction, electrolyte, and fluid replacement.

Fistulas

Vesicovaginal fistula may follow cesarean or traumatic vaginal deliveries. Injuries to the urinary tract must be recognized and repaired at the time of the procedure. If these injuries are diagnosed after surgery, intravenous pyelography, cystoscopy, or retrograde pyelography may be needed to make the diagnosis. If appropriate drainage is used, such as a bladder catheter or ureteral stent, spontaneous closure may result. Falk described delayed closure of up to 6 months to allow inflammation to subside, thereby allowing for a better repair.[18] Repair can be initiated from a week to 6 months after injury; however, early repair does appear to increase the risk of recurrence. It is important that appropriate drainage be used after repair to allow healing.

Intestinal injuries may result in a small or large bowel fistula. The injuries in obstetric procedures tend to occur while entering the abdominal cavity, during hysterectomy, or at the time of closure. Most fistulas are either enterovaginal or enterocutaneous. Initial treatment includes fluid and electrolyte balance and appropriate diagnosis. Spontaneous closure is common in the small bowel, whereas fistulas in the colon and rectum usually need surgical closure together with a colostomy. Patients are placed on a low-residue diet when spontaneous closure is expected. Prevention is the best policy; however, recognition of injury and appropriate repair at surgery decrease formation of fistulas. (Definitive repairs are described in Chapter 23.)

Postoperative Fever

Puerperal fever may on occasion occur from breast engorgement. This is usually because of blocked ducts, which result in a low-grade fever. Either manual expression or a pump can be used, with good success.

If mastitis is present, cellulitis that starts in nipple cracks and erythema are usually seen. Flu-like symptoms with chills may be present. The common bacterium recovered from the mouth and newborn pharynx is *Staphylococcus aureus.* Oral penicillinase-resistant penicillin, such as nafcillin or erythromycin, is effective in treatment. In serious and mixed-flora infections, clindamycin may be indicated. Failure to treat or respond can result in the formation of a breast abscess that may need surgical draining. Continued nursing is advised, since emptying the breast can be therapeutic and need only be stopped if drugs are used that may be harmful to the newborn.

Urinary tract infection is a cause of post-cesarean febrile morbidity, and the reported incidence is 2 to 16%.[5] This complication often coexists with endometritis. The indwelling catheter is the usual reason for urinary tract infection and should be removed as soon as possible. In most cesarean section cases, there is no need for the catheter to be present after 12 hours or once the patient is ambulating. Common bacteria are enterococci and gram-negative bacilli, which respond well to cephalosporin antibiotics. Persistent fever not related to the uterus indicates the possibility of urinary tract obstruction from trauma, ligation of the ureter, or urolithiasis. An intravenous pyelogram and ultrasound studies may be useful in determining the cause of fever.

The risk of endomyometritis is increased if a surgical procedure was necessary for the delivery or for correction of a complication. Infection is also increased in the presence of prolonged rupture of the membranes, prolonged labor, and fetal manipulation at delivery. In addition, the trauma to the vagina and vulva that usually accompanies deliveries by forceps raises the incidence of infection. The incidence of endomyometritis varies from institution to institution and has been reported to vary from 5 to 50%.[11] The highest rate is usually reported in young women of low socioeconomic status. It is, however, apparent that when these patients are treated in private institutions, the rate of infection is much lower. The use of prophy-

lactic antibiotics has sharply reduced the risk of infection.[12]

Endomyometritis can lead to bacteremia, septicemia, pelvic abscess, septic shock, and septic thrombophlebitis. The advent of appropriate antibiotics and atraumatic surgical technique has reduced serious complications to less than 5%.[11-13]

Common bacteria found in endomyometritis include aerobic *Streptococcus,* groups B and D, anaerobic gram-positive *Peptococcus,* and *Peptostreptococcus.*[13] The most predominant aerobic gram-negative organism is *Escherichia coli;* however, *Klebsiella pneumoniae* and *Proteus* species may be isolated in cultures. Gram-negative anaerobic bacteria include *Bacteroides* species and *Gardnerella vaginalis.* In addition, *Mycoplasma hominis* and *Chlamydia trachomatis* appear to be playing an increasing role in endomyometritis.[13]

Appropriate evaluation by culture of the endometrium and blood is important. Treatment should be started after cultures are taken. The most effective regimens include either clindamycin-gentamicin, extended broad-spectrum cephalosporins and penicillins, or metronidazole-penicillin-gentamicin combinations. Antibiotics can be changed as indicated by culture results or if there is no response within 36 hours.

If antibiotic treatment is not effective and an abscess develops, drainage may be required. Diagnosis of pelvic abscess or pyometra can be made by ultrasonography. Pyometra may result from premature cervical closure causing obstruction. Treatment consists of cervical dilatation and evacuation of the purulent contents. Addition of an oxytocic keeps the uterus contracted and helps in resolution of the problem. An extraperitoneal pelvic abscess can be drained through a colpotomy or abdominal incision. In either case, loculations must be broken down and appropriate continued drainage instituted. On rare occasions hysterectomy and bilateral salpingo-oophorectomy may be necessary.[12]

Wound Complications

Wound infection may be seen after a cesarean delivery, an episiotomy, or an abdominal procedure.[5, 10] The causative factors include prolonged labor and rupture of membranes, bacterial inoculum, and local wound conditions. Wound infection can be prevented by adequate nutrition, correction of anemia and hypovolemia, and the use of prophylactic antibiotics. It is very important that atraumatic surgery be performed using sterile technique with adequate hemostasis.

Wound infections usually result from contamination from the skin or uterus; therefore, it is important to use antiseptic agents to cleanse the vagina and skin. Again, the skin hair is better removed with clippers than by shaving. The latter opens skin pores and allows entry of *Staphylococcus aureus* into the exposed wound. The bacteria most often isolated from wound infections are *S. aureus, E. coli, Proteus mirabilis,* and species of *Bacteroides.*

The use of drains to prevent infection is controversial. They should be used when blood, serum, or infected fluids are not completely removed from the wound. Should a drain be necessary, it should be placed through a separate stab wound. Drains can be avoided by meticulous layer by layer closure and by avoiding dead space. In infected wounds or markedly obese patients, the fat and skin can be left open and closed secondarily once the wound is clean and granulating.

Wound infection must be recognized by the cardinal signs of inflammation, often accompanied by draining of purulent material. Once a wound infection is recognized, it must be opened, cultured, and drained. Sharp débridement of dead tissue may be needed. Cleansing with hydrogen peroxide or Dakin solution should be continued until clean granulation tissue is present. When granulation tissue forms, it should not be made to bleed or be removed, since this is needed for revascularization. Sterile packing should be used to keep the wound open during healing by secondary intention. Secondary closure is often used and, on occasion, skin grafts may be needed. Systemic antibiotics are rarely needed in wound infection, since drainage suffices.

Perhaps the most serious wound complication is necrotizing fasciitis. It takes the form of muscle necrosis as a result of clostridia or more generalized necrosis from synergistic infection of multiple organisms. Extensive débridement of all damaged tissue is needed in conjunction with high doses of penicillin, an aminoglycoside, and either clindamycin or metronidazole (Flagyl). In addition, hyperbaric oxygen may be needed.

Wound dehiscence can be superficial and is usually secondary to infection or seroma formation. Drainage and cleaning result in good healing, and secondary closure can be anticipated. The drainage of a serosanguineous material from the wound usually heralds a fascial dehiscence and necessitates inspection in the operating room. Early recognition is important to prevent evisceration, which carries with it mortality rates in excess of 19%.[18] When wound disruption is recognized, fluid and electrolytes should be replaced and the bowel contents protected with moist lap pads.

At surgery, the bowel must be carefully replaced and trauma avoided. The wound edges should be cleaned and débrided. Closure can be effected with through and through permanent sutures or by the Smead-Jones technique. The latter is favored by most surgeons and has proved superior to other closures. Postoperative gastrointestinal suction and adequate balanced fluid replacement are needed. Broad-spectrum antibiotics should be continued until secondary healing is complete. Blood transfusion may aid in the patient's recovery. A high calorie, protein, and vitamin diet should be started when bowel sounds have returned.

Thromboembolism

Thromboembolic problems in pregnancy are uncommon. Pregnancy, however, is a hypercoagulable state, and risk of thrombosis is increased because of increased levels of coagulation factors accompanied by a decrease in fibrinolysis. The incidence of lower extremity deep vein thrombosis is reported in 0.24% of all vaginal deliveries.[4] The risk after a cesarean delivery or other surgical procedure is three to five times greater. Fifteen to twenty-four percent of untreated deep vein thromboses develop a pulmonary embolus, and 12 to 15% of patients have a fatal complication.[15] The risk for pulmonary embolus and death is decreased to 4.5% and 0.7%, respectively, if the patient has appropriate treatment.[15]

The diagnosis of postpartum thrombophlebitis is often difficult. The clinical signs are pain, edema, color change, and, if advanced, a palpable umbilical cord. The clinical test used is the Homans sign (calf pain on dorsiflexion of the foot) and the Löwenberg test (pain distal to a blood pressure cuff inflated to 180 mm Hg). Symptoms and signs may be deceiving. Only one half of clinically diagnosed patients eventually have proven thrombosis.

Iliofemoral vein obstruction may result in swelling and cyanosis of the involved leg. The arterial blood flow can be compromised, resulting in decreased pulses and a cold extremity.

Pulmonary embolism may be the first sign of deep vein thrombosis. Symptoms of embolism include dyspnea, pleuritic chest pain, and cough. Tachypnea, however, is the most consistent sign. Physical examination may elicit tachycardia, chest rales, fever, diaphoresis, pleural friction rub, cyanosis, hemoptysis, and accentuated second heart sound. If immediate therapy is not started, cardiac arrest may result, usually within 2 to 3 hours.

The diagnosis of deep vein thrombosis includes the use of Doppler ultrasonography, impedance plethysmography, venography, ^{125}I-labeled fibrinogen scanning, and radionucleotide scanning using ^{99m}Tc.[10]

Doppler studies relate to blood flow and show either a decrease or a total absence of flow. This technique misses 50% of thromboses in the calf. It is most effective in the iliofemoral area.[16] Plethysmography depends on blood flow after sudden deflation of a thigh cuff. Impaired outflow is indicated by flow impedance or an increase in electrical resistance.

The most accurate test for phlebothrombosis is ascending venography. Complications from the procedure include pain, tenderness, and thrombosis. Iodine 125–labeled fibrinogen is also very accurate; however, it should not be used in breast-feeding patients, since iodine may affect the fetal thyroid. The ^{99m}Tc scan necessitates a gamma counter and is therefore seldom used.[10] In my opinion, ultrasonography, together with color flow Doppler mapping, is the most accurate noninvasive test.

The diagnosis of postsurgical pulmonary embolus is made by signs and symptoms, lung scan, or pulmonary angiography. Baseline laboratory studies should include arterial blood gases, chest radiograph, electrocardiogram, and clotting profile. An arterial blood partial pressure of oxygen of less than 85 mm hg on room air in most cases suggests pulmonary embolism. A ventilation lung scan is performed by intravenous injection of ^{99m}Tc-labeled albumin particles, which are trapped in the precapillary arteriolar bed.[16] This is performed in conjunction with ^{133}Xe perfusion scan. This results in a typical ventilation-perfusion scan, which is examined for segmental defects. The results are reported as low, intermediate, or high probability of pulmonary embolus. A normal scan essentially excludes the possibility of a pulmonary embolus.[15, 16]

Should the lung scan and clinical findings differ, a pulmonary arteriogram should be performed. This procedure may be necessary to avoid unnecessary anticoagulation. Best results are obtained in the first 12 hours of the diagnosis; however, specificity remains high as long as a segmental ventilation-perfusion defect is present.

Treatment with heparin is required in both deep vein thrombosis and pulmonary embolism. Heparin works by increasing the anticoagulation effect of antithrombin III.[16] The half-life of heparin is about 2 hours, and the higher the dose, the higher the peak effect and the longer the half-life. Heparin can be used by either the intravenous or the subcutaneous route. Baseline activated prothrombin time and clotting time should be obtained. Complications of heparin are bleeding, thrombocytopenia, hypersensitivity, and osteoporosis. Osteoporosis is most common when therapy is used for more than 6 months during pregnancy.

Heparin therapy begins with an initial intravenous bolus of 70 to 100 units/kg followed by 15 to 20 units/kg/hr. A therapeutic range is reached when the partial thromboplastin time is 1.5 to 2.5 times controls. Once stabilization has taken place, daily testing of partial thromboplastin time is sufficient. Intravenous therapy should be used from 2 to 10 days, followed by subcutaneous injection at intervals of 8 to 10 hours. Effectiveness is followed by partial thromboplastin time (1.5–2 × controls) or heparin levels. Six hours after injection, levels should be 0.2 to 0.3 units/mL. Therapy should be continued for 6 weeks, using either heparin or oral warfarin. Breast-feeding can be continued using either drug.

If septic thrombophlebitis is encountered, antibiotics should be added. It is important to treat early if ovarian vein thrombosis is present, since extension into the vena cava may cause left renal vein thrombosis or bilateral renal flow compromise. Surgical intervention may be necessary by vena cava ligation, Teflon clips, umbrella filter, or Greenfield filters.

Prevention of thromboembolic disease can reduce the incidence of postoperative thromboembolism. The use of support hose during pregnancy in patients who have varicosities can be of help. In addition, use of elastic stockings prior to and during surgery in patients at risk for thrombosis is of value. Good anesthesia, minimization of lower extremity trauma, prevention of circulatory retardation during the procedure, and early ambulation can also decrease the incidence of thrombosis.

The use of prophylactic anticoagulants is controversial. For patients at risk, or for those who will need to be confined to bed for a prolonged period of time, use of an anticoagulant is preferred. The use of 5000 to 10,000 units of heparin subcutaneously twice daily can be helpful in decreasing lower extremity thrombosis.

Hematomas

Vulvar hematomas can occur spontaneously after traumatic vaginal deliveries or hurried episiotomy repairs. They are caused by rupture of blood vessels, and because they are superficial to the pelvic diaphragm, they are usually self-limited. Small hematomas can be controlled by pressure and cold packs, whereas large hematomas need evacuation, suturing, and primary closure or packing.

Paravaginal and pararectal hematomas are usually discovered late during the postpartum course.[17] Some need incisional evacuation, suturing, and drains. Care must be taken not to injure the adjacent ureters or bowel.[18] Broad ligament hematomas may present in severe shock, and crystalloid solution and blood are often needed.[18, 19] If stable, they are best left alone, although infection may complicate the problem. Evacuation and vessel ligation may be attempted, but often hysterectomy may have to be performed to save the patient's life. Broad ligament hematoma is usually a complication of forceps rotation or cesarean section, and it may become an increased complication as vaginal birth after cesarean birth becomes more popular (see complete discussion in Chapter 23).

Uterine Rupture

Uterine rupture can be spontaneous after a previous cesarean delivery, traumatic delivery by forceps, or version and extraction. Treatment is to avoid shock, with adequate fluid and blood replacement and definitive repair (see Chapter 13).

Acute Renal Failure

Acute renal failure is a syndrome of rapidly developing impairment of kidney excretion that results from a compromise in renal vascular circulation with development of glomerular or tubular degeneration, or both.[20] Shock secondary to hemorrhage often accompanies this syndrome, and rapid azotemia may develop.[20] Tubular necrosis, renal cortical necrosis, or renal vessel infarction is the usual result. Almost all obstetric cases of acute renal failure result from reversible acute tubular necrosis. Diagnosis can be made by serum and urine studies. On occasion, intravenous pyelography may be needed to rule out obstruction.

Usually oliguria (less than 400 ml of urine output per day) is followed by anuria (less than 100 ml of urine output per day). The oliguria phase of acute renal failure lasts 6 to 12 days, during which time congestive heart failure and pulmonary edema are common. Laboratory tests reveal decreased serum sodium, chloride, and bicarbonate levels and elevated osmolarity. Hyperkalemia is of great concern because the myocardium can be affected. The oliguric phase is followed by a diuretic stage with low urine osmolality. General management includes restriction of fluids to avoid overhydration, balancing of electrolytes, and administration of glucose. The last is used for protein-sparing effect. Cation exchange resins can lower potassium levels, but they tend to produce acidosis and edema.

Dialysis by either the peritoneal or the extracorporeal route allows the kidney to heal, and a good outcome can be expected in a high percentage of cases.[20]

Prevention of hypovolemic shock by aggressive blood and fluid replacement is the key. The prognosis depends on the severity of the insult to the kidney, and physiologic management usually results in a good outcome.

SUMMARY

Postsurgical complications in pregnancy are not rare. They need immediate diagnosis with aggressive management. Shock and infection are the most common problems and need quick, appropriate management with fluid, blood, and antibiotics. This makes other definitive procedures easier to complete with a better prognosis. In all cases of complication, prevention is the key.

References

1. Rebulla P, Giovanetti AM, Petrini G, et al.: Autologous blood predeposit for elective surgery: A program for better use and conservation of blood. Surgery 97:463, 1985.
2. Sandler SG, Beyth L, Laufer N, et al.: Autologous blood transfusions and pregnancy. Obstet Gynecol 53:625, 1979.
3. Martin C: Physiologic changes during pregnancy: The mother. In Quilligan EJ, Kretchmer N (eds.): Fetal and Maternal Medicine. New York: John Wiley & Sons, Inc, 1980, pp. 140–180.
4. Wilcox CF, Hunt AB, Owen CA: The measurement of blood loss during cesarean section. Am J Obstet Gynecol 77:772, 1959.
5. Farrell SJ, Anderson HF, Work BA Jr: Cesarean section: Indication and post operative morbidity. Obstet Gynecol 56:696, 1980.
6. Clark SL, Horenstein JM, Phelan JP, et al.: Experience with pulmonary artery catheter in obstetrics and gynecology. Am J Obstet Gynecol 152:374, 1985.
7. Rosen MA, Hughes SC, Shnider SM: Epidural morphine for relief of postoperative pain after cesarean delivery. Anesth Analg 62:166, 1983.
8. Bartlett RH, Brennan ML, Gazzonigia AB, et al.: Studies on the pathogenesis and prevention of postoperative pulmonary complications. Surg Gynecol Obstet 137:925, 1973.
9. Cohen SE: The aspiration syndrome. Clin Obstet Gynecol 9:235, 1982.
10. Phelan JP, Clark SL (eds.): Cesarean Delivery. New York: Elsevier Science Publishing Co., 1988, pp. 299–459.
11. Duff P: Pathophysiology and management of post cesarean endomyometritis. Obstet Gynecol 67:269, 1986.
12. Cartwright PS, Pittaway DE, Jones HW, et al.: The use of prophylactic anti-biotics in obstetrics and gynecology: A review. Obstet Gynecol 39:357, 1984.
13. Hoyme UB, Kiviat N, Eschenbach DA: Microbiology and treatment of late postpartum endomyometritis. Obstet Gynecol 68:226, 1986.
14. Villasanta U: Thromboembolic disease in pregnancy. Am J Obstet Gynecol 93:142, 1965.
15. Stead RB: Regulation of hemostasis. In Goldhaber SZ (ed.): Pulmonary Embolism and Deep Venous Thrombosis. Philadelphia: W.B. Saunders Co., 1985, pp. 27–40.
16. Kipper MS, Moser KM, Kortman KE, et al.: Long term follow up of patients with suspected pulmonary embolism and normal lung scan. Perfusion scans in embolic subjects. Chest 82:411, 1982.
17. Hamilton HG: Post partum labial or paravaginal hematomas. Am J Obstet Gynecol 39:642, 1940.
18. Douglas RG, Stromme WI: Postoperative complications. In Quilligan EJ, Zuspan FP (eds.): Douglas-Stromme Operative Obstetrics, 4th Edition. New York: Appleton-Century-Crofts, 1982, pp. 843–890.
19. Fliegner JRH: Post partum broad ligament hematomas. J Obstet Gynaecol Br Common 78:184, 1971.
20. Merril JP: Acute renal failure. In Straus MB, Welt LG (eds.): Disease of the Kidney. Boston: Little, Brown & Co., Inc., 1971, Chapter 7.

5

Anesthesia for Obstetrics

Fred J. Spielman
Robert C. Cefalo

Well-administered obstetric anesthesia is not simply the performance of epidural and spinal blocks for cesarean delivery, nor is it merely precisely extubating the patient at the end of the operation and quickly transporting her to the recovery room. Well-conducted obstetric anesthesia is safe anesthesia in which the best technique is employed after careful consideration of the patient's and the obstetrician's needs, as well as the concerns of the anesthesiologist. The practice of obstetric anes-

thesia necessitates knowledge of the clinical implications of the physiologic changes induced by pregnancy and an understanding of the side effects and possible complications from administering obstetric medications and anesthetic agents at the same time. Care of the critically ill parturient demands a thorough mastery of drugs employed for heart failure as well as those used to significantly raise or lower blood pressure. Seriously ill women often require invasive monitoring; the indications, advantages, and disadvantages of these monitoring techniques are therefore essential. Information about massive blood loss and the best methods to treat hemorrhage is mandatory. Finally, knowledge of obstetric anesthesia should include the etiology of and ways to reduce maternal mortality. This chapter addresses these important topics. The obstetrician who is knowledgeable in these areas is more able to work with the obstetric anesthesiologist as a team member and deliver the best possible care to his or her patient.

PHYSIOLOGIC CHANGES OF PREGNANCY

Successful management of the high-risk parturient necessitates a thorough understanding of the major physiologic changes, particularly those related to the cardiovascular and pulmonary systems, that accompany pregnancy, labor, and delivery. These changes can represent a major challenge to the parturient patient if they are superimposed on other systemic disease states.

Capillary engorgement of the mucosa throughout the respiratory tract causes swelling of the nasal and oral pharynx, larynx, and trachea. As a result, the parturient patient frequently appears to have the symptoms of an upper respiratory tract infection. These changes may be markedly exacerbated by a respiratory infection or a fluid overload, which may lead to airway obstruction.[1]

Starting at about 12 weeks' gestation, minute ventilation increases so that by term it is about 50% above prepregnancy levels, primarily because of an increased tidal volume (40%) with little change in respiratory rate (10%).[2] Hormonal changes, specifically progesterone levels, are the stimuli for the respiratory alterations. As a result of the increased alveolar ventilation, maternal arterial carbon dioxide pressure is decreased to about 30 to 34 mm Hg, but there is little change in pH because of a compensatory decrease in serum bicarbonate (Table 5–1). In labor, without adequate analgesia, however, maternal minute ven-

Table 5–1. CHANGES IN THE RESPIRATORY SYSTEM AT TERM

Measurement	Change	Percent Average Change
Minute ventilation	Increased	50
Tidal volume	Increased	40
Respiratory rate	Increased	10
Arterial pH	No change	
Arterial P_{CO_2}	Decreased	20
Serum bicarbonate	Decreased	20
Functional residual capacity	Decreased	20
Expiratory reserve volume	Decreased	20
Oxygen consumption	Decreased	20

Table 5–2. CHANGES IN CARDIOVASCULAR SYSTEM AT TERM

Measurement	Change	Percent Average Change
Blood volume	Increased	50
Plasma volume	Increased	45
Red blood cell volume	Increased	20
Cardiac output	Increased	40
Stroke volume	Increased	30
Heart rate	Increased	15
Total peripheral resistance	Decreased	15
Systolic blood pressure	Decreased	0–15 mm Hg
Diastolic blood pressure	Decreased	10–20 mm Hg

tilation may increase by as much as 300%, producing significant maternal hypocarbia and alkalemia. This marked respiratory alkalosis may cause hypoventilation between contractions, resulting in maternal and fetal hypoxemia. Effective epidural analgesia can significantly reduce hyperventilation.[3] The tidal volume and the respiratory rate return to normal 1 to 3 weeks after delivery.

Starting after the fifth month of gestation, there is a reduction in functional residual capacity (20%) and expiratory reserve volume (20%). For many women, as the pregnancy progresses, abdominal breathing diminishes and the supine position impairs respiratory function. Up to one half of pregnant women in the supine position develop airway closure during normal ventilation, making the parturient patient more susceptible to hypoxemia.[4]

Oxygen consumption during pregnancy is markedly increased both at rest and during exercise, as compared with that which occurs during the nonpregnant state. This change is a result of both increases in metabolism and increased work of breathing. With painful contractions, oxygen consumption is increased an additional 60 per cent. Regional analgesia, however, eliminates this additional increase in oxygen consumption.[5]

At as early as 6 to 8 weeks of pregnancy, blood volume begins to increase, reaching a maximal value at 28 to 32 weeks, when it is 50% higher than that of the nonpregnant woman.[6] (Table 5–2). The increase in plasma volume (45%) is greater than the increase in red blood cell mass (20%), which leads to reduced hemoglobin concentration. The mechanism responsible for the hypervolemia of pregnancy is complex, but appears to be related primarily to the increased production of aldosterone under the influence of estrogen. Cardiac output begins a progressive rise in the first trimester and peaks by 20 to 24 weeks of gestation, when it is 40 to 50% higher than that of the nonpregnant woman.[7] Increases in stroke volume (30%) and heart rate (15%) are responsible for these changes in cardiac output. Because of a fall in systemic vascular resistance, systolic and diastolic blood pressures fall slightly and a widening of pulse pressure occurs. These changes are mediated in part by prostacyclin, aldosterone, and the decrease in the vascular resistance of the uteroplacental and pulmonary circulation. No change in central venous pressure occurs.

Up to 15% of pregnant patients in the latter part of gestation develop hypotension, nausea, vomiting, and diminished cerebral functioning when they assume the supine position.[8] These symptoms are produced by vena caval and aortic compression by the gravid uterus. This uterine compression begins to develop during the second trimester and is greatest at 36 to 38 weeks. With the descent of the fetal head into the pelvis, the effects become somewhat attenuated. Women who have large uteri (multiple gestations, hydramnios), who are obese, who are hypovolemic, or who have been given narcotics or either general or regional anesthesia are particularly susceptible to supine hypotension syndrome.

In addition to the cardiovascular stress imposed by pregnancy, additional demands are made during labor and delivery, particularly in the parturient who is anxious and who is experiencing discomfort. Catecholamine release accompanies painful labor. These hormones produce tachycardia and an increase in the contractile state of the heart. With the onset of each contraction, there is an addition of 300 to 500 ml of venous blood returning to the heart. The above factors produce a significant elevation in cardiac output, stroke volume, left ventricular workload, and myocardial oxygen demand above prelabor values. The normal heart tolerates these alterations without problems. Cardiac patients, however, may decompensate during labor unless the stress is reduced. Regional anesthesia prevents the marked increase in cardiac output during the late stages of labor and delivery.[9] The hemodynamic aberrations seen during labor continue into the postpartum period. Often the most striking changes occur soon after delivery, when cardiac output may increase by 60 to 80%.[10] This is because of the autotransfusion of blood from the contracted uterus into the central circulation and of a decrease in aortocaval compression, allowing an increase in venous return to the heart. The increase in cardiac output seen in pregnancy remains for up to several weeks post partum.

The cardiorespiratory alterations during pregnancy often make it difficult to correctly diagnose lung disease and heart disease. Certain complaints and physical findings associated with cardiac and pulmonary disease in the nonpregnant patient are often present in the healthy parturient patient. Dyspnea, orthopnea, dizzy spells, and syncope are common in pregnancy. Chest radiographs taken during normal pregnancy often show increased lung markings that may stimulate mild congestive heart failure. Physical examination may reveal peripheral edema, distended neck veins, and systolic murmurs.[11] A mild amount of pulmonary atelectasis from the enlarging uterus adjacent to the diaphragm occasionally leads to the presence of basilar rales. Some heart lesions, which were not evident on physical examination before pregnancy, become detectable, whereas others are less impressive. The heart sounds louder, with accentuated first apical and second pulmonic heart sounds. Sinus tachycardia, premature contractions, and atrial tachycardia are common in parturient patients. The presence, however, of any one of the following criteria confirms the diagnosis of heart disease in pregnancy:[12] (1) diastolic, presystolic, or continuous murmur; (2) unequivocal cardiac enlargement; (3) a loud, harsh, systolic murmur, especially a thrill; or (4) severe arrhythmia. In addition, attention should be paid to the occurrence of hemoptysis, angina, cyanosis, and clubbing.

ANESTHESIA FOR CESAREAN SECTION

The question of which anesthetic technique is best for cesarean section has provided more continuous controversy than for almost any other operative procedure. The anesthetic technique must ensure sufficient placental transport of oxygen and carbon dioxide, and central nervous system and cardiovascular depression resulting from placental drug transfer and impaired placental perfusion must be avoided. The anesthetic technique should provide optimal operating conditions for the obstetrician.

Successful anesthesia for cesarean section can be accomplished in a number of ways; no one ideal method exists. The choice depends on the indications for and the degree of urgency of the cesarean section, maternal preference, and the experience and skills of the anesthesiologist.[13]

General anesthesia is the method of choice for emergency situations in which there is fetal distress or maternal bleeding because the anesthesia can be induced quickly and support of the maternal cardiovascular system can be accomplished.[14] The choice is less obvious when the patient is to undergo cesarean section for more common and less urgent indications, such as dystocia, repeat cesarean section, and breech presentation.

At the present time, regional anesthesia for elective cesarean section is the most common technique (Table 5–3). However, this has not always been the case. In an analysis of cesarean sections in Seattle from 1950 to 1959, Lamkee and colleagues[15] found that 93.9% were performed with general anesthesia. Increased interest in regional anesthesia by obstetricians, anesthesiologists, and patients and increased knowledge of the physiology of spinal and epidural anesthesia in the parturient have led to an increased use of regional

Table 5–3. ANESTHETIC TECHNIQUES FOR CESAREAN SECTION

Percent	Private 1950–1956	Private and Teaching 1971	Teaching 1976	Private and Teaching 1979
Local infiltration	0.1	1.0	1.0	0
Spinal anesthesia	3.8	53.0	24.0	36.0
Epidural anesthesia	0	3.0	32.0	26.0
General anesthesia	96.3	32.0	43.0	38.0
Combination	0.8	10.0	0	0

From Spielman FJ, Corke BC: Advantages and disadvantages of regional anesthesia for cesarean section. A review. J Reprod Med 30:832, 1985.

anesthesia. The popularity of regional anesthesia in the United States is paralleled by similar changes in Europe.[16]

Regional anesthesia for cesarean section can be accomplished by local infiltration or by spinal or epidural anesthesia. Local infiltration has never been a popular technique because of the difficulty in providing adequate analgesia and the possibility of a toxic reaction from the large amounts of local anesthetic required.[17] The relative merits of spinal and epidural anesthesia for cesarean section are summarized in Table 5–4. The advantage of spinal anesthesia is that the procedure is simple, quick, and reliable, with minimal exposure of the fetus to the drug. When compared with epidural anesthesia, spinal anesthesia is associated with a higher incidence of hypotension, nausea, vomiting, and lumbar puncture headache. Epidural anesthesia can be used for prolonged postoperative analgesia, is associated with less maternal hypotension, and lessens the chance of lumbar puncture headache unless a dural tap is performed accidentally. However, when compared with a spinal procedure, the epidural procedure entails such disadvantages as increased complexity of technique, a greater chance of inadequate block, and measurable maternal and neonatal blood levels of local anesthetics.[17]

General and regional anesthesia for cesarean section have been compared thoroughly. In some areas, particularly that of maternal mortality, the results appear clear and undeniable. In other areas, such as the effects of anesthesia on the neonate, the data are conflicting and often confusing. The disparate results are mostly because of

Table 5–4. COMPARISON BETWEEN EPIDURAL AND SPINAL ANESTHESIA FOR CESAREAN SECTION

Epidural	Spinal
Advantages	
Avoids dural puncture	Simplicity, speed
Lowers incidence of hypotension	Reliability
Relieves postoperative pain	Minimal drug exposure
Disadvantages	
Complexity of technique	Hypotension
Longer onset time	Headache
High doses of local anesthetic required	Limited duration of action

From Spielman FJ, Corke BC: Advantages and disadvantages of regional anesthesia for cesarean section. A review. J Reprod Med 30:832, 1985.

investigators' use of experimental designs, anesthetic techniques, and tools of measurement that are not comparable. Table 5–5 shows the proposed advantages and disadvantages of regional anesthesia, which is discussed in detail here.

The effects of anesthesia on the fetus during cesarean section have been evaluated with the Apgar score, acid-base status, time to sustained respiration, and neurobehavioral examinations. Neonatal depression may occur secondary to the placental passage of drugs or indirectly from maternal hypotension, which decreases blood flow, causing fetal and neonatal hypoxia and acidosis.

Studies in the 1960s and early 1970s suggested that 1-minute Apgar scores were higher for regional anesthesia than for general anesthesia.[18] Shnider and Levinson[13] believe that the poor Apgar scores at 1 minute resulted from transient sedation from nitrous oxide rather than asphyxia. Nitrous oxide rapidly crosses the placenta. After 3 minutes, the fetal to maternal concentration ratio is 0 to 8; after 15 minutes, the umbilical artery to vein concentration ratio is almost 0 to 0.9.[19] Therefore, as the induction-to-delivery interval increases, the fetus is exposed to significant amounts of nitrous oxide and therefore is delivered "anesthetized," with poor 1-minute Apgar scores.[13] Assisted ventilation and stimulation of the newborn provide excellent 5-minute Apgar scores in infants, depressed respiration at 1 minute. An advantage of regional anesthesia is that neonatal respiration is not depressed after a long induction-to-delivery time. Therefore, if general anesthesia is chosen, the delivery needs to be expeditious, and if a prolonged delivery is anticipated, regional anesthesia should be administered.

Joyce[18] reviewed five studies that compared general anesthesia with epidural anesthesia and noted that the acid-base status of the neonates was essentially the same. However, for both regional and general anesthesia, a prolonged uterine incision to delivery interval is a factor contributing to fetal hypoxia and acidosis. Datta and colleagues[20] and Crawford and colleagues[21] studied patients receiving general and regional anesthesia for cesarean section. They found that in both groups a long uterine incision to delivery interval correlated with low Apgar scores and a poor acid-base balance. Prolonged and vigorous uterine manipula-

Table 5–5. PROPOSED ADVANTAGES AND
DISADVANTAGES OF REGIONAL ANESTHESIA

Advantages

Decreased incidence of maternal morbidity
Decreased maternal requirement for drugs
Decreased incidence of neonatal respiratory depression
Maternal- and paternal-neonatal bonding
Ability to administer 100% oxygen
Decreased maternal blood loss
Reduced incidence of deep venous thrombosis and embolism
Postoperative pain control
Quicker return of gastrointestinal function
Less maternal stress
Avoiding possibility of awareness of operation with general
    anesthesia
Fewer postoperative infections

Disadvantages

Maternal hypotension
Nausea and vomiting
Pain during cesarean section
Lumbar puncture headache
Backache
Neurologic complications
Cardiotoxicity of local anesthetics

tion may decrease the placental and uterine blood flow and also cause aortic and inferior vena caval compression. The longer period needed for extraction of the fetus perhaps causes an increased amount of amniotic fluid to be inhaled.[20]

Examining respiratory function in the fetus is another method of comparing fetal outcome after use of different anesthetic techniques. The time to sustained respiration after delivery is thought to be normal if it is less than 60 seconds.[18] Early studies showed that time to sustained respiration was quicker after regional anesthesia than after general anesthesia[22]; however, in these investigations, the duration of fetal exposure to anesthesia was often prolonged (mean induction-to-delivery time, 20.9 minutes), and, therefore, the fetal respiratory center was depressed as a result of high levels of nitrous oxide. Recognizing that anesthetic agents alter breathing parameters, Fisher and colleagues[23] investigated 19 infants delivered under epidural anesthesia and 9 delivered under general anesthesia; measurements were made of the newborn's pattern of breathing, including tidal volume, total breath duration, minute ventilation, inspiratory and expiratory times, and mouth occlusion pressure. The results were similar in both groups, and the author concluded that both epidural and general anesthesia were suitable for cesarean section.

Apgar scores, acid-base balance, and time to sustained respiration can measure only significant depression of the respiratory center of the newborn. These tests are not sensitive to the subtle or delayed effects of obstetric medication.[24] Used in the first 48 hours after delivery, the neurobehavioral examination is an index of neonatal depression. The most popular neurobehavioral scale is the early neonatal neurobehavioral score (ENNS),

which was adapted by Scanlon and colleagues[25] from earlier work done by Brazleton.[26] It consists of observations of primary reflexes, muscle tone, decrement response to stimulation, and state of consciousness. In the neurobehavioral examination, the individual drugs and amounts employed appear to be more important than the anesthetic technique. For epidural anesthesia, bupivacaine, etidocaine, lidocaine, and 2-chloroprocaine do not produce adverse changes in the ENNS.[27] The effects of mepivacaine are less favorable; however, its effects on neurobehavior are minimal and transient.[24] Holleman and co-workers[28] compared the neurobehavioral effects of epidural and general anesthesia and noted no significant difference between the two groups. Warren and co-workers[29] and Abboud and co-workers[30] found that when used for general anesthesia, halothane, enflurane, and isoflurane did not affect ENNS scores. When both general and regional anesthesia are administered optimally, there is little difference in the infant's neurobehavioral score.[31] Regardless of the way in which the anesthetic drugs are administered, appropriate doses and concentrations should be employed, and the causes of neonatal depression must be avoided.

Moir[32] has shown that decreased blood loss occurs when using epidural anesthesia instead of general anesthesia at cesarean section. He compared epidural anesthesia with three general anesthesia techniques. The mean blood loss associated with regional anesthesia (378 ± 146 ml) was about one half that associated with general anesthesia. In addition, no patient receiving an epidural blockade lost more than 1 L. The sympathectomy that accompanies epidural anesthesia results in lower mean arterial and venous pressure, producing less arterial and venous bleeding.[17]

The immediate postpartum period is associated with an increased risk of deep venous thrombosis, especially after cesarean section. The traditional attempt to prevent deep venous thrombosis includes early ambulation and use of compression stockings. An epidural block continued into the postoperative period may reduce the incidence of deep venous thrombosis and pulmonary embolism.[33–35] A comparison of epidural anesthesia and general anesthesia for patients undergoing total hip replacement showed that the use of epidural anesthesia in the postoperative period was associated with a lower incidence of deep venous thrombosis and pulmonary embolism. The reasons for reduced thrombosis with regional anesthesia as compared with general anesthesia are many. As measured by venous occlusion plethysmography, epidural anesthesia produces better arterial inflow and venous emptying and increased venous capacity than does general anesthesia.[33] An analysis of fibrinolysis inhibition and plasminogen activity in the immediate postoperative period proved that there is significantly better fibrinolytic function in patients receiving epidural anesthesia than in those who have received general anesthesia.[32] The improved fibrinolysis and lower tendency toward clotting associated with regional anesthesia should offer an advantage for patients at risk of thromboembolic disease who are undergoing cesarean section.

Epidural anesthesia continued into the postoperative period has been shown to be beneficial in restoring gastrointestinal function. Narcotics given to relieve pain are responsible for delayed gastric emptying, nausea, and vomiting. Using acetaminophen absorption as an indirect index of the rate of gastric emptying, Nimmo[36] studied patients after abdominal hysterectomy. There was only a moderate delay in gastric emptying in patients who had received local anesthesia and extradural analgesia, but gastric emptying was inhibited markedly in those receiving intramuscular narcotics.

The maternal stress response to cesarean section is less when regional anesthesia is used rather than general anesthesia. Namba[37] studied the effects of epidural anesthesia and general anesthesia on the adrenocortical response to elective cesarean section. Plasma cortisol concentrations were measured before surgery, at delivery, and at 30 and 60 minutes after the skin incision. The cortisol levels in patients under epidural anesthesia did not change significantly from the presurgery levels at any time; however, those under general anesthesia had significantly increased concentrations from the presurgery values at 30 and 60 minutes. Irestedt and colleagues[38] found that the plasma norepinephrine and epinephrine concentrations were lower in women undergoing elective cesarean section with epidural anesthesia than in those undergoing the procedure with general anesthesia. Abboud and colleagues[39] observed that plasma-β-endorphin increased on induction of general anesthesia, but that there was no significant change in plasma β-endorphin in those women who underwent cesarean section with spinal or epidural anesthesia. It appears that regional anesthesia plays a major role in modifying the stress response to cesarean section; however, it is unclear what the benefits of this reduction are in terms of perioperative morbidity.

Regional anesthesia is not without contraindications. Refusal of the patient, local or general sepsis, bleeding disorders, and use of anticoagulants by the patient are considered by most anesthesiologists to be absolute contraindications to regional anesthesia. The relative contraindications are less easily defined and agreed on. However, the patient who is unsophisticated, apprehensive, or poorly informed may not be able to tolerate the pulling sensations and pressure that accompany surgery with regional anesthesia. Active central nervous system diseases are considered by many anesthesiologists to be a relative contraindication to regional anesthesia, but there are no reliable data to show that regional anesthesia exacerbates pre-existing disease. In fact, Crawford[40] has provided continuous epidural analgesia without sequelae for patients with spina bifida, a history of subarachnoid hemorrhage, spastic paraplegia, myasthenia gravis, muscular dystrophy, multiple sclerosis, and many other neurologic disorders. He stated that "epidural analgesia, employed with the approved standard of care, has no deleterious effects upon the course of chronic neurologic disease." Potential technical difficulties, such as obesity and scoliosis or the patient's lack of cooperation, often make regional anesthesia more difficult to administer.

A common, potentially dangerous complication of regional anesthesia is maternal hypotension, commonly defined as a 20 to 30 mm Hg fall in systolic blood pressure or a systolic pressure of less than 100 mm Hg. The etiology of the cause of the hypotension is the blockade of sympathetic vasomotor activity, which is often aggravated by hypovolemia or aortocaval compression. Hypotension occurs more often with spinal anesthesia because the sympathectomy is rapid and there is less time for upper-body vasoconstriction or fluid administration. A fluid preload with 1500 to 2000 ml of crystalloid and lateral uterine displacement should be used to reduce the incidence or severity of hypotension. Datta and colleagues[41] have shown that intravenous ephedrine given as soon as any fall in blood pressure is detected prevents a further decline and reduces the incidence of maternal nausea and vomiting and neonatal acidosis.

Brownridge[42] stated, "Cesarean section in an awake patient is undoubtedly a major test of regional anesthesia. The operation may be lengthy, profound blockade of many nerves is required, strong visceral stimulation is present. . . . The patient herself is likely to be apprehensive, excited, and expectant." Therefore, it is no surprise to those who have witnessed many cesarean sections under regional anesthesia that it is common for some patients to experience considerable discomfort. Up to 20% of patients under epidural anesthesia experience some pain.[43] From over 1500 cesarean births, Shnider and Levinson[13] found that between 12 and 14% of patients require supplemental analgesia before the birth. Often the pain is localized to the shoulder tip or subcostal area and caused by traction on the uterus or by air or blood under the diaphragm. Inadequate concentrations or amounts of local anesthetics and poor spread of drugs in the epidural space often contribute to insufficient analgesia. Because an inadequate spinal or epidural procedure often necessitates the immediate induction of general anesthesia under circumstances that are less safe than those at the outset,[16] it is best to assess the level and quality of the regional anesthesia prior to making the skin incision.

The remaining complications of regional anesthesia fall into the category of neurologic sequelae. These complications include direct neurologic trauma from needles or catheters, subarachnoid or epidural hematoma, infection, and chemical contamination. Although these are the most feared and serious of all adverse reactions to regional anesthesia, they are extremely rare. Usubiaga[44] found an incidence of 1 in 11,000 neurologic complications in a survey of 780,000 epidural blocks. Hellman[45] observed no complications in over 20,000 epidural procedures for obstetrics, and Ostheimer[46] reported no major neurologic sequelae from over 27,000 epidural procedures for delivery. In fact, the more common nerve lesions in obstetrics are unrelated to anesthesia and include spontaneous epidural hematoma and compression of peripheral nerves as they cross the pelvic brim.[47] Neurotoxicity has occurred following the accidental injection of large doses of 2-chloroprocaine into the subarachnoid space.[48, 49] The neurologic complications include cauda equina syndrome and progressive adhesive arachnoiditis. The use of sodium bisulfate as an antioxidant in 2-chloroprocaine and the low pH of the drug may be responsible in part for the observed neural damage.

Cardiotoxicity leading to cardiac arrest and death has occurred following accidental injection of bupivacaine into an epidural vein.[50] Bupivacaine, highly protein-bound and lipid-soluble, is more cardiotoxic than local anesthetics, such as lidocaine, which are less protein-bound and lipid-soluble. With bupivacaine, the onset of cardiac depression is sudden and quite resistant to resuscitative measures.[51]

There is no doubt that both minor and serious complications can occur during and after regional anesthesia. Careful selection of patients; thorough knowledge of fetal and maternal physiology; and employment of meticulous technique, sterile equipment, and safe drug concentrations contribute greatly to the low incidence of adverse effects and complications.

It is clear that there is no ideal anesthetic method for cesarean section, but that either regional or general anesthesia, when used correctly, has very insignificant deleterious effects on the mother and fetus. Regardless of the type of anesthesia administered, the anesthesiologist must be skilled at using it and comfortable with it. A team approach must be instituted, with cooperation among the anesthesiologist, obstetrician, pediatrician, and paramedical personnel, and there must be a well-organized and well-equipped operating room.

HEMODYNAMIC MONITORING IN PREGNANCY

Cardiovascular monitoring may identify correctable physiologic alterations before they become life-threatening, as well as provide objective physiologic measurements for therapeutic decision making.

This section summarizes the usefulness, indications, advantages, and disadvantages of various monitoring modes, from routine noninvasive techniques to those that are highly invasive.

Electrocardiogram

The electrocardiogram is useful in detecting cardiac dysrhythmias, myocardial ischemia, and electrolyte abnormalities, particularly potassium abnormalities. It has become a standard monitor for all anesthetized patients; in addition, all parturient patients with cardiorespiratory disease should be monitored continuously during labor, delivery, and the postpartum period. Continuous graphic electrocardiographic display provides the earliest recognition of electrical changes associated with disorders of the cardiac muscle. Hard copy readings should be available for high-risk patients in order to better analyze the electrocardiogram.

Although any lead can be used to detect cardiac dysrhythmias, lead II is particularly useful because it makes the P wave easy to identify and can, therefore, facilitate differentiation between supraventricular and ventricular dysrhythmias. The V_5 position is employed when the goal is to monitor for myocardial ischemia, since the ST segments are more clearly identifiable. It should be remembered that the electrocardiogram reflects only the electrical activity occurring in the heart and is in no way a measure of heart function. For example, a normal electrocardiographic complex in the absence of an effective cardiac output is possible (electromechanical dissociation).[52]

Temperature

Hypothermia may occur in small numbers of patients with septic shock, reduced metabolism, and malnutrition. In addition, body temperature may decline 1 to 4° during surgery. Although this decrease in body temperature is usually not serious, postoperative shivering may increase oxygen consumption by as much as 400%.[52]

Temperature elevations are most often associated with infection, tissue necrosis, late-stage carcinomatosis, hyperthyroidism, and other hypermetabolic states. Low-grade fever is also present with hematomas, foreign bodies, and obstruction of the urinary and bronchial tracts.[53] There are several sites that can be utilized to monitor body temperature. The most accurate area is the lower one third of the esophagus; its disadvantage is obvious, except for patients undergoing general anesthesia. The rectum is a common site, but accuracy as a reflection of core temperature depends on adequate rectal blood flow. The temperature of the skin and the axilla varies with subcutaneous blood flow, sweating, radiation, and conduction of heat to and from other objects.[52] Oral temperatures may reflect the temperature of the inhaled gases; this may present a problem when the patient is breathing humidified gases.

Blood Pressure Monitoring

Blood pressure can be monitored noninvasively or by direct intra-arterial measurement. Noninvasive methods offer simplicity, reasonably reliable measurement, and freedom from complications. Automatic blood pressure machines have become increasingly popular and are capable of measuring every 15 seconds. The disadvantage of noninvasive monitoring is that auscultated readings of blood pressure often underestimate the pressure in hypovolemic patients, those in shock, or those with vasoconstriction, and they are not able to give moment-to-moment data.[54] In addition, errors in measurement may result if the size and position of the blood pressure cuff are incorrect. The width of the cuff should be greater than one third of the circumference of the limb. The bladder should cover at least one half of the circumference of the arm while positioned directly over the artery. If an aeroid manometer is employed, it should be calibrated against a mercury manometer.[52]

Continuous measurement of blood pressure, ready access to arterial blood for the purposes of blood gas determinations, hematocrit level, electrolyte balance, and accurate blood pressure measurement in critically ill patients, particularly those who are hypotensive and vasoconstricted, are the advantages provided by direct arterial catheterization. Arterial cannulation may be performed at many sites, but the radial artery is the most frequently used because it is accessible and has a generous blood supply in the event of thrombosis. Use of the femoral artery makes nursing care difficult, limits the ability of the patient to move, and increases the risk of infection. The catheters used for cannulation should be small in diameter, 20- or 22-gauge. The smaller the catheter, the less the likelihood of thrombosis and occlusion of the artery. Accidental disconnection and blood loss are among the major and most frequent complications of arterial catheters. Other complications are less frequent but may include hematoma and bleeding, embolism, arterial injury, and infection. Another consideration is the time required for placement and cost.[55]

Pulse Oximetry

The use of the pulse oximeter is now standard for all anesthetics and is highly recommended for the care of patients in the post-anesthesia recovery room. In addition, parturient patients with significant cardiac and respiratory disease should be monitored with this device. Pulse oximeters provide valuable information about blood oxygenation in a continuous manner without elaborate equipment, pain, or complications. They reduce the need for arterial blood sampling. Pulse oximetry employs spectrophotometric determination of arterial oxygenation, using a probe that can be placed on any pulsatile arterial bed (finger, toe, nose, bridge of nose). Light of a specific wavelength is directed across the pulsating artery. Changes in light transmission during each pulse are detected and analyzed and displayed on a monitor as the percent oxygen saturation.

Pulse oximeters have few disadvantages. However, they are frequently not useful for patients who are in shock states with diminished cutaneous blood flow. Because the device measures oxygen saturation and not oxygen tension, and because the oxygen-hemoglobin dissociation curve is nearly flat, considerable changes in partial pressure of oxygen greater than 70 mm Hg cause negligible changes in saturation. Intravenously administered dyes, such as methylene blue, indigo carmine, and indocyanine green, decrease the accuracy of the pulse oximeter. Abnormal hemoglobins, such as methemoglobin and carboxyhemoglobin, cause the oximeter to generate erroneous readings.

Central Venous Pressure

The central venous catheter is an important tool for estimation of central blood volume, long-term intravenous feedings, especially hyperalimentation, and safe administration of vasoactive drugs.

The four veins commonly utilized for catheterization are the brachial, subclavian, and external and internal jugular veins. The relative advantages and disadvantages of using each vessel are summarized in Table 5–6. Cannulation of the brachial vein is associated with a small complication rate, but advancement of the catheter is often unsuccessful. The subclavian vein is easily cannulated and allows the catheter to be securely fixed on the chest wall, but complications occur much more frequently than with any other route. Use of the internal jugular vein has minimal complications, but nursing management may be difficult.[52]

The central venous pressure measurement has its limitations. In addition to cardiac function and blood volume, there are many different factors that influence central venous pressure, values such as vasopressor administration, intraperitoneal and intrathoracic pressures, and intrinsic lung disease. The central venous pressure may be elevated for reasons independent of volume status and may not reflect simultaneous filling pressures on the left

Table 5–6. ADVANTAGES OF DIFFERENT APPROACHES TO CENTRAL VEIN CATHETERIZATION

	Vein			
	Brachial	*Subclavian*	*External Jugular*	*Internal Jugular*
Ease of insertion	+	+	+ +	+ +
Success rate	+	+ +	+ + +	+ +
Complications	+ + +	+	+ +	+
Ability to insert pulmonary artery catheter	−	−	+	+ +

Key: + + +, marked advantage; + +, moderate advantage; +, minimal advantage; −, no advantage.
From Stoelting RK, Miller RD: Basics of Anesthesia. New York: Churchill Livingstone, 1984, p. 213.

side of the heart. Some of these conditions may be seen in obstetric patients, for example, pulmonary embolism and amniotic fluid embolism. In other instances, the central venous pressure may not be elevated even though the left ventricular pressures are high, such as in patients with severe pre-eclampsia and mitral stenosis.[54] When there are discrepancies in the functional status of the right and left ventricles, the central venous pressure values and even trends may provide misleading information. Complications of central venous catheter placement are numerous, including venous and arterial injury, pneumothorax and hemothorax injury, thoracic duct injury, thrombosis, embolism, sepsis, and cardiac arrhythmias.

Pulmonary Artery Catheter

A flow-directed, balloon-tipped pulmonary artery catheter enables the following information to be obtained: measurement of intracardiac pressures, cardiac output, systemic and pulmonary vascular resistances, and calculation of shunt. It also enables atrial and ventricular pacing and electrocardiographic studies to be performed. A modification of the pulmonary artery catheter makes possible continuous monitoring of mixed venous oxygen saturation. Mixed venous oxygen saturation is best thought of as a measure of the balance between total body oxygen consumption and supply. Saturation may decline with hemorrhage, decreases in arterial oxygenation of cardiac output, or increases in metabolic rate. The average mixed venous oxygen saturation is 40 mm Hg; patients with a saturation of less than 25 mm Hg are most likely to be critically ill.[56] Cardiac output is determined by the thermodilution method. An exact quantity of fluid at a controlled temperature

is injected into the proximal port (right atrium). A thermistor is located in the distal port (pulmonary artery). A bedside computer calculates the cardiac output from the rate of change in temperature of the fluid as it passes from the right side of the heart to the left side of the heart.[54] Indications for the pulmonary artery catheter include massive blood loss and transfusion, septic shock with hypotension and oliguria, severe pregnancy-induced hypertension with oliguria that is unresponsive to fluid challenge, amniotic fluid embolism, and severe cardiac and lung disease, such as mitral stenosis or adult respiratory distress syndrome. Pulmonary artery catheter placement is an invasive procedure that entails both the risks of central venous pressure monitoring and the hazards unique to the pulmonary artery catheter (Table 5–7). These risks can be modified by the experience of the physician performing the procedure, the patient's condition, and the vigilance of the nursing staff.

MATERNAL CARDIOVASCULAR EFFECTS OF DRUGS THAT ALTER UTERINE ACTIVITY

All drugs that modify uterine activity have cardiovascular effects. These changes, which include alterations in blood pressure, heart rate, cardiac output, and the peripheral vascular resistance, can have a significant impact on both mother and fetus. The intensity of these effects is dependent on the concentration of the agent, its infusion rate, and the additive effects of other drugs administered concomitantly. A knowledge of these potentially adverse cardiovascular properties of medications that alter uterine activity is required for compe-

Table 5–7. COMPLICATIONS OF THE PULMONARY ARTERY CATHETER

Insertion	Passage of the Catheter	Maintenance of the Catheter
Carotid artery puncture	Cardiac arrhythmias	Cardiac arrhythmias
Pneumothorax	Intracardiac knotting	Pulmonary infarction
Hemothorax	Damage to heart valves and muscle	Pulmonary embolism
Neurologic injury	Perforation of cardiac chambers	Bacteremia
		Balloon rupture

tent management of preterm and term labor and delivery.

Uterine Stimulants

Oxytocin has a direct relaxing effect on vascular smooth muscle and in high doses can cause a transient, but serious, decrease in systolic and diastolic blood pressures.[57] The degree and duration of the vasodilation are proportionate to the dose of the drug and the rate of injection. A constant infusion of less than 10 mIU/min, a level commonly used for the induction of labor, has minimal vasodilating effects and therefore little effect on the cardiovascular system. However, when higher doses are administered for therapeutic abortion or postpartum uterine atony, significant cardiovascular effects can be appreciated. Weis and co-workers,[58] investigating the hemodynamic effects of oxytocin, 0.1 mIU kg intravenous bolus, during general anesthesia in women undergoing first trimester dilatation and curettage, found a 25 to 68% decrease in mean arterial pressure and noted a 31 to 70% fall in systolic blood pressure that lasted about 4 minutes. Tachycardia occurs 5 to 10 seconds after the onset of the fall in blood pressure and is secondary to baroreceptor stimulation from vasodilation and decrease in venous return to the heart. Despite a fall in peripheral vascular resistance, the tachycardia and increase in stroke volume elevate the cardiac output above control values so that the overall flow to organs is well maintained in healthy individuals.[58] Sympathetic or ganglionic blockade or both during regional or general anesthesia may augment oxytocin-induced hypotension.[59]

When oxytocin is given as a rapid intravenous injection, electrocardiographic changes can include premature ventricular contractions, ST-T wave changes, flattening of the T wave, and prolongation in the Q-T interval. The changes in the T wave are possibly an indication of some interference with myocardial blood flow and evidence of temporary coronary insufficiency.

Oxytocin is generally considered a model drug with an excellent therapeutic index and few side effects.[58] However, if it is administered incorrectly, disastrous consequences may occur. To avoid water intoxication in both fetus and mother, large quantities of intravenous electrolyte-free solution should not be infused when higher concentrations of oxytocin are needed. Increasing the dose of oxytocin should be accomplished by increasing the concentration of the drug, not by increasing the volume of infusion. Although young, healthy women subjected to bolus injections can usually tolerate vasodilation and a fall in blood pressure well, bolus oxytocin administration is especially dangerous in hypovolemic parturient patients or in those with cardiac disease and limited cardiac output. The hypotensive effect of oxytocin can be minimized or eliminated by ensuring that the patient is in the lithotomy or Trendelenburg position when the drug is given intravenously as a bolus. These positions ensure venous return to the heart and maintain the cardiac output and blood pressure during the period of vasodilation.[60] In practice, intravenous oxytocin should never be given by bolus injection but always in dilute solution.

Semisynthetic ergonovine maleate (Ergotrate) and methylergonovine maleate (Methergine) are the two amine alkaloids used for uterine stimulation. It is the intravenous administration of ergots that is responsible for their significant cardiovascular effects and complications. Ergot preparations, in contrast to oxytocin, cause intense vasoconstriction through direct stimulation of both arterial and venous vessels. Hypertension following intravenous use may be associated with nausea, vomiting, blurred vision, headache, and convulsions. The vasoconstriction produced by amine alkaloids becomes manifest in 3 to 7 minutes and may last for several hours after intramuscular administration. Blood pressure rises in about 50% of patients following administration of ergonovine and in 20% after methylergonovine. However, in only 2% of patients is there a rise in blood pressure greater than 25 mm Hg systolic pressure and 20 mm Hg diastolic pressure.[60]

The cardiovascular effects of the ergot alkaloids are significantly modified by route and speed of administration, prior vasopressor use, and ongoing regional or general anesthesia. Life-threatening hypertension occurs most often after intravenous injection; such episodes are rare after intramuscular administration.

Blood pressure elevation following administration of ergot alkaloids is particularly pronounced after use of ephedrine and other vasopressors. In a study of 741 women who received ephedrine and an oxytocic drug 3 to 6 hours apart, 4.6% had a rise in systolic blood pressure greater than 40 mm Hg.[61] The sudden, extreme hypertensive episodes associated with prior vasopressor use have caused cerebral edema and hemorrhage, retinal detachment, convulsions, and coronary artery vasoconstriction leading to myocardial infarction.[61, 62] All commonly used vasopressors, including ephedrine, have been found to cause significant elevations of blood pressure when combined with ergot alkaloids. Patients susceptible to coronary artery spasm may experience constriction with intravenous doses of ergonovine as low as 0.05 mg. Coronary artery spasm may be more common in patients with other vasospastic disorders, such as migraine headaches or Raynaud disease.[62]

Adequate hydration prior to regional anesthesia and lateral uterine displacement decreases the need for vasopressors. If the parturient has received a vasopressor, ergot alkaloids are best avoided in favor of a dilute, slow infusion of oxytocin.[63] Epinephrine should not be added to local anesthetics when ergot administration is anticipated.[59]

Routine use of ergot alkaloids to prevent uterine atony is not recommended. If excessive blood loss occurs post partum as a result of uterine atony, 0.2 mg of methylergonovine maleate can be given intramuscularly. In particular, ergonovine maleate (Ergotrate) should be avoided in patients who have received ephedrine or other vasopressors and in those with pregnancy-induced or chronic hypertension. Caution is advised for patients with hepatic or renal disease. Chlorpromazine and hydralazine have been effective in treating hypertensive episodes produced by ergot alkaloids. The occurrence of chest pain in a patient recently treated with ergot alkaloids is an indication for a prompt clinical evaluation and electrocardiogram in order to rule out myocardial ischemia.[63, 64]

Although many prostaglandins exist, only dinoprostone (PGE$_2$, Prostin E$_2$), dinoprost tromethamine (PGF$_{2\alpha}$, Prostin F$_{2\alpha}$), and carboprost tromethamine (15-methyl PGF$_{2\alpha}$, Prostin 15 m) are used in obstetrics. Dinoprostone vaginal suppositories are employed in second-trimester abortions and in the management of missed abortions or intrauterine fetal death at or before 28 weeks. Dinoprost tromethamine administered by intra-amniotic instillation is widely used for abortions in the second trimester when the uterus is large enough for amniocentesis to be performed.[65] Systemic absorption is minimal with this route of administration; however, low levels may be detected in the maternal plasma. Carboprost tromethamine, a synthetic analogue of PGF$_{2\alpha}$, can be given by intramuscular injection.

Prostaglandins are effective in treating postpartum hemorrhage secondary to uterine atony. Dinoprost tromethamine, 1 mg, or 15-methyl PGF$_{2\alpha}$, 250 μg, can be given intramuscularly or, in divided doses, can be injected directly into the uterine corpus. Dinoprost tromethamine vaginal suppositories can be used as well, but blood flow from the uterus may dislodge the suppository from the upper vagina, thereby decreasing its effectiveness. Whether given as a suppository or an intramuscular injection, the dose can be repeated at 15-minute intervals if the bleeding does not diminish.

All prostaglandins used in obstetrics are commonly associated with diarrhea, nausea, and vomiting as a result of stimulation of the smooth muscle of the alimentary tract. Both PGE$_2$ and PGF$_{2\alpha}$ have cardiovascular effects. These drugs are vasodilators and, therefore, blood pressure decreases slightly. However, because of reflex tachycardia, cardiac output actually increases. Dinoprost tromethamine can cause vasoconstriction of the pulmonary circulation and elevate pulmonary artery pressure[59] and therefore should be used with caution in patients with a history of hypertension or cardiovascular disease. In addition, prostaglandins may induce bronchospasm and should not be administered to patients with asthma. In high-risk patients undergoing abortion in the second trimester, surgical dilatation and evacuation should be considered, since this method may impose fewer cardiovascular changes than would prostaglandins.

Uterine Relaxants

Excess magnesium is known to have several direct and indirect effects on the heart. Various electrocardiographic changes are associated with increases in plasma magnesium concentration. An increase in the PR interval, intraventricular conduction defects, and increased QRS and QT intervals occur at plasma concentrations of 5 to 10 mEq/L. Diminution of P-wave voltage and some T-wave peaking have also been reported. Bradycardia has been observed, even at relatively small elevations. Complete heart block may occur at levels greater than 15 mEq/L.[66] Changes in the electrocardiogram with excess magnesium are variable, and no classic electrocardiographic changes have been described.

The effects of magnesium on myocardial contractility and peripheral vascular resistance are minimal, provided that calcium concentration is normal. However, Bourgeois and colleagues[67] reported that two pre-eclamptic women with serum magnesium levels of 6 to 8 mEq/L became severely hypotensive. The combination of hypovolemia and magnesium-induced vasodilatation were thought responsible for the decrease in blood pressure. Although it is commonly believed that magnesium sulfate is an antihypertensive agent, studies in chronically monitored ewes and women with pre-eclampsia reveal that a magnesium bolus followed by a constant infusion causes a mild and transient decrease in blood pressure that is associated with a fall in peripheral vascular resistance.[68, 69]

Patients undergoing tocolytic therapy with magnesium should have their deep tendon reflexes, respiratory rate, and urine output monitored closely. Patellar tendon reflexes disappear when the plasma magnesium concentration reaches 8 to 10 mEq/L. Respiratory arrest occurs when levels are approximately 12 to 15 mEq/L. Calcium gluconate, 1 g intravenously, should be administered along with oxygen if respiratory depression occurs. Intubation and ventilation occasionally may be necessary.[70] Excessive concentrations of magnesium are extremely rare in the case of normal renal function and correct administration of the drug. If there is any doubt that the plasma magnesium concentration is elevated above therapeutic levels, a plasma magnesium concentration must be obtained.

Beta-adrenergic agents cause a dose-related decrease in uterine muscle tone and a decrease in the frequency and intensity of uterine contractions without altering uterine blood flow. Beta-adrenergic receptors are divided into two types: β-1 and β-2. The β-1 receptors are present in the heart and cause positive inotropic and chronotropic effects. The β-2 receptors are present in vascular smooth muscle, bronchi, liver, and myometrium and cause vasodilation, bronchodilation, glycogenolysis, and uterine relaxation. The basic site of action of these tocolytic drugs is the stimulation of β-2 receptors in the myometrium, an effect mediated by production of cyclic adenosine monophosphate.[71] Ritodrine is the only β-agonist approved for tocolytic therapy by the Federal Drug Administration. However, many obstetricians employ terbutaline, an agent used for years in treating asthmatic patients. Terbutaline and ritodrine are equally effective.

The cardiovascular effects of β-adrenergic drugs in pregnant women have been thoroughly investigated.[71, 72] All β-agonist tocolytic agents have both β-1 and β-2 properties, but in differing proportions. Circulatory side effects vary from one agent to another, depending on the degree of β-1 stimulation.[71] The newer drugs, such as ritodrine and terbutaline, are more β-2 specific than the earlier tocolytic agents isoxsuprine and metaproterenol and, therefore, are the ones used as labor-inhibiting agents at the present time. Bieniarz and colleagues,[73] using a dye dilution technique, measured cardiac output, arterial pressure, and maternal heart rate in five women in premature labor who were receiving ritodrine and found a rise in systolic blood pressure and a decrease in diastolic blood pressure. The fall in diastolic pressure resulted from decreased peripheral resistance because of the vasodilation produced by β-adrenergic drugs on smooth muscle. A significant increase in maternal heart rate, cardiac output, and stroke volume, which elevated the systolic pressure, was also evident. The increase in heart rate is because of the chronotropic effects of β-adrenergic stimulation and because of the vasodilation-activating baroreceptor reflexes. Hendricks, Keroes, and Katz[74] studied the electrocardiograms of patients in preterm labor before, during, and after ritodrine therapy. Only two of the 112 patients developed serious cardiovascular symptoms during therapy. However, 96% developed sinus tachycardia, 70% had ST segment depression, and 55% developed T-wave flattening or inversion. No patient showed a significant change in QRS interval or axis deviation. There was no statistical correlation between the rate of ritodrine administration or the concentration of serum potassium and the incidence of electrocardiographic changes. The increase in cardiac output is produced by both an increase in heart rate and an increase in stroke volume. The rise in stroke volume is caused by increased venous return.

Wagner and colleagues[75] used M-mode echocardiography in 16 pregnant women to evaluate the effects of terbutaline on left ventricular size and performance. Heart rate, ejection fraction, and cardiac output increased significantly, whereas diastolic blood pressure decreased. Hosenpud and colleagues,[76] also using M-mode echocardiography, evaluated the effects of ritodrine and also found increases in heart rate, stroke volume, ejection fraction, and cardiac output. Schwarz and Retzke[71] found similar cardiovascular effects when investigating fenoterol and nylidrin. It is important to understand that the cardiovascular effects of β-adrenergic drugs are dose-related. It should be remembered that the increase in cardiac output secondary to β-2 stimulation is superimposed on the already elevated cardiac function of pregnancy, and it is not unusual for cardiac output to reach 10 L/min.[73]

Beta-agonists can also stimulate antidiuretic hormone release, which reduces urine output and stimulates the renin-aldosterone system.[77] Shortly after initiation of therapy, a decrease in hematocrit, hemoglobin, and serum albumin levels is often observed as a result of expansion of intravascular volume.[78] The decrease in albumin can reduce the colloid osmotic pressure and contribute to the onset of pulmonary edema associated with beta stimulants.

Adverse cardiovascular reactions to the β-adrenergic drugs are varied and have been frequently reported. Arrhythmias, including atrial fibrillation,[79] supraventricular tachycardia with severe hypotension,[80] premature ventricular contractions, and premature nodal contractions,[81] have been described. Chest pain with electrocardiographic signs of ischemia has also been documented.[73, 82, 83] Many patients who became symptomatic were later found to have underlying cardiac pathologies, such as conduction abnormalities, obstructive cardiomyopathy, and atrial septal defects. Aggravating factors include anemia, which reduces the oxygen-carrying capacity of the blood, and hypokalemia, which can impair myocardial contraction and electrical conduction. Cardiac stimulation caused by β-adrenergic agents increases the demands already placed on the heart in pregnancy. Discontinuation of the tocolytic agent and administration of supplemental oxygen usually reverse the adverse symptoms.

A rare but potentially life-threatening complication of β-adrenergic tocolytic therapy is the occurrence of pulmonary edema. It has been reported to occur in as many as 5% of patients who were given terbutaline.[84] The precise mechanism leading to pulmonary edema is not known at the present time, and no absolute pharmacologic basis has been identified. It has also occurred with salbutamol, ritodrine, and fenoterol. Initially, it was thought that pulmonary edema was secondary to myocardial failure and fluid overload.[81] However, measurements of cardiac output and left ventricular function have not revealed depressed myocardial contractility.[85] Beta-agonists may increase pulmonary artery and venous pressure in addition to increasing pulmonary vascular permeability in women with hypervolemia who already have hyperdynamic cardiovascular systems.[86] In fact, increased protein levels in the edema fluid have led some investigators to conclude that pulmonary edema may develop on a noncardiogenic basis.[81] Although many cases of pulmonary edema have occurred in women also receiving corticosteroids to enhance fetal lung development, there is no convincing evidence that steroid administration is a key factor in the development of pulmonary edema. Underlying cardiac abnormalities have been found in some patients who developed pulmonary edema.[72, 87] Risk factors for the development of pulmonary edema include excessive fluid administration, multiple gestation, prolonged duration of therapy, and infections.[81] Successful treatment consists of discontinuing the β-agonist, administering supplemental oxygen, and placing the patient in an upright position. Recent fluid balance should be calculated and furosemide administered unless the patient is hypovolemic. Subsequent intravenous fluids should be infused at a rate of 50 to 75 mL/hr. A pulmonary artery catheter is required if the patient develops pulmonary edema that has not responded to the traditional therapy as described. No further tocolytic agents should be given, even if all evidence of pulmonary edema clears.

In an effort to reduce the frequency and intensity of the ill effects of β-adrenergic drugs, it is important to adhere to strict guidelines for the initiation of treatment and monitoring during therapy. Identification of the patient at high risk for complications should be accomplished by the use of medical history, physical examination, and laboratory studies. Correction of anemia, hypokalemia, or hyperglycemia prior to therapy should be considered. All patients should receive a baseline electrocardiogram, which should be repeated as indicated. In addition, serum electrolyte, glucose, and hematocrit levels should be obtained. Meticulous attention should be paid to fluid balance, daily weights, frequent auscultation of the lungs, and serial hematocrit and electrolyte level determinations. Rational use of the β-agonists is required; discontinue or reduce dosage for maternal heart rate greater than 140 beats/min or if intravenous therapy is longer than 24 to 48 hours.[77] The drug should be stopped if the patient has chest pain or shortness of breath; to ascribe these symptoms to "anxiety" without complete evaluation is unwise. The infusion should be at the lowest rate that adequately inhibits labor. Beta-adrenergic agents should not be used in patients with cardiac disease, hyperthyroidism, uncontrolled hypertension, or diabetes, or in patients with hypovolemia or asthma.

Treatment of a patient with β-agonists in premature labor requires personnel, necessary equipment to evaluate both the mother and the fetus, and close access to a neonatal intensive care facility.[88] Finally, it should be understood that β-agonists may potentiate the effects of other adrenergic amines and may have an additive hypotensive effect with anesthetics.

Nifedipine (Procardia) belongs to the class of drugs known as calcium antagonists, which block calcium entry into the smooth muscle cell, thereby interfering with excitation and contraction. Use of calcium antagonists in cardiology has generally been in the treatment of angina pectoris and hypertension, since they cause vasodilation of the coronary vessels and a reduction of vascular smooth muscle tone. Preliminary investigations have found that nifedipine safely and successfully serves as a tocolytic agent. Nifedipine has been shown to inhibit uterine contractions in the premenstrual period and those induced by prostaglandins in the first and second trimester. Nifedipine also inhibits oxytocin-induced contractions.[89] Read and Wellby[90] compared the effects of nifedipine and ritodrine with no treatment in 60 women with singleton pregnancies and intact membranes between 20 and 35 weeks' gestation who were having contractions at least once every 10 minutes. Nifedipine was more successful in stopping labor than either ritodrine or no treatment.

Nifedipine, at present, is available only in an oral-sublingual preparation. It is almost completely absorbed from the gastrointestinal tract, undergoing extensive first-pass hepatic metabolism. It is strongly protein-bound.[91] After oral or sublingual administration, peak plasma concentrations are reached in 30 to 60 minutes.[92]

Patients receiving nifedipine often experience dizziness, flushing, and headaches. The most commonly observed hemodynamic effects after oral administration of nifedipine are a slight fall in blood pressure, an increase in heart rate, a facilitation of atrioventricular conduction, an increase in cardiac output, and a reduction in left ventricular filling pressure. Siimes and Creasy,[93] studying sheep, found that a nifedipine infusion during labor at a rate sufficient to decrease uterine activity as measured by Montevideo units 76%, increased maternal heart rate 42%, mean arterial pressure 9%, cardiac output 9%, and decreased peripheral vascular resistance 16%. Veille and coworkers,[94] using pregnant goats, observed that the fall in maternal blood pressure and rise in maternal heart rate return to baseline 5 to 30 minutes after bolus administration of nifedipine. A slightly greater increase in cardiac output, decrease in blood pressure, and fall in peripheral vascular resistance were noted with ritodrine as compared with nifedipine.[92] Unlike ritodrine, nifedipine also decreases myocardial oxygen requirement and is a potent coronary artery dilator.[91]

EFFECTS OF VASOPRESSORS AND ANTIHYPERTENSIVE MEDICATIONS ON FETAL, NEONATAL, AND MATERNAL HEALTH

There is little available information regarding the adverse effects of most cardiac medications on the fetus and the neonate. This is because there are a limited number of cases available for analysis, multiple drugs are usually administered to the parturient, and maternal cardiac failure often produces altered placental blood flow and oxygenation, which adversely affect the fetus and the neonate.[95] In most instances, the maternal disease process itself generally carries more of a risk to the mother and fetus than does the medication, which should not be withheld simply because the patient is pregnant.[96]

Vasopressors

Vasopressors are used most frequently in obstetrics to prevent or treat hypotension resulting from spinal and epidural anesthesia, bleeding, or shock (Table 5–8). They act primarily by constricting arteries and arterioles, increasing the rate and force of cardiac muscle function, and constricting veins and venules. The uterine vasculature is considered to be maximally dilated at rest, such that perfusion varies passively with changes in maternal blood pressure. Hypotension, therefore, decreases uterine perfusion.[97] Unfortunately, vasopressors not only maintain or increase arterial blood pressure, but also may increase uterine vascular and myometrial tone, thereby increasing uterine vascular resistance. The uterine vessels have both α- and β-adrenergic receptors, and stimulation of the α-receptors causes constriction, producing marked reduction of uterine blood flow. Vasopressors with predominant α-adrenergic action include methoxamine, phenylephrine, angiotensin, and norepinephrine.[97] These drugs produce a rise in uterine vascular resistance that exceeds the rise in maternal blood pressure so that uterine blood flow is diminished and the uterine vasocon-

striction persists after the blood pressure returns to control levels. Epinephrine has significant effects on both α- and β-adrenergic receptors. If given in high doses by accidental intravascular injection of epinephrine-containing local anesthetics, the effects are maternal hypertension and increase in total peripheral resistance and uterine vasoconstriction, producing a decrease in uterine blood flow.

Studies of sheep and primates have shown that when hypotension occurs, uterine blood flow is most effectively restored by ephedrine (acting primarily on β-adrenergic receptors as well as producing venoconstriction). It increases cardiac output and has minimal α-agonist properties, which cause no fetal problems. The recommended dose is 5 to 10 mg at a time.

Antihypertensives

Drugs such as hydralazine, beta-blockers, nitroglycerin, and nitroprusside are drugs commonly employed to treat hypertensive disorders of pregnancy, to minimize the noxious stimulation of intubation, and to reduce blood pressure during intracranial aneurysm surgery. The choice of a specific drug depends on desired onset of action, potency, whether afterload or preload reduction is desired, and length of action. Ideally, drugs used to treat maternal blood pressure should also reduce uterine vascular resistance so that uterine blood flow is either unchanged or increased.[98]

Hydralazine is a slow-acting antihypertensive drug that has been shown to reduce blood pressure but maintain cardiac output and heart rate. Frequent, small, incremental doses, 5 to 10 mg, minimize the chance of a profound and dangerous reduction in blood pressure. It easily crosses the placenta; serum concentrations are equal to or greater than those in the mother.[95] All the β-adrenergic antagonists cross the placenta and produce signs of blockage in the neonate. Propranolol administered prior to delivery has been responsible for causing neonatal bradycardia and hypoglycemia, which may persist up to 72 hours after delivery. It may also impair the newborn's response to hypoxia.[99–100] Labetalol, a combined α- and β-an-

Table 5–8. PHARMACOLOGIC EFFECTS AND THERAPEUTIC DOSES OF CATECHOLAMINES

Catecholamine	MAP	HR	CO	SVR	RBF	Preparation (mg/500 ml)	Intravenous Dose (μg/kg/min)
Dopamine	+	+ +	+ + +	+	+ + +	400	2–20
Norepinephrine	+ + +	−	−	+ + +	− − −	8	0.05–0.2
Epinephrine	+ +	+ +	+ +	+ +	− −	8	0.05–0.2
Isoproterenol	−	+ + +	+ + +	− −	−	2	0.03–0.3
Dobutamine	+	+	+ + +	±	±	500	2–2.0

Abbreviations: MAP—mean arterial pressure; HR—heart rate; CO—cardiac output; SVR—systemic vascular resistance; RBF—renal blood flow.
Symbols: +, mild increase; + +, moderate increase; + + +, severe increase; −, mild decrease; − −, moderate decrease; − − −, severe decrease.
From Stoelting RK, Miller RD: Basics of Anesthesia. New York: Churchill Livingstone, 1984, p. 27.

tagonist, appears to be safer than propranolol in its ability to cause minimal neonatal adrenergic blockage. Nitroglycerin is a rapidly acting, short-duration vasodilator used to treat angina and severe hypertension. It has been shown to cause no fetal or neonatal harm. Sodium nitroprusside crosses the placenta and theoretically may result in fetal cyanide toxicity. Employing the standard recommended dose of this drug, however, does not pose a risk of excessive accumulation of cyanide in the fetal liver.[95]

TRANSFUSION THERAPY

Life-threatening bleeding can occur during or immediately after a cesarean section. No other obstetric complication is as serious and dramatic as hemorrhage severe enough to cause hypovolemic shock. In order of frequency, the three most common causes of postpartum hemorrhage are uterine atony, lacerations of the vagina and cervix, and retained placenta (including placenta accreta). Perioperative blood transfusion is often a lifesaving procedure that improves hemodynamic function and critical organ perfusion. This section discusses blood component transfusion therapy, the risks and complications of transfusing blood products, and methods to reduce the need for homologous blood transfusion.

Component Therapy

Although transfusions can be lifesaving, advances in the use of blood components have made whole blood transfusion rarely necessary. Blood component therapy provides the patient with only those products that are necessary, thereby helping to conserve blood resources. Components from one unit of blood can be used to treat several patients.[101] Approximately 86% of the 12 million units of blood collected annually in the United States is used for component therapy.[102]

Packed red blood cells are a cost-effective way to provide increased volume and oxygenation. They are prepared from whole blood by removing 200 to 250 ml of plasma. Each unit of packed red blood cells contains 250 ml and has a hematocrit of 70 to 80%, thus providing the same increase in hemoglobin as one unit of whole blood but at approximately half the volume.[103] Transfusing one unit of packed red blood cells increases the hemoglobin by 1 g/dl and the hematocrit by 2 to 3% in an average, 70-kg woman. The decision to transfuse a specific patient should include consideration of the duration of the anemia, the intravascular volume, the extent of the operation, and the presence of coexisting diseases, such as impaired pul-

monary function or myocardial ischemia.[104] Packed red blood cells should not be transfused solely for volume expansion, to enhance wound healing, or to improve general well-being.[101] Although there has been a long-standing tradition that patients undergoing elective surgery should have a hemoglobin level of at least 10 gm/dl, there is no scientific basis for this.

Fresh frozen plasma contains 7% protein, all the clotting factors, small amounts of carbohydrates and lipids, and 90% water. Fresh frozen plasma can be stored frozen for up to one year.[103] Laboratory tests should be used to monitor the patient who is suspected of having a clotting disorder, and fresh frozen plasma should be transfused only when coagulation factors are known to be below normal. If the prothrombin time and partial thromboplastin time are less than 1.5 times normal, fresh frozen plasma transfusion is usually not indicated. Fresh frozen plasma may be useful in reversing the effects of warfarin sodium or in patients with antithrombin III deficiency and thrombotic thrombocytopenic purpura. Fresh frozen plasma should not be given to correct hypovolemia, as a nutritional supplement, or prophylactically with a massive blood transfusion.[101]

One unit of platelets increases the platelet count by 5000 to 10,000 mL in the average adult woman and can be stored for 72 hours at 20° C. Platelets should be transfused only to control and correct bleeding associated with a known decrease in platelet concentration or function or both. Platelet transfusions should not be used for patients with immune thrombocytopenic purpura or prophylactically with massive blood transfusions. A patient undergoing an operation is unlikely to benefit from a platelet transfusion unless the concentration is less than 50,000 mL. Each platelet concentrate contains a small amount of red blood cells; therefore, there is the potential for sensitization and the blood bank usually provides platelets from a blood group- and rhesus-compatible donor.

Infection, alloimmunization, and the effects of massive transfusion, which arise from changes in blood caused by storage, constitute most of the complications associated with transfusion of blood products.

Recently, greater attention has been focused on the risk of transfusion of viruses, which include human immunodeficiency virus, hepatitis B, non-A, non-B hepatitis, and cytomegalic inclusion disease. There is a relationship between these risks and the number of donor exposures (Table 5–9).

Table 5–9. INCIDENCE OF TRANSFUSION RISKS PER UNIT

Non-A, Non-B hepatitis	1:100
Fever, chills, urticaria	1:100
Hemolytic transfusion reaction	1:6000
Fatal hemolytic transfusion reaction	1:100,000
Human immunodeficiency virus	1:40,000 to 1,000,000

Table 5–10. CHEMICAL AND HEMATOLOGIC CHANGES IN CITRATE PHOSPHATE DEXTROSE BLOOD WITH STORAGE TIME

Test	Day			
	1	7	14	21
Blood pH	7.1	7.0	7.0	6.9
Blood P_{CO_2} (mm Hg)	48	80	110	140
Blood lactate (mEq/L)	41	101	145	179
Plasma bicarbonate (mEq/L)	18	15	12	11
Plasma potassium (mEq/L)	3.9	12	17	21
Plasma dextrose (mg/100 ml)	345	312	181	231
Plasma hemoglobin (mg/100 ml)	1.7	7.8	13	19
2,3-DPG* (μM/ml)	4.8	1.2	>1	>1
Platelets (%)	10	0	0	0
Factors V and VII (%)	70	50	40	20

*2,3-DPG—2,3-diphosphoglycerate
From Miller RD, Brzica SM Jr: Anesthesia. New York: Churchill Livingstone, 1986, p. 1335.

The overall risk of contracting acquired immune deficiency syndrome from blood collected since routine testing for human immunodeficiency virus was implemented is extremely low.[105] Patients who received blood between 1981 and 1985 are at the highest risk because this was the period between disease identification and the onset of routine donor screening.

Viral hepatitis is the most frequent and most important infection associated with transfusion. Although screening of blood for hepatitis B surface antigen has helped, at least 90% of transfusion-related hepatitis is non-A, non-B. Although non-A, non-B hepatitis may not be clinically evident for several months following the transfusion, 30 to 50% of those infected develop chronic active hepatitis, and 10% of these people later develop cirrhosis. There is no way of screening blood for this form of hepatitis at present.

Cytomegalovirus infection occurs as a result of blood transfusion with considerable frequency. Except for low-grade fever, most of these infections are asymptomatic. Immunocompromised patients develop more serious complaints. The virus is very prevalent; probably 40% of Americans have it and received it during the perinatal period via maternal transmission.[106] Donor screening is impractical because of the high prevalence of the virus.

Fatal transfusion reactions are almost always caused by blood group incompatibility due to errors in blood product labeling or patient identification. Three fourths of the reported transfusion-related deaths are caused by these errors. These mishaps produce an acute intravascular hemolytic reaction. The clinical manifestations include fever, chills, hypotension, disseminated intravascular coagulation, hemoglobinemia, hemoglobinuria, acute renal failure, and cardiac arrest. Unfortunately, the classic signs of chills, fever, chest and flank pain, and nausea are masked by anesthesia. Immediate supportive care should include stopping the transfusion, administering diuretics, alkalinization of the urine, and the treatment of hypotension and hyperkalemia. Assays for urine and plasma hemoglobin concentration should be performed, as well as coagulation studies, complete blood count, and antibody screen.

The complications of massive blood transfusion result from changes in blood caused by storage (Table 5–10). Plasma potassium concentration slowly increases; however, if the patient maintains adequate perfusion and oxygenation, hyperkalemia does not occur, because the potassium moves intracellularly. Rapid infusion of blood maintained at 4° C can lower the core temperature by several degrees, especially if the patient is anesthetized and in a cold operating room. If the temperature of the blood is less than 30° C, ventricular irritability and even cardiac arrest may occur. This can be prevented by warming the blood to be transfused.[107] The anticoagulant employed for blood collection and storage contains a large amount of citrate to maintain adequate anticoagulation. The citrate binds the ionized calcium. Citrate is metabolized in the liver, usually without difficulty. In patients who are cold or have liver disease, however, citrate may accumulate and cause a decrease in ionized calcium. The signs of citrate intoxication are hypotension, elevated central venous pressures, and a widened pulse pressure. As blood is stored, it becomes more acidic. The decrease in pH is caused by the addition of citrate phosphate dextrose and accumulation of lactic and pyruvic acids as a result of red blood cell metabolism and glycolysis. Despite the significant change in pH, transfusion of large amounts of stored blood usually does not lead to acidosis. Both platelets and coagulation factors V and VIII are lower in transfused blood. However, only 5 to 20% of these factors are required for adequate hemostasis, so that even with massive transfusion, fresh frozen plasma is rarely required. Dilutional thrombocytopenia is more commonly the problem than a deficiency of factors V and VIII. Storage of blood also causes a qualitative defect. Bleeding after massive transfusion may also occur secondary to disseminated intravascular coagulopathy, and it may be prudent to monitor the prothrombin time, the partial thromboplastin time, the fibrinogen, and the fibrin split–product concentrations.

Autologous Transfusion

Up to 70% of red blood cell transfusions are given in the perioperative period; the demand for blood products has increased dramatically in the last decade. The goal of newer management strategies is to reduce the risk of homologous transfusion and to conserve resources. In the past several years, autologous blood transfusion has emerged as a significant transfusion modality. There are three methods of autologous transfusion: intraoperative salvage, transfusion associated with normovolemic hemodilution, and predeposited blood with intra- or postoperative administration.

Intraoperative blood salvage is employed when there is heavy bleeding into the operative field. The blood is collected, washed, filtered, and then infused into the patient. Most often, this process occurs during vascular surgery. To date, this approach has not been used for obstetrics. Because it does require technicians and expensive equipment, to be cost-effective, 2 to 3 units should be salvaged and infused.

Acute normovolemic hemodilution is the removal of whole blood and its concurrent replacement with cell-free substitutes, such as lactated Ringer's solution, albumin, or dextran. The blood is stored for a short term and is reinfused after cessation of the blood loss. At present, it is employed for open-heart surgery and for major reconstructive surgery for scoliosis. Preoperative removal and storage of blood has been employed with success in pregnant women.[108, 109] Parturients tolerate the blood donation without difficulty. Vital signs are unchanged, and the fetal monitoring during and after the procedure suggests no deleterious effects. Women with placenta previa who are not bleeding, those with a history of postpartum hemorrhage, and those with multiple gestations are excellent candidates. The process involves removing blood from the patient by gravity drainage; the blood bank then separates and removes the plasma. The packed red blood cells can be maintained for up to 6 weeks. If two or more units are required, the succeeding ones are taken 4 to 7 days apart. It must be remembered that predonation does not avoid the greatest single cause of severe transfusion reaction: human error that results in blood group incompatibility.

POSTOPERATIVE ANALGESIA

Effective control of postoperative pain is one of the most important issues in obstetrics. For too many patients, pain is inadequately controlled. Significant discomfort after a cesarean section can have many detrimental physiologic effects. It can slow the patient's recovery from surgery and contribute to postoperative morbidity. The incidence and severity of pain experienced after a cesarean section are influenced by the duration of the operation, the type of incision, and the amount of intraoperative trauma, as well as the physiologic and psychologic makeup of the patient, the presence of complications related to the operation, and, most important, the quality of the postoperative care. Pain can impede the return of normal pulmonary function. Splinting, inability to cough, and bronchospasm can promote atelectasis and pneumonia.[110] Pain causes an increase in cardiac output, blood pressure, and oxygen consumption. Pain reduces gastrointestinal motility and increases nausea and vomiting. There is also marked increase in the secretion of catecholamines, cortisol, glucagon antidiuretic hormone, and adrenocorticotropic hormone.[111] Thrombus formation in the lower extremities occurs with increased frequency in the postoperative patient whose pain is inadequately relieved and who reduces physical activity because of fear of aggravating her pain.[112] Women undergoing cesarean section usually desire considerable interaction with their newborn and other family members, early discharge from the hospital, and minimal side effects from analgesic medications. Analgesia should be highly effective while being safe for the mother and the child.[113]

Intravenous and Intramuscular Narcotics

The traditional method of postoperative pain control for cesarean section has been intermittent injections of intravenous or intramuscular narcotics. These approaches have significant side effects and, in addition, are often inadequate in delivering consistent pain relief. Although intravenous injections are effective in achieving rapid blood levels, the analgesic effect is relatively short, as the plasma levels rapidly decline because of redistribution and elimination. In addition, a high dose may result in toxic plasma concentrations.[114] Although intramuscular injections have been the most common method of postoperative pain control, research has indicated that up to 75% of patients reported that they experienced significant pain in the postoperative period.[115] Wide variations in patients' requirements for analgesia sometimes lead to overdose, but this occurs more commonly under medication when standard postoperative pain orders are employed. Patients receiving intramuscular injections may have very high blood levels of narcotics soon after administration, which results in sedation and inadequate blood levels much before the next injection is scheduled to be given. Finally, considerable variability in the onset times as well as in the duration of action is common with intramuscular injections.

Patient-Controlled Analgesia

Patient-controlled analgesia avoids many of the disadvantages of postoperative pain relief by intramuscular injection. The objectives of patient-controlled analgesia are to achieve effective analgesia as rapidly as possible with a minimum amount of drug so that the side effects are minimized while constant and effective analgesia is maintained for prolonged periods of time. Patient-controlled analgesia systems consist of a syringe-type infusion pump with a microprocessor, which is piggy-backed into the intravenous line. After achieving adequate analgesia in the recovery room, the patient is instructed to press a button when she experiences pain, and a preset dose of narcotic is administered. After the bolus, the machine enters a lockout period. The dose, agent, and lockout period are variable and can be altered to meet the patient's changing analgesic requirements. The lockout period is usually the time it takes for an intravenous dose to achieve a peak effect, 5 to 10 minutes. In addition to the intermittent-demand bolus, patient-controlled analgesia devices can also be programmed to provide a constant, fixed, background infusion.[116] Although there are a large number of narcotics that can be employed for patient-controlled analgesia, morphine and meperidine have been used the most (morphine 0.5 to 1.5 mg/bolus, meperidine 5 to 15 mg/bolus). Patient-controlled analgesia is more effective than intramuscular narcotic administration because blood concentrations remain fairly constant, and the continuous infusion permits patients to titrate their own analgesic requirements. The psychologic benefit of patient-controlled analgesia is that it gives patients the ability to control their own analgesia and a feeling of security in being able to obtain pain relief quickly without the need to involve other people in helping them. There is less of the oversedation and risk of respiratory depression that is associated with large intramuscular injections, which is particularly advantageous for the patient who desires to interact with her newborn. With patient-controlled analgesia, there is none of the discomfort that is associated with repeated intramuscular injections. The evidence suggests that the use of patient-controlled analgesia, as compared with the use of intramuscular injections, results in earlier mobilization, a shorter hospital stay, and fewer pulmonary complications.[113] Patient-controlled analgesia also appears to place fewer demands on the nursing staff and can be employed by the vast majority of women undergoing cesarean section. Its use, however, does require the patient to be alert, oriented, and able to understand the concept.

When comparing the effects of epidural narcotics and intramuscular injections in 60 post-cesarean section patients, Eisenach and co-workers[117] found that the epidural narcotic gave more profound analgesia but that the patients favored patient-controlled analgesia the most. In addition, less pruritus was experienced with patient-controlled analgesia than with epidural morphine. Rayburn and colleagues[118] found similar results with 130 patients, using patient-controlled analgesia and intramuscular injections of meperidine. The patient-controlled analgesia technique does have disadvantages. The most common problems are related to operator error, such as misprogramming the device, improper loading of the syringe, or inability to respond to the safety alarm. Patient errors include failure to understand the patient-controlled analgesia device.[119] Patient-controlled analgesia machines are expensive, costing about $2000 to $5000 each, and some devices require expensive disposable accessories.

Epidural and Subarachnoid Narcotics

The aim of epidural and subarachnoid narcotic administration is to deliver the narcotics to the opioid receptors on the spinal cord, which are involved in pain transmission. Since the early 1980s, research has demonstrated that preservative-free morphine, 4 to 5 mg, placed in the epidural space provides excellent, long-lasting (16 to 27 hours) pain relief after cesarean section and is associated with fewer side effects than are intramuscular narcotics or regional anesthesia with local anesthetics.[120, 121] A 1987 survey of members of the Society for Obstetric Anesthesia and Perinatology found that 71% of the members used epidural narcotics for analgesia after cesarean section.[122] The onset of analgesia is usually 30 to 60 minutes after injection. It is important, therefore, to administer the morphine as soon as possible after clamping the umbilical cord so that analgesia occurs prior to the regression of the local anesthetic blockade. Most of the regional anesthesia for cesarean section in the United States is spinal anesthesia, and therefore the use of subarachnoid narcotics is ideal. Studies have shown that employing as little as 0.1 to 0.25 mg of morphine, injected with the local anesthetic, provides analgesia for 18 to 28 hours.[123, 124] Intrathecal morphine doses are so small that low maternal blood concentrations are achieved; this minimizes the potential for narcotic exposure to the fetus and nursing newborn. Most patients given a single dose of epidural or subarachnoid morphine do not require additional analgesics in the first 12 to 24 hours; many then only need oral medications, and if parenteral narcotics are required, only a low dose is usually needed.

The side effects of epidural and subarachnoid narcotics mainly result from their action on the brain stem, especially the fourth ventricle, following cephalad movement in the cerebrospinal fluid.

Pruritus, nausea, vomiting, and urinary retention can be unpleasant or troublesome. Respiratory depression is more serious. Pruritus is the most frequent complication seen in patients after cesarean section. The incidence may be as high as 60 to 90%. However, treatment with diphenhydramine or a dilute naloxone infusion reduces the incidence and severity considerably. Naloxone, if carefully titrated, does not usually reverse the analgesia. The mechanism responsible for causing pruritus has not been elucidated.

The incidence of nausea and vomiting in patients receiving epidural and subarachnoid narcotics may be higher than in those receiving parenteral narcotics. This may be a result of the rostral migration of the narcotic in the spinal fluid and direct stimulation of the chemoreceptor trigger zone in the medulla.[113] Antiemetic therapy reduces the incidence dramatically. Urinary retention is most common and troublesome in men. Although poorly understood, the mechanism may result from direct effect on the sacral spinal area, which inhibits the micturition reflex. Urinary retention in patients having a cesarean section is usually not a problem because a urinary catheter is in place for the first 24 hours, the period of time when retention is most common.

Patients who receive epidural or subarachnoid narcotics are at risk for respiratory depression for 6 to 24 hours after administration. This is because of the cephalad movement of the narcotic in the cerebrospinal fluid and subsequent depression of the respiratory center in the medulla. A number of factors increase the chance of respiratory depression, including the administration of supplemental parenteral narcotics and decreased pulmonary function. The decrease in ventilation is not sudden; it occurs slowly over a 1- to 2-hour period. Recovery of the patient in the intensive care unit is not necessary. The nursing staff, however, must be instructed in the physiology, signs, symptoms, and treatment of respiratory depression. Several thousand obstetric patients have been observed and monitored after administration of epidural and subarachnoid narcotics; only rarely has a patient been identified as having a significant decrease in ventilation. It has been postulated that the parturient may be particularly resistant to ventilatory depression because of the increased drive to breathe that occurs in pregnancy.[113] The decrease in ventilation is associated with a generalized central nervous system depression, manifested in somnolence. Recent evidence suggests that respiratory depression with epidural and subarachnoid narcotics is less than that occurring with parenteral narcotics. If necessary, intravenous or intramuscular naloxone reverses respiratory depression.

MATERNAL MORTALITY

Although the overall death rate for the parturient has been steadily declining, improvements in anesthesia have unfortunately not kept pace with those in obstetrics. Anesthesia is responsible for an increasing percentage of deaths.[125] The most frequent obstetric causes of mortality are embolism (thrombotic and amniotic), pre-eclampsia and eclampsia, hemorrhage, and infection. The majority of deaths related to anesthesia are caused by aspiration, failure to intubate the trachea, regional anesthesia, and misuse of drugs and equipment. Much of the data on anesthesia-related maternal mortality is derived from the Confidential Inquiry into Maternal Deaths in England and Wales, a government-sponsored program that began in 1928. Each maternal death is reviewed carefully to ascertain if additional or different action might have given the mother a better chance of survival.[126] The reports are published every 3 years. The system of reporting is voluntary, and the costs of the project are supported by the Department of Health and Social Services. Deaths are classified by referees (obstetricians and anesthesiologists) as "avoidable" or not.[127] Avoidable factors during emergency cesarean section are responsible for the vast majority of deaths. Unlike Great Britain and Wales, the United States does not have an organized review of maternal mortality. However, various case reports and state medical audits show that anesthesia is a major cause of maternal mortality in the United States.

Aspiration of Gastric Contents

The parturient is at increased risk of aspiration of gastric contents, and, if it occurs, has a greater chance of serious sequelae than does the nonpregnant patient. Decreased gastrointestinal peristalsis, diminished sphincter tone, and delayed gastric emptying may occur; in addition, the gastric contents, even in the fasting state, often have large volumes and decreased pH. This situation mainly results from the hormonal changes of pregnancy and from the effects of pain and narcotic administration. Aspiration of gastric juice causes irritation of bronchial mucosa, bronchospasm, focal hemorrhages, and necrosis. Aspiration of food results in airway obstruction and collapse. All pregnant women should be told to avoid food and drink when in labor. After admission to the hospital, intravenous fluid administration helps avoid dehydration and ketosis. Clear, nonparticulate antacids should elevate the pH of gastric secretions to a safe level. Further gastric secretion can be minimized by the administration of H_2-blocking drugs, such as cimetidine and ranitidine.

On induction of anesthesia, cricoid pressure (Sellick maneuver) must be applied. This procedure consists of pressure on the cricoid, the only complete tracheal ring, onto the esophagus, which functionally seals the esophagus until the endotracheal tube is securely placed in the trachea.[128]

Cricoid pressure must be applied by a skilled assistant because incorrectly placed pressure makes intubation quite difficult.

Intubation

Difficulty or inability to intubate usually can be managed without serious consequences to the surgical patient. This may not be possible for the parturient who has a rapidly declining oxygen content because of increased consumption and diminished functional residual capacity. All pregnant women who are at risk for surgery must undergo a careful evaluation of their airways. Those patients who are morbidly obese, have a severe overbite, limited neck extension, or a short, fat neck are at risk for difficult intubation and mask ventilation, and added consideration should be given to regional anesthesia or an awake fiberoptic intubation. Rapid verification of proper tracheal tube placement is essential. Although observation of the endotracheal tube pass between the vocal cords is helpful, auscultation of both lungs and stomach, the use of end-tidal carbon dioxide monitoring, and pulse oximetry are also mandatory in order to ensure safety of the patient.

Despite the most careful evaluation and the most experienced anesthesiologists, there are women in whom intubation is very difficult or impossible. Unless the surgery is anticipated to be lifesaving for the patient and the fetus, the patient should be allowed to regain consciousness while the 100% oxygen and cricoid pressure are administered, at which time regional anesthesia or an awake fiberoptic intubation can be performed. The anesthesiologist must realize that prolonged and misguided attempts at intubation result in significant maternal and fetal morbidity and mortality.

Regional Anesthesia

Although the exact risk of death attributable to regional anesthesia is unknown, the two most common fatal complications are total spinal and systemic local anesthetic overdose. Excessive amounts of local anesthetic in the subarachnoid space may occur during the progress of a spinal anesthetic when an inappropriately high dose is administered or during an attempted epidural block, with accidental drug injection into the subarachnoid space. This results in a rapid and profound decrease in maternal blood pressure, bradycardia, depressed level of consciousness, and apnea, which may progress rapidly to cardiopulmonary arrest. The parturient is particularly susceptible to this phenomenon because of a decrease in the local anesthetic requirements associated with pregnancy and because of aortocaval compression, which produces decreased venous return and cardiac output.

Accidental intravenous injection of a large quantity of local anesthetic into an epidural vein causes significant systemic toxicity. Inadvertent injection into the vein is most likely to occur via an epidural catheter. The physiologic changes of pregnancy induce marked dilation of epidural veins and increase the risk of cannulation. Verification of correct needle or catheter placement is imperative. Venous placement may be identified by aspiration of blood through the catheter or by administration of a "test dose" of local anesthetic that induces minor central nervous system symptoms (jitteriness, tinnitus, metallic taste in mouth) or both. Subsequent doses should be low, and careful questioning of the patient for signs of subarachnoid or intravenous local anesthetic placement is essential.

Misuse of Drugs and Equipment

The misuse of drugs and equipment is almost always avoidable. The anesthesiologist must be aware of the pharmacology and potential complications of obstetric and anesthetic drug interactions, such as tocolytic and uterotonic agents, neuromuscular blockers, vasopressors, and sedatives. Their interactions may produce significant, severe, and persistent muscle paralysis, hypertension, or hypotension. All machinery and monitoring equipment must be repeatedly checked and calibrated. Regular servicing is essential. This is particularly vital in the instance of ventilator and breathing circuits.

In order to reduce the number of maternal deaths, the following guidelines should be adhered to:

1. Early consultation between the obstetricians and anesthesiologists is necessary. It is especially important to give the anesthesia team as much time as possible to evaluate the patient and formulate a safe plan.

2. Obstetric anesthesia equipment and operating room facilities must be the same quality as those in the main operating room.

3. Anesthesiology staff who work in obstetrics should not be junior members of the department but have adequate training and experience in regional and general anesthesia, resuscitation, and intubation.

4. The post-anesthesia recovery room must be adequately equipped and staffed with well-trained and motivated nurses.

5. Every obstetric unit should have an established drill for dealing with patients in whom intubation is not possible. In addition, there should be a plan to manage parturients who require emergency cesarean sections, as well as those who need sudden, massive blood replacement.

The safe practice of perinatal medicine includes consultation with obstetric anesthesiologists. The well-being of both the mother and fetus can be promoted by early consultation with anesthesiologists who are knowledgeable of maternal physiology and pharmacology, skillful in the care of the critically ill parturient, and proficient at general and regional anesthesia.

References

1. Cheek TG, Gutsche BB: Maternal physiologic alterations during pregnancy. In Shnider SM, Levinson G (eds.): Anesthesia for Obstetrics. Baltimore: Williams & Wilkins, 1987, p. 3.
2. Prowse CM, Gaensler EA: Respiratory acid base changes during pregnancy. Anesthesiology 26:381, 1965.
3. Curtis J, Shnider SM, Saitto C, et al.: The effect of painful contractions, position and epidural anesthesia on maternal transcutaneous oxygen tension (TcPo₂). Anesthesiology (suppl) 53:315, 1980.
4. Russell IF, Chambers IF: Closing volume in normal pregnancy. Br J Anaesth 53:1043, 1981.
5. Hagerdal M, Morgan CW, Sumner AE, Gutsche BB: Minute ventilation and oxygen consumption during labor with epidural analgesia. Anesthesiology 59:425, 1983.
6. Pritchard JA: Changes in the blood volume during pregnancy and delivery. Anesthesiology 26:393, 1965.
7. Lees MM, Taylor SH, Scott DB, Kerr MG: A study of cardiac output at rest throughout pregnancy. J Obstet Gynecol Brit Comm 74:319, 1967.
8. Marx GF: Aortocaval compression: Incidence and prevention. Bull NY Acad Med 50:443, 1974.
9. Albright GA, Joyce TH III, Ferguson JE II, Jones MM: Physiology of pregnancy. In Albright GA, Joyce TH III, Ferguson JE II, Stevenson DK (eds.): Anesthesia in Obstetrics: Maternal, Fetal, and Neonatal Aspects. Boston: Butterworth Publishers, 1986, p. 41.
10. Joyce TH III: Cardiac disease. In James FM III, Wheeler AS (eds.): Obstetric Anesthesia: The Complicated Patient. Philadelphia: FA Davis Co., 1982, p. 87.
11. McAnulty JH, Metcalfe J, Ueland K: General guidelines in the management of cardiac disease. Clin Obstet Gynecol 24:773, 1981.
12. Pritchard JA, MacDonald PC: Williams Obstetrics. New York: Appleton-Century-Crofts, 1980, p. 730.
13. Shnider SM, Levinson G: Anesthesia for cesarean section. In Shnider SM, Levinson G (eds.): Anesthesia for Obstetrics. Baltimore: Williams & Wilkins, 1979, p. 254.
14. James FM, Crawford JS, Hopkinson R, et al.: A comparison of general anesthesia and lumbar analgesia for elective cesarean section. Anesth Analg 56:228, 1977.
15. Lamkee MJ, Donaldson LB, de Alvarez RR: Analysis of cesarean sections in a teaching and a nonteaching hospital. Am J Obstet Gynecol 83:619, 1962.
16. Davis AG: Anaesthesia for caesarean section: The potential for regional block. Anaesthesia 37:748, 1982.
17. Datta S, Alper MH: Anesthesia for cesarean section. Anesthesiology 53:142, 1980.
18. Joyce TH III: Regional versus general anesthesia. Any advantage? Semin Anesth 1:125, 1982.
19. Marx GF, Joshi CW, Orkin LR. Placental transmission of nitrous oxide. Anesthesiology 32:429, 1970.
20. Datta S, Ostheimer GW, Weiss JB, et al: Neonatal effect of prolonged anesthetic induction for cesarean section. Obstet Gynecol 58:331, 1981.
21. Crawford JS, James FM, Crawley M: A further study of general anaesthesia for cesarean section. Br J Anaesth 48:661, 1976.
22. Fox GS, Houle GL: Acid-base studies in elective caesarean sections during epidural and general anaesthesia. Can Anaesth Soc J 18:60, 1971.
23. Fisher JT, Mortola JP, Smith B, et al.: Neonatal pattern of breathing following cesarean section: Epidural versus general anesthesia. Anesthesiology 59:385, 1983.
24. Dailey PA, Baysinger CL, Levinson G, et al.: Neurobehavioral testing of the newborn infant: Effects of obstetric anesthesia. Clin Perinatol 9:191, 1982.
25. Scanlon JW, Brown WV Jr, Weiss JB, et al.: Neurobehavioral responses of newborn infants after maternal epidural anesthesia. Anesthesiology 40:121, 1974.
26. Brazelton TB: Neonatal behavioral assessment scale. Philadelphia: J. B. Lippincott Co., 1973, p. 27.
27. Datta S, Corke BC, Alper MH, et al.: Epidural anesthesia for cesarean section: A comparison of bupivacaine, chloroprocaine, etidocaine. Anesthesiology 52:48, 1980.
28. Hollmen AI, Jouppila R, Kovisto M, et al.: Neurologic activity of infants following anesthesia for cesarean section. Anesthesiology 48:350, 1978.
29. Warren TM, Datta S, Ostheimer GW, et al.: Comparison of the maternal and neonatal effects of halothane, enflurane, and isoflurane for cesarean delivery. Anesth Analg 62:516, 1983.
30. Abboud T, Henriksen E, Kim SH, et al.: Enflurane and halothane: Effects on placental transfer. Anesthesiology (suppl) 51:306, 1979.
31. Corke BC, Ostheimer GW, Alper MH: Neurobehavioral assessment of the neonate. Anesth Rev 6:16, 1979.
32. Moir DD: Anaesthesia for caesarean section. An evaluation of a method using low concentration of halothane and 50 per cent of oxygen. Br J Anaesth 42:136, 1970.
33. Modig J: Thromboembolism and blood loss: Continuous epidural block versus general anesthesia with controlled ventilation. Reg Anesth 7(suppl):84, 1982.
34. Modig J, Borg T, Karlstrom G, et al.: Thromboembolism after total hip replacement: Role of epidural and general anesthesia. Anesth Analg 62:174, 1983.
35. Modig J, Borg T, Bagge L, et al.: Role of extradural and of general anaesthesia in fibrinolysis and coagulation after total hip replacement. Br J Anaesth 55:625, 1983.
36. Nimmo WS: Gastrointestinal function following surgery. Reg Anesth 7(suppl):105, 1982.
37. Namba Y, Smith JB, Challis JRG: Plasma cortisol concentrations during caesarean section. Br J Anaesth 52:1027, 1980.
38. Irestedt L, Lagercrzntz H, Hjemdahl P, et al.: Fetal and maternal plasma catecholamine levels at elective cesarean section under general or epidural anesthesia versus vaginal delivery. Am J Obstet Gynecol 142:1004, 1982.
39. Abboud TK, Noveihed R, Khoos S, et al.: Effects of induction of general and regional anesthesia for cesarean section on maternal plasma β-endorphin levels. Am J Obstet Gynecol 146:927, 1983.
40. Crawford JS. Epidural analgesia for patients with chronic neurologic disease. Anesth Analg 62:620, 1983.
41. Datta S, Alper MH, Ostheimer GW, et al.: Method of ephedrine administration and nausea and hypotension during spinal anesthesia for cesarean section. Anesthesiology 56:68, 1982.
42. Brownridge P: Central neural blockade and caesarean section: Part I. Review and case series. Anaesth Intensive Care 7:33, 1979.
43. Brownridge P: Central neural blockade and caesarean section: II. Patient assessment of the procedure. Anaesth Intensive Care 7:163, 1979.
44. Usubiaga JE: Neurologic complications following epidural analgesia. Int Anesthesiol Clin 13:2, 1975.
45. Hellman K: Epidural anaesthesia in obstetrics: A second look at 26,127 cases. Can Anaesth Soc J 12:398, 1965.
46. Ostheimer GW: Obstetric anesthesia. In American Society of Anesthesiologists Annual Refresher Course Lecture Book, 1983.
47. Bromage PR: Neurologic complications of regional analgesia for obstetrics. In Shnider SM, Levinson G (eds.):

Anesthesia for Obstetrics. Baltimore: Williams & Wilkins, 1979, p. 301.

48. Ravindram RS, Bond VK, Tasch MP, et al.: Prolonged neural blockade following regional analgesia with 2-chloroprocaine. Anesth Analg 59:446, 1980.

49. Reisner LS, Hockman BN, Plumber MH: Resistant neurological deficit and adhesive arachnoiditis following intrathecal 2-chloroprocaine injection. Anesth Analg 59:452, 1980.

50. Albright GA: Cardiac arrest following regional anesthesia with etidocaine or bupivacaine. Anesthesiology 51:285, 1979.

51. Liu P, Feldman HS, Covino BM, et al.: Acute cardiotoxicity of intravenous amide local anesthetics in anesthetized ventilated dogs. Anesth Analg 61:317, 1982.

52. Stoelting RK, Miller RD: Basics of Anesthesia. New York: Churchill Livingstone, 1984, p. 213.

53. Shoemaker WC: Monitoring of the critically ill patient. In Shoemaker WC, Thompson WL, Holbrook PR (eds.): Textbook of Critical Care. Philadelphia: W. B. Saunders Co., 1984, p. 105.

54. Harrelson E, Cohen WR: Critical care of the parturient. In Cohen WR, Acker DB, Friedman EA (eds.): Management of Labor. Rockville, Maryland: Aspen Publications, 1989, p. 479.

55. Civetta JM. Invasive catheterization. In Shoemaker WC, Thompson WL (eds.): Critical Care: State of the Art. Society of Critical Care Medicine, 1980. Fullerton, California.

56. Kirshon B, Cotton DB: Invasive hemodynamic monitoring in the obstetric patient. Clin Obstet Gynecol 30:579, 1987.

57. Hendricks CH, Brenner, WE: Cardiovascular effects of oxytocic drugs used postpartum. Am J Obstet Gynecol 134:399, 1979.

58. Weis FR, Markeuo R, Mo B, Bochiechio P: Cardiovascular effects of oxytocin. Obstet Gynecol 46:211, 1975.

59. James FM III: Interactions between obstetric medications and anesthetic agents. American Society of Anesthesiologists Refresher Course. 1982, p. 123.

60. Johnstone M: The cardiovascular effects of oxytocic drugs. Br J Anaesth, 44:8261, 1972.

61. Casady GN, Moore DC, Bridenbaugh LD: Postpartum hypertension after use of vasoconstrictor and oxytocic drugs. JAMA 172:1011, 1960.

62. Taylor GJ, Cohen B: Ergonovine-induced coronary artery spasm and myocardial infarction after normal delivery. Obstet Gynecol 66:821, 1985.

63. Alper MH: In Smith NT, Miller RD, Corbascio AN (eds.): Agents in Obstetrics: Mother, Fetus, and Newborn. Drug Interactions in Anesthesia. Philadelphia: Lea & Febiger, 1981, p. 305.

64. Abouleish E: Postpartum hypertension and convulsion after oxytocic drugs. Anesth Analg 55:813, 1976.

65. Russ JS, Rayburn WF, Samuel MJ: Uterine Stimulants. In Rayburn WF, Zuspan FP (eds.): Drug Therapy in Obstetrics and Gynecology. Norwalk, Connecticut: Appleton-Centry-Crofts, 1982:123.

66. Shine KF: Myocardial effects of magnesium. Am J Physiol 237:413, 1979.

67. Bourgeois FJ, Thiagarajah S, Harbert GM, Difazio C: Profound hypotension complicating magnesium therapy. Am J Obstet Gynecol 154:919, 1986.

68. Cotton DB, Gonik B, Dorman KF: Cardiovascular alterations on severe pregnancy induced hypertension: Acute effects of intravenous magnesium sulfate. Am J Obstet Gynecol 148:162, 1984.

69. Dandavido A, Woods, JR Jr., Murayama K, Brinkman CR III, Assali NS: Circulatory effects of magnesium sulfate in normotensive and renal hypertensive pregnant sheep. Am J Obstet Gynecol 127:770, 1977.

70. McCubbin JH, Sibai BM, Abdella TN, Anderson GD: Cardiopulmonary arrest due to acute maternal hypermagnesemia. Lancet 1:1058, 1981.

71. Schwarz R, Retzke U: Cardiovascular effects of terbutaline in pregnant women. Acta Obstet Gynecol Scand 62:419, 1983.

72. Sudinio S, Olkonen H, Lahtinen T: Maternal circulatory response to a single dose of ritodrine hydrochloride during orthostasis in normal and hypertensive late pregnancy. Am J Obstet Gynecol 130:745, 1978.

73. Bieniarz J, Ivankovich A, Scommegna A: Cardiac output during ritodrine treatment in premature labor. Am J Obstet Gynecol 118:910, 1974.

74. Hendricks SK, Keroes J, Katz M: Electrocardiographic changes associated with ritodrine-induced maternal tachycardia and hypokalemia. Am J Obstet Gynecol 154:921, 1986.

75. Wagner JM, Morton MJ, Johnson KA, et al.: Terbutaline and maternal cardiac function. JAMA 246:2697, 1981.

76. Hosenpud JD, Morton MJ, O'Grady JP: Cardiac stimulation during ritodrine hydrochloride tocolytic therapy. Obstet Gynecol 62:52, 1983.

77. Jacobs MM, Arias F: Cardiopulmonary complication associated with beta-adrenenrgic tocolytic therapy. In Berkowitz RL (ed.): Critical Care of the Obstetric Patient. New York, Churchill Livingstone, 1981, p. 505.

78. Philipson T, Eriksen PS, Lynggard F: Pulmonary edema following ritodrine-saline infusion in premature labor. Obstet Gynecol 58:304, 1981.

79. Frederiksen MC, Toig RM. Depp III R: Atrial fibrillation during hexoprenoline therapy for premature labor. Am J Obstet Gynecol 145:108, 1983.

80. Grospietsch G, Fenske M, Dietrich B, Ensink FBM, Holzl M, Kuhn W: Effects of the tocolytic agent fenoterol on body weight, urine excretion, blood hematocrit, hemoglobin, serum protein, and electrolyte levels in nonpregnant rabbits. Am J Obstet Gynecol 143:667, 1982.

81. Beneditti TJ: Maternal complications of parental B-sympathomimetic therapy for premature labor. Am J Obstet Gynecol 145:1, 1983.

82. Michalak D, Klein V, Marquette GP: Myocardial ischemia: A complication of ritodrine tocolysis. Am J Obstet Gynecol 146:861, 1983.

83. Ying YK, Tejani NA: Angina pectoris as a complication of ritodrine hydrochloride therapy in premature labor. Obstet Gynecol 60:385, 1982.

84. Creasy RK: Side effects of beta-mimetic administration: Tocolytic agents. Proceedings of a Symposium on Tocolytic Therapy. New Orleans: The Society of Perinatal Obstetricians, 1980, p. 87.

85. Schreyer P, Caspi E, Arielv S, Herzianu I, User P, Gilbda Y, Zaidman JL: Metabolic effects of intravenous ritodrine infusion during pregnancy. Eur J Obstet Gynec Reprod Biol 9:97, 1979.

86. Haller DL: The use of terbutaline for premature labor. Drug Intell Clin Pharm 14:757, 1980.

87. Pou-Martinez A, Kelly SH, Newell FD, Culbert CM: Postpartum pulmonary edema after ritodrine and betamethasone use. J Reprod Med 27:428, 1982.

88. Lipshitz J: Beta-adrenergic agents. Semin Perinatol 5:252, 1981.

89. Ulmsten U, Andersson K-E, Wingerup L: Treatment of premature labour with the calcium antagonist nifedipine. Arch Gynaecol 229:1, 1980.

90. Read MD, Wellby DE: The use of calcium antagonist (nifedipine) to suppress preterm labour. Br J Obstet Gynecol 93:933, 1986.

91. Kates RA, Kaplan JA: Calcium Channel Blocking Drugs. In Kaplan JA (ed.): Cardiac Anesthesia. Vol. 2: Cardiovascular Pharmacology. New York: Grune and Stratton, 1983, p. 209.

92. Golichowski AM, Hathaway DR, Fineberg N, Peleg D: Tocolytic and hemodynamic effects of nifedipine in the ewe. Am J Obstet Gynecol 151:1134, 1985.

93. Siimes ASI, Creasy RK: Cardiac and uterine hemodynamic responses to ritodrine hydrochloride administrations in pregnant sheep. Am J Obstet Gynecol 133:19, 1979.

94. Veille JC, Bissonnette JM, Hohimer AR: The effect of a calcium channel blocker (nifedipine) on uterine blood flow in the pregnant goat. Am J Obstet Gynecol 154:1160, 1986.

95. Garite TJ, Briggs GG: Effects on the fetus of drugs used in critical care. In Clark SL, Phelen JP, Cotton DB (ed.): Critical Care Obstetrics. Oradell, New Jersey: Medical Economics Books, 1987, p. 487.

96. Little BB, Gilstrap LC: Cardiovascular drugs during pregnancy. Clin Obstet Gynecol 32:13, 1989.

97. Eisenach JC: Fetal stress/distress. Probl in Anesth 3:19, 1989.

98. Cosmi EV, Shnider SM: Obstetric anesthesia and uterine blood flow. In Shnider SM, Levinson G (ed.): Anesthesia for Obstetrics. Baltimore: Williams & Wilkins, 1987, p. 22.

99. Turnstall ME: The effects of propranolol on the onset of breathing at birth. Br J Anaesth 41:792, 1969.

100. Habib A, McCarthy JS: Effects on the neonate of propranolol administered during pregnancy. J Pediatr 91:808, 1977.

101. Transfusion Alert: Indications for the use of red blood cells, platelets, and fresh frozen plasma. U.S. Department of Health and Human Services, Public Health Service, National Institutes of Health, 1989.

102. Polesky HF: Blood banking in the United States: 1981. Transfusion 25:304, 1985.

103. Kilpatrick SJ, Lards RJ Jr.: Transfusion therapy. In Parer J (ed.): Antepartum and Intrapartum Management. Philadelphia: Lea & Febiger, 1989, p. 121.

104. Perioperative Red Cell Transfusion. National Institute of Health Consensus Development Conference Statement, 1988.

105. FDA Drug Bulletin: Progress on AIDS, 15:27, 1985.

106. Rader DL: Cytomegalovirus infection in patients undergoing noncardiac surgical procedures. Surg Gynecol Obstet 160:13, 1985.

107. Miller RD, Brzica SM Jr.: Blood, Blood Components, Colloids and Autotransfusion Therapy. In Miller RD (ed.): Anesthesia. New York: Churchill Livingstone, 1986, p. 1329.

108. Kruskall MS, Leonard S, Klapholz H: Autologous blood donation during pregnancy: Analysis of safety and blood use. Obstet Gynecol 70:938, 1987.

109. Herbert WNP, Owen HG, Collins ML: Autologous blood storage in obstetrics. Obstet Gynecol 72:166, 1988.

110. Craig DB: Postoperative pulmonary function. Anesth Analg 60:46, 1981.

111. Kehlet H: The modifying effect of general and regional anesthesia on the endocrine-metabolic response to surgery. Reg Anesth 7:38, 1982.

112. Modig J: Thromboembolism and blood loss: Continuous epidural block versus general anesthesia with controlled ventilation. Reg Anesth 7:84, 1982.

113. Chadwick HS, Ross BK: Analgesia for post-cesarean delivery pain. Anesth Clin NA 7:133, 1989.

114. Brown JG: Systemic opioid analgesia for postoperative pain management. Anesth Clin NA 7:51, 1989.

115. Utting JE, Smity JM: Postoperative analgesia. Anaesth 34:320, 1979.

116. Thompson CC, Bailey MK, Conroy JM, Baker JD III, Cooke JE: Patient controlled analgesia. Advances in the last five years. Anesth Rev 16:14, 1989.

117. Eisenach JC, Grice SC, Dewan DM: Patient-controlled analgesia following cesarean section: A comparison with epidural and intramuscular narcotics. Anesthesiology 68:444, 1988.

118. Rayburn WF, Geranis BJ, Ramadei CA, Woods RE, Patil KD: Patient-controlled analgesia for post-cesarean section pain. Obstet Gynecol 72:136, 1988.

119. White PF: Use of patient-controlled analgesia for management of acute pain. JAMA 259:243, 1988.

120. Cohen SE, Woods WA: The role of epidural morphine in the postcesarean patient: Efficacy and effects on bonding. Anesthesiology 58:500, 1983.

121. Chadwick HS, Ready LB: Intrathecal and epidural morphine sulfate for postcesarean analgesia—a clinical comparison. Anesthesiology 68:925, 1988.

122. Knapp RM, Writer D: Epidural narcotics in obstetrics: survey of SOAP members (Abstract). Society for Obstetric Anesth Perinatol, 1988, p. 66.

123. Abboud TK, Dror A, Mosaad P: Mini-dose intrathecal morphine for the relief of post-cesarean section pain: Safety, efficacy and ventilatory responses to carbon dioxide. Anesth Analg 67:137, 1988.

124. Abouleish E, Rawal N, Fallon K, Hernandez D: Combined intrathecal morphine and bupivacaine for cesarean section. Anesth Analg 67:370, 1988.

125. Pelerossi JM: Maternal mortality. In Ostheimer GW (ed.): Manual of Obstetric Anesthesia. New York: Churchill Livingstone, 1984, p. 373.

126. Morgan M: Anaesthetic contribution to maternal mortality. Br J Anaesth 59:842, 1987.

127. Hunter AR, Moir DD: Confidential enquiry into maternal deaths. Br J Anaesth 55:367, 1983.

128. Marx GF, Berman JA: Anesthesia-related maternal mortality. Bull NY Acad Med 61:323, 1985.

6

Clinical Pelvimetry

Sterling E. Sightler

Pelvimetry is the measurement of the dimensions and capacity of the pelvis. This is most accurately accomplished by radiographic pelvimetry. Because of radiation hazards to mother and fetus and of failure to demonstrate an improvement in pregnancy outcomes with its use, radiographic pelvimetry has largely been abandoned except in cases of contemplated vaginal breech delivery.

Clinical pelvimetry entails using the hands to measure certain pelvic diameters, to assess the pelvic architecture, and to predict the adequacy of the pelvis for a particular fetus if done during labor or for a certain-sized fetus if done early in pregnancy. As a diagnostic tool, clinical pelvimetry is rapidly and easily performed at the time of pelvic examination, requires little or no equipment, is inexpensive, and incurs no risks or side effects other than minimal discomfort to the patient. With experience, the clinician can achieve a practical degree of accuracy in separating the adequate pelvis from the pelvis that is suspected to be inadequate.

It has been truly said that the fetal head is the best pelvimeter. It is never possible to determine by pelvimetry that the fetus will, in fact, pass safely through the pelvis. The obstetrician uses the information obtained with pelvimetry to aid decisions about the induction and conduct of labor. Evaluation of cephalopelvic relationships is necessary for clinical management decisions in protraction and arrest disorders of labor. Pelvimetry is important when considering vaginal delivery of presentations other than vertex, obstetric fetal manipulations, or forceps operations. The final test of whether safe passage can occur is progressive dilatation of the cervix and descent of the presenting part, accompanied by careful monitoring and evaluation of fetal and maternal parameters.

NORMAL PELVIC ANATOMY

The pelvis is composed of four bones: the two innominate bones, the sacrum, and the coccyx (Fig. 6–1). Each *innominate bone* has three parts: the ilium, the ischium, and the pubis. These three parts come together at the *acetabulum*, the fossa that articulates with the head of the femur. The *ilium* is the superior wing-shaped portion of the innominate bone, with a concavity on the medial surface termed the *iliac fossa*. Its upper curved border is the *iliac crest*, the terminal points of which form the *anterior superior* and *posterior superior iliac spines*. The *ischium* is the posterior inferior portion of the innominate bone, which forms most of the pelvic side wall. Its lowermost portion is the *ischial tuberosity*, the large prominence on which the body rests when in a sitting position. The *ischial spine* separates the *greater sciatic notch* from the *lesser sciatic notch* and is the landmark used to assess the station of the presenting part during labor. The *pubis* is the anterior inferior portion of the innominate bone and consists of a body, a *superior ramus*, and an *inferior ramus*. The two pubic bones meet in front to form the symphysis pubis, and the two inferior rami form the *pubic arch*. The superior border of the body is the *pubic crest*, which ends laterally in an elevation called the *pubic tubercle*. The sharp edge of the superior surface of the superior ramus forms the anterior portion of the *iliopectineal line*, and where it meets the ilium is found a small protuberance of the pelvic brim termed the *iliopectineal eminence*.

The *sacrum* is a wedge-shaped bone formed by the fusion of five sacral vertebrae; in rare cases, there are four or six. The anterior superior edge of the first sacral vertebra is the *sacral promontory*, and the lateral portions on each side are known as the *alae*, or wings. The *coccyx* is formed by the fusion of four (sometimes three or five) rudimentary vertebrae. In rare cases, the sacrum and the coccyx are fused, with resultant limitation of mobility of the sacrococcygeal joint.

There are four joints in the adult pelvis: the symphysis pubis, the sacrococcygeal joint, and two sacroiliac synchondroses. The *sacroiliac joint* is formed by the articulation of the sacrum with the ilium. This joint is partly cartilaginous and partly synovial, allowing for a limited backward and forward movement of the sacrum. The *sacrococcygeal joint* is a synovial hinge joint between the fifth sacral and the first coccygeal vertebrae. Extension of this joint allows the coccyx to bend backward during the delivery of the fetal head; overextension during delivery may result in fracture of the joint or of the coccyx itself. The *symphysis pubis* is a cartilaginous joint formed by the junction of the two pubic bones anteriorly. Normally, little movement occurs at this joint. During pregnancy, increased flexibility of all the pelvic joints occurs, which is thought to be a result of hormonal changes. The pubic bones may separate by 1.0 to 12.0 mm, leading to pain and difficulty in walking.[1]

Two accessory ligaments of the pelvis are of obstetric significance. The *sacrotuberous ligament* connects the sacrum with the ischial tuberosity, and it forms part of the lateral boundary of the pelvic outlet. The *sacrospinous ligament* connects the sacrum with the ischial spine; it spans the width of the greater sciatic notch.

For obstetric purposes, the pelvis is divided by the linea terminalis into the false pelvis above this demarcation and the true pelvis below it. The *linea terminalis*, or pelvic brim, includes the pubic crests, the iliopectineal lines, the alae of the sacrum, and the sacral promontory. The *false pelvis* is bounded by the lumbar vertebrae posteriorly, the iliac fossae laterally, and the lower portion of the anterior abdominal wall anteriorly. Its only obstetric function is to support the enlarging uterus during pregnancy and to direct the presenting part downward. The *true pelvis*, or pelvic cavity, is the bony canal through which the baby must pass to be born vaginally. It is shaped like a bent cylinder, with its anterior wall measuring about 5.0 cm and its posterior wall measuring about 10.0 cm. It is bounded superiorly by the linea terminalis; inferiorly by the ischial tuberosities and the tip of the coccyx; posteriorly by the anterior surface of the sacrum and the coccyx; laterally by the inner surface of the ischial bones and the sacrosciatic notches and ligaments; and anteriorly by the posterior surface of the symphysis pubis, the pubic bones, the obturator foramina, and the ascending rami of the ischial bones.

The normal *pelvic inclination* in the upright position is with the anterior superior iliac spine in the same vertical plane as the pubic tubercle. The plane of the pelvic brim thus makes an angle of about 60 degrees with the horizontal. With the pelvis thus oriented, the axis of force of the uterine contractions during labor is directed perpendicular to the inlet. In cases in which the pelvis is inclined considerably more posteriorly with the symphysis directly beneath the sacral promontory, labor is likely to be inefficient, with the force of the con-

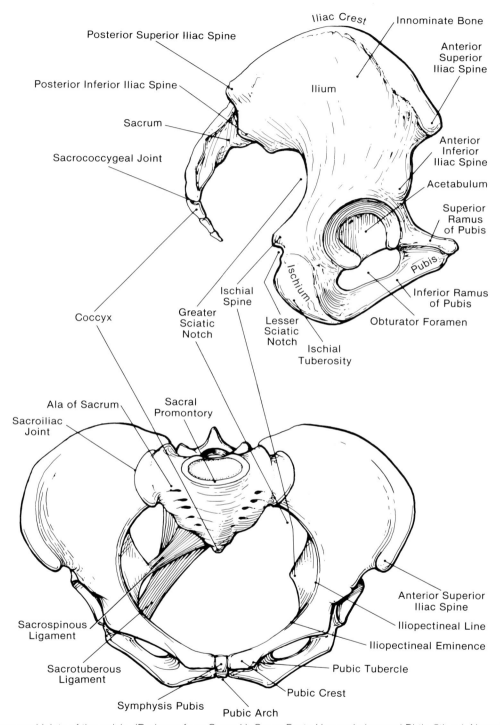

Figure 6–1. Bones and joints of the pelvis. (Redrawn from Oxorn H: Oxorn-Foote Human Labor and Birth, 5th ed. Norwalk, CT, Appleton-Century-Crofts, 1985.)

tractions directed against the pubis rather than into the inlet.

The *axis of the birth canal*, or pelvic curve, which is also known as the curve of Carus, is a curved line determined by drawing a perpendicular to each plane of the pelvis from inlet to outlet. It is the path taken by the presenting part as it passes through the pelvis. This curve corresponds to the pelvic curve of the forceps blades, and it is the curved path that must be reproduced in performing a forceps delivery. The station of the presenting part is measured along the pelvic curve.

Planes and Diameters of the Pelvis

The true pelvis has three planes of obstetric significance: the inlet, the plane of least dimensions, or the midplane, and the outlet. The pelvic cavity, or midpelvis, extends from the inlet to the outlet. Many planes at right angles to the pelvic axis can be constructed through this cavity, and all are anatomic midplanes. The largest of all the possible midplanes is called the *plane of greatest dimensions*; it is of no obstetric significance. The smallest of all the possible midplanes is called the *plane of least dimensions*. It is highly significant, as it is the smallest of the pelvic planes through which the baby must pass. The obstetric term *midplane* denotes the plane of least dimensions.

INLET. The *inlet*, also known as the superior strait, is the upper entrance into the true pelvis (Fig. 6–2). Its boundaries are the pubic crests anteriorly, the iliopectineal lines laterally, and the alae and promontory of the sacrum posteriorly. Six diameters of the inlet are customarily described: one transverse, two obliques, and three anteroposterior. The *anatomic conjugate*, or *true conjugate*, or *conjugata vera* is the anteroposterior diameter extending from the middle of the sacral promontory to the middle of the upper margin of the symphysis pubis. It normally measures 11.5 cm, and it is of no obstetric significance. The obstetrically important anteroposterior diameter is the *obstetric conjugate*, which is the shortest distance between the sacral promontory and the symphysis pubis. It is generally drawn from the middle of the sacral promontory to the closest point on the convex posterior surface of the symphysis pubis, and it usually measures 11.0 cm. If, however, there is a point on the upper sacrum or on the fifth lumbar vertebra that is closer to the symphysis than the sacral promontory, the posterior endpoint of the obstetric conjugate should be taken at that point.[2] Thus, the obstetric conjugate represents the actual space available to the fetus in negotiating the inlet. If the obstetric conjugate measures less than 10.0 cm, it is considered contracted.

The *diagonal conjugate* extends from the midpoint of the sacral promontory to the midpoint of the inferior margin of the symphysis pubis. It is

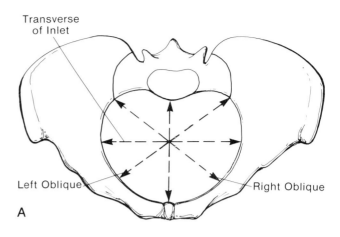

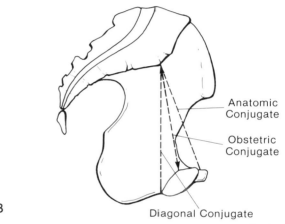

Figure 6–2. Pelvic inlet. *A*, Anteroposterior view. *B*, Sagittal section. (Redrawn from Oxorn H: Oxorn-Foote Human Labor and Birth, 5th ed. Norwalk, CT, Appleton-Century-Crofts, 1985.)

approximately 12.5 cm in length, and it is the only diameter of the inlet that can be measured clinically. By subtracting 1.5 cm from the diagonal conjugate, the approximate length of the obstetric conjugate can be obtained. This relationship between the obstetric conjugate and the diagonal conjugate was first recognized by Smellie in 1752. Radiographic studies have subsequently demonstrated that the difference between these two diameters actually varies from 0.1 to 3.1 cm.[2, 3]

The *transverse diameter of the inlet* is the widest distance between iliopectineal lines, which is perpendicular to the anteroposterior diameters, and it generally measures 13.5 cm. Each *oblique diameter* of the inlet extends from one sacroiliac synchondrosis to the opposite iliopectineal eminence and is designated right or left according to the sacroiliac synchondrosis from which it originates. Each oblique diameter averages 12.75 cm in length.

MIDPLANE. The *midplane*, or the plane of least dimensions, is bounded anteriorly by the inferior margin of the symphysis pubis, laterally by the ischial spines, and posteriorly by the level at which the plane determined by these three points intersects the sacrum, which is usually at the junction of the fourth and fifth sacral vertebrae (Fig. 6–3). The transverse diameter, called the *interspinous* or *bispinous diameter*, is the distance between the ischial spines. It is normally 10.5 cm in length. Less than 9.5 cm is considered contracted. The *anteroposterior diameter* of the midplane extends from the inferior margin of the pubic symphysis through the midpoint of the interspinous diameter to the point on the sacrum dictated by this angle. It measures about 12.0 cm and can be divided by the transverse diameter into *anterior sagittal* and *posterior sagittal segments*. The posterior sagittal diameter averages 4.5 to 5.0 cm in length. Less than 4.5 cm is considered inadequate.

OUTLET. The pelvic *outlet*, also known as the inferior strait, is not a single plane but is composed of two triangles with a common base, giving it the shape of a bent diamond (Fig. 6–4). The common base is the *bituberous diameter*, the distance between the inner aspects of the ischial tuberosities. This transverse diameter of the outlet measures

Table 6–1. SUMMARY OF PELVIC MEASUREMENTS

Pelvic Plane	Diameter	Average Length (cm)	Contracted Length (cm)
Inlet	Anatomic conjugate	11.5	
	Obstetric conjugate	11.0	10.0
	Diagonal conjugate	12.5	11.5
	Transverse of inlet	13.5	12.0
	Oblique diameters	12.75	
Midplane	Interspinous	10.5	9.5
	Anteroposterior of midplane	12.0	
	Posterior sagittal	4.5–5.0	4.5
Outlet	Anteroposterior of outlet	11.5	
	Bituberous	11.0	8.0*

*This is a clinical rather than an actual measurement.

approximately 11.0 cm. A clinical measurement of less than 8.0 cm is considered contracted. The apex of the anterior triangle is the inferior margin of the symphysis pubis. Its sides are the pubic rami and the ischial tuberosities. The apex of the posterior triangle is the tip of the sacrum, and its sides are the sacrotuberous ligaments. The *anteroposterior diameter of the outlet*, from the inferior margin of the symphysis to the sacrococcygeal joint, measures 11.5 cm. Because the coccyx is usually pushed out of the way by the advancing presenting part, it is not included in measurements of the outlet for obstetric purposes. The outlet is the only pelvic plane in which the anteroposterior diameter does not transect the transverse diameter. Table 6–1 summarizes the average and contracted values for the pelvic measurements.

Aspects of Pelvic Architecture

HEIGHT, INCLINATION, AND THICKNESS OF THE SYMPHYSIS

In the normal pelvis, the longitudinal axis of the symphysis is parallel to the longitudinal axis of the sacrum. If the inferior margin of the symphysis is inclined forward, it is called *anterior inclination of the symphysis* (Fig. 6–5). If the inferior margin of the symphysis is inclined backward, it is called *posterior inclination of the symphysis*. Anterior inclination increases the length of the diagonal conjugate relative to the obstetric conjugate, and it is necessary to subtract more than 1.5 cm from the diagonal conjugate to get the approximate length of the obstetric conjugate. Posterior inclination decreases the length of the diagonal conjugate relative to the obstetric conjugate, and it is necessary to subtract less than 1.5 cm.

The height of the symphysis is normally about 5.0 cm. Symphysial height of more than 6.0 cm increases the length of the diagonal conjugate relative to the obstetric conjugate, and it is necessary to subtract 2.0 to 2.5 cm from the diagonal

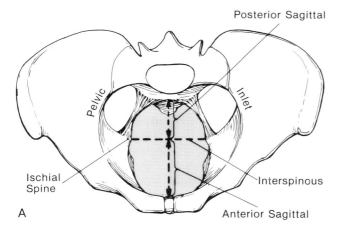

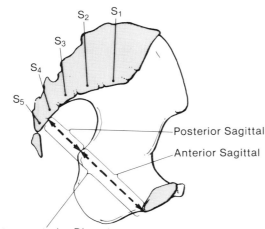

Figure 6–3. Pelvic midplane (plane of least dimensions). *A,* Anteroposterior view. *B,* Sagittal section. (Redrawn from Oxorn H: Oxorn-Foote Human Labor and Birth, 5th ed. Norwalk, CT, Appleton-Century-Crofts, 1985.)

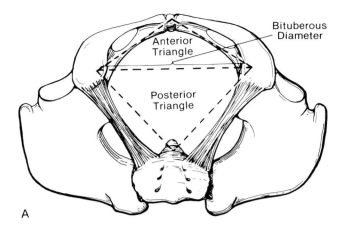

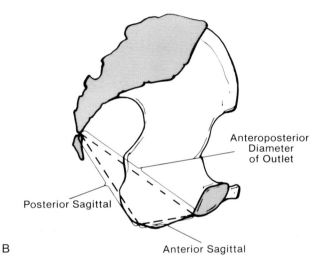

Figure 6–4. Pelvic outlet. *A,* Inferior view. *B,* Sagittal section. (Redrawn from Oxorn H: Oxorn-Foote Human Labor and Birth, 5th ed. Norwalk, CT, Appleton-Century-Crofts, 1985.)

conjugate to obtain the approximate length of the obstetric conjugate (Fig. 6–5). An unusually thick symphysis decreases the length of the obstetric conjugate relative to the diagonal conjugate, and

it may be necessary to subtract as much as 3.0 cm from the diagonal conjugate (Fig. 6–5).[4]

SIZE AND SHAPE OF THE PUBIC ARCH

The pubic arch is formed by the inferior margin of the symphysis pubis and the descending rami of the pubic bones. The angle formed by the pubic bones should be at least 90 degrees in a normal female pelvis. When the arch is wide and round, the fetal head fits easily under the symphysis, and the entire anteroposterior diameter of the outlet can be utilized by the fetal head. When the pubic arch is narrow, the fetal head is forced posteriorly and the usable portion of the anteroposterior diameter of the outlet is shortened.[5] In addition, when the head is forced posteriorly by a narrow arch, the incidence of perineal tears is increased unless a wide episiotomy is performed.[6]

SHAPE OF THE FOREPELVIS

The shape of the inner aspect of the forepelvis may be wide and round, narrow and oval, or narrow and angulated. When the forepelvis is wide and round, the larger transverse diameter of the fetal head (the biparietal rather than the bitemporal) can be accommodated in the forepelvis, and engagement usually occurs in the transverse or occiput anterior position. When the forepelvis is narrow and angulated, the biparietal diameter is forced posteriorly, and occiput posterior positions are more likely to occur.[7]

ANGLE OF THE PELVIC SIDE WALLS

The pelvic side walls extend from the pelvic brim at the point of the widest transverse diameter of the inlet in a downward and forward line to the inner aspects of the ischial tuberosities. In the normal pelvis, the side walls converge slightly. If the planes of each were extended beyond the pelvis, they would meet at about the level of the knees.[8] However, normal pelvic side walls are described as parallel or straight. Convergent side walls are associated with a funnel pelvis and often predict midplane or outlet contraction. The pelvis with

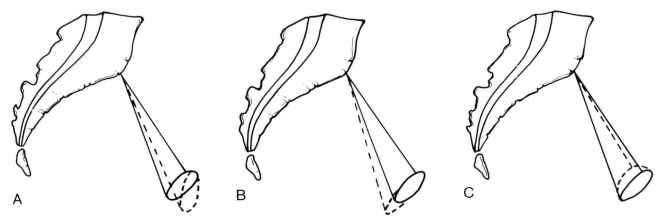

Figure 6–5. Variations in the height, inclination, and thickness of the symphysis pubis. *A,* Anterior inclination. *B,* Height greater than 6.0 cm. *C,* Unusual thickness. (Redrawn from Oxorn H: Oxorn-Foote Human Labor and Birth, 5th ed. Norwalk, CT, Appleton-Century-Crofts, 1985.)

divergent side walls is infrequently seen. It has been called the "blunderbuss" type of pelvis because of its association with precipitous delivery once the fetal head has negotiated the inlet.[9]

SACROSCIATIC NOTCH

The sacrospinous ligament lies between the lateral border of the sacrum and the ischial spine, and the width of the sacrosciatic notch is measured along this ligament. The width of the sacrosciatic notch is important because it affects the posterior sagittal diameters of the midplane and the outlet. The width of this notch, along with the shape and inclination of the sacrum, determines the amount of room in the posterior pelvis. If the notch is wide, the sacrum is inclined backward or its curve is deep, thus increasing the anteroposterior diameter of the midplane. A narrow notch indicates forward inclination of the sacrum, a flat sacrum, or both. In this situation, the anteroposterior diameter of the midplane is decreased and, particularly in association with very prominent spines, midplane contraction can be anticipated.

SHAPE OF THE SACRUM

The shape of the sacrum may be a gentle curve, a deep curve, flat, or J-shaped. Marked curvature of the sacrum in a shallow pelvis may bring the sacral tip in close proximity to the ischial spines, thereby decreasing the space available in the posterior midpelvis.[9] A J-shaped sacrum with a "fish-hook coccyx" that is angulated sharply forward may result in delay at the outlet if the coccyx does not fracture, and considerable discomfort in the postpartum period if it does.

CLASSIFICATION OF PELVIC TYPES

The classification system of pelvic types that is in current use was first described by two investigators, Caldwell and Moloy, in 1933. The Caldwell-Moloy classification is based on the shape of the pelvic inlet. Four pure or parent types were originally described: gynecoid, android, anthropoid, and platypelloid.[10] The majority of pelves are of mixed types and do not correspond exactly to one of the four pure types.[11, 12]

The *gynecoid* pelvis is the normal female pelvis. It occurs in about 50% of women, and it is the ideal pelvis for childbearing. It has a round or transverse oval inlet with the transverse diameter equal to or slightly greater than the anteroposterior diameter. The forepelvis is wide and round, the side walls are straight, the ischial spines are blunt, and the pubic arch is wide with a concave inward "Norman arch" configuration. The sacrum usually has an average curvature and an average or backward inclination with a medium to wide sacrosciatic notch, creating roominess throughout the midpelvis and the lower pelvis. Typically, engagement occurs in the transverse or oblique anterior position, followed by descent, anterior rotation, and spontaneous vaginal delivery.

The *android* pelvis is the typical male-type pelvis. It occurs in about 20% of all women, with an incidence of 25 to 35% in white women and 10 to 15% in black women. The bone structure is heavy in comparison with the other three pelvic types. The inlet is heart-shaped or wedge-shaped; this is created by the narrow and angulated forepelvis, coupled with a prominent sacral promontory that indents the shallow posterior segment of the inlet. The pubic arch is narrow with long, straight rami, simulating a "Gothic arch." The side walls are convergent, producing a funnel pelvis. The ischial spines are very prominent, often encroaching on the midplane. The sacrum is long, flat, and inclined forward, and the sacrosciatic notch is narrow, thus limiting the posterior sagittal diameters throughout the pelvis. Engagement usually occurs in the transverse or posterior position. A frequent outcome is deep transverse arrest or arrest as an occiput posterior with failure of rotation, leading to cesarean section or difficult midforceps rotation. If vaginal delivery occurs, the narrow pubic arch may lead to major perineal tears.

The *anthropoid* pelvis is known as the ape-like pelvis, resembling in shape that of the anthropoid apes. Its incidence is 25% in white women and 40 to 45% in black women. The inlet is oval, with the anteroposterior diameter much longer than the transverse diameter. In the anthropoid pelvis, all the anteroposterior diameters are longer and all the transverse diameters are shorter in comparison with the average gynecoid pelvis. The forepelvis is oval and more narrow than in the gynecoid pelvis. The side walls are generally straight, the spines are usually not encroaching, and the pubic arch is normal or relatively narrow but well shaped. The sacrum has an average curvature and an average or slightly backward inclination with a wide sacrosciatic notch, creating increased space in the posterior pelvis. Engagement usually occurs in the anteroposterior or an oblique diameter, and posterior positions are common. Fetuses in occiput posterior positions usually descend and deliver without rotating to an anterior position. The prognosis is good for spontaneous vaginal delivery, with an increased frequency of occiput posterior deliveries.

The *platypelloid* or flat pelvis is rare, occurring in less than 3% of women. The inlet is a transverse oval, with the transverse diameter much longer than the anteroposterior diameter. The characteristics of the platypelloid pelvis are those of a gynecoid pelvis that has been compressed in the anteroposterior direction; all the transverse di-

Table 6–2. CLASSIFICATION OF PELVIC TYPES

	Gynecoid	Android	Anthropoid	Platypelloid
Sex type	Normal female	Male	Ape-like	Flat female
Incidence	About 50%	About 20% 25–35% in white women 10–15% in black women	25% in white women 40–45% in black women	Less than 3%
Inlet				
Shape of inlet	Round, or transverse oval, with transverse diameter slightly greater than anteroposterior diameter	Heart-shaped, wedge-shaped, or triangular	Oval, with anteroposterior diameter much longer than transverse	Transverse oval, with transverse diameter much longer than anteroposterior diameter
Forepelvis	Well rounded and wide	Narrow and angulated	Oval, more narrow than the gynecoid pelvis	Very wide and round
Midpelvis				
Side walls	Straight	Convergent (funnel pelvis)	Straight or somewhat convergent	Straight or occasionally divergent
Ischial spines	Blunt	Very prominent, frequently encroaching on midplane	Blunt apex with broad base	Variable, somewhat prominent but not significant because transverse diameter very wide
Midpelvis				
Sacrum	Average width, average curvature, and average inclination	Long, flat, of average width, and inclined forward; limits posterior sagittal diameters throughout pelvis	Long, narrow, average curvature, frequently has 6 segments; average or backward inclination with increased space in posterior pelvis throughout	Wide and short, with average to deep curve and average inclination
Sacrosciatic notch	Medium to wide, at least 3 fingerbreaths	Narrow, 2 to 2.5 fingerbreadths, high-arched	Wide, about 4 fingerbreadths	Wide and flat
Outlet				
Pubic arch	Wide and round, >90°, Norman arch effect	Narrow, <90°, with long, straight rami, Gothic arch effect	Normal or relatively narrow but well shaped	Very wide

ameters are long, and all the anteroposterior diameters are shortened. If engagement can occur, it is in the transverse position, often with marked asynclitism. Frequently, however, there is disproportion at the inlet, leading to early cesarean section. Gradual extension of the head at the inlet may occur, creating brow presentations.

The characteristics of the four pelvic types are summarized in Table 6–2.[1]

TECHNIQUE OF CLINICAL PELVIMETRY

Clinical pelvimetry is generally performed during the first prenatal visit. The finding of a borderline or small pelvis alerts the clinician to the increased likelihood of disproportion during labor. Sharing these findings with the patient helps her to prepare for such a possibility. If a trial of labor after previous cesarean section is being considered, assessment of the pelvic capacity may figure prominently in the decision to allow or proscribe trial labor. In cases of known or suspected pelvic deformity, radiographic evaluation of the pelvis may be appropriate later in pregnancy (Fig. 6–6).

Some clinicians prefer to delay clinical evaluation of the pelvis until early in the third trimester or until 36 weeks' gestation. Relaxation and softening of the pelvic tissues reach a maximum about 1 month before term, so that late in pregnancy the examination can be performed with greater accuracy and less discomfort to the patient. If delivery occurs prior to 36 weeks, bony disproportion is not likely to be a problem. When the assessment is performed near term, some information about the size of the presenting part is available for comparison with the pelvis, particularly if engagement has occurred in a primigravid woman.[7] Although clinical pelvimetry need not be repeated during labor on all patients, it is indicated as part of the evaluation of dysfunctional labor when there is a question of disproportion.

Each practitioner should develop a routine for clinical pelvimetry so that the examination proceeds as quickly and smoothly as possible and so that no steps of the procedure are omitted. The examiner should bear in mind throughout the examination the effects of the soft tissues, tightness or looseness of the vaginal outlet, and the degree of relaxation of the patient on the findings. The results recorded should reflect the contour of and the distances between the bones, not the resistance of the perineal muscles or the general difficulty of the examination.

Hand Measurements

Before performing clinical pelvimetry, it is necessary to take several measurements of the hands for use in estimating certain diameters. First, the length of the reach of the examining fingers is taken from the tip of the longest (middle) finger to the junction of the index finger and thumb (Fig. 6–7). This is the reach that is used to obtain the diagonal conjugate; therefore the ruler should be pressed against the base of the thumb with the same degree of force that is exerted against the patient's symphysis to obtain the measurement.

Second, the width of the closed fist is measured from outer aspect to outer aspect of the knuckles of the four fingers (Fig. 6–8). This hand measurement is used in estimating the bituberous diameter. If an 8.0 cm fist can be inserted between the ischial tuberosities, the outlet is considered adequate. If the fist does not measure 8.0 cm, a third measurement should be taken by positioning the flexed thumb next to the first knuckle and adding the width of the thumb knuckle into the measurement (Fig. 6–9). This yields a second "pelvimeter" for use in estimating the bituberous diameter, although if it measures more than 10.0 cm, it rarely fits between the ischial tuberosities.[13]

Width of the Pubic Arch

The first step in clinical pelvimetry is to measure the width of the pubic arch by placing two fingers

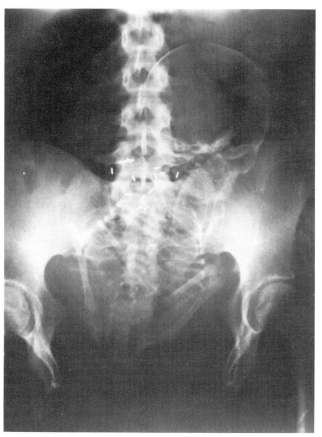

Figure 6–6. Pelvic radiograph in last trimester of pregnancy—breech presentation in a patient with congenital exstrophy of the bladder. Note absence of pubic bones and symphysis.

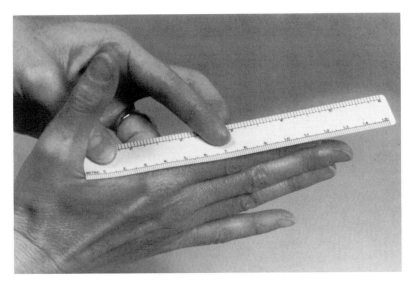

Figure 6–7. Measuring the hand for manual estimation of the diagonal conjugate.

directly under the symphysis pubis (Fig. 6–10). If the fingers rest comfortably beneath the bone and can be separated slightly, the arch is considered adequate, or greater than 90 degrees.

Height, Inclination, and Thickness of the Symphysis

Next, the index and middle fingers of the examining hand slide up along the posterior surface of the symphysis to the pelvic brim. The height of the symphysis is noted, as well as its thickness. The position of the symphysis is also noted for comparison with the position of the sacrum, which is to be assessed later; this determines whether there is anterior or posterior inclination of the

pubis. It is necessary to subtract 2.0 to 2.5 cm from the diagonal conjugate to obtain the length of the obstetric conjugate if the height of the symphysis is more than 6.0 cm, if the symphysis is unusually thick, or if there is anterior inclination of the symphysis. Although evaluation of the height, inclination, and thickness of the symphysis adds finesse to the evaluation of the pelvis, it is one of the more difficult and least essential aspects of the procedure and is omitted by many, if not most, examiners.

Forepelvis

The next step is to palpate the forepelvis to determine its curvature. The middle and index fingers are moved as far laterally as possible (to the patient's left if the examiner is right-handed) along the pelvic brim (Fig. 6–11). Then the fingers palpate back along the pelvic brim to the sym-

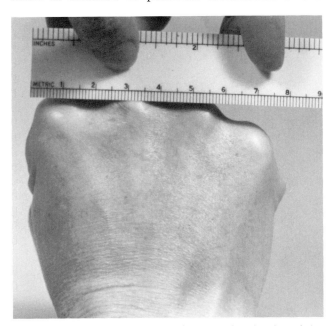

Figure 6–8. Measuring the hand for manual estimation of the bituberous diameter of the pelvis—the four-knuckle fist.

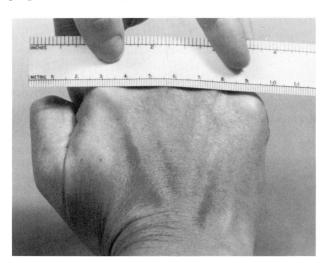

Figure 6–9. Measuring the five-knuckle fist for estimation of the bituberous diameter.

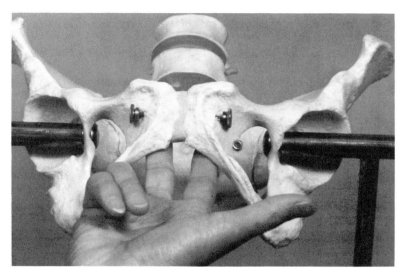

Figure 6–10. Manual estimation of the width of the pubic arch.

physis, across the symphysis, and as far as possible to the opposite side, following the anterior curvature of the pelvic brim.[13] As this maneuver is performed, note whether the forepelvis is smooth and round, or angulated, causing the fingers to dip into a V behind the symphysis and back out of the V on the opposite side. It is very important during this maneuver to lift the fingers away from the bone posteriorly as the urethra is crossed, as direct pressure on the urethra is extremely painful for the patient.

Side Walls

The pelvic side wall is next palpated to determine whether it is straight, convergent, or divergent. Starting from the right lateral pelvic brim where the assessment of the forepelvis ended, the fingers palpate straight down the pelvic side wall to the base of the ischial spine, in the direction of the ischial tuberosity. The endpoint of the palpa-

tion is the base of the ischial spine, not the tip of the spine, which projects inward and makes many normal pelves feel convergent if the palpation is continued inward to the tip.

A helpful maneuver in evaluating the side walls is to place the thumb of the other hand on the ischial tuberosity and note its relationship to the examining fingers located at the base of the ischial spine. If the thumb on the ischial tuberosity is medial to the fingertips on the base of the ischial spine, the side walls converge; if it is lateral, they diverge.[14]

Ischial Spines

The ischial spine is then palpated and assessed as to whether it is blunt (difficult to identify at all), prominent (easily felt but not large), or very prominent (large and encroaching on the midplane). If identification of the ischial spine is dif-

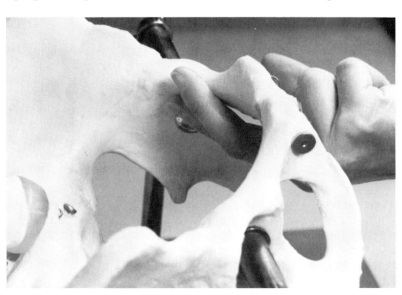

Figure 6–11. Manually estimating the curvature of the forepelvis.

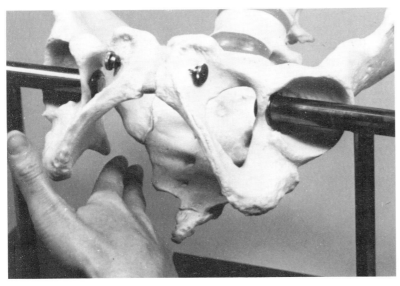

Figure 6–12. Estimating the width of the sacrosciatic notch (sacrospinous ligament).

ficult, it can be located by following the sacrospinous ligament to its lateral end.

Sacrosciatic Notch

The sacrospinous ligament is followed medially from the ischial spine to the edge of the sacrum. An estimate is made of how many fingers could be placed side by side along the length of the ligament between the spine and the sacrum (Fig. 6–12). Two and a half fingerbreadths or more is considered adequate.

Mobility of the Coccyx

From the edge of the sacrum the fingers move to the tip of the coccyx and press firmly on it several times to determine whether it gives. If it does, it is movable. If it does not, it is fixed. If mobility is difficult to determine, one or two fingers of the other hand may be placed against the posterior aspect of the coccyx externally and an attempt made to move it to and fro between the fingers of the two hands. Note should be made if the coccyx juts forward, forming a sharp angle with and creating a J-shaped sacrum.

Shape and Inclination of the Sacrum

After testing the coccyx, the examining fingers move up the sacrum toward the promontory by palpating progressively higher along its anterior surface. The shape is assessed by noting whether the fingers follow a flat plane or whether they move progressively in a posterior direction into a gentle or deep curve. The inclination of the sacrum

is forward if it is easy to reach and backward if it is difficult to reach. An attempt is also made to compare the longitudinal axis of the sacrum with the position of the symphysis, which was estimated earlier, to determine whether they are parallel, or whether there is anterior or posterior inclination of the symphysis.

Diagonal Conjugate

The diagonal conjugate, the distance from the sacral promontory to the inferior aspect of the symphysis, is measured next. If contact can be maintained with the sacrum throughout its whole length, the fingers simply keep moving upward until the promontory is reached, and the measurement is easily taken. In many cases, however, the fingers lose contact with the sacrum if it has a deep curve or a posterior inclination. Should this occur, the fingers should continue moving upward because the sacrum may be re-encountered just below or at the promontory as it curves forward. In reaching for the promontory, the wrist of the examining hand should be dropped so that the direction of the fingers is at a 45-degree angle with the horizontal. Maximal pressure can be exerted against the perineum by bracing the elbow of the examining arm on the examiner's hip or thigh, with the foot elevated on the step of the examining table.[13]

If the promontory is touched, contact with it is maintained while raising the hand until it touches the undersurface of the symphysis pubis (Fig. 6–13). The point where the examining hand touches the symphysis is marked with a finger of the other hand. After the hand is withdrawn from the vagina, the distance from the tip of the middle finger to the mark is measured, and this distance is recorded as the diagonal conjugate. If the promontory is not reached, the diagonal conjugate is

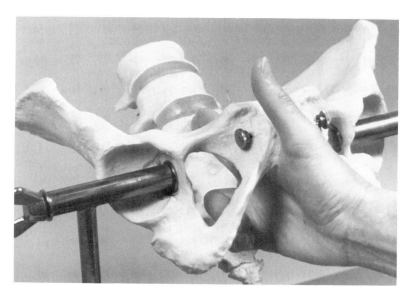

Figure 6–13. Manual estimation of the diagonal conjugate.

recorded as being greater than the number of centimeters of the examiner's previously measured reach.

Interspinous Diameter

The next step is estimation of the interspinous diameter, which is probably the most difficult and least accurate part of clinical pelvimetry. First, the patient's left ischial spine is located and then the right spine, which has been previously felt, is relocated. The two examining fingers are then spread as far apart as possible, and an attempt is made to place one finger on each spine. This is rarely possible, no matter how far apart the fingers can be spread in unrestricted space, as the introitus limits the finger spread that can be achieved within the vagina. If both spines can be touched simultaneously, the interspinous diameter is about 9.5 cm or less and is therefore inadequate for an average-sized baby.

If the spines are not touched simultaneously, the distance between them is estimated by sweeping the fingers across the pelvic cavity from one ischial spine to the other and back again several times. Considerable experience is required to develop accuracy at this maneuver.

While this maneuver is being performed, the examiner's impression of the adequacy of the pubic arch can be confirmed by noting whether the arch constricts the knuckles of the index and middle fingers as they are pronated and supinated beneath it. If it is difficult to turn the fingers over to cross the pelvic cavity, the arch is probably narrow. If the knuckles turn easily, it is probably adequate. To appreciate this, it is necessary that the fingers remain extended in alignment with the forearm and not be permitted to flex while performing this maneuver.[15]

Other Side of the Pelvis

Some practitioners believe that both sides of the pelvis should be palpated and evaluated completely. To do this, it is necessary either to turn the examining hand over to measure the notch and palpate the side wall on the opposite side or to withdraw the hand and use the other hand to do this. Most clinicians feel that unless there is some reason to suspect that the pelvis is asymmetric, such as a history of pelvic fracture or an obvious physical deformity, it is sufficient to palpate only one side and to assume that the two sides of the pelvis are similar.[13]

Anteroposterior Diameter of the Outlet

Although it is not usually done, it is possible to measure the anteroposterior diameter of the outlet clinically. To do so, the tips of the examining fingers are placed on the tip of the sacrum, which is the last rigid part of the sacrum above the movable coccyx. The examining hand is raised until it touches the undersurface of the symphysis, and the point of the contact is marked with a finger of the other hand. This distance can be measured after withdrawing the hand in the same manner as for the diagonal conjugate.

Shape of the Pubic Arch

After the hand is withdrawn, the shape of the pubic arch is evaluated by placing the thumbs of both hands beneath the symphysis and palpating downward along the descending rami to the ischial

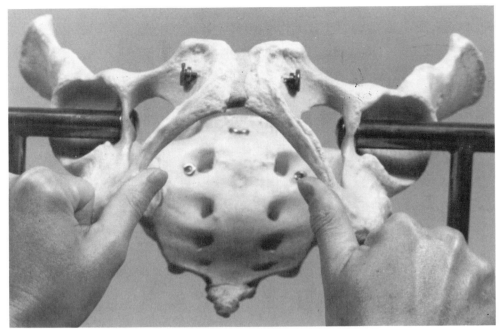

Figure 6–14. Evaluating the shape of the pubic arch.

tuberosities, noting the width and curvature of the path taken by the thumbs (Fig. 6–14).

Bituberous Diameter

Last, the bituberous diameter is estimated by placing the previously measured closed fist be-tween the inner aspects of the ischial tuberosities (Fig. 6–15). For examiners with small hands, a second estimate can be made by attempting to place the previously measured five-knuckle fist between the tuberosities. The actual bituberous diameter will be one or two centimeters greater than the width of a fist that exactly fits between the tuberosities, because one or more centimeters

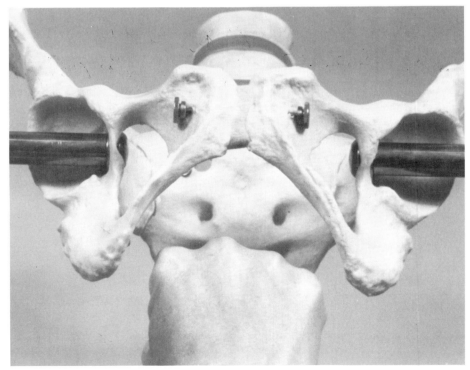

Figure 6–15. Manual estimation of the bituberous diameter.

Table 6–3. CLINICAL PELVIMETRY PROTOCOL WITH FINDINGS INDICATING AN ADEQUATE PELVIS

Width of pubic arch	≥90°
*Height, inclination, and thickness of symphysis	Thickness: average Inclination: parallel to sacrum
Forepelvis	Round
Side walls	Straight
Ischial spines	Blunt
Sacrosciatic notch	2.5–3 fingerbreadths
Coccyx	Movable
Curvature and inclination of sacrum	Hollow, average inclination
Diagonal conjugate	≥11.5 cm
Interspinous diameter	≥10.0 cm
*Anteroposterior diameter of outlet	≥11.0 cm
Shape of pubic arch	Well rounded
Bituberous diameter	>8.0 cm
Prognosis:	Adequate for a 7.5-lb baby

*These items are optional.

of space are occupied by the soft tissue, depending on the weight of the patient. When measured clinically, the bituberous diameter is recorded as greater than the number of centimeters of the fist used as the pelvimeter (or less than, if the fist did not fit).

Confirmation by Rectovaginal Examination

If evaluation of the midpelvic and lower pelvic structures was difficult, these structures can be re-evaluated by rectovaginal examination. The coccyx, ischial spines, sacrosciatic notch, and lower sacrum are felt more easily through the rectum than vaginally.

Table 6–3 summarizes the clinical pelvimetry protocol, along with the findings accepted as indicating an adequate pelvis. It is recommended that the record of the clinical pelvimetry findings conclude with a summary statement of the examiner's overall impression, such as "Adequate for 9-lb baby;" "Android tendencies—watch for cephalopelvic disproportion in the midpelvis;" or "Short obstetric conjugate—watch for cephalopelvic disproportion at the inlet."

CONCLUSIONS

Clinical pelvimetry has been largely ignored as a field of obstetric competence in the past decade.

As attempts are made to reduce the rate of cesarean sections by carefully considering vaginal delivery for many cases, knowledge of the architecture of the maternal pelvis and estimates of the size of critical pelvic diameters assume increasing importance.

The obstetrician must diligently practice this elusive skill. The reward is better decisions about induction of labor, management of prolonged and arrested labor, and safer outcomes for fetal manipulations and vaginal operative deliveries.

Careful clinical pelvimetry is an important component of the physical examination of every pregnant woman.

References

1. Oxorn H: Oxorn-Foote Human Labor and Birth, 5th edition. Norwalk, Connecticut: Appleton-Century-Crofts, 1986, pp. 1–6; 23–39.
2. Kaltreider DF: The diagonal conjugate. Am J Obstet Gynecol 61:1075–1086, 1951.
3. Dippel AL: The diagonal conjugate versus x-ray pelvimetry. Surg Gynecol Obstet 1939; 68:642–647.
4. Greenhill JP: Principles and Practice of Obstetrics. 10th edition. Philadelphia: W. B. Saunders Co., 1951, pp. 108–116.
5. Wallace JT: Practical manual pelvimetry. GP 36:121–127, 1967.
6. Iffy L, Kaminetzky HA: Principles and practice of obstetrics and perinatology. New York: John Wiley and Sons, 1981, pp. 733–745.
7. Danforth DN, Scott JR, DiSaia PJ, Hammond CB, Spellacy WN, eds.: Obstetrics and Gynecology, 5th edition. Philadelphia: J. B. Lippincott Co., 1986, pp. 43–48; 629–646.
8. Cunningham GF, MacDonald PC, Gant NF: Williams Obstetrics. 18th edition. Norwalk, Connecticut: Appleton and Lange, 1989, pp. 163–175.
9. Grody MH: Clinical and radiologic pelvimetry in obstetrics. GP 7:34–36, 1953.
10. Caldwell WE, Moloy HC: Anatomical variations in the female pelvis and their effect in labor with a suggested classification. Am J Obstet Gynecol 26:479–505, 1933.
11. Caldwell WE, Moloy HC, D'Esopo DA: Further studies on the pelvic architecture. Am J Obstet Gynecol 28:482–497, 1934.
12. Caldwell WE, Moloy HC, D'Esopo DA: The more recent conceptions of the pelvic architecture. Am J Obstet Gynecol 40:558–565, 1940.
13. Varney H: Nurse-Midwifery, 2nd edition. Boston: Blackwell Scientific Publications, Inc., 1987, pp. 729–743.
14. Danforth DN: Clinical pelvimetry, Chapter 51, 1977. In Sciarra JJ (ed.): Gynecology and Obstetrics, Vol. 2: Clinical Obstetrics. Philadelphia: Harper & Row Publishers, Inc., 1977.
15. Steer CM: Moloy's evaluation of the pelvis in obstetrics, 3rd edition. New York: Plenum Medical Book Co., 1975.

II

Surgical Problems of Early Pregnancy

7

Pregnancy Termination

Haywood Brown

Abortion is the most frequent outcome of human conception. Abortions are divided into two general categories: (1) spontaneous abortions, in which there is expulsion of products of conception without deliberate interference and (2) induced abortions, in which a deliberate effort to terminate the pregnancy has occurred. The actual incidence of spontaneous abortion is unknown. This is primarily because of the difficulty in recognition of very early conception and wastage. Many pregnancy losses occur before the woman is aware of the pregnancy. However, it is estimated that the overall rate of spontaneous abortion in recognized pregnancy is approximately 10 to 15%. More simply stated, one in every six women with a known pregnancy has a spontaneous abortion.

Legal abortion in the United States occurs 1.5 million times annually. When legal and spontaneous abortion are added together, it is clear that there are as many abortions in the United States as live births.

The Committee on Terminology of the American College of Obstetricians and Gynecologists defines abortion as termination of pregnancy prior to the twentieth completed week of gestation (139 days), calculated from the first day of the last normal menstrual period. The World Health Organization classifies abortions as early or late, depending on

119

whether they occur before 12 weeks or between 12 and 20 weeks of gestation. In some instances, fetal weight may also figure into this definition of abortion if the weight of the fetus is less than 500 g.

SPONTANEOUS AND INDUCED ABORTIONS

Spontaneous abortion can be subdivided into the following categories:

1. *Threatened*—the condition in which bleeding of intrauterine origin occurs with or without uterine colic, without expulsion of the products of conception, and without dilation of the cervix.

2. *Inevitable*—the condition in which bleeding of intrauterine origin occurs with continuous and progressive dilation of the cervix but without expulsion of the products of conception.

3. *Incomplete*—expulsion of some but not all products of conception.

4. *Complete*—expulsion of all products of conception.

5. *Missed*—abortion in which the embryo or fetus dies but is retained in utero for 8 weeks or more.

6. *Habitual*—the occurrence of three or more consecutive spontaneous abortions.

7. *Septic*—an infected abortion in which there is dissemination of microorganisms and their products into the maternal systemic circulation.

Induced abortion can also be subdivided into the following:

1. *Therapeutic*—interruption of pregnancy for medically approved indication.

2. *Nontherapeutic*—interruption of pregnancy without medical indication by any means.

3. *Criminal or illegal abortion*—although these are not appropriate medical terms, they refer to interruption of pregnancy under circumstances not legally acceptable in the state in which the abortion is performed.

Threatened Abortion

In threatened abortion, the likelihood of spontaneous abortion is approximately 50%.[1] The bleeding associated with threatened abortion is usually scanty and occurs repeatedly over many days. Vaginal bleeding may vary from bright red spotting to a dark brownish discharge. There is no good evidence that drugs or other therapy affect the course of threatened abortion.

With accurate dating of conception, the lack of fetal cardiac activity on real-time ultrasonography after 8 weeks' gestation is the best predictor of outcome. A poor prognosis warrants therapeutic intervention. The validity of hormonal assays such as human chorionic gonadotropin, human placental lactogen, estradiol, and progesterone varies widely in predicting outcome in threatened abortion.

Inevitable and Incomplete Abortion

Hemorrhage in inevitable and incomplete abortion can be brisk, and in many circumstances it may be life-threatening. In both instances, there is no opportunity for fetal salvage, and attempts at preservation of pregnancy are contraindicated. Inevitable abortion is signaled by gross rupture of membranes and cervical dilation. In this situation, no tissue may pass for hours or even days. On rare occasions, leakage or rupture of membranes occurs in the first trimester and early second trimester without serious consequences. In fact, genetic amniocentesis carries a significant risk of rupture of membranes which, when managed conservatively, is associated with an overall good outcome. However, in spontaneous and unprovoked situations, the majority of women with rupture of membranes in early pregnancy ultimately have bleeding, cramping, or even fever, which necessitates immediate uterine evacuation.

Prior to 10 weeks' gestation, fetal and placental tissue are likely to be expelled completely in cases of abortion. However, after 10 weeks, it is not unusual to see retention of all or part of the products of conception accompanied by significant uterine bleeding, indicating an incomplete abortion. Bleeding in an incomplete abortion, especially in more advanced gestations, can be profuse, leading to hypovolemia and even shock. A partially separated placenta can usually be blamed for this brisk bleeding. The partially separated placenta interferes with normal myometrial contractility in the area of detachment, leaving exposed vessels at the placental site that do not have the ability to vasoconstrict because of poor myometrial contractility.

Suction curettage is the primary method of uterine evacuation in the first trimester and early second trimester in inevitable abortions. After 14 weeks' gestation, evacuation by prostaglandin E vaginal suppositories is more appropriate in inevitable abortions. However, in incomplete abortion, bleeding is often more significant, and suction curettage is the safest and most efficient option for prompt uterine evacuation.

Complete Abortion

It is often difficult to distinguish between complete abortion and those in which the products of conception are incompletely expelled. In both instances, the cervix may be open or closed, uterine size similar, and bleeding absent or present. Curettage in women with complete abortion is controversial. It has been suggested that as many as

30% of women with a recognized complete abortion do not require curettage. However, necrosis of decidua remaining in the uterus after complete abortion is a common cause of postabortion bleeding and infection. Therefore, curettage has been advocated, even in cases where the conceptus has been passed intact, to shorten recovery time. Nevertheless, it is not our practice to routinely perform or recommend curettage in complete abortion, especially in situations in which an intact gestational sac with placental or decidual tissue is confirmed to be present and the patient has a normal examination without signs of continued bleeding.

HISTORY OF INDUCED ABORTION

Since the Supreme Court ruling on January 22, 1973, legal pregnancy termination has become one of the most frequently performed operations in the United States. In 1987, 1.3 million legal abortions were reported to the Centers for Disease Control from the 50 states and the District of Columbia.[2] In 1987, there were 24 abortions per 1000 women, ages 15 to 44, or 356 abortions per 1000 live births. This rate is less than the 25 abortions per 1000 women reported for 1980 by the Centers for Disease Control. In the 1980 report, 29% of abortions were in teenagers, 36% in women 20 to 24 years of age, and 35% in older women.[2] In 1987, the number of teenagers obtaining abortions decreased to 26%, 33% occurred in women 20 to 24 years of age, and 41% occurred in women over 24 years of age. In addition, women who obtained abortions were usually white (65%) and unmarried (73%).[2]

Techniques for attempting abortion are evident in the artifacts of ancient civilizations. Even today, various folk medicines and techniques are used throughout the world to induce abortion. These include oral abortifacients derived from various plant substances and various objects and instruments that can be inserted through the cervix into the uterus. In the nineteenth century and first two thirds of the twentieth century, illegal abortions were common in the United States.

In spite of the current widespread availability of legal abortion in the United States, a small number of illegally performed abortions continue to occur. Estimates by Binkin and colleagues[3] for the late 1970s of the number of illegal abortions in the United States ranged from 5000 to 23,000 per year. Before 1970, as many as 200,000 to 1.2 million illegal procedures were performed in the United States annually.[4] Polgar and Fried[5] reported the most frequently used oral substances for inducing abortion in the 1960s in New York City. These included such caustic agents as turpentine, laundry bleach, and quinine, and intrauterine substances such as soap, phenol disinfectants, and insertable foreign objects.

The complications of illegally performed abortions in the United States and competition from lay abortionists concerned the medical societies to such degree in the late 1800s that laws were passed making abortion illegal in most states by the end of the nineteenth century.[8] However, many procedures continued to be performed illegally even after the 1973 Supreme Court decision.

Only seventeen women were reported dead from illegal abortion in the United States between 1975 and 1979.[3] However, illegal abortion leads to complications that cause 115,000 to 200,000 maternal deaths each year worldwide.[6] Infection and hemorrhage from uterine or cervical lacerations cause the majority of deaths. In Bangladesh alone, an estimated 5000 and 7800 women die from illegal abortions each year.[7] In Mexico, where 1.5 million illegal abortions are performed annually, approximately 140,000 women die of complications. In the 17 illegal abortion deaths in the United States between 1975 and 1979, sepsis (10 cases) and air embolism (3 cases) accounted for the majority.[3] Embolism resulted from intrauterine manipulation, injection of cleaning solutions, or insertion of foreign bodies, such as catheters or coat hangers.

PREGNANCY TERMINATION

In recent years, there has been much debate on the pros and cons of legalized abortion in the United States. Recent legislation on the Federal and State levels has threatened women's reproductive rights with regard to legal abortion. In this author's opinion, a woman's right to legalized abortion is essential if for no other reason than the implication illegal abortion has for medical care and society.

PREGNANCY TERMINATION METHODS

The various techniques for pregnancy termination can be subdivided into two broad categories: surgical evacuation and labor-induced evacuation (Table 7–1).

The choice of method for pregnancy termination

Table 7–1. METHODS FOR PREGNANCY TERMINATION

Surgical Evacuation
Menstrual regulation (minisuction)
Vacuum suction curettage
Dilation and evacuation
Hysterotomy/hysterectomy
Labor Induction
Intrauterine instillation
($PGF_{2\alpha}$, hypertonic saline, urea)
(vaginal)
15-methyl PGF_2 (intramuscular)
Antiprogesterones
Mifepristone (RU-486)
Epostane

is largely dependent on the duration of pregnancy (weeks of gestation) and the skill of the clinician. In 1987, over 93% of pregnancy terminations were accomplished by suction curettage and over 50% were performed at 8 weeks' gestation or less. Less than 1% of abortions were performed after 21 weeks' gestation.[2]

Surgical Evacuation

The most frequently used and by far the safest method for abortion is suction curettage. Vacuum aspiration was first described by two Chinese physicians in 1954.[9] Prior to this time, most procedures were performed by dilation and curettage (D and C) or by scraping the uterus with a sharp curette after manual cervical dilation. In comparison to sharp curettage, vacuum procedures are felt to be less traumatic, quicker, much safer, and associated with less blood loss. Suction curettage is the method of choice for first trimester abortion.

Preoperative evaluation of patients for abortion by suction evacuation should include counseling, which may be best performed a day or so preceding the operation to ensure that the patient is emotionally committed to undergoing the abortion. At this time, informed consent should be obtained and a brief history and physical examination performed focusing on gynecologic and medical problems that may complicate the operation.

Appropriate laboratory tests should include a hematocrit or hemoglobin level or both, Rh type, and possibly a cervical culture for gonorrhea.

MENSTRUAL EXTRACTION PROCEDURE

Menstrual extraction, or menstrual regulation, or minisuction, is a suction aspiration abortion technique that was first described in the early 1970s.[10, 11] This procedure can be performed 42 to 50 days from the first day of the last menstrual period (6 weeks' gestation). The procedure employs a small-bore, flexible vacuum cannula 4 mm to 6 mm in diameter, as described by Karman and Potts,[11] and a 50-ml syringe as a vacuum source and requires minimal to no dilation.

Menstrual regulation was originally seen as a safe and cost-effective means of early pregnancy termination, with many advantages when properly performed.[12] However, it is important that this procedure not be performed until a positive pregnancy test is confirmed. This should not pose a problem, considering the sensitivity of modern pregnancy tests. The reason for such caution comes from years of experience that demonstrated several shortcomings with minisuction, such as attempted abortion in women who were not pregnant and failure to abort a very early gestation. Because the procedure was originally performed before a positive pregnancy test was confirmed, between 27% and 59% of menstrual extraction procedures were performed on women who were not pregnant. Failure tests, defined by incomplete evacuation or continuing pregnancy, were as high as 11 to 12%.[13, 14]

Anesthesia is not usually required for minisuction, although mild preoperative sedation with pentobarbital sodium or a mild analgesic, such as 25 to 50 mg of meperidine administered intramuscularly, relieves anxiety and the cramping that normally occurs at the end of the evacuation procedure.

After proper pelvic examination has confirmed the shape and position of the uterus and a gestation of less than 7 weeks, the cervix is exposed with a speculum and cleansed with an appropriate antiseptic, such as povidone-iodine solution. A cannula 4 to 5 mm in diameter can then be atraumatically placed through the cervical canal as a dilator, if necessary. This step is usually not required in the parous female. A 5- to 6-mm flexible plastic cannula is then inserted into the uterine cavity and attached to a 50-mL syringe, and the pinch valve is released to establish suction.

The cannula is rotated with gentle strokes to different areas of the uterine cavity and pushed in and out while staying within the uterine cavity until no more tissue is returned. A gritty feel of the endometrial cavity as the cannula scrapes against the uterine wall and the appearance of bubbles in the syringe are good indications that the cavity is empty. The plastic cannula should then be removed from the uterine cavity, exposing the tip, which should be cleared in a sterile manner. The cannula tip can be cleared manually by extracting tissue with forceps or by aspirating saline through the cannula. Once cleared, the plastic cannula can be reinserted and the vacuum re-established to confirm that the uterus has indeed been emptied. Care should be taken not to remove the cannula while it is under vacuum and not to advance the syringe plunger while it is connected to the cannula within the uterine cavity, because air embolism can result.

The tissue specimens obtained should be inspected. This can be accomplished by floating the aspirated tissue in a clear container of saline and carefully visualizing the specimen over a light source until the gestational sac is identified.

Careful inspection of the aspirated tissue, histologic examination, and follow-up pregnancy test and pelvic examination reduce the possibility of a failed or incomplete abortion's going unnoticed.[15]

VACUUM SUCTION CURETTAGE

Suction or vacuum curettage (Fig. 7–1), or suction D and C, is similar to minisuction but requires dilation of the cervix prior to aspiration of the uterine cavity and employs larger cannulas, from 7 to 12 mm in diameter. The procedure is reserved

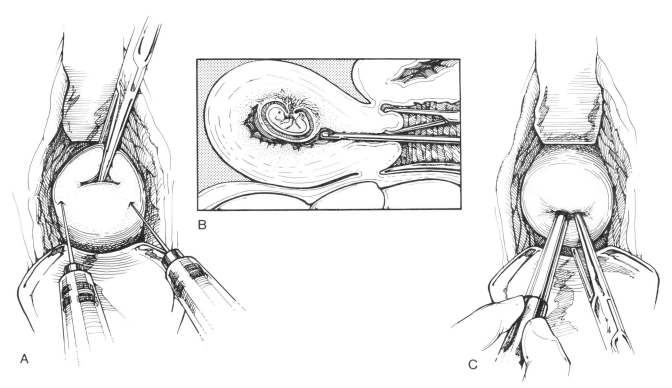

Figure 7–1. Vacuum suction curettage. *A*, Administration of paracervical block anesthesia. *B*, Cannula inserted to the level of the lower uterine segment. *C*, Suction is applied at 60 cm Hg as the cannula moves in piston-like fashion through 360 degrees of rotation.

for patients 7 to 12 weeks from the first day of the last menses. Up to 12 weeks' gestation, virtually all pregnancy terminations in the United States are performed using this method.[16] Although in some hands suction curettage can safely be employed in gestations of up to 15 weeks, between 13 and 20 weeks, the more complicated dilation and evacuation (D and E) technique is the most frequently used.[16]

Vacuum curettage procedures are usually performed in an outpatient setting unless the patient's medical history dictates hospitalization and medical consultation (e.g., in the case of cardiac disease). The patient should have fasted on the day of the procedure. Review her history and physical examination prior to beginning the surgery.

The woman should empty her bladder before being placed in dorsal lithotomy position, or a catheter should be used to drain the bladder when the patient is in position.

Anesthesia for vacuum curettage depends on gestational age and must be individualized based on the degree of patient anxiety or apprehension. For most patients, a paracervical block anesthetic is sufficient, especially if the pregnancy is of less than 10 weeks' gestation. General anesthesia can be used, but local anesthesia such as paracervical block is safer and less expensive and its use is predominant in the United States in suction abortions.[17]

Paracervical block anesthesia can be performed after insertion of the speculum and appropriate cleansing of the vagina and cervix with an anti-septic solution such as povidine-iodine. Local anesthetics, such as 0.5 to 1% lidocaine hydrochloride, 0.25% bupivacaine hydrochloride, or 2% chloroprocaine hydrochloride, are most commonly used for the procedure. A small volume of the lowest concentration of anesthetic should be used. The use of a local anesthetic with a vasoconstrictor, such as epinephrine, 1:200,000, slows absorption of the drug and often results in the need for a higher total dose. If lidocaine hydrochloride, 0.5% or 1%, is used, the total dose should not exceed 300 mg.

Using a 21-gauge spinal needle, a total of approximately 10 mL of anesthetic is used and injected superficially just under the vaginal epithelium at the lateral margins of the cervix into two to four sites: 3 and 9 o'clock or 3, 5, 7, and 9 o'clock (Fig. 7–1A). Usual aspiration precautions should be observed, making sure the needle is subepithelial and thereby avoiding intravascular injection. A small amount of anesthetic may also be injected at 12 o'clock prior to placing the tenaculum. Wait at least 3 minutes after the last site is injected for the anesthetic to take effect.

After adequate anesthesia is obtained, slowly dilate the cervix by serially inserting tapered dilators up to a diameter of 1 mm less than the estimated menstrual weeks of gestation or just enough to allow insertion and rotation of the desired plastic cannula. Use of the uterine sound to determine the depth of the uterus is not indicated and only increases the risk of perforation.

Pratt dilators require less force to dilate the

cervix than Hegar dilators and are preferable for suction-type abortions. Carefully dilate the cervix to avoid cervical laceration or uterine perforation. Irreparable cervical injury may occur with overzealous dilation, resulting in an incompetent cervix and infertility.

Proper technique for cervical dilation includes holding the dilator between the thumb and the index finger. If more than the force of two fingers is required to dilate the cervix, the clinicain should consider other options rather than risk cervical injury from too much force. Options to be considered at this point include using a smaller plastic cannula or packing the cervix with laminaria and completing the procedure after appropriate dilatation has occurred.

Laminaria are often used prior to abortion procedures as an alternative to the standard forcible dilation with tapered rods that is most commonly employed in abortion techniques (Fig. 7–2).

Several types of preabortion laminaria substances are currently being used for cervical dilation. Several hours are usually needed for laminaria to exert their effect, and they may be left in overnight. The number of laminaria used depends on the size of the cervical canal. Place as many laminaria as the cervix will accommodate.

Laminaria tents *L. japonicum* and *L. digitata,* the hygroscopic stems of dried seaweed, have a complicated mode of action. When placed in the cervical canal as small, dry twigs, laminaria take up water from the cervix over several hours and slowly swell. They exert gentle pressure on the cervical canal, forcing it to soften and open. Stubblefield[18] has suggested the principal mechanism of action of laminaria to be desiccation of the cervix, altering the ratio of collagen to ground substance. Laminaria may also have an effect via

elaboration or degradation of uterine prostaglandin $F_{2\alpha}$ ($PGF_{2\alpha}$). Other synthetic laminaria-like substances currently being used include Lamicel, which is a magnesium sulfate sponge, and Dilipan, which is manufactured from polyacrylate-based hydrogel.

Pretreatment with laminaria prior to first trimester abortion has definite advantages. Schulz[19] reported a fivefold reduction in cervical lacerations when pretreatment laminaria were used. The Joint Program for the Study of Abortion reported the risk for uterine perforation to be reduced threefold.[20] Therefore, organic laminaria or synthetics, such as Dilipan, can provide adequate preoperative dilatation or facilitate further dilatation of the cervix, making it less painful for the patient as well as reducing the risk of cervical trauma from forcible mechanical dilation. Although pretreatment with laminaria has been thought to increase the risk of post-abortion infection, this risk is minimal. In fact, the Joint Program for the Study of Abortion report failed to show increased risk of post-abortion infection when pretreatment with laminaria was used.[20]

Disadvantages of pretreatment with laminaria include the need for insertion by a skilled practitioner and waiting for hours for the cervical dilatation to occur. Synthetic laminaria, such as Dilipan or Lamicel, have the advantage of more rapid cervical softening and dilatation than conventional laminaria tents, as well as a shortening of induction-abortion time interval in women undergoing intra-amniotic instillation–type abortions.[21] Grimes and co-workers,[22] in a comparison of Lamicel with natural laminaria for pretreatment cervical dilation prior to early second trimester abortion, found Lamicel to be associated with a significantly lower rate of bleeding on removal and

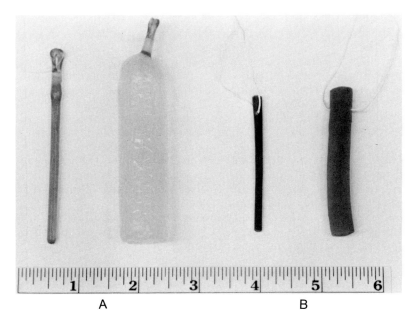

A   B

Figure 7–2. Laminaria. Hygroscopic laminaria materials swell when exposed to body fluids. *A,* Synthetic polyacrylate. *B,* Natural seaweed *Laminaria.*

to be more convenient, less costly, and comparably efficacious.

Alternatives to laminaria include various analogues of vaginally administered prostaglandin E (PGE) and $PGF_{2\alpha}$, both of which have been reported to produce significant cervical dilatation in as few as 3 hours.[23–25]

After appropriate dilatation of the cervix has been obtained, a plastic vacuum cannula the same outside diameter as the last inserted dilator or a cannula 1 mm less than the menstrual weeks of gestation is inserted into the uterine cavity. For example, for a patient with 10 weeks' gestation, a 9-mm suction cannula is used. Plastic suction cannulas used for abortion in the United States can be rigid or flexible, curved or straight. Rigid, angulated cannulas are superior to flexible cannulas. The choice of using a straight or curved cannula depends on uterine position; however, in most instances an angulated cannula suffices and is preferable.

The cannula is inserted to the level of the lower uterine segment and connected to the vacuum control swivel handle and plastic tubing, which are attached to the port on the collecting jar on the suction machine (see Figs. 7–1B and 7–1C). The suction machine is turned on to begin evacuation of the uterine contents. At least 60 cm Hg suction pressure is required to safely and effectively evacuate the uterus. As with minisuction, rotation of the plastic cannula 360 degrees is employed in a piston-like, clockwise fashion. Minimal in and out motions are required. Larger excursions increase the risk of uterine perforation with the suction cannula.

Products of conception are seen flowing into the connected tubing. Amniotic fluid appears first, followed by pale white fetal tissue and pink to red placental tissue. Removal of the cannula tip from the uterine cavity may be required for clearing of tissue. Suction should be off prior to removal and reinsertion of the cannula tip to prevent cervical or vaginal trauma. Suction is continued until bubbles appear in the cannula and the uterine cavity feels empty. After suction aspiration is complete, a sharp curette is gently placed in the uterus to explore the cavity and ensure that it is empty. Curettage or scraping of the uterine cavity is unnecessary and may result in perforation or damage to the underlying decidua basalis. The suction cannula is reintroduced a final time to remove any additional tissue.

The aspirated tissue should be examined as with minisuction to confirm the presence of fetal tissue or villi. If fetal tissue cannot be confirmed, either the procedure is not complete and the uterus needs to be re-evacuated or the possibility of ectopic pregnancy exists. The uterine contents in such a situation should have prompt pathologic assessment. If no villi or products of conception are identified, the patient is notified to return for immediate re-evaluation to rule out the possibility of ectopic pregnancy. A gestation of 9 weeks or more has definitive fetal parts, and earlier gestations have identifiable chorionic villi. The characteristic appearance of villi is of soft, feathery tissues with finger-like projections that float in water, whereas decidua appears coarse and shaggy.

Prophylactic Antibiotics in Suction Abortion

Prophylactic administration of antibiotics before suction abortion is probably unwarranted. However, it has been almost routine practice in most outpatient abortion clinics to administer oral antibiotics, such as tetracycline, 500 mg, four times a day for 3 to 5 days after an uncomplicated suction abortion. Tetracycline is potentially effective in treating any asymptomatic undiagnosed gonococcal or chlamydial infection. Some studies examining the use of oral antibiotics for prevention of post-abortion infection have shown benefits.[36, 37] Other randomized trials failed to show any differences in post-abortion infection in treatment versus no treatment groups.[38]

Complications Associated with Suction Abortion

Although legal abortion is a safe procedure, serious complications and mortality can result (Table 7–2). Between 1972 and 1982, 186 women died as a result of legal abortions in the United States; however, the death rate dropped from 4.1 per 100,000 women in 1972 to 0.8 per 100,000 women in 1982.[39] Women who were older, black, of high parity, and at a later gestation at the time of abortion were at a greater risk for mortality. Mortality rates increase 30% with each passing week of gestation, with a rate of 0.4 in 100,000 at 8 weeks or less and 14 in 100,000 after 21 weeks.[40] The lowest mortality for abortion is in that group obtaining suction abortion, and the highest mortality is in the group undergoing abortions performed by hysterotomy and hysterectomy.

The major causes of death related to abortion in the United States are infection (23%), embolism (23%), hemorrhage (20%), and complications of anesthesia (16%).[40]

The most common immediate complications during suction curettage abortion are cervical lacerations, uterine perforation, uterine hemorrhage, and anesthesia-related accidents.

Table 7–2. COMPLICATIONS OF SUCTION CURETTAGE

Uterine perforation
Cervical injury
Hemorrhage
Intestinal injury
Retained placenta
Infection
Post-abortion febrile reaction

Gestational age is the most significant determinant of abortion morbidity, followed by the pregnancy termination method. Women receiving abortions by suction methods whose gestations are between 7 and 10 weeks have the lowest incidence of serious complications, even when compared with women whose gestations are of 6 weeks or less. Thereafter, complications for suction abortion increase as gestational age advances.

CERVICAL INJURY. Cervical laceration is a frequent complication with suction abortion. The incidence of cervical injury requiring suture repair was reported by Cates and colleagues[41] to be 1 per 100 suction curettage abortion procedures. The most common type of cervical injury is superficial lacerations caused by the tenaculum pulling away from the cervical lip during cervical dilation. More serious injury to the cervix can also occur, including tearing off of the full thickness of the cervical wall and longitudinal lacerations ascending to the level of the uterine vessels. Cervicovaginal fistulas can result from severe lacerations.

Cervical lacerations can usually be avoided by slow and gradual dilation using rod dilators, or by laminaria pretreatment. Firmly grasping the cervix full thickness with a single-toothed tenaculum placed vertically with one branch into the cervical canal usually prevents injury from tenaculum pulls. Cervical injury is also less likely in women having suction abortion under local rather than general anesthesia.[40]

UTERINE PERFORATION. Uterine perforation is a very serious and potentially life-threatening complication of suction curettage abortion. The incidence of perforation with suction abortion reported by Cates and colleagues[41] was 0.2 per 100 suction curettage abortions. Lauersen and Birnbaum[42] and Nathanson[43] reported that a large percentage of perforations occur when the uterus is sounded. For this reason, the uterine cavity should not be sounded during abortion. If necessary, a sound may be used in the endocervix only to determine its direction.

Risk of perforation with suction abortion increases as gestational age advances. Parous women are at greater risk of perforation than are nulliparous women.

Perforation may lead to significant hemorrhage and damage to intra-abdominal contents, such as the bowel and the bladder. Lateral perforation at the level of the cervicoisthmic junction can cause injury to major blood vessels that lie in close proximity, giving rise to intra-abdominal bleeding, broad ligament hematoma, and pain. Perforations of this severity are likely to come to the immediate attention of the clinician (Fig. 7–3). In these instances, laparotomy must be performed.

Management of uterine perforation depends on the state of emptiness of the uterus at the time of perforation, the type of instrument causing the

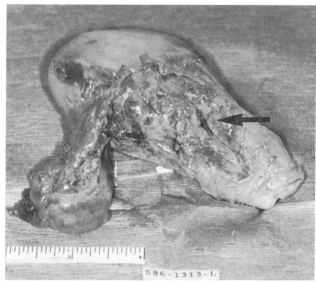

Figure 7–3. Uterine laceration from a dilation and curretage for abortion. The arrow points to a large lateral laceration in the lower uterine segment that required hysterectomy to control hemorrhage and an expanding broad ligament hematoma. (Courtesy Shaila Raj, M.D.; photographed by Rita L. Letellier.)

perforation, and the possibility that the perforation has caused damage to other viscera.

Perforation with a dilator or sound is not likely to cause serious damage, especially if the perforation occurs in the area of the fundus of the uterus. However, perforation with a suction cannula under pressure or with forceps can lead to significant damage to abdominal viscera, necessitating laparotomy.

When perforation is recognized prior to completion of the suction abortion, the operation should be terminated. Laparoscopy is then necessary to assess the damage, and if no injury or hemorrhage has occurred, the abortion can be completed under direct laparoscopic observation. If the abortion is complete when the perforation is recognized and there is no unusual bleeding, the patient may be observed for several hours and then discharged for next day follow-up examination if she remains asymptomatic.

Perforations such as those that can occur with the suction cannula necessitate laparotomy to thoroughly inspect the bowel for injury and to repair viscera and ligate damaged vessels. The uterus can usually be repaired, and hysterectomy is not needed.

Risk of uterine perforation decreases with the experience of the physician, with pretreatment cervical dilation with laminaria, and with use of local rather than general anesthesia.

HEMORRHAGE AND POST-ABORTION HEMATOMETRA. Acute and excessive vaginal bleeding during suction curettage abortion may result from uterine atony, trauma, or low placental implantation. Rates of hemorrhage ranging from 0.05 to 4.9 per 100 abortions have been reported.[41]

However, hemorrhage requiring transfusion occurs in 0.06 per 100 suction curettage abortions and 0.26 per 100 D and E abortions.

Management of acute hemorrhage should include reassessment of gestational age and inspection of the uterus for injury. Uterine massage and intravenous oxytocin usually correct uterine atony. Persistent bleeding suggests either trauma or retained clot or tissue and necessitates more aggressive measures, including repeat curettage or more aggressive surgical intervention.

Hematometra, or post-abortion syndrome, is a type of uterine atony that usually occurs within 2 hours after the suction abortion. The syndrome was first recognized in 1974 and is seen in 0.2 to 1 per 100 suction curettage procedures.[44] Symptoms include severe lower abdominal cramping and possibly tachycardia and diaphoresis, with minimal vaginal bleeding. On examination, the uterus is large, globular, and tense. Treatment includes immediate repeat uterine suction curettage with evacuation of clot followed by intravenous oxytocin to keep the uterus firm. Pretreatment of abortion patients with ergot alkaloids, 0.1 mg intramuscularly, or routine use of oxytocin during abortion may reduce the incidence of hematometra.[44]

Delayed complications after suction abortion include retained tissue, infection, bleeding, and anemia. Delayed complications occur at a rate of 2.4% at 8 weeks to 5% at 15 weeks.

Retained tissue occurs in less than 1 per 100 suction abortion procedures and can lead to hemorrhage and infection. Symptoms include cramping and bleeding, accompanied by fever, several days after the procedure. Prompt suction curettage is needed to evacuate the uterus and resolve the problem.

Fever after abortion usually indicates retained products of conception. Post-abortion fever, a temperature of 38°C or higher, occurs in less than 1 per 100 suction abortions. Post-abortion endometritis is caused by indigenous vaginal organisms, such as group B β-hemolytic streptococci, *Bacteroides* species, *Neisseria gonorrhoeae*, *Escherichia coli*, and *Staphylococcus aureus*.[45]

Management includes curettage and intravenous or oral antibiotics effective against vaginal flora. Prophylactic antibiotics, such as tetracycline, may be beneficial in preventing post-abortion endometritis.[46]

DILATATION AND EVACUATION

The most popular technique for abortion in the United States after 13 weeks is dilation and evacuation, or D and E. Dilation and evacuation has a lower morbidity than instillation techniques.[26–28] In gestations of 13 to 15 weeks, D and E is the procedure of choice for pregnancy termination and

has lower mortality than instillation abortions at or after 16 weeks' gestation.[29]

Dilation and evacuation becomes increasingly difficult with advancing gestational age. In D and E abortion in particular, the complication rate is directly related to the skill of the clinician. A properly trained individual can perform the operation with relative safety.

The patient scheduled for D and E, especially after 15 weeks' gestation, should have pretreatment laminaria inserted as previously described. Although not mandatory, confirmation of gestational age by ultrasonography can avoid the serious complications associated with underestimation of gestational age.

Laminaria are necessary to obtain the wider cervical dilatation required for D and E. Hern[30] developed a multistage pretreatment abortion laminaria technique whereby laminaria are inserted and removed in three separate steps over a 40-hour period. Current practice in the United States uses either the one-stage forcible rod dilation and evacuation approach without pretreatment laminaria as described by Finks,[31] or the two-stage procedure of Hanson,[32] which utilizes one set of laminaria left in for at least 5 hours or overnight. In patients with more than 20 weeks' gestation, a modification of the Hern pretreatment method using two-stage laminaria insertion over 48 hours before the evacuation has advantages. Patients for D and E should have an intravenous line for slow administration of diazepam, 5 mg, and fentanyl, 0.05 mg, or an equivalent.

In addition to the usual instruments used for standard suction abortion, curettage and forceps instruments are usually required to aid in removal of larger fetal parts. Commonly used forceps include Förster forceps for 13- to 15-week abortions and Hern, Bierer, or Sopher forceps for more advanced procedures.

After laminaria are removed, prepare the cervix and vagina for the evacuation using an antiseptic, such as povidone-iodine (Betadine). Perform paracervical block using approximately 30 ml of 0.5% or 1% lidocaine with epinephrine, 1:200,000. General anesthesia increases the risk for cervical laceration, perforation, and hemorrhage in D and E.[33]

Insert a large vacuum cannula into the uterine cavity to rupture the membranes and drain the amniotic fluid. Pregnancies of 13 to 16 weeks' gestation can usually be evacuated using the 12- to 14-mm vacuum cannula with vacuum aspiration alone. However, liberal forcep extraction can be employed as needed. After 16 weeks, forceps extraction is usually required to remove large fetal parts and placenta with primary utilization of the large-bore, 16-mm vacuum cannula system. The vacuum cannula is removed and reinserted repeatedly to pull down tissue and alternated with the forceps, which then grasp and remove tissue from the lower segment. When the procedure is felt to be complete, a medium to large sharp curette can be used to explore the uterine cavity and confirm complete evacuation.

The fetal calvarium poses the most difficulty in the evacuation and is the fetal part most often retained in the initial evacuation. Fetal tissue should be inspected before concluding the procedure. If the calvarium is not identified, exploration of the fundus with forceps aids in location and removal. The use of intraoperative real-time ultrasonography can be of major benefit not only in first-trimester termination, but also as a routine in D and E, especially after 16 weeks, to facilitate location and removal of hard to obtain fetal tissues such as the calvarium.[34, 35]

In situations where tissue is still hard to remove, the procedure should be discontinued and intravenous oxytocin given over 2 to 3 hours. The oxytocin causes uterine contractions and usually pushes the fetal tissue to the level of the cervical os, allowing it to be grasped with forceps and easily removed.

The use of oxytocin as a facilitative measure for suction curettage and evacuation abortions is probably not warranted on a routine basis, especially since the majority of these procedures are performed using local anesthesia. Abortion under general anesthesia is associated with greater blood loss, and oxytocin may have some benefit in reducing blood loss in these women.

Similarly, ergot alkaloid derivatives, which are often given orally for 48 to 72 hours after suction abortions, are probably not warranted and have no proven benefit.

ABORTION BY ABDOMINAL HYSTEROTOMY

Hysterotomy and hysterectomy have been infrequently employed in the past as methods for pregnancy termination and have little use in modern abortion practices. In 1973, of 610,250 legal abortions in New York City, only 0.4% were by hysterotomy. From 1984 to 1987, less than 0.05% of abortions were performed using hysterotomy or hysterectomy.[2] Present indictions for hysterotomy abortion might include failed induced abortion and advanced gestation with a placenta previa. Hysterotomy may be the method of choice for abortion in those women with a permanent cerclage in place, such as may be the case in cerclages placed abdominally. Abortion by hysterectomy should be reserved for a pre-existing uterine pathology, such as cancer. These procedures are not only more expensive than conventional abortion methods but are also associated with a much greater morbidity and mortality.

Hysterotomy Technique

An appropriate abdominal incision is made, as has been outlined in Chapter 3, exposing the anterior surface of the uterus.

Prior to making the uterine incision, 5 to 10 units of dilute oxytocin can be injected subserosally at the proposed low vertical (midline) incision site. Intravenous oxytocin can also be used throughout the procedure to further minimize bleeding. The uterine incision should be only as large as is necessary to remove the products of conception. For gestations between 16 and 22 weeks, an incision of 5 to 7 cm or less should be adequate. The vertical incision should be carried through uterine serosa and muscularis until the gestational sac is exposed and swells into the incision. Decidua and placental tissue may be visualized first. With the index finger placed between the gestational sac and the uterine wall, the fetus can be stripped away and the sac and the placenta lifted out of the uterine incision in toto without rupturing membranes. Artificial or accidental rupture of the sac increases hemorrhage and should be avoided. After inspection of the gestational sac and uterine cavity to ensure that all tissue has been removed, the incision can be closed.

A layered closure similar to that employed for a cesarean section can be used. We prefer 2–0 polyglycolate delayed absorbable suture for closure. The first layer of closure utilizes sutures approximately 0.5 to 1 cm apart that encompass the majority of the uterine muscularis. The second layer of closure gathers the remainder of the muscularis, reapproximating the serosal edges, and is placed in a continuous fashion. The third and final layer closes the serosa in a continuous subcuticular fashion. The abdominal incision is closed in a manner previously outlined.

Complications of hysterotomy are similar to those encountered in cesarean sections and include hemorrhage, endomyoparametritis, thrombophlebitis, and embolism.

LABOR INDUCTION ABORTION METHODS

Abortion by labor induction may be accomplished by intrauterine instillation techniques employing prostaglandin $F_{2\alpha}$, or hypertonic solutions of saline, urea, or a combination of all three, and by vaginally or intramuscularly administered uterotonics, such as prostaglandin E and 15-methyl analogue of $PGF_{2\alpha}$. In 1987, 1.3% of all abortions in the United States were performed by intrauterine instillation methods, compared with 3.1% in 1980 and 10.4% in 1972.[2]

Prostaglandins

Prostaglandins were the first abortifacient drugs proved to be both effective and safe. Prostaglandins act directly on the uterine myometrium to stimulate contractions but also dilate the cervix. In the United States, three prostaglandins have been approved for clinical use to induce abortion. Prostaglandin $F_{2\alpha}$ is used primarily by intra-amniotic instillation in midtrimester abortions. Successful abortion with $PGF_{2\alpha}$ was reported by Karim[47] in 1970, and it was the first prostaglandin approved by the United States Food and Drug Administration for abortion. Prostaglandin E_2 placed vaginally induces abortion and at present is the most commonly used prostaglandin for second trimester abortion. The most recently licensed prostaglandin for midtrimester abortion, the 15-methyl analogue of $PGF_{2\alpha}$ (Prostin 15 M), induces abortion when administered by gluteal intramuscular injection.

Intra-amniotic instillation of $PGF_{2\alpha}$ requires amniocentesis. Amniocentesis is usually performed under direct ultrasound guidance using a 20-gauge needle. Amniotic fluid need not be removed prior to the instillation of $PGF_{2\alpha}$; however, it has been common practice to remove approximately 100 to 200 mL of amniotic fluid prior to other instillation techniques. Usually a single dose of 40 to 50 mg of $PGF_{2\alpha}$ is placed in the amniotic cavity.

The average injection-abortion interval with intra-amniotic $PGF_{2\alpha}$ ranges between 19 and 22 hours, and the placenta is retained in approximately one third of patients.[45] Borten[48] found that the injection to abortion interval could be shortened by adding 50 mL of hypertonic saline to the $PGF_{2\alpha}$ infusion. The addition of saline also reduced transient fetal survival in gestations of 20 weeks and greater. Intravenous infusion of oxytocin may be added if labor fails to occur or if the placenta does not deliver within 2 hours after delivery of the fetus.

Prostaglandin E_2 suppositories placed vaginally are now the most common labor induction method for abortion in the second trimester. A 20-mg suppository is placed every 3 to 4 hours until the products of conception are expelled. Induction to abortion interval is approximately 13.4 hours, and 90% of patients abort by 24 hours.[49] When the patient is found to be fully dilated, gentle uterine massage without rupturing membranes usually helps immediate expulsion of the placenta along with the fetus. Pretreatment laminaria may further shorten the induction-abortion interval.

Induction of abortion with Prostin 15 M is highly effective. Prostin 15 M is given as 250 μg intramuscularly every 2 hours. The mean induction-abortion interval is 15 to 17 hours, with about 80% of patients aborting by 24 hours.[50]

Gastrointestinal side effects, including nausea, vomiting, and diarrhea, are common in prostaglandin-induced abortions. Another commonly encountered side effect is hyperpyrexia. Prostaglandin E is associated with fewer gastrointestinal side effects. We find it helpful to pretreat patients with an antidiarrhea preparation, such as oral diphenoxylate and atropine (Lomotil) and antipyretics, such as acetaminophen suppositories. Pretreatment with transdermal scopolamine in the time-release patch form approximately 6 to 8 hours

before beginning the prostin induction helps to minimize nausea and vomiting.

Abortion By Hypertonic Instillation

Abortion by instillation of hypertonic saline is one of the oldest labor induction methods of abortion. The procedure calls for 200 ml of a 20% sodium chloride solution to be slowly injected into the intra-amniotic cavity. Kerenyi and colleagues[51] reported on 5000 consecutive saline abortions without serious morbidity and no maternal deaths. Even when this method is augmented with intravenous oxytocin, the mean induction to abortion time is 25 to 26 hours.[52] When used without oxytocin, hypertonic saline abortion is associated with a higher number of failed abortions, retained placentas, increased blood loss, and infection. Significant complications that have been associated with hypertonic saline instillation abortion include cardiovascular collapse, pulmonary and cerebral edema, renal failure, and disseminated intravascular coagulation.

Hyperosmolar urea can also be used for instillation abortion and has the advantage over hypertonic saline and $PGF_{2\alpha}$ of a shorter induction to abortion interval. Abortion by urea instillation utilizes 80 mg in 135 mL of 5% dextrose in water, making a 60% solution of urea for injection into the amniotic cavity. A 5-mg dose of $PGF_{2\alpha}$ is injected into the amniotic cavity after placing the urea solution. The mean injection to abortion interval with urea-$PGF_{2\alpha}$ is 17.5 hours, with 80% of patients aborting within 24 hours.[53, 54] Delivery of a live fetus with this abortion method is rare; however, the percentage of retained placentas is approximately 35 to 46%.[53]

Mifepristone (RU-486)

Mifepristone (RU-486) is an antiprogesterone 19-norsteroid that competitively inhibits progesterone binding at the receptor level.[55] Mifepristone was synthesized in 1980.[56] The drug was first used to terminate pregnancies in humans in 1982.[57] The advantage of mifepristone is that it can be used as a medical alternative to surgical abortion procedures in the early first trimester, i.e., 49 days of amenorrhea or less. The hypothesized mechanism of action for mifepristone involves interruption of progesterone action, thereby causing irreversible damage to the decidualized endometrium that leads to evacuation of the conceptus.[58] Mifepristone has been used alone or in combination with prostaglandin for pregnancy termination.[59] In the experience of French investigators, the protocol calls for a 600-mg oral dose of mifepristone, followed in 36 to 48 hours by the administration of a low dose of synthetic prostaglandin analogue as a vaginal suppository or by intramuscular injection.[60] The overall efficacy rate for complete pregnancy expulsion was 95%, with expulsion taking place within 4 hours in more than 60% of cases. Approximately 3% to 4% of pregnancies were incompletely aborted and 1% uninterrupted with this protocol and required subsequent surgical intervention to complete the pregnancy termination.

Mifepristone appears to be a safe and effective method of early pregnancy termination. The drug is currently under investigation in the United States, and Grimes and colleagues[61] have reported similar favorable results with mifepristone. However, mifepristone has not yet been approved by the Food and Drug Administration for early first trimester pregnancy termination.

Termination of early pregnancy by the oral administration of the 3β-hydroxysteroid dehydrogenase inhibitor epostane, which reduces progesterone synthesis, has also been reported.[62]

CONCLUSIONS

Legal pregnancy termination is one of the safest operations in the United States. Gestational age is the most important determinant for pregnancy termination method. The short-term complications of legal abortion are low. The potential for long-term morbidity as measured by secondary infertility, ectopic pregnancy, and cervical incompetence in women undergoing uncomplicated first-trimester induced abortion has not been shown to be significantly increased. However, repeated sharp curettage or multiple induced abortions may be associated with increased long-term morbidity. A World Health Organization study group concluded that pregnancy termination has frequent psychologic benefits and a low level of adverse reaction. However, abortion is a serious operation both medically and socially and should never be taken lightly.

References

1. Sande HA, Reiertsen O, Fonstelien E, et al.: Evaluation of threatened abortion by human chorionic gonadotropin levels and ultrasonography. Int J Gynaecol Obstet 18:123, 1980.
2. Centers for Disease Control: Abortion Surveillance: Preliminary Analysis—United States, 1986 and 1987. MMWR 37:662–663, 1989.
3. Binkin N, Gold J, Cates W Jr: Illegal-abortion death in the United States: Why are they still occurring? Fam Plann Perspect 14:163, 1982.
4. Cates W Jr, Rochat RW: Illegal abortions in the United States: 1972–1974. Fam Plann Perspect 8:86, 1976.
5. Polgar S, Fried ES: The bad old days: Clandestine abortions among the poor in New York City before liberalization of the abortion law. Fam Plann Perspect 8:125, 1976.
6. Royston E, Armstrong S: Preventing maternal deaths. Geneva: World Health Organization (1988). Population Reports XV1(2)(7):4–5, 1988.
7. Khan AR, Jahan FA, Begum SF: Maternal mortality in rural Bangladesh: the Jamalpur District. Studies in Family Planning 7(1):7–12, 1986.
8. Mohr JC: Abortion in America: The origin and revolution of national policy. Oxford University Press: New York, 1978.
9. Wu YT: Suction in artificial abortion: 300 cases. Chin J Obstet Gynecol 6:447, 1958.
10. Goldsmith S, Margolis AJ: Aspiration abortion without cervical dilatation. Am J Obstet Gynecol 110:580, 1971.
11. Karman H, Potts M: Very early abortion using a syringe as a vacuum source. Lancet 1:1051, 1972.
12. Laufe LE: The menstrual regulation procedure. Stud Fam Plann 8:253, 1977.
13. Hodgson JE: A reassessment of menstrual regulation. Stud Fam Plann 8:263, 1977.
14. Atienza MF, Burkmann RT, King TM, et al.: Menstrual extraction. Am J Obstet Gynecol 121:490, 1975.
15. Burnhill MS, Armstead JW: Reducing the morbidity of vacuum aspiration abortion. Int J Gynecol Obstet 16:204, 1975.
16. Binkin NJ, Lang PRH, Rhodenhiser EP, et al.: Abortion surveillance, 1981, MMWR CDC Surveill Summ 33:1ss, 1985.
17. Peterson HB, Grimes DA, Cates W Jr, et al.: Comparative risk of death from induced abortion at <12 weeks' gestation performed with local versus general anesthesia. Am J Obstet Gynecol 141:763, 1981.
18. Stubblefield PG: Present techniques for cervical dilatation. In Naftolin F, Stubblefield PG (eds.): Dilatation of the Uterine Cervix. New York: Raven Press, 1980, p. 335.
19. Schulz KF, Grimes DA, Cates W Jr: Measures to prevent cervical injury during suction curettage abortion. Lancet 1:1182, 1983.
20. Gold J, Schulz KR, Cates W Jr, Tyler CW: The safety of laminaria and rigid dilators for cervical dilatation prior to suction curettage for first trimester abortion: A comparative analysis. In Naftolin F, Stubblefield PG (eds.): Dilatation of the uterine cervix: Connective tissue biology and clinical management. New York: Raven Press, 1980, p. 363.
21. Blumenthal PD: Prospective comparison for pretreament of the cervix in second-trimester induction abortion. Obstet Gynecol 72:243–246, 1988.
22. Grimes DA, Ray IG, Middleton CJ: Lamicel versus laminaria for cervical dilation before second-trimester abortion: A randomized clinical trial. Obstet Gynecol 69:887–889, 1987.
23. Ganguli AC, Green K, Bygdeman M: Preoperative dilatation of the cervix by single vaginal administration of 15 methyl PGF$_{2\alpha}$ methyl ester. Prostaglandins 14:779, 1977.
24. Hulka JF, Chepko M: Vaginal prostaglandin E1 analogue (ONO-802) to soften the cervix in first trimester abortion. Obstet Gynecol 69:57–60, 1987.
25. Natrajan P, Tzingounis VA: Cervical dilation with prostaglandin F$_{2\alpha}$ for first trimester abortion. South Medical J 79:830–831, 1986.
26. Grimes DA, Schulz KF, Cates W Jr, et al.: Midtrimester abortion by dilatation and evacuation: A safe and practical alternative. N Engl J Med 296:1141, 1977.
27. Grimes DA, Hulka JF, McCutchen ME: Midtrimester abortion by dilatation and evacuation versus intra-amniotic instillation of prostaglandin F$_{2\alpha}$: A randomized clinical trial. Am J Obstet Gynecol 137:785, 1980.
28. Kafrissen ME, Schulz KF, Grimes DA, et al.: Midtrimester abortion. JAMA 251:916, 1984.
29. Cates W Jr, Grimes DA: Deaths from second trimester abortion by dilatation and evacuation: Causes, prevention, facilities. Obstet Gynecol 58:401, 1981.
30. Hern WM: Abortion practice. Philadelphia: J.B. Lippincott Co., 1984.
31. Finks AI: Midtrimester abortion. Lancet 1:263, 1973.
32. Hanson MS: D and E midtrimester abortion preceded by laminaria. Presented at the sixteenth annual meeting of the Association of Planned Parenthood Physicians, San Diego, Calif., Oct. 26, 1978.
33. Mackay HT, Schulz KR, Grimes DA: The safety of local

versus general anesthesia for second trimester dilatation and evacuation abortion. Obstet Gynecol 66:661, 1985.

34. Darney PD: Midtrimester abortion under ultrasound guidance. Post Graduate Course, National Abortion Federation, Tampa, Fla., Jan. 31, 1983.

35. Fakih MH, Barney ER, Yarkoni S, DeCherney AH: The value of real-time ultrasonography in first trimester termination. Contraception 33:533–538, 1986.

36. Sonne-Holm S, Heisterberg L, Hebjorn S, et al.: Prophylactic antibiotics in first trimester abortions: A clinical controlled trial. Am J Obstet Gynecol 139:693, 1981.

37. Levallois P, Rioux JE: Prophylactic antibiotics for suction curettage abortion: Results of a clinical controlled trial. Am J Obstet Gynecol 139:693, 1986.

38. Westrom L, Svensson L, Wolner-Hanssen P, et al.: A clinical double-blind study on the effect of prophylactically administered single dose tinidazole on the occurrence of endometritis after first trimester legal abortion. Scand J Infect Dis 26(suppl):104, 1981.

39. Atrash HK, Mackay T, Binkin NJ, Hogue CJ: Legal abortion mortality in the United States: 1972 to 1982. Am J Obstet Gynecol 156:605–612, 1987.

40. Tietz C: Induced abortion. A World Review, 1983. New York: The Population Council, 1983, p. 83.

41. Cates W Jr, Schulz KF, Grimes DA, et al.: Short-term complications of uterine evacuation techniques for abortion at 12 weeks' gestation or earlier. In Zatuchini GI, Sciarra JJ, Speidel JJ (eds.): Pregnancy Termination: Procedures, Safety, and New Developments, Hagerstown, New Jersey, Harper and Row, 1979, p. 127.

42. Lauersen NH, Birnbaum S: Laparoscopy as a diagnostic and therapeutic technique in uterine perforation during first trimester abortions. Am J Obstet Gynecol 117:522, 1973.

43. Nathanson BN: Management of uterine perforations suffered at elective abortion. Am J Obstet Gynecol 114:1054, 1972.

44. Sands RX, Burnhill MS, Hakim-Elahi E: Post-abortal uterine atony. Obstet Gynecol 43:595, 1974.

45. Burkman RT, Atienza MF, King TM: Culture and treatment results in endometritis following elective abortion. Am J Obstet Gynecol 128:556, 1977.

46. Grimes DA, Schulz KF, Cates W Jr: Prophylactic antibiotics for curettage abortion. Am J Obstet Gynecol 150:689, 1984.

47. Karim SM, Filshie GM: Therapeutic abortion using prostaglandin $F_{2\alpha}$. Lancet 1:157, 1970.

48. Borten M: Use of combination prostaglandin $F_{2\alpha}$ and hypertonic saline for midtrimester abortion. Prostaglandins 12:625–629, 1976.

49. Surrago EJ, Robin J: Midtrimester pregnancy termination by intravaginal administration of prostaglandin E_2. Contraception 26:285, 1982.

50. Robins J, Mann LT: Second generation prostaglandins: Midtrimester pregnancy termination by intramuscular injection of a 15 methyl analog of prostaglandin $F_{2\alpha}$. Fertil Steril 27:104, 1976.

51. Kerenyi TD, Nathan M, Sherman DH: Five thousand consecutive saline inductions. Am J Obstet Gynecol 116:593–600, 1973.

52. Berger GS, Edelman DA: Oxytocin administration, instillation to abortion time, and morbidity associated with saline instillation. Am J Obstet Gynecol 121:941, 1975.

53. Burkman RT, King TM, Atienza MF: Second trimester termination of pregnancy. In Symonds EM, Zuspan FP (eds.): Clinical and Diagnostic Procedures in Obstetrics and Gynecology. Part B. Gynecology, New York: Marcel Dekker, Inc., 1984, p. 241.

54. Binkin NJ, Schulz KF, Grimes DA, Cates W: Urea-prostaglandin versus hypertonic saline for instillation abortion. Am J Obstet Gynecol 146:947, 1983.

55. Moguilensky M, Philibert D: Biochemical profile of RU-486. In Banlieu EE, Segal SJ (eds.): The antiprogestin steroid RU-486 and human fertility control. New York: Plenum Press, 1985, p. 87–97.

56. Teutsch G: Analogues of RU-486 for the mapping of the progestin recepton. In Baulieu E-E, Segal SJ (eds.): The antiprogestin steroid RU-486 and human fertility control. New York: Plenum Press, 1985, pp. 27–47.

57. Hermann W, Wyss R, Riondel A, et al.: Effet d'un stéride antiprogesterone chez la femme: Interruption du cycle menstruel et de la grossesse au début. CR Acad Sci (111) 294:933–938, 1982.

58. Capso AI, Erdos T: The critical control of progesterone levels and pregnancy by anti-progesterone. Am J Obstet Gynecol 126:598, 1976.

59. Cameron IT, Michie AF, Baird DT: Therapeutic abortion in early pregnancy with antiprogesterone RU-486 alone or in combination with prostaglandin analogue (Gemeprost). Contraception 34:459–468, 1986.

60. Silvestre L, Dubois C, Renault M, et al.: Voluntary interruption of pregnancy with mifepristone (RU-486) and a prostaglandin analogue. N Engl J Med 322:645–658, 1990.

61. Grimes DA, Mishell DR, Shoupe D, Lacarra M: Early abortion with a single dose of the antiprogestin RU-486. Am J Obstet Gynecol 158:1307–1312, 1988.

62. Crooji MT, Nooyer CCA, Rao BR, et al.: Termination of early pregnancy by the 3-β-hydroxysteroid dehydrogenase inhibitor epostane. N Engl J Med 319:813–817, 1988.

8

Management of Tubal Pregnancy

Bryan D. Cowan
John C. Morrison

EPIDEMIOLOGY

Ectopic pregnancy has become a surgical epidemic during the last 2 decades (Figs. 8–1A, 8–1B).[1-6] This condition is a significant cause of maternal mortality; it adversely affects future reproductive prospects and contributes significantly to the economic burden of health care for women. From 1970 to 1986, the incidence of ectopic pregnancy in the United States increased every year. A small reduction in both the number and the incidence of ectopic gestations has occurred in the last 4 years. More than 70,000 ectopic pregnancies occur annually, and the incidence is nearly 20 per 1000 live births. The National Hospital Discharge Survey conducted by the National Center for Health Statistics obtains comprehensive data regarding ectopic pregnancies. These data are compiled by the Centers for Disease Control and are presented in Table 8–1.

The reasons for the increased frequency of ectopic pregnancy over the last 2 decades are not

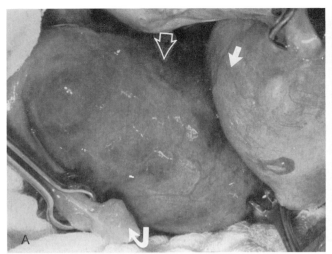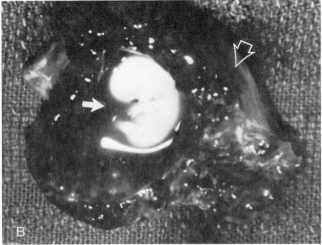

Figure 8–1. *A,* Twelve-week tubal ectopic gestation. Intraoperative photograph of ectopic pregnancy in midportion of fallopian tube. *Closed arrow*—uterus. *Open arrow*—ectopic. *Curved arrow*—fimbriated end of fallopian tube. *B,* Twelve-week tubal ectopic gestation. Opened surgical specimen from patient *A. Open arrow*—fallopian tube. *Closed arrow*—fetus in amniotic sac.

clearly understood[4, 7, 8] but can be attributed in part to better reporting, improved diagnostic tools for the detection of this condition, and acquired risks for this disease in the reproductive population of women (Table 8–2).[9–17] The most significant risk factor is scarring of the pelvic viscera from previous infection. Pelvic infection not only increases the chance of ectopic pregnancy but also greatly reduces subsequent fertility. The incidence of pelvic infection has increased during recent years. *Chlamydia* and *Neisseria gonorrheae* represent the most important and frequently occurring genital tract pathogens. Reparative pelvic surgery, previous sterilization, gamete technology

(gamete-zygote intrafallopian or intrauterine placement), congenital tubal anomalies, diethylstilbestrol exposure in utero, and transperitoneal migration of the ovum also contribute to the pool of ectopic pregnancies (see Table 8–2) (Figs. 8–2A and 8–2B show a rare accessory tube anomaly). However, these factors are much less important than acquired pelvic disease, prior infection, surgery, or endometriosis. Finally, as a national trend, many women are deferring childbirth until late in their reproductive lives. The risk for ectopic gestation is greatest in older women, and this sociologic shift has occurred with sufficient magnitude to become an important contributor to the incidence of ectopic pregnancy.

Complications from ectopic pregnancy remain a leading cause of maternal death in the United States today.[6, 18] However, the death rate decreased dramatically in the years from 1970 to 1976 and has continued to fall in the years from 1977 to 1986. Thirty-nine women died in 1984 as a result of ectopic pregnancy, 33 died in 1985, and 36 died in 1986. The case-fatality rates for these 3 years ranged between 4.2 and 5.2 deaths per 10,000 ectopic pregnancies. A study of 86 deaths among 102,100 cases of ectopic pregnancy that occurred in the United States between 1979 and 1980 revealed that 77% of these women sought medical

Table 8–1. NUMBERS AND RATES OF ECTOPIC PREGNANCIES BY YEAR, UNITED STATES, 1970–1986

		Rates		
Year	**No.***	**Reported pregnancies†**	**Live births‡**	**Females ages 15–14§**
1970	17,800	4.5	4.8	4.2
1971	19,300	4.8	5.4	4.4
1972	24,500	6.3	7.5	5.5
1973	25,600	6.8	8.2	5.6
1974	26,400	6.7	8.4	5.7
1975	30,500	7.6	9.8	6.5
1976	34,600	8.3	11.0	7.2
1977	40,700	9.2	12.3	8.3
1978	42,400	9.4	12.8	8.5
1979	49,900	10.4	14.3	9.9
1980	52,200	10.5	14.5	9.9
1981	68,000	13.6	18.7	12.7
1982	61,800	12.3	17.0	11.5
1983	69,600	14.0	19.2	12.6
1984	75,400	14.9	20.6	13.6
1985	78,400	15.2	20.9	14.0
1986	73,700	14.3	19.7	12.8
TOTAL	790,800	10.3	13.4	9.3

*Rounded to nearest 100.
†Rate per 1000 reported pregnancies.
‡Rate per 1000 live births.
§Rate per 10,000 females.

Table 8–2. RISK FACTORS FOR ECTOPIC PREGNANCY

Prior pelvic infection
Adhesions
Pelvic or abdominal surgery
Endometriosis
Failed sterilization
Prior or concomitant intrauterine contraceptive device use
Gamete technology
External migration of the ovum
Congenital tubal anomalies (including exposure to diethystilbestrol)

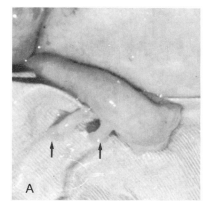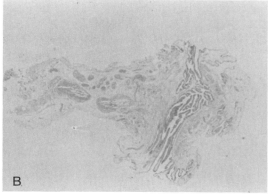

Figure 8–2. *A,* Anomalous accessory fallopian tubes *(arrows). B,* Anomalous fallopian tube. Microscopic section of specimen from *A.*

care, that 100% complained of pain, and that the cause of death was acute hemorrhage in 85% of the cases.[1] Error in diagnosis occurred in 49% of the cases; diagnosis was commonly confused with gastrointestinal disorders, intrauterine pregnancy, or pelvic inflammatory disease. More than half of these deaths might have been prevented if patients or providers had acted more expeditiously.

HISTOPATHOLOGY

Approximately 90% of ectopic pregnancies occur in the oviduct,[8] and most of these are ampullary implantations (Figs. 8–3*A* and 8–3*B*). Regardless of the implantation site, the invading trophoblast usually mimics the same biologic responses as a trophoblast invading the decidua of the endometrium (Fig. 8–4).[19–23] Thereafter, the trophoblast destroys the epithelium and invades the muscularis. Controversy concerning the penetration limits of the muscularis by the invading trophoblast confuses possible explanations of tubal rupture. Most of the invading trophoblast proliferates below the mucosa of the lumen within the muscularis. Penetration of the muscularis to the peritoneum

is rare because trophoblast growth is usually restricted by the muscularis. Focal bleeding and hemorrhage into the implantation site are common sequelae of oviductal nidation and are believed to be responsible for distension, intermittent pelvic pain, and ultimate rupture.

The ampullary muscularis is considerably thinner than the corresponding sites of the isthmus and the interstitium. The depth of the "submucosal" area that can be invaded is therefore considerably less in ampullary ectopic gestations compared with those occurring in isthmic sites. As such, ampullary gestations are amenable to conservative removal of the ectopic pregnancy without tubal resection. Those pregnancies arising in the isthmus or the interstitium are more difficult to remove without resecting the tube. Additionally, isthmic and interstitial implantations commonly injure the narrow lumen,[24] and extraction of these gestations without resection of the tube leads to a high incidence of repeat ectopic pregnancies.[25]

DIAGNOSIS

Prior to the last 2 decades, most women (85%) with ectopic pregnancies were diagnosed only after

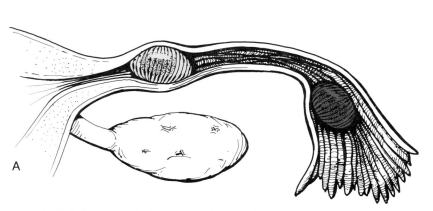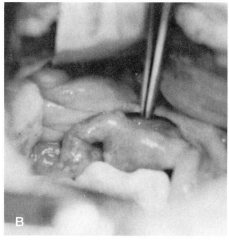

Figure 8–3. *A,* Common tubal pregnancy implantation sites. Approximately 85% of tubal pregnancies attach to the distal half of the tube (ampullary), and 15% attach to the proximal portion (isthmus). *B,* Ectopic pregnancy, midportion of the fallopian tube, 7 weeks' gestation *(arrow).*

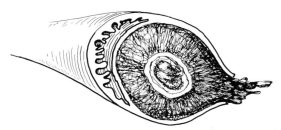

Figure 8–4. Implantation of tubal pregnancy. The trophoblast penetrates the mucosa and proliferates within the submucosal connective tissue. Focal bleeding into the implantation site distends and necroses the tube.

tubal leakage or rupture occurred.[8] Quantitation of human chorionic gonadotropin (hCG) and serum progesterone combined with pelvic sonography can now diagnose tubal pregnancy prior to rupture. Abdominal pain occurs in 85 to 100% of women with ectopic pregnancy symptoms. The cause of pain is peritoneal stretching from the expanding fallopian tube or blood in the peritoneal cavity from tubal regurgitation or rupture. Unfortunately, abdominal pain is a common gynecologic complaint. In a review of 119 women with suspected ectopic gestation, 94% of the patients who did not have a tubal pregnancy also had abdominal pain.

The second most common symptom associated with extrauterine pregnancy is abnormal vaginal bleeding. The bleeding occurs in over 60% of women as the result of insufficient hormonal support of the decidualized endometrium. The triad of pelvic pain, abnormal vaginal bleeding, and an adnexal mass represents the classic hallmark of an ectopic pregnancy. Unfortunately, the severity of the symptoms and their common association with ectopic pregnancy are dependent on the duration of the gestation at the time the patient seeks medical attention. This triad is present in only one third of ectopic gestations and most commonly occurs in advanced gestations. In general, the adnexal mass of an ectopic pregnancy develops late, and its detection by manual vaginal examination is made difficult because of patient discomfort.

Human Chorionic Gonadotropin Excretion in Ectopic Pregnancy

Human chorionic gonadotropin is secreted differently in normal and abnormal gestations (Figure 8–5). The hCG doubles in a normal pregnancy at approximately 2-day intervals during the first 42 days of gestation.[26–30] Tubal pregnancies have a slower doubling time, and 85% show less than a 66% increase in hCG concentration within the 48-hour interval.[31] A slow doubling time, however, is not uniformly associated with abnormal gestations. Fifteen percent of normal intrauterine pregnancies have slow hCG doubling. The amount of hCG produced varies with the gestational age. The hCG doubling is more rapid in early gestation (1.4 to 1.5 days to double) than in the pregnancy approaching 7 to 8 weeks' gestation (3.3 to 3.5 days to double). After approximately 7 to 8 weeks of gestation, the hCG titer peaks and declines. As a consequence, hCG doubling is generally not helpful after 7 to 8 weeks of gestation.[32]

The interpretation of quantitative hCG titers is somewhat confused by the development of two reference standards for hCG.[32, 33] In 1964, the second international standard for hCG titers was developed. This was followed in 1974 by the development of the international reference preparation. The international reference preparation is a highly purified hCG, and the hCG molecule is referenced as CR119. It is difficult to convert one standard to the other because the second international standard refers to a bioassay and the international reference preparation quantitates the mass of hormone. For estimates of conversion, 1 ng of hCG (CR119) is approximately equivalent to 5 mIU of the second international standard, or 9.3 mIU of the international reference preparation.

In addition to the abnormal hCG doubling times associated with ectopic pregnancies, subunit secretion is aberrant.[34] Ectopic pregnancies secrete significantly more free alpha subunit than normal gestations. Although not generally applied clinically, quantitation of the free alpha subunit may provide an additional valuable adjunct for the early diagnosis of this condition.

Sonography

Pelvic sonography is used to visualize the pelvic structures and locate the gestation. The applica-

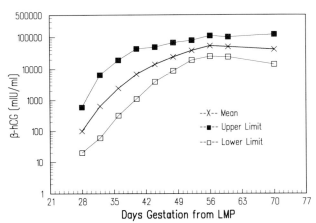

Figure 8–5. Serum β-hCG concentrations in normal pregnancies during the first 80 days of gestation. The mean, upper, and lower limits of hCG concentrations are plotted for each interval of increasing gestation. Note that hCG begins to decline at about 56 days (Modified from Ooi DS, et al.: Serum human chorionic gonadotropin levels in early pregnancy. Clin Chim Acta 181:201, 1989).

tion of this technique is dependent on the recognition of "discriminatory hCG zones," which define a threshold level for the sensitivity and predictive value of the test.[35-45] The initial discriminatory zone of hCG for transabdominal sonography was reported by Kadar and colleagues in 1981.[35] They showed that a concentration of hCG greater than 6500 mIU/mL was highly correlated with the ability to visualize an intrauterine gestational sac by transabdominal sonography. Furthermore, ectopic pregnancy existed in 86% of women with an hCG titer above that discriminatory zone in which an intrauterine gestational sac was not detected by transabdominal sonography. Unfortunately, transabdominal sonography is unable to detect a normal gestational sac when the hCG value is less than 6500 mIU/mL. Women with ectopic pregnancies commonly present when the hCG titer is less than 6000 mIU/mL. Therefore, an additional time interval is required before the hCG titer exceeds 6500 mIU/mL for sonography to be diagnostic.

The development of transvaginal sonography[38-40] greatly improved the ability to discriminate accurately between intrauterine and extrauterine gestations. The sensitivity of transvaginal sonography has consistently been superior to that of transabdominal sonography. An intrauterine gestational sac can be visualized by transvaginal technology when the hCG titer is as low as 2000 mIU/mL (Fig. 8–6). In addition, the transvaginal approach can detect adnexal pathology more commonly than can transabdominal methods (Fig. 8–7). Transvaginal sonography confirmed the presence of an adnexal mass consistent with ectopic pregnancy in 26 of 29 women with low hCG titers (below the transabdominal discriminatory threshold) and ectopic pregnancies.[40] By comparison, an adnexal mass could only be located in 12 of the same 29 patients using the transabdominal technique. Thus, the ability to detect intrauterine gestational sacs at low hCG levels[42-44] and the better resolution

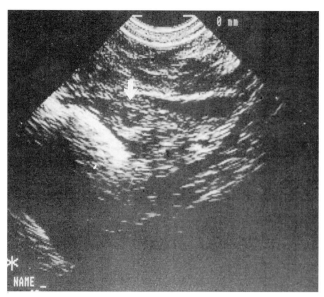

Figure 8–7. Transvaginal sonogram demonstrating a tubal pregnancy *(arrow)*. A moderate amount of fluid is present in the posterior cul-de-sac. The amniotic sac and the trophoblast are easily seen. Serum β-hCG was 2320 mIU/mL.

of adnexal pathology[45] have made transvaginal sonography the method of choice for detecting abnormal and ectopic gestations.

Progesterone

Serum progesterone concentrations are low in ectopic pregnancies when compared with intrauterine gestations of the same gestational age.[46-53] Most ectopic pregnancies are associated with a progesterone concentration of less than 15 ng/mL (Fig. 8–8). In an emergency room environment that assessed 582 pregnancies, Stovall and colleagues[52] reported that all normal pregnancies had a progesterone concentration of more than 6.5 ng/mL. Unfortunately, progesterone measurements are a poor predictor of normal gestations. There is no agreement as to the "discriminatory value of progesterone," which defines an abnormal gestation. Furthermore, a progesterone determination can only predict that the gestation is abnormal but cannot distinguish between an abnormal intrauterine gestation (a missed abortion) and an ectopic pregnancy. Thus, progesterone monitoring during early gestation can identify pregnancies at risk but cannot predict normalcy or discriminate between abnormal intrauterine and ectopic gestations.

Figure 8–9 outlines a systematic evaluation of early pregnancy. This diagnostic algorithm utilizes the contemporary tools of serial hCG monitoring and vaginal sonography. In the absence of pain, evaluation of the patient in an ambulatory setting can be performed. Hospitalization is necessary if pain is a presenting complaint. Culdocentesis de-

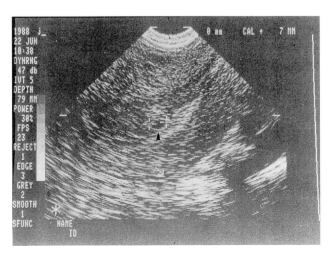

Figure 8–6. Transvaginal sonogram of a 7-mm intrauterine gestational sac *(arrowhead)*. The hCG titer was 1420 mIU/mL.

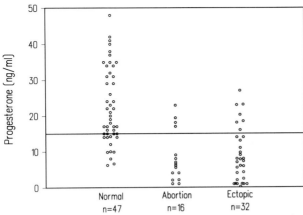

Figure 8–8. Progesterone concentrations categorized by diagnostic groups. A value of 15 ng/ml segregates most ectopic gestations from normal gestations and all but four abnormal intrauterine gestations.

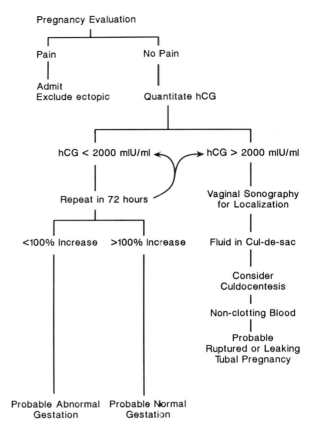

Figure 8–9. Evaluation of early pregnancy using serial hCG monitoring and vaginal sonography. An important aspect of this algorithm is the hospitalization of patients who have pain and suspected ectopic pregnancy.

termines the presence of hemoperitoneum. It is 90% predictive of blood in the abdomen when the test is positive and just as reliable when the test is negative.[17] However, culdocentesis is invasive and painful. If fluid is not seen in the cul-de-sac on vaginal sonography, culdocentesis is usually nondiagnostic and not indicated.

SURGICAL TREATMENT

Prior to the development of safe anesthesia for surgical treatment, expectant management of ectopic pregnancies resulted in a mortality rate of nearly 70%.[54] Salpingectomy for surgical treatment was first described in 1884,[55] and its remarkable effectiveness in reducing maternal mortality from ectopic pregnancy made extirpative surgery standard treatment. In 1953, the first case of conservative surgical treatment for ectopic pregnancy was reported in the English literature.[56] Since then, many methods for the conservative treatment of ectopic pregnancy have been introduced.[57–70] During the last decade, advances in endoscopic instrumentation and techniques have allowed successful surgical treatment via endoscopy.[71–77] This surgical approach has reduced operative morbidity and hospital costs and has allowed patients to return to normal activities in a shorter time than those recovering from laparotomies.

Conservative or nonconservative tubal surgery for treatment of the patient with an ectopic pregnancy must be individualized for each patient and surgeon. The patient should desire future fertility, be hemodynamically stable, and have an unruptured gestation and an accessible tube. Appropriate equipment and instruments must be available (Table 8–3), and the surgeon as well as the operating room team must be properly trained. If the fallopian tube is ruptured or if the patient is hemodynamically unstable, more urgent and nonconservative surgical treatment is usually required for expeditious management of the patient. The selection of the operation is guided by the location of the ectopic pregnancy, the capabilities of the surgeon, and the availability of operating room resources.

Operations for Distal Tubal Pregnancy

Salpingostomy is commonly used to treat unruptured ampullary gestations. In this technique, a linear incision is performed in the antimesenteric portion of the fallopian tube, and the ectopic gestation is expressed through this incision (Fig. 8–10A–E). To minimize bleeding and optimize suc-

Table 8–3. INSTRUMENTS FOR SALPINGOSTOMY

Unipolar cutting needle (e.g., Corson)
Scissors
CO_2 laser
KTP laser
Argon laser fiber
Sapphire Nd:YAG* contact tip laser

*Nd:YAG—neodymium-yttrium-aluminum-garnet.

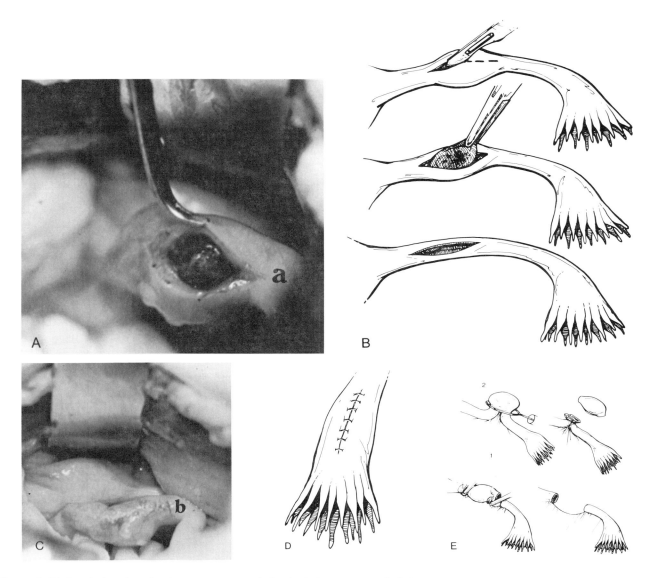

Figure 8–10. Surgical options for the management of distal tubal pregnancy. *A, B,* Linear salpingostomy—a small incision along the length of the tube directly over the ectopic pregnancy (a). The pregnancy is extruded, bleeding points are controlled, and the edges of the incision are not approximated (photo courtesy Sebastian Faro, M.D.). *C, D,* Salpingotomy—the incision is placed over the ectopic pregnancy as in *A* and *B*. After the gestation is extruded, the incision is reapproximated with 4–0 or 5–0 polyglycolic acid sutures (photo courtesy Sebastian Faro, M.D.). *E,* Partial salpingectomy: (1) removal of the ectopic gestation and the affected portion of the tube. The tube is cauterized or sutured on each side of the ectopic pregnancy to establish hemostasis. The tubal segment containing the pregnancy is resected. The mesosalpinx directly beneath the ectopic pregnancy is cauterized or sutured. (2) An alternative method is to apply a loop suture that incorporates the pregnancy and excise the affected tubal segment.

cess of this procedure, cauterization of the serosal vessels at both sides of the anticipated incision is often performed. Additionally, a dilute solution of vasopressin (20 U/mL mixed with 10 to 20 mL normal saline) can be injected into the mesosalpinx below the ectopic pregnancy. The vascular supply of the conceptus arises here, and constriction of these vessels with dilute vasopressin prior to evacuation of the conceptus significantly reduces bleeding. After the incision has been performed, small bleeding vessels can be ligated or cauterized.

To perform salpingostomy through the laparo-

scope, a three-puncture technique is usually required (Table 8–4). Two suprapubic punctures are used for operative instruments to stabilize and manipulate the ectopic gestation. An atraumatic, grasping forceps should be used to evaluate and stabilize the pregnancy. If vasopressin is used, injection should be directed into the mesosalpinx by laparoscopic visualization. Generally, 4 to 8 ml of the dilute solution is injected. Instruments used to create the tubal incision include the CO_2 laser, argon or potassium-tungsten-phosphate (KTP) fibers, neodymium-yttrium-aluminum-garnet con-

Table 8–4. ESSENTIAL INSTRUMENTS FOR SUCCESSFUL ENDOSCOPIC REMOVAL OF ECTOPIC PREGNANCY

Atraumatic grasping forceps to stabilize the tube
Long needle for vasopressin injection
Cutting source or instrument for salpingostomy
Endocoagulation-electrocautery-loop sutures for hemostasis
Spoon grasping forceps for removal of ectopic gestation and tube
Two suprapubic trochars
Irrigation-aspiration system

tact laser tips, electrocautery, endocoagulation, and operative scissors. There is no evidence that any of these techniques is superior to the others. The decision as to which method to use is the preference of the individual surgeon.

A 2 to 4 cm incision is created, and the ectopic gestation is gently teased from its decidual bed. The surgeon should avoid excessive grasping at the bed of the ectopic gestation because this usually leads to tubal damage and increases bleeding. Once the gestational sac has been removed, an irrigation system is introduced to copiously lavage both the pelvis and the tubal site. Bleeding can be recognized at the time of irrigation and controlled with bipolar forceps or needle-point unipolar electrocautery. Finally, the ectopic gestation is removed from the abdomen with the 5- or 10-mm biopsy forceps. Large ectopic pregnancies are removed by morcellation until all of the tissue has been withdrawn.

Salpingotomy is performed in the same fashion as salpingostomy, but in this technique the edges of the incision are approximated with fine, interrupted suture. The incision is generally closed in one layer, using 5–0 or 6–0 synthetic polyglycolic acid sutures. Despite the aesthetic appeal of reapproximating the serosal edges, there is no evidence that salpingotomy is superior to salpingostomy, and the additional surgery at the site of the ectopic pregnancy may increase adhesions in the fallopian tube.[78]

Fimbrial expression of the ectopic pregnancy has been reported as treatment for distal ampullary ectopic pregnancies to avoid opening the oviduct. However, this approach may be associated with a higher incidence of persistent trophoblast tissue. It should be reserved for those patients with fimbrial pregnancies that are already in the process of spontaneous abortion.

Tubal rupture and overt hemorrhage commonly necessitate salpingectomy (complete or partial) to provide rapid treatment and prevent serious morbidity and mortality (Fig. 8–11). The removal of the ovary is not recommended, as was once the common practice,[68] unless the ovary is involved with the ectopic pregnancy or other ovarian pathology exists.

Operations for Proximal Tubal Pregnancy

Segmental resection has been the preferred operation for tubal pregnancies located in the isth-

mus of the fallopian tube (see Fig. 8–8C). The tubal lumen is narrow, and the site of the ectopic pregnancy is difficult to identify. The muscularis is commonly invaded by the ectopic gestation at this site, and the subsequent inflammatory response after salpingostomy leads to an increased rate of proximal tubal obstruction.[24] The incidence of repeat ectopic pregnancy in patients with isthmic ectopic pregnancies treated with linear salpingotomy is nearly 50%.[25]

Therefore, removal of the tubal segment containing the gestation is advised when the ectopic pregnancy is found in this location. The smallest portion of fallopian tube necessary to include the gestation is resected. The area of the tube that contains the ectopic gestation is elevated to expose the mesosalpinx. The proximal and distal segments of the tube are ligated with a transfixing suture passed below the tube and into the mesosalpinx. The tube is then divided, liberating the involved segment with its attachment to the mesosalpinx. The mesosalpinx is ligated with absorbable suture and the segment resected. Endoscopically directed procedures use endocoagulation or electrocautery of the tubal segments prior to transecting the tube or placement of a preformed loop of absorbable suture material around the ectopic gestation. Excision can be accomplished by surgical dissection with either scissors or unipolar electrocautery.

Although tubal anastomosis has been performed at the time of resection, most surgeons prefer to perform a second operation after edema and inflammation from the ectopic pregnancy have resolved.[66, 71] If primary anastomosis is selected, rather than ligate the proximal and distal ends of

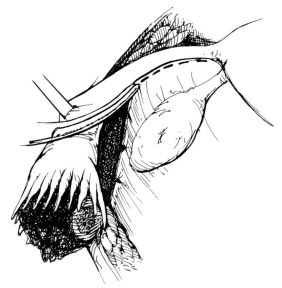

Figure 8–11. Salpingectomy: the ectopic pregnancy and tube have been identified. The mesosalpinx is successively clamped and divided along the indicated resection line. Each successive pedicle is divided and ligated with an absorbable suture. The proximal end of the tube is clamped, the tube is excised, and the clamp is replaced with an absorbable suture.

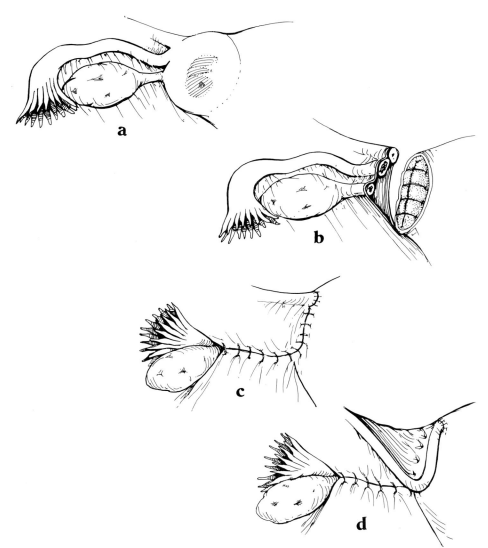

Figure 8–12. Cornual resection of an interstitial pregnancy. (a) The interstitial pregnancy, tube, and ovary are identified. (b) The interstitial (cornual) pregnancy and surrounding myometrium are resected. The deep edges of the resected portion of the uterus are approximated with interrupted 0 chromic sutures. The serosa is approximated with a continuous stitch. (c) Partial or tubal salpingectomy is performed as in Figure 8–9. The ovary is spared when possible. (d) The round ligament is reattached and swung over the myometrium (as in a modified Coffey suspension) to help support the uterus and cover the surgical site.

the tube, a Babcock clamp is placed on either side immediately adjacent to the pregnancy. Prior to excision of the ectopic pregnancy, a stabilizing suture is placed lateral to each resection plane in the mesosalpinx and tied after resection. This method provides hemostasis of the mesosalpinx as well as partial approximation of the tubes. Tubal anastomosis is performed, using 3 or 4 interrupted sutures placed in the muscularis and peritoneum to approximate the anastomosis in a single layer. Additional interrupted sutures can be placed to provide a smooth peritoneal approximation. This technique is somewhat different than the procedure utilized with nonpregnant women, in which the tubal anastomosis is usually closed in two layers (muscularis and serosa).

The surgical treatment of cornual (interstitial) ectopic pregnancies risks hemorrhage that may require hysterectomy (Fig. 8–12). The cornual gestation is better protected in the interstitium than in the remainder of the tube, and as a result, such pregnancies are usually much more advanced than

tubal pregnancies when diagnosed. Cornual resection and repair can only be performed in about 50% of such cases, and hysterectomy is required for the remainder. In general, hysterectomy is recommended for multiparous women over 35 years old, and conservative treatment is recommended for nulliparous women or women under 35. The surgical technique requires a V-shaped wedge of uterine tissue to be removed. The myometrial bed of the resection is closed with interrupted or circular 2–0 or 0 chromic sutures. Then the muscularis is approximated, and the serosa is closed with an inverted "baseball" stitch. Attachment of the round ligament over the incision is an effective method to prevent adhesions to the resection area (Coffey suspension).

COMPLICATIONS

Conservative treatment for ectopic pregnancy, whether by salpingotomy or fimbrial expression, has the potential to preserve fertility and reduce operative morbidity.[78-88] The major problems associated with nonextirpative surgery are hemorrhage at the implantation site and persistent trophoblast proliferation. Hemorrhage after removal of the gestation is usually managed with compression of the site or injection of the mesosalpinx with dilute vasopressin. Occasionally, small bleeding vessels can be identified within the implantation bed and cauterized or ligated. If these therapies fail, salpingectomy or resection of the involved segment is performed.

Women who undergo surgical removal of the ectopic pregnancy without removal of the affected tube are at risk for "persistent ectopic pregnancy," or "persistent ectopic trophoblast."[89-97] Although the etiology of this condition is not clear, it is generally believed that the trophoblast continues to grow within the tube from which it was incompletely removed at the time of surgical extraction or that trophoblast implants develop at sites within the pelvis that the ectopic pregnancy touched during surgical excision.

The incidence of this complication is difficult to obtain from the medical literature. The largest study is that of Pouly and colleagues,[76] who reported 15 cases of persistent ectopic trophoblast tissue in 321 tubal pregnancies (4.7%) that were treated conservatively with laparoscopic techniques. Undoubtedly, conservative surgery results in incomplete removal of the gestation or dissemination of trophoblast cells within the pelvis. If the tissue is aggressive and persists, repeat treatment is required. To confirm that surgical treatment for ectopic pregnancy was successful, all patients who have salpingostomy or ampullary expression of an ectopic pregnancy should be monitored with hCG titers.[89-93] In general, if the trophoblast tissue is completely resected, hCG titers disappear in approximately 12 to 24 days.[89, 92] If left untreated, the clinical course for women with persistent ectopic trophoblast is unclear. However, the cases reported in the literature are often associated with pain, adnexal mass, tubal rupture, hypotension, and hemoperitoneum.[94-97] Therefore, treatment for persistent trophoblast should be initiated if hCG titers persist or rise. Therapy for persistent trophoblast has been limited to surgery or medical therapy. Therapy has involved laparoscopy with fulguration or removal of the affected area of the tube, fulguration or laser vaporization of trophoblast implants on the peritoneum, laparotomy with excision of the involved areas, or treatment with methotrexate.[93-99]

SUBSEQUENT REPRODUCTION

Subsequent reproduction after ectopic pregnancy is independent of the technique of management (Table 8–5). DeCherney and Kase[100] compared in-

Table 8–5. PREGNANCY AFTER SALPINGOSTOMY FOR ECTOPIC PREGNANCY*

	Year	Patients	Intrauterine Pregnancy (%)	Ectopic Pregnancy (%)
Laparotomy				
Timonen[67]	1967	185	53	12
Stromme[88]	1973	45	71	15
DeCherney[65]	1980	9	55	0
Sherman[84]	1982	43	81	7
Hallatt[70]	1986	174	56	14
Laparoscopy				
Bruhat[74]	1980	25	72	12
Pouly[76]	1986	62	86	16
		56	41	29
DeCherney[77]	1987	79	62	16

*Only first authors have been cited.

trauterine and ectopic pregnancy rates in women treated with salpingostomy with those treated with salpingectomy. There was not a significant difference between the groups. Approximately 40% in both groups had a subsequent intrauterine gestation, and 12% in each group had a recurrent ectopic pregnancy. This information is different from that reported for conservative surgery a decade ago, in which the incidence of ectopic pregnancy was greater in those women who had conservative management of their tubal pregnancies rather than salpingectomy. At that time, conservative surgical treatment of tubal pregnancies was only performed on patients with abnormal or absent contralateral tubes. This operation was "a rescue" surgical procedure to save reproductive function, since a salpingectomy would sterilize the patient. In recent years, the indications for conservative surgery have been expanded to include women with normal contralateral anatomy, and recent data reflect these trends. Intrauterine pregnancy rates consistently range from 35 to 50%, and ectopic pregnancy rates range between 3 and 17%.[76, 77, 84, 85, 100-102] Postoperative infertility after conservative surgery is significantly associated with previous sterility, coexistent periadnexal adhesions or tubal disease, rupture of the ectopic pregnancy, and older age.[70, 76, 103]

NONSURGICAL TREATMENT

Tubal pregnancies may resolve spontaneously without the need for medical or surgical intervention.[3] This has been particularly well documented in recent clinical series in which patients with ectopic gestations confirmed by laparoscopy had resolution of the disease without the need for surgical management.[104-109] However, one must remember that 70% of patients so affected subsequently died before surgery was practical for ectopic pregnancy. This high mortality occurred because only the most advanced ectopic gestations were clinically recognizable. In the modern era of early detection of this condition, many ectopic

Table 8–6. TREATMENT OF ECTOPIC PREGNANCY WITH METHOTREXATE: INITIAL TREATMENT OUTCOMES

Author*	Year	Site	Patients	Resolved	Route
Tanaka[112]	1982	Cornual	1	1	IM†
Farabow[113]	1983	Cervix	1	1	IM
Chotiner[114]	1985	Tube	1	1	IM
Ory[115]	1986	Tube	6	5	IM
Rodi[116]	1986	Tube	7	7	IM
Cowan[98]	1986	Persistent	1	1	IM
Cheng[117]	1986	Cervix	1	0	IM
Higgins[99]	1986	Persistent	1	1	IM
Brandes[118]	1986	Cornual	1	1	IM
Goldstein[119]	1986	Tube	13	12	IM
Feichtinger[120]	1987	Tube	1	1	Sac
Ichinoe[121]	1987	Tube	23	22	IM
Kenigsberg[122]	1987	Tube	1	1	IM
Sauer[123]	1987	Tube	21	20	IM
Haans[124]	1987	Tube	1	1	IM
Sauer[125]	1988	Tube	5	5	IM
Patsner[126]	1988	Persistent	1	1	Oral
Leeton[127]	1988	Tube	2	2	Sac
Stovall[127]	1989	Tube	36	34	IM
Clark[129]	1989	Tube	1	1	Sac
Pansky[130]	1989	Tube	27	24	Sac
Zakut[131]	1989	Tube	10	10	Sac
Skannal[132]	1989	Cervix	1	1	IM
Cairns[133]	1989	Persistent	1	1	Oral
Kojima[134]	1990	Tube	9	9	Sac
TOTALS			173	163	

*Only first authors have been cited.
†IM—intramuscular.

gestations undergo spontaneous resolution before becoming clinically apparent. In 1955, Lund studied 285 patients with ectopic pregnancies treated by surgery or expectant management.[97] He treated 116 patients with salpingectomy, whereas the remainder (119 patients) were managed expectantly. Patients who were observed experienced spontaneous resolution in 57% of cases. In the 1980s, six series reported the results of expectant management of presumed ectopic pregnancies.[104–109] In all, 59 patients, who were rigorously selected, had an intact fallopian tube, confirmed by laparoscopy, and no intra-abdominal bleeding. Spontaneous absorption of the ectopic pregnancy occurred in 83% of these patients, and all demonstrated declining hCG titers during the study interval. The remaining 17% had either rising hCG concentrations or clinical deterioration that required laparotomy for surgical management. Unfortunately, declining hCG titers do not always represent resolution of the disease.[110, 111] Case reports of tubal rupture during rapidly declining hCG titers or of low hCG titers associated with chronic ectopic pregnancies emphasize the need for caution in the clinical management of these patients.

Recently, there has been an interest in the development of medical therapy for the treatment of unruptured tubal pregnancy. This treatment avoids surgical intervention, potentially preserves reproductive potential, and reduces the cost of medical care. Methotrexate, a folinic acid antagonist, was the first drug used to treat tubal pregnancies nonsurgically.[112–134] To date, the outcome of over 170 patients treated with methotrexate has been reported in the literature (Table 8–6). The cure rate with this therapy is over 90%, and little toxicity occurs.

In general, candidates for methotrexate therapy should have an unruptured ectopic pregnancy, an hCG titer of less than 15,000 to 20,000 mIU/ml, a desire for future reproduction, or a severe medical disease that would be compromised by surgery. In addition to the primary treatment of ectopic pregnancy with methotrexate, this agent has been advocated as the treatment of choice for persistent trophoblast after conservative tubal surgery for ectopic pregnancy.[98, 99, 122, 133]

Several routes of methotrexate treatment have been used. The most common is intramuscular injection. Most physicians are familiar with this route of administration; the technique is not associated with vesication complications, and the drug is readily available. The dosage of methotrexate used to treat ectopic pregnancies has been determined empirically, principally modeled after the experience with treatment of gestational trophoblastic disease.[135–140] The most common regimen used in this country has been 1 mg methotrexate per kilogram body weight (1 mg/kg) administered every other day for three or four doses. To reduce systemic toxicity, leukovorum rescue has been commonly used at a dose of 0.1 mg/kg on days when methotrexate is not given. In addition to intramuscular injection, oral methotrexate has been successfully used.[126] Direct injection of the ectopic pregnancy at laparoscopy and ultrasound-guided needle aspiration and injection of the gestational sac have shown promising results.[120, 127, 129–131, 134] Thus far, only cases of transvaginal ultrasound-guided injection of the ectopic gestations have been reported. However, Pansky and colleagues[130] reported the treatment of 27 women with laparoscopically confirmed ectopic pregnancy with laparoscopically directed injections of the gestation. They used a dose of 12.5 mg of methotrexate and required that the ectopic pregnancy be less than 3 cm, with an intact serosa. In his series, 24 of 27 women had resolution of the pregnancy within 35 days. Three women required laparotomy for rising hCG titers. Only two women in this series had an hCG titer of more than 1000 mIU/ml, and both of these failed. The dose of 12.5 mg of methotrexate appears sufficient only for low-titer ectopic gestations (less than 1000 mIU/ml). Kojima and colleagues[134] used 25 mg of methotrexate for laparoscopically directed treatment of nine unruptured ectopic pregnancies. All patients in his series were cured without complications. Lastly, transvaginal aspiration of tubal pregnancies with injection of potassium chloride has cured tubal pregnancies as well.[141, 142]

Eight patients were treated with methotrexate at the University of Mississippi (Table 8–7). Four received therapy to avoid surgery and preserve reproductive capacity; two had significant pulmonary disease; and the remaining two patients had rising hCG titers after conservative surgical treatment of an ectopic pregnancy. Seven patients were treated with 1 mg/kg of methotrexate every other day for three doses, and the eighth patient had transvaginal ultrasound-guided amniotic sac aspiration with injection of 25 mg of methotrexate. In all patients, the ectopic pregnancies were resolved.

In addition to methotrexate, two other agents have been utilized to treat ectopic pregnancy. An antiprogestin (RU-486) was used by Kenigsberg and colleagues[122] to treat a patient with an unruptured ectopic pregnancy. The pregnancy failed to respond to this antiprogestin and was subsequently treated with methotrexate. Vejtorp and colleagues[143] treated 11 women with local injection of prostaglandin $F_{2\alpha}$ at the time of laparoscopy. Prostaglandin was injected under laparoscopic guidance if (1) the tube was visualized; (2) the transverse diameter of the oviduct over the conceptus was less than 2.5 cm; (3) the serosa over the site of the pregnancy was intact; and (4) there was no fresh bleeding for the tubal ostium. In 10 women, the serum concentration of hCG decreased to nonpregnant levels after treatment. One woman required surgery 6 days after treatment because of abdominal pain and unchanged hCG titers.

SUMMARY

The incidence of ectopic pregnancy increased steadily between 1970 and 1984. Since that time, the incidence has remained constant at nearly 20 per 1000 live births. Approximately 70,000 tubal pregnancies and slightly more than 30 deaths occur annually. Historically, most ectopic gestations were diagnosed late in their course, often only after rupture occurred, before the development of readily available hCG and progesterone assays. The addition of transvaginal sonography to the diagnostic armamentarium of the clinician has further improved our ability to detect ectopic pregnancies before symptoms or rupture occurs. Early detection and a desire to conserve reproductive potential in women affected with tubal pregnancies have led to the application of conservative surgery and medical treatment for this condition. Nearly 45% of women treated with conservative surgery or methotrexate subsequently carry a pregnancy to term.

References

Epidemiology and Risk Factors

1. Dorfman SF, Grimes DA, Cates W Jr, et al.: Ectopic pregnancy mortality, United States, 1979 to 1980: Clinical aspects. Obstet Gynecol 64:386, 1984.
2. Coupet E: Ectopic pregnancy: The surgical epidemic. J Natl Med Assoc 81:567, 1989.
3. Makinen JI: Increase of ectopic pregnancy in Finland: Combination of time and cohort effects. Obstet Gynecol 73:21, 1989.
4. Makinen JI: Erkkola RU, Laippala PJ: Causes of the increase in the incidence of ectopic pregnancy. A study on 1017 patients from 1936 to 1985 in Turku, Finland. Am J Obstet Gynecol 160:642, 1989.
5. Leach RE, Ory SJ: Modern management of ectopic pregnancy. J Reprod Med 34:324, 1989.
6. Ectopic pregnancy: United States, 1984 and 1985. MMWR 37:637, 1988.
7. James WH: A hypothesis on the increasing rates of ectopic pregnancy. Paediatr Perinat Epidemiol 3:189, 1989.
8. Breen JL: A 21 year survey of 645 ectopic pregnancies. Am J Obstet Gynecol 106:1004, 1979.
9. Russel JB: The etiology of ectopic pregnancy. Clin Obstet Gynecol 30:181, 1987.
10. Uotila J, Heinonen PK, Punnonen R: Reproductive outcome after multiple ectopic pregnancies. Int J Fertil 34:102, 1989.

Table 8–7. PATIENTS TREATED FOR TUBAL PREGNANCIES WITH METHOTREXATE AT THE UNIVERSITY OF MISSISSIPPI

Condition	Initial hCG	Route	Days to Resolve
Persistent	142	IM	22
Primary	3660	IM	55
Primary	1250	IM	27
Primary	3890	IM	44
Primary	2360	IM	47
Primary	519	IM	53
Persistent	17,957	IM	77
Primary	14,229	Sac	60
Persistent	4520	IM	32

*IM—intramuscular.

11. Mitchell DE, McSwain HF, Peterson HB: Fertility after ectopic pregnancy. Am J Obstet Gynecol 161:576, 1989.
12. Scott JR: Ectopic pregnancy. Danforth's Obstetrics and Gynecology, 6th Edition. Philadelphia: J.B. Lippincott Co., 1990, p. 221.
13. Puri P, McGuinness EPJ, Guiney EJ: Fertility following perforated appendicitis in girls. J Pediatr Surg 24:547, 1989.
14. Ory SJ: Ectopic pregnancy: Current evaluation and treatment [Editorial]. Mayo Clin Proc 64:874, 1989.
15. Kjer JJ, Knudsen LB: Ectopic pregnancy subsequent to laparoscopic sterilization. Am J Obstet Gynecol 160:1202, 1989.
16. Fedele L, Acaia B, Parazzini F, Ricciardiello O, Bandiani GB: Ectopic pregnancy and recurrent spontaneous abortion: Two associated reproductive failures. Obstet Gynecol 73:206, 1989.
17. Easley HA, Olive DL, Holman JF: Contemporary evaluation of suspected ectopic pregnancy. J Reprod Med 32:901, 1987.
18. Ectopic Pregnancy: United States, 1986. MMWR 38:481, 1989.

Histopathology

19. Parmley TH: The histopathology of tubal pregnancy. Clin Obstet Gynecol 30:119, 1987.
20. Stock RJ: Histopathology of fallopian tubes with recurrent tubal pregnancy. Obstet Gynecol 75:9, 1990.
21. Budowick M, Johnson TRB Jr, Genadry R, et al.: The histopathology of the developing tubal ectopic pregnancy. Fertil Steril 34:169, 1980.
22. Stock RJ: Histopathologic changes in tubal pregnancy. J Reprod Med 30:923, 1985.
23. Green LK, Kott ML: Histopathologic changes in ectopic tubal pregnancy. Int J Gynecol Pathol 8:255, 1989.
24. McClausland AM: Endosalpingosis ("endosalpingoblastosis") following laparoscopic tubal coagulation as an etiologic factor of ectopic pregnancy. Am J Obstet Gynecol 143:12, 1982.
25. Hallatt S: Tubal conservation in ectopic pregnancy: A study of 200 cases. Am J Obstet Gynecol 154:1216, 1986.

hCG and Diagnosis

26. Pittaway DE, Reish RL, Wentz AC: Doubling times of human chorionic gonadotropin increase in early viable intrauterine pregnancies. Am J Obstet Gynecol 152:299, 1985.
27. Pittaway D: Diagnosis of ectopic pregnancy. Obstet Gynecol 68:440, 1986.
28. Holman FJ, Tyrey EL, Hammond CB: A contemporary approach to suspected ectopic pregnancy with use of quantitative and qualitative assays for the beta subunit of human chorionic gonadotropin and sonography. Am J Obstet Gynecol 150:151, 1984.
29. Milwidsky A, Adoni A, Segal S, et al.: Chorionic gonadotropin and progesterone levels in ectopic pregnancy. Obstet Gynecol 50:145, 1977.
30. Batzer FR, Weiner S, Corson SL: Landmarks during the first forty-two days of gestation demonstrated by the b-subunit of human chorionic gonadotropin and ultrasound. Am J Obstet Gynecol 146:973, 1983.
31. Pittaway D, Wentz AC, Maxson W, et al.: The efficacy of early pregnancy monitoring with serial chorionic gonadotropin determinations and relay-time sonography in an infertility population. Fertil Steril 44:190, 1985.
32. Ooi DS, Perkins SL, Claman P, Muggah HF: Serum human chorionic gonadotropin levels in early pregnancy. Clin Chim Acta 181:281, 1989.
33. Storring PL, Gaine-Des RE, Bangham DR: International reference preparation of human chorionic gonadotropin for immunoassay: Potency estimates in various bioassays and protein binding assay systems and international reference preparation of the alpha and beta subunits of human chorionic gonadotropin for immunoassay. J Endocrinol 84:295, 1980.
34. Kauppila A, Rantakyla P, Huhtaniemi I, et al.: Trophoblastic markers in the differential diagnosis of ectopic pregnancy. Obstet Gynecol 55:560, 1980.
35. Kadar N, DeVore G, Romero R: Discriminatory hCG zone: Its use in the sonographic evaluation for ectopic pregnancy. Obstet Gynecol 58:156, 1981.
36. Kadar N, Caldwell BV, Romero R: A method of screening for ectopic pregnancy and its indications. Obstet Gynecol 58:162, 1981.
37. Romero R, Kadar N, Philipe J, et al.: Diagnosis of ectopic pregnancy: Value of the discriminatory human chorionic gonadotropin zone. Obstet Gynecol 66:357, 1985.
38. Funk A, Hubner F, Fendel H: The use of a vaginal probe in the diagnosis of ectopic pregnancy. Arch Gynecol Obstet 244:163, 1989.
39. Timor-Tritsch IE, Yeh MN, Peisner DB, Lesser KB, Slavik TA: The use of transvaginal ultrasonography in the diagnosis of ectopic pregnancy. Am J Obstet Gynecol 161:157, 1989.
40. Cacciatore B, Stenman UH, Ylostalo P: Comparison of abdominal and vaginal sonography in suspected ectopic pregnancy. Obstet Gynecol 73:770, 1989.
41. Bryson SCP: B-subunit of human chorionic gonadotropin, ultrasound, and ectopic pregnancy: A prospective study. Am J Obstet Gynecol 146:163, 1983.
42. Mahony B, Filly R, Nyberg D, et al.: Sonographic evaluation of ectopic pregnancy. J Ultrasound Med 4:221, 1985.
43. Fossum G, Davajan V, Kletzky O: Early detection of pregnancy with transvaginal ultrasound. Fertil Steril 49:788, 1988.
44. Shapiro B, Cullen M, Taylor K, et al.: Transvaginal ultrasonography for the diagnosis of ectopic pregnancy. Fertil Steril 50:425, 1988.
45. Romero R, Kadar N, Castro D, et al.: The value of adnexal sonographic findings in the diagnosis of ectopic pregnancy. Am J Obstet Gynecol 158:52, 1988.
46. Radwansaka E, Frankenberg V, Allen E: Plasma progesterone levels in normal and abnormal early human pregnancy. Fertil Steril 30:398, 1978.
47. Hubinot CJ, Thomas C, Schwers JF: Luteal function in ectopic pregnancy. Am J Obstet Gynecol 156:669, 1987.
48. Norman RJ, Buck RH, Kemp MA, et al.: Impaired corpus luteum function in ectopic pregnancy cannot be explained by altered human chorionic gonadotropin. J Clin Endocrinol Metab 66:1166, 1988.
49. Matthew CP, Coulson PB, Wild RA: Serum progesterone levels as an aid in the diagnosis of ectopic pregnancy. Obstet Gynecol 68:390, 1986.
50. Yeko T, Gorrill M, Hughes L, et al.: Timely diagnosis of early ectopic pregnancy using a single blood progesterone measurement. Fertil Steril 48:1048, 1987.
51. Buck RH, Joubert SM, Worman RJ: Serum progesterone in the diagnosis of ectopic pregnancy: A valuable diagnostic test? Fertil Steril 50:752, 1988.
52. Stovall TG, Ling FW, Cope BJ, Buster JE: Preventing ruptured ectopic pregnancy with a single serum progesterone. Am J Obstet Gynecol 160:1425, 1989.
53. Riss PA, Radivojevic K, Bieglmayer C: Serum progesterone and human chorionic gonadotropin in very early pregnancy: Implications for clinical management. Eur J Obstet Gynecol Reprod Biol 32:71, 1989.

Surgery

54. Parry JS: Extrauterine pregnancy: Its causes, species, pathologic anatomy, clinical history, diagnosis, prognosis, and treatment. Philadelphia: Lea and Febiger, 1876.
55. Tait RL: Five cases of extrauterine pregnancy operated upon at the time of rupture. Br Med J 1:1250, 1884.
56. Stromme WB: Salpingotomy for tubal pregnancy: Report of a successful case. Obstet Gynecol 1:472, 1953.
57. DeCherney AH, Romero R, Naftolin F: Surgical manage-

ment of unruptured ectopic pregnancy. Fertil Steril 35:21, 1981.

58. DeCherney A, Boyers A: Isthmic ectopic pregnancy: Segmental resection as the treatment of choice. Fertil Steril 44:307, 1985.

59. Vermesh M, Silva PD, Rosen GF, et al.: Management of unruptured ectopic gestation by linear salpingostomy: A prospective, randomized clinical trial of laparoscopy versus laparotomy. Obstet Gynecol 73:400, 1989.

60. Langer R, Bukovsky I, Herman A, et al.: Conservative surgery for tubal pregnancy. Fertil Steril 38:427, 1982.

61. Henderson SR: Ectopic tubal pregnancy treated by operative laparoscopy. Am J Obstet Gynecol 160:1462, 1989.

62. Novy M: Surgical alternatives for ectopics: Is conservative treatment best? Contemp OB/GYN 21:91, 1983.

63. Stangel JJ, Reyniak JV, Stone ML: Conservative surgical management of tubal pregnancy. Obstet Gynecol 48:241, 1976.

64. Shinfeld J, Reedy G: Mesosalpingeal vessel ligation for conservative treatment of ectopic pregnancy. J Reprod Med 28:823, 1983.

65. DeCherney AH, Polan ML, Kort H, et al.: Microsurgical technique in the management of tubal ectopic pregnancy. Fertil Steril 34:324, 1980.

66. Stangel JJ, Gomel V: Techniques in conservative surgery for tubal gestation. Clin Obstet Gynecol 23:1221, 1985.

67. Timonen S, Nieminen U: Tubal pregnancy: Choice of operative method of treatment. Acta Obstet Gynecol Scand 46:327, 1967.

68. Jeffcoate TN: Salpingectomy or salpingo-oophorectomy. J Obstet Gynecol 135:74, 1955.

69. Abrams J, Farrel D: Salpingectomy and salpingoplasty for tubal pregnancy: Survey of the literature. Obstet Gynecol 24:281, 1964.

70. Hallatt JG: Tubal conservation in ectopic pregnancy: a study of 200 cases. Am J Obstet Gynecol 154:1216, 1986.

71. Schenker JG, Evron S: New concepts in the surgical management of tubal pregnancy and the consequent postoperative results. Fertil Steril 40:709, 1983.

72. Mecke H, Semm K, Lehmann-Willenbrock E: Results of operative pelviscopy in 202 cases of ectopic pregnancy. Int J Fertil 34:93, 1989.

73. Brumstead J, Kessler C, Gibson C, et al.: A comparison of laparoscopy and laparotomy for the treatment of ectopic pregnancy. Obstet Gynecol 71:889, 1988.

74. Bruhat MA, Manhes H, Mage G: Treatment of ectopic pregnancy by means of laparoscopy. Fertil Steril 33:411, 1980.

75. Shapiro H, Adler D: Excision of an ectopic pregnancy through the laparoscope. Am J Obstet Gynecol 117:290, 1983.

76. Pouly J, Mahnes H, Mage G, et al.: Conservative laparoscopic treatment of 321 ectopic pregnancies. Fertil Steril 46:1093, 1986.

77. DeCherney A, Diamond M: Laparoscopic salpingostomy for ectopic pregnancy. Obstet Gynecol 70:948, 1987.

78. Tulandi T, Falcone T, Kafta I: Second-look operative laparoscopy 1 year following reproductive surgery. Fertil Steril 52:421, 1989.

79. Makinen JI, Salmi TA, Nikkanen VP, Koskinen EYJ: Encouraging rates of fertility after ectopic pregnancy. Int J Fertil 34:46, 1989.

80. Plowman L, Wicksell F: Fertility after conservative surgery in tubal pregnancy. Acta Obstet Gynecol Scand 39:143, 1960.

81. Kucera E, Mack F, Novak J, et al.: Fertility after operations of extra uterine pregnancy. Int J Fertil 14:127, 1969.

82. Schenker J, Eyal Z, Polishuk W: Fertility after tubal surgery. Surg Gynecol Obstet 135:74, 1972.

83. Franklin E, Ziederman A: Tubal ectopic pregnancy: Etiology and obstetric and gynecologic sequelae. Am J Obstet Gynecol 117:220, 1973.

84. Sherman D, Langer R, Sadovsky G, et al.: Improved fertility following ectopic pregnancy. Fertil Steril 37:497, 1982.

85. Badawy S, Taymoar E, Shaykh M, et al.: Conservative treatment of tubal pregnancy: Factors affecting future fertility. Int J Fertil 31:187, 1986.

86. Vehaskari A: The operation of choice for ectopic pregnancy with references to subsequent fertility. Acta Obstet Gynecol Scand 39(Suppl 3):1, 1960.

87. Jaruinen PA, Nummi S, Pietila K: Conservative operative treatment of tubal pregnancy with postoperative hydrotubation. Acta Obstet Gynecol Scand 51:169, 1972.

88. Stromme WB: Conservative surgery for ectopic pregnancy: A twenty year review. Obstet Gynecol 41:215, 1973.

Persistent Trophoblast

89. Johnson TRB, Sanborn JR, Wagner KS, Compton AA: Gonadotropin surveillance following conservative surgery for ectopic pregnancy. Fertil Steril 33:207, 1980.

90. Thatcher SS, Grainger DA, True LD, DeCherney AH: Pelvic trophoblastic implants after laparoscopic removal of tubal pregnancy. Obstet Gynecol 74:514, 1989.

91. Reich H, DeCaprio J, McGlynn F, Wilkie WL, Longo S: Peritoneal trophoblastic tissue implants after laparoscopic treatment of tubal ectopic pregnancy. Fertil Steril 52:337, 1989.

92. Kamrava MM, Taymor ML, Berger MJ, et al.: Disappearance of human chorionic gonadotropin following removal of ectopic pregnancy. Obstet Gynecol 62:486, 1983.

93. Richards BX: Persistent trophoblast following conservative operation for ectopic pregnancy. Am J Obstet Gynecol 150:100, 1984.

94. Rivlin M, Meeks GR, Cowan BD, et al.: Persistent trophoblastic tissue following salpingostomy for unruptured ectopic pregnancy. Fertil Steril 43:323, 1985.

95. Bell O, Awadalla S, Mattox J: Persistent ectopic syndrome: A case report and literature review. Obstet Gynecol 69:521, 1987.

96. DiMarchi J, Kosasa T, Kobara T, et al.: Persistent ectopic pregnancy. Obstet Gynecol 70:555, 1987.

97. Lund J: Early ectopic pregnancy: Comments on conservative treatment. J Obstet Gynecol Br Emp 62:70, 1955.

98. Cowan BD, McGehee RP, Bates GW: Treatment of persistent ectopic pregnancy with methotrexate and leukovorum rescue: A case report. 67(suppl):50, 1986.

99. Higgins KA, Schwartz MB: Treatment of persistent trophoblastic tissue after salpingostomy with methotrexate. Fertil Steril 45:427, 1986.

100. DeCherney A, Kase N: The conservative surgical management of unruptured ectopic pregnancy. Obstet Gynecol 54:451, 1979.

101. Swolin K, Fall M: Ectopic pregnancy. Acta Eur Fertil 3:147, 1972.

102. Bruhat M, Manhes H, Mage G, et al.: Treatment of ectopic pregnancy by means of laparoscopy. Fertil Steril 33:411, 1980.

103. Langer R, Bukovsky I, Herman A, et al.: Conservative surgery for tubal pregnancy. Fertil Steril 38:427, 1982.

104. Ohel G, Katz M, Blumenthal B: Complete abortion of early ectopic pregnancy. Int J Gynaecol Obstet 17:596, 1980.

105. Masiach S, Carp H, Serr D: Nonoperative management of ectopic pregnancy. A preliminary report. J Reprod Med 27:127, 1982.

106. Carp HJ, Oelsner G, Serr D, et al.: Fertility after nonsurgical treatment of ectopic pregnancy. J Reprod Med 31:119, 1986.

107. Dericks T, Scholtz C, Tauber H: Spontaneous recovery of ectopic pregnancy: A preliminary report. Eur J Obstet Gynecol Reprod Biol 25:181, 1987.

108. Garcia A, Aubert J, Sama J, et al.: Expectant management of presumed ectopic pregnancy. Fertil Steril 48:395, 1987.

109. Fernandez H, Rainhorn J, Pariernik E, et al.: Spontaneous

resolution of ectopic pregnancy. Obstet Gynecol 71:171, 1988.

110. Grets G, Quagliarello J: Declining serum concentrations of the beta subunit of hCG and ruptured ectopic pregnancy. Am J Obstet Gynecol 156:940, 1987.

111. Uribe MA, Dunn RC, Buttram VC: Tubal pregnancy with normal hysterosalpingogram and negative pregnancy test. Obstet Gynecol 75:483, 1990.

New Frontiers and Methotrexate

112. Tanaka T, Hayashi H, Kutsuzawa T, et al.: Treatment of interstitial ectopic pregnancy with methotrexate: report of a successful case. Fertil Steril 37:851, 1982.

113. Farabow WS, Fulton JW, Fletcher V Jr, Velat CA, White JT: Cervical pregnancy treated with methotrexate. NCMJ 44:91, 1983.

114. Chotiner HC: Nonsurgical management of ectopic pregnancy associated with severe hysterstimulation syndrome. Obstet Gynecol 66:740, 1985.

115. Ory SJ, Villanueva AL, Sand PK, and Tamura RK: Conservative treatment of ectopic pregnancy with methotrexate. Am J Obstet Gynecol 154:1299, 1986.

116. Rodi IA, Sauer MV, Gorrill MJ, et al.: The medical treatment of unruptured ectopic pregnancy with methotrexate and citrovorum rescue: Preliminary experience. Fertil Steril 46:811, 1986.

117. Cheng YT, Chang FM, Hsieh FJ, et al.: Cervical pregnancy: Report of a case with unsuccessful treatment of methotrexate. J Formosan Med Assoc 85:1000, 1986.

118. Brandes MC, Youngs DD, Goldstein DP, Parmley TH: Treatment of cornual pregnancy with methotrexate: Case report. Am J Obstet Gynecol 155:655, 1986.

119. Goldstein DP: Treatment of unruptured ectopic pregnancy with methotrexate with folinic acid rescue (MTX-FA). Presented at the 34th Annual Clinical Meeting, American College of Obstetricians and Gynecologists, New Orleans, May 1986.

120. Feichtinger W, Kemeter P: Conservative treatment of ectopic pregnancy by transvaginal aspiration under sonographic control and methotrexate injection. Lancet (February 14):381, 1987.

121. Ichinoe K, Wake N, Shinkai N, et al.: Nonsurgical therapy to preserve oviduct function in patients with tubal pregnancies. Am J Obstet Gynecol 156:484, 1987.

122. Kenigsberg D, Porte J, Hull M, Spitz IM: Medical treatment of residual ectopic pregnancy: RU 486 and methotrexate. Fertil Steril 47:702, 1987.

123. Sauer MV, Gorrill MJ, Rodi IA, et al.: Nonsurgical management of unruptured ectopic pregnancy: An extended clinical trial. Fertil Steril 48:752, 1987.

124. Haans LCF, van Kessel PH, Kock HCLV: Treatment of ectopic pregnancy with methotrexate. Eur J Obstet Gynecol Reprod Biol 24:63, 1987.

125. Sauer MV, Gorrill MJ, Rodi IA, et al.: Nonsurgical treatment of unruptured isthmic ectopic pregnancy: Preliminary experience. Int J Fertil 33:116, 1988.

126. Patsner B, Kenigsberg D: Successful treatment of persistent ectopic pregnancy with oral methotrexate. Fertil Steril 50:982, 1988.

127. Leeton J, Davison G: Nonsurgical management of unruptured tubal pregnancy with intra-amniotic methotrexate: Preliminary report of two cases. Fertil Steril 50:167, 1988.

128. Stoval TG, Ling FW, Buster JE: Outpatient chemotherapy of unruptured ectopic pregnancy. Fertil Steril 51:435, 1989.

129. Clark L, Raymond S, Stanger J, Jackel G: Treatment of ectopic pregnancy with intraamniotic methotrexate: A case report. Aust N Z J Obstet Gynaecol 29:84, 1989.

130. Pansky M, Bukovsky I, Golan A, et al.: Local methotrexate injection: A nonsurgical treatment of ectopic pregnancy. Am J Obstet Gynecol 161:393, 1989.

131. Zakut H, Sadan O, Katz A, et al.: Management of tubal pregnancy with methotrexate. Br J Obstet Gynaecol 96:725, 1989.

132. Skannal D, Burkman RT: Cervical pregnancy treated with methotrexate: A case report. J Reprod Med 34:496, 1989.

133. Cairns JD, Xuereb D: Persistent ectopic syndrome. Can J Surg 32:387, 1989.

134. Kojima E, Abe Y, Morita M, et al.: The treatment of unruptured tubal pregnancy with intratubal methotrexate under laparoscopic control. Obstet Gynecol 75:723, 1990.

135. Berkowitz RS, Goldstein DP, Bernstein MR: Ten years' experience with methotrexate and folinic acid as primary therapy for gestational troploblastic disease. Gynecol Oncol 23:111, 1986.

136. Stanhope CR, Smith JP: Germ cell tumours. Clin Obstet Gynecol 10:357, 1983.

137. Rustin GJS, Booth M, Dent J, et al.: Pregnancy after cytotoxic chemotherapy for gestational trophoblastic tumours. Br Med J 288:103, 1984.

138. Pektasides D, Rustin GJS, Newlands ES, et al.: Fertility after chemotherapy for ovarian germ cell tumours. Br J Obstet Gynecol 94:477, 1987.

139. Golbus MS: Oocyte sensitivity to induced meiotic nondisjunction and its relationship to advanced maternal age. Am J Obstet Gynecol 146:435, 1983.

140. Gates AH, Donaldson CH, Ley MD: Oocyte aneuploidy screening using superovulating prepubertal mice: effect of methotrexate. Teratology 24:321, 1981.

141. Robertson DE, Moye MA, Hansen JN, et al.: Reduction of ectopic pregnancy by injection in patients with ultrasound control. Lancet (April 25):974, 1987.

142. Timor-Tritsch I, Baxi L, Peisner DB: Transvaginal salpingocentesis: a new technique for treating ectopic pregnancy. Am J Obstet Gynecol 160:459, 1989.

143. Vejtorp M, Vejerslev LO, Ruge S: Local prostaglandin treatment of ectopic pregnancy. Human Reprod 4:464, 1989.

144. Feichtinger W, Kemeter P: Treatment of unruptured ectopic pregnancy by needling of sac and injection of methotrexate or PG E_2 under transvaginal sonography. Arch Gynecol Obstet 246:85, 1989.

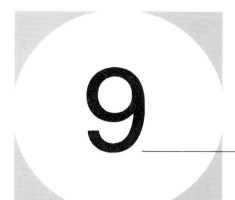

9

Extratubal Ectopic Gestation

Warren C. Plauché

- GENERAL DISCUSSION
  Incidence
  Morbidity and Mortality
- SPECIFIC EXTRATUBAL ECTOPIC
  GESTATIONS
  Ovarian Pregnancy
  Abdominal (Peritoneal) Pregnancy
  Rudimentary Horn Pregnancy

Intraligamentous Pregnancy
Pregnancies Within the Uterine Wall
  Cornual Pregnancy
  Intramural Pregnancy
  Cervical Pregnancy
  Pregnancy in Uterine Sacculations
- SUMMARY

GENERAL DISCUSSION

Ninety-two to 97% of ectopic gestations occur in the fallopian tube.[1] The remaining 3 to 8% of cases are among the most interesting and unusual of all pregnancy complications. Extratubal ectopic pregnancy is usually thought of as "abdominal pregnancy." The subject is much more complex and covers pregnancies at several sites.

Ectopic pregnancies that occur on the peritoneal surface of the pelvic organs are the common true abdominal pregnancies. The fetus develops within the peritoneal cavity in these cases and may reach advanced gestational age.

Extratubal ectopic pregnancies also develop within the ovary, in the broad ligament, or within the wall of the normal uterus or cervix. The fertilized ovum can settle in an isolated rudimentary horn of the uterus or in a uterine sacculation. Ectopic gestations occur in organs as remote from the pelvis as the liver, the spleen, and the omentum.

A small number of abdominal pregnancies are primary implantations of fertilized eggs. Most cases are secondary implantations, the result of pregnancies that continue to develop after tubal abortions or uterine ruptures.

There was once controversy in the obstetric literature about the existence of both primary and secondary implantations. This argument led to the establishment of strict criteria for the diagnosis of primary peritoneal pregnancy.[2] We are drawn to the probability of primary implantations by abdominal gestations in patients with previous total vaginal or abdominal hysterectomies. Niebyl[3] and Nehra and Loginsky[4] collected 29 such cases. Milosevic and Toth[5] published the microscopic findings of a pregnancy localized entirely within an ovarian follicle, confirming a primary extratubal gestation site.

Nicholas,[6] in 1934, found it experimentally impossible to transfer implanted ova to sites other than the original implantation. This work, with rat embryos, appeared to discredit the hypothesis of secondary peritoneal implantations. The finding proved to be species-specific. Ectopic gestation is indeed a rare phenomenon in lower mammals. Displaced human embryos often develop at implantation sites other than the endometrial cavity. Figure 9–1 illustrates the potential sites of ectopic gestation.

Extratubal ectopic pregnancies occasionally survive to advanced gestational age. There are several reports of term abdominal pregnancies with delivery of living children.[7–10] Badawy[11] stated that advanced ectopic gestations, though rare, are some of the most dangerous complications of childbearing. The outcome for the fetus is very poor. The mother is at some risk of death and at high risk for extensive and prolonged morbidity. Advanced ectopic gestation challenges the diagnostic ability and surgical skills of the most seasoned obstetricians.

This chapter discusses the diagnosis and clinical management of the broad spectrum of extratubal ectopic gestation.

Incidence

Table 9–1 displays a classification of ectopic implantation sites, with an estimate of the occur-

Table 9–1. FREQUENCY OF ECTOPIC IMPLANTATION SITES

Site	% of Ectopic Pregnancies	
	%	%
Primary tubal		92–97
Primary ovarian		0.5–2
Peritoneal (abdominal)		1.6
Primary	(0.2)	
Secondary	(1.4)	
Primary hepatic, splenic, and omental	(0.01)	
Uterine		4.9–5.6
Interstitial	(4.1)	
Cornual	(0.3–0.7)	
Cervical	(0.1–0.2)	
Intramural	(0.3–0.5)	
Sacculation	(0.1)	
Rudimentary horn	(0.08)	
Intraligamentous		0.3–0.5

rence rate at each site. It is difficult to determine the true incidence of many of these entities because of their infrequent occurrence.

The worldwide incidence of ectopic pregnancies approaches 1 in 200 pregnancies. The number of ectopic pregnancies increased sharply in the past 2 decades.[1] Makinen[12] spoke of an epidemic of ectopic pregnancy in Scandinavian countries that report the highest incidences of ectopic gestations.

Figure 9–2 outlines the age-related occurrence rate for ectopic gestation in Finland between the years 1968 and 1984. The slope of the curve of rising incidence is steep and shows no tendency to moderation. This curve could be extrapolated, with only slight modification, to describe the prevalence of ectopic gestation in most Western countries.

The fallopian tube traps most (92 to 97%) of the wayward fertilized eggs destined to be ectopic

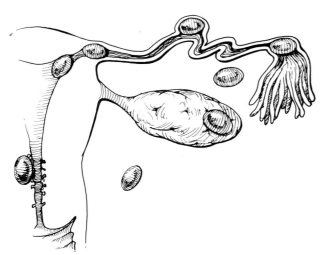

Figure 9–1. Sites of ectopic gestations: fallopian tube, uterine cornu, cervix, broad ligament, ovary, and peritoneal cavity.

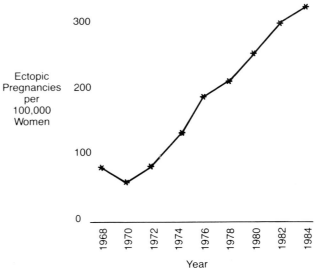

Figure 9–2. Incidence of ectopic pregnancy in Finland, age group 25 to 35 years. Modified from Makinen JI: Obstet Gynecol 73:21, 1989.

pregnancies. The preceding chapter discussed tubal ectopic gestations. The most common sites of ectopic gestation other than the fallopian tube are uterine sites outside the endometrial cavity (4.9 to 5.6%). The fertilized egg may implant in a uterine cornu (0.3%) or in the interstitial portion of the tube (4.1%).[7, 13] It may float down and become lodged in the cervix (0.1 to 0.2%).[14] It may burrow within the wall of the myometrium (0.3 to 0.5%)[5] or find itself in a congenital sacculation of the uterine wall (0.1%). The rarest of uterine implantations is in the blind pouch of a rudimentary uterine horn (0.08%).[15]

The peritoneal cavity supplies an adequate, though ascetic, implantation site for human embryos.[3, 8, 10] Peritoneal gestations constitute 1.6% of extratubal ectopic pregnancies. Primary peritoneal gestations implant on peritoneal surfaces throughout the coelomic cavity. Even the liver, spleen, bowel, and omentum support an occasional ectopic pregnancy.[16–18]

Secondary peritoneal implantations favor the surfaces of the broad ligament, the posterior surface of the uterus, and the pouch of Douglas.[1] The trophoblastic elements of these pregnancies often spread to involve the adnexal structures, the lateral pelvic wall, and the large and small bowel in search of sustaining blood supply. Because no decidual layer separates the ectopic trophoblast from the organs it invades, the placenta becomes a dangerous, invasive parasite.

The ovary is the primary site of implantation in 0.5% of ectopic gestations.[19–21] The criteria required to make the diagnosis of primary ovarian pregnancy are strict. The observation of a gestation within an ovarian follicle proves the existence of ovarian pregnancy as an entity separate from peritoneal pregnancies affixed to the ovary.[5]

A rare form of ectopic gestation grows between the leaves of the broad ligament (0.3 to 0.5%).[22, 23] Intraligamentary gestation is particularly dangerous because of the proximity of large uterine and iliac vessels and the ureter.

Heterotopic gestation combines extrauterine and intrauterine pregnancies. Reports of over 500 heterotopic pregnancy cases appear in the literature.[15, 24]

Fewer than 100 cases of trophoblastic neoplasias, hydatidiform mole or choriocarcinoma, are reported in ectopic gestations.[15, 25] Teratomatous chorionepithelioma is among the most unusual manifestations of ectopic gestation. The literature contains only a dozen such tumors.[15]

Morbidity and Mortality

Ware,[9] in a 1948 survey of 249 cases from the world's literature on abdominal pregnancy, quoted a maternal mortality rate of 14.5%. Beacham and colleagues[10] surveyed 65 cases from Charity Hospital of New Orleans in 1962 and recorded a maternal mortality rate of 6%. More recent studies quote maternal mortality rates varying from 0 to 20%.[26–28]

The fetus does not fare as well as the mother. Recent papers quote fetal mortality rates of 50[29] to 95%.[10] Tan and colleagues[30] found deformities of the fetus in 20 to 40% of abdominal pregnancies. These are mostly pressure-induced deformities. The frequency of deformities related to genetic chromosomal abnormalities is no higher than that of intrauterine pregnancies.[31]

Clark and Jones[32] estimated the overall fetal salvage rate with abdominal pregnancy to be 11%. They stated that any improvement of this outcome would only come at significant and increased risk to the mother.

SPECIFIC EXTRATUBAL ECTOPIC GESTATIONS

Ovarian Pregnancy

Ovarian pregnancy constitutes 0.5 to 2% of ectopic gestations. The incidence has been estimated from 1 per 5000 to 1 per 50,000 pregnancies.[33] Table 9–2 outlines the incidence reported in several studies over the last 3 decades.[19, 33–42] The mean incidence is one ovarian pregnancy per 17,820 deliveries (0.006%). One of 141 ectopic gestations fulfills the criteria for ovarian pregnancy (0.7%).

Table 9–2. INCIDENCE OF OVARIAN PREGNANCY

Author	Year	Incidence Per No. of Deliveries	Incidence Per No. of Ectopic Pregnancies
Hertig[34]	1951	1/33,000	1/110
Bercovici et al.[35]	1958	1,5,900	1/24
Bacile and Nagler[37]	1959	1/11,156	
Dowling et al.[37]	1960	1/55,316	1/486
Malkasian et al.[20]	1963	1/14,185	1/208
Boronow et al.[21]	1965	1/9229	1/36
Lehfeldt et al.[38]	1970	1/40,000	1/143
Ellis[39]	1978	1/5,641	
Gray and Ruffolo[40]	1978	1/2,034	1/21.5
Hallatt[19]	1981	1/11,300	1/97
Grimes and Nosal[33]	1983	1/8263	
MEAN		1/17,820	1/141

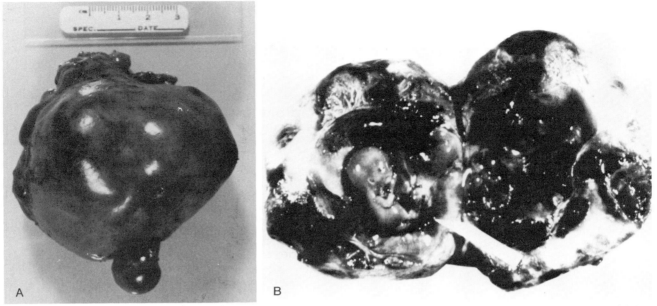

Figure 9–3. A, Ovarian pregnancy. Surgical gross specimen, intact. B, Specimen from A opened. Fetus of crown-rump length of 3½ cm is seen entirely within the ovary. (Reprinted with permission from the American College of Obstetricians and Gynecologists. Grimes HG, Nosal RA, Gallagher JC: Ovarian pregnancy: A series of 24 cases. Obstet Gynecol 61:176, 1983.)

Ovarian pregnancy was first recognized in the late seventeenth century. There are many individual reports of unusual ovarian gestations. Grimes and Nosal[33] recorded an ovarian pregnancy occurring years after the mother had a vaginal hysterectomy (Fig. 9–3). There have been cases of twin ovarian pregnancies and molar ovarian pregnancies.[18, 21] Pregnancy has been recorded within an ovarian follicle[5] and in an ovarian endometrial cyst[35] (Fig. 9–4). Williams and colleagues[41] recorded a pregnancy that originated in the ovary and went to term.

The English language literature lists fewer than 500 ovarian pregnancies. Some historic cases were not verified primary ovarian pregnancies but abdominal pregnancies that involved the ovary.

Spiegelberg[42] set strict criteria for the diagnosis of primary ovarian pregnancy. The tube must be intact on the involved side. The fetus and membranes must be near the ovary. The pregnancy site must be traceable to the uterus via the utero-ovarian pedicle. There must be ovarian tissue in the wall of the gestation sac. Quilligan and Zuspan[15] added the requirement of chorionic villi within the ovary. Rubin[43] insisted on removal of the tube with the ovary to establish the true site of the pregnancy. Baden and Heins[44] believed that ovarian tissue must form an intact tissue layer around the gestation to qualify as a true primary ovarian pregnancy. Table 9–3 summarizes the criteria for the diagnosis of ovarian pregnancy.

Ovarian pregnancies rarely become advanced. Symptoms usually appear early and mimic tubal ectopic gestation. Williams and colleagues,[41] how-ever, reported a term ovarian pregnancy with delivery of a living female infant.

CLASSIFICATION OF OVARIAN PREGNANCY

Baden and Heins[44] classified ovarian pregnancy as outlined in Table 9–4. This classification has more teleologic and pathologic than clinical significance. The clinical picture and management decisions are similar for all classes.

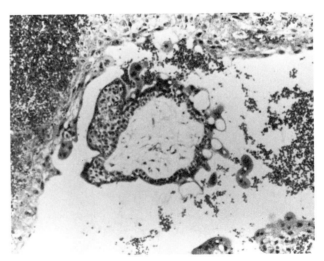

Figure 9–4. Ovarian pregnancy, very early gestation. Chorionic vesicle with surrounding trophoblast within a hemorrhagic ovarian cyst surrounded by ovarian cortex. (From Gray CL, Ruffolo EH: Ovarian pregnancy associated with intrauterine contraceptive devices. Am J Obstet Gynecol 132:135, 1978.)

Table 9–3. CRITERIA FOR THE DIAGNOSIS OF
OVARIAN PREGNANCY

Fallopian tube on the involved side is intact
Fetus and membranes are located in the region of the ovary
Pregnancy site is traceable to the uterus via the utero-ovarian
   pedicle
Ovarian tissue in the wall of the gestation sac is histologically
   proved
Trophoblastic tissue and villi are histologically identified within
   the ovary

ASSOCIATED CONDITIONS

Lehfeldt and colleagues,[38] in 1970, described the association between ovarian pregnancies and the use of intrauterine contraceptive devices. More than two dozen studies from the 1970s confirmed this relationship. Intrauterine contraceptive devices coexisted with one tenth of all of the cases of ovarian pregnancy. This relationship is beyond the realm of chance. Five of the last eight patients with ovarian pregnancies in Hallatt's[19] large series used intrauterine contraceptive devices, and yet this author did not emphasize the use of these devices as being an important etiologic factor.[19] Hallatt emphasized the relationship between ovarian pregnancy and pelvic inflammatory disease and previous tubal ligation.

Boronow and colleagues[21] listed a number of potential causes of ovarian implantation varying from likely to fanciful (Table 9–5). It is difficult to demonstrate that ovulation is impeded by sticky granulosa cells or low follicular pressure. Parthenogenesis seems an unlikely proposal. The presence of positive chromatin bodies within the nuclei of cells of fetuses in ovarian pregnancies militates against the possibility of virginal ovarian pregnancy.

Pure accident is a plausible explanation. The ubiquitous sperm must very occasionally fertilize a mature egg near the surface of the ovary just after ovulation. If the tube fails to entrap this fertilized egg, the developing trophoblast invades any contiguous tissue available, ovarian or otherwise.

Retrograde peristalsis and flow of particles in the fallopian tube have been demonstrated. It is conceivable that a fertilized egg in the tube might occasionally be regurgitated into the peritoneal cavity to seek a secondary target of opportunity for implantation.

The most attractive hypothesis is obstructed ovulation resulting from the residual effects of

Table 9–4. CLASSIFICATION OF OVARIAN PREGNANCY

Primary ovarian pregnancy—ovarian tissue completely around
   pregnancy
   Intrafollicular
   Extrafollicular—juxtafollicular, interstitial, cortical, superficial
Combined ovarian pregnancy—ovary forms a portion of
   pregnancy wall

Table 9–5. POSSIBLE CAUSES FOR OVARIAN
IMPLANTATION

Obstructed ovulation
   Inflammation and adhesions
   Tenacious granulosa cells
   Low intrafollicular pressure
Ineffective tubal function
   Inflammation
   Adhesions
   Idiopathic
   Retrograde tubal peristalsis
Favorable surface phenomena
   Decidualization
   Endometriosis
Parthenogenesis
Chance

Modified from Boronow RC, McElin TW, West RH: Ovarian pregnancy: Report of 4 cases and 13 year review of English literature. Am J Obstet Gynecol 91:1095, 1965.

pelvic inflammatory disease. A fallopian tube with an endothelial lining destroyed by inflammation or containing fimbria distorted by adhesions rejects a fertilized egg but ensnares it long enough to allow surface implantation on the ovary. Neither decidual reaction nor endometriotic glands are necessary on the ovarian surface for implantation.

CLINICAL FINDINGS

Few clinical features distinguish ovarian pregnancy from the common tubal ectopic gestation. Hallatt[19] pointed out the clinical features shared by the two entities, as outlined in Table 9–6. Patients with ovarian pregnancies seldom have histories of preceding infertility. This could be because a large number of ovarian pregnancies are first pregnancies. The incidence of primigravidas in collections of ovarian pregnancies is actually about 27%, not an unusual number for any sampling of pregnant women.[21] In contrast, tubal ectopic pregnancy patients often give histories of infertility, previous tubal surgery, or previous ectopic gestation.

The association with intrauterine contraceptive devices appears with both ovarian and tubal ectopic pregnancies. Patients with ovarian pregnancies become symptomatic as early in gestation as those with tubal implantations. An average of only

Table 9–6. CLINICAL FEATURES: OVARIAN VERSUS TUBAL
ECTOPIC PREGNANCY

	Tubal	Ovarian
Average age (yr.)	30	28
Multiparous (%)	68	84*
Infertility (%)	28	4*
Amenorrhea (%)	17	16
Intrauterine contraceptive device (%)	14	20
Average days from last menstrual period to operation	58	55

*Statistically significant difference at p<0.05
From Hallatt JG: Primary ovarian pregnancy: A report of 25 cases. Am J Obstet Gynecol 143:56, 1982.

55 days elapsed between the last normal menstrual period and operation in Hallatt's large series of ovarian pregnancies.

Incorrect preoperative diagnosis occurs in 30 to 70% of ovarian pregnancies.[19, 21] The most common incorrect preoperative diagnoses are ruptured corpus luteum, tubal ectopic pregnancy, and ovarian cyst. Only a high index of suspicion when approaching a patient with suspected ectopic gestation permits the diagnosis of ovarian pregnancy. Only pathologic examination of material obtained by wedge resection or enucleation of a bleeding ovarian mass confirms or rules out this diagnosis.

Obstetricians currently manage many cases of hemorrhagic corpus luteum by laparoscopic identification of the lesion followed by simple observation of the patient. Those lesions that are actively bleeding are often managed without biopsy or enucleation. These management methods fail to diagnose many of the fortunately rare ovarian pregnancies.

The principal clinical manifestations of ovarian pregnancy are abdominal pain and signs of peritoneal irritation. A history of irregular vaginal bleeding is an inconstant feature. Specific preoperative diagnosis is uncommonly difficult.[21]

Table 9–7 outlines surgical features associated with ovarian pregnancy. All cases were located in the immediate vicinity of the corpus luteum. Eighty-four per cent of cases had hemoperitoneum. The amount of blood exceeded 500 mL in 81% of cases.[19] Sixty-four per cent of cases were managed by enucleation or wedge resection. The remainder required oophorectomy.

SURGICAL MANAGEMENT

The patient receives supportive medications, hydration, and transfusion, as with any ectopic gestation. Ultrasonographic evaluation is useful in stable patients. Ultrasound studies show a complex mass in the region of the ovary, separate from the uterus in most cases. Very early cases often display no ultrasonographic abnormality. Fluid in the cul-de-sac of Douglas helps confirm and quantitate hemoperitoneum.

Table 9–7. SURGICAL FEATURES OF PRIMARY OVARIAN PREGNANCY

Surgical Feature	%
Hemoperitoneum	84
Surgical diagnosis	
Ovarian pregnancy	7
Ruptured corpus luteum	18
Tubal ectopic pregnancy	75
Surgical procedure	
Oophorectomy	36
Wedge or enucleation	64
Location adjacent to corpus luteum	100

From Hallatt JG: Primary ovarian pregnancy: A report of 25 cases. Am J Obstet Gynecol 143:56, 1982.

The presence of hemoperitoneum demonstrated by ultrasonography or by culdocentesis leads to prompt laparoscopy or laparotomy. Laparoscopic demonstration of a hemorrhagic ovary is useful but not definitive. An ovarian pregnancy may be missed and may create further problems if the surgeon chooses simple observation.

Laparotomy with enucleation or wedge resection and repair of the ovary is definitive treatment for early ovarian pregnancy.[19, 20] Resection of an early corpus luteum raises some concern about the fate of a possible intrauterine gestation. This concern is legitimate only in the first few weeks of gestation.

Boronow and colleagues[21] rejected the idea of resecting the tube for serial pathologic studies to prove pure ovarian gestation. They suggested conservation of the tube and as much ovarian tissue as possible in patients who wish further pregnancies.

Ovarian pregnancy rarely progresses to advanced gestation. Seventy-five to 90% of these gestations terminate in the first trimester.[21] Advanced cases resemble abdominal pregnancies because trophoblastic tissue invades nearby organs. Management of this situation is described in the following section on abdominal pregnancy.

Abdominal (Peritoneal) Pregnancy

Obstetric historians recorded abdominal or peritoneal pregnancy as early as the tenth century. The removal of an advanced extrauterine pregnancy by swine gelder John Nufer in 1500 is quintessential obstetric history. Mother and child lived, but confirmation of the pathologic findings is missing. John Bard of New York operated in 1759 for advanced extrauterine pregnancy before anesthesia or aseptic techniques existed.[4] The carefully documented case of Galbin in 1896 begins our real knowledge about this pregnancy aberration.[46]

CLASSIFICATION OF ABDOMINAL PREGNANCY

Studdiford[2] provided detailed criteria for the classification of abdominal or peritoneal pregnancies. He identified primary and secondary types. Primary abdominal pregnancies meet the criteria shown in Table 9–8: The tubes and ovaries must be normal; there must be no uteroperitoneal fistula; and there must be an exclusive relationship to the peritoneal surface early in gestation. Emil Novak of Johns Hopkins believed the last criterion could never be met and labeled all abdominal pregnancies secondary ones.[50] More recent authors support this view.[27]

Secondary implantations are certainly the most common manifestation of abdominal pregnancy (Fig. 9–5). These occur after tubal abortion or occasionally after expulsion of a normal implan-

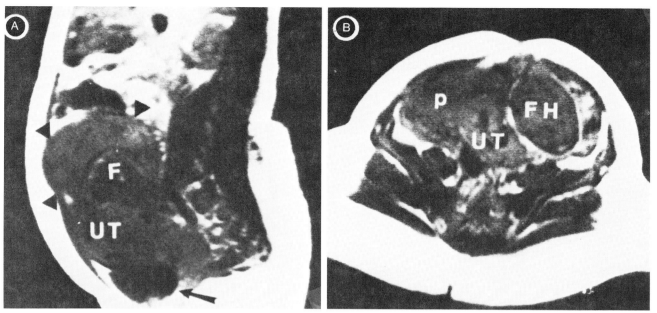

Figure 9–5. *A, B,* Magnetic resonance imaging of an abdominal pregnancy. UT—uterus; F—fetus; P—placenta; FH—fetal head. (From Spanta R, et al.: Abdominal pregnancy: Magnetic resonance identification with ultrasonographic follow-up of placental involution. Am J Obstet Gynecol 157:888, 1987.)

tation through a uterine rupture.[11] Abdominal pregnancies confined to organs very distant from the pelvis are likely to be primary implantations. It is of little clinical concern whether an abdominal pregnancy is primary or secondary.

A more useful clinical classification relates to the location of the extrauterine pregnancy. Table 9–9 outlines the reported sites of implantation of extratubal abdominal (peritoneal) gestations. Abdominal pregnancies most commonly implant in the pouch of Douglas or on the posterior surface of the uterus.[48] The posterior surface of the broad ligament and the lateral pelvic wall are the next most favored sites. Abdominal pregnancies frequently involve segments of the large and small bowels. Advanced abdominal pregnancies often attach to several of these organs, making resection difficult and hazardous.

Peritoneal surface pregnancies can involve distant extrapelvic organs, such as the liver,[16] the spleen,[17] the omentum,[18] and the inferior surface of the diaphragm (Fig. 9–6).[48]

Table 9–8. CLASSIFICATION OF ABDOMINAL (PERITONEAL) PREGNANCIES

Primary Type
Tubes and ovaries normal
No uteroperitoneal fistula
Pregnancy related exclusively to the peritoneal surface, early enough to preclude primary nidation elsewhere

Secondary Type
Post-tubal abortion
Post-uterine rupture

INCIDENCE

Abdominal pregnancy occurs in 0.9 to 5% of ectopic gestations and 1 in 3000 to 1 in 26,000 deliveries.[45, 47] Beacham and colleagues[10] reported one of the highest incidences of abdominal pregnancies at Charity Hospital of New Orleans: 1 in 3161 deliveries. Atrash and colleagues[47] reviewed 5221 abdominal pregnancies reported in the United States from 1970 to 1983. They estimated that abdominal pregnancy occurred once in 9174 pregnancies. There were 9.2 abdominal pregnan-

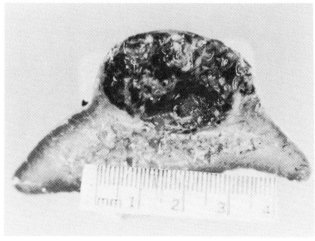

Figure 9–6. Splenic pregnancy. (Reprinted with permission from The American College of Obstetricians and Gynecologists. Yackel DB et al.: Splenic pregnancy: A case report. Obstet Gynecol 71:472, 1988.)

Table 9–9. REPORTED SITES OF IMPLANTATION OF ABDOMINAL (PERITONEAL) PREGNANCY

Intrapelvic Locations
Pouch of Douglas
Posterior surface of uterus
Posterior surface of broad ligament
Lateral pelvic wall
Extrapelvic Locations
Large bowel
Small bowel
Omentum
Liver
Spleen
Diaphragm

From Martin et al.: Abdominal pregnancy: Current concepts of management. Obstet Gynecol 71:549, 1988.

Table 9–10. MORTALITY RISK IN ABDOMINAL PREGNANCY

	Years	Cases	% Mortality
Aggregated reports	1937–1961	169	5.32
Recent reports	1970–1982	2147	0.51

From Atrash HK et al.: Abdominal pregnancy in the United States: Frequency and maternal mortality. Obstet Gynecol 69:333, 1987.

cies among every 1000 ectopic gestations (0.92%) cited in the review by Atrash and colleagues. For the average obstetrician, abdominal pregnancy is a once in a lifetime experience.

MORBIDITY AND MORTALITY

Table 9–10 summarizes maternal mortality risks from abdominal pregnancy as organized by Atrash and colleagues. Individual studies reported deaths varying from 0 to 10% of mothers with abdominal gestations.[28, 32] The mean mortality rate of the historic series was 5.32%. Atrash and co-workers' collection of 2147 cases from the modern era had a mean mortality rate of only 0.51%. Mortality risk has decreased tenfold because of improved early diagnosis, better management decisions, blood transfusions, antibiotics, and access to improved surgical facilities.

Patients with abdominal pregnancy rarely die if the condition is recognized and treated early in gestation. Among all deaths related to abdominal pregnancy, only 13% of patients presented in the first trimester. Nine of the 11 deaths in Atrash and co-workers' modern series were first seen after 12 weeks' gestation.[47] The middle trimester and early last trimester are the times of instability and highest maternal mortality risk in abdominal pregnancies.

The maternal mortality risk for patients reaching term with abdominal gestations is 19%. Intra-abdominal hemorrhage causes most of the maternal deaths.[47] Abdominal and pelvic infections are the next leading causes of death.

The perinatal mortality risk for fetuses of abdominal pregnancies varies from 40 to 95%. Thirty to 90% of these infants have severe malformations.[47] Most malformations are compression disorders, not chromosomal abnormalities (Fig. 9–7).

CLINICAL FINDINGS

The clinical picture of patients with abdominal pregnancy varies with the gestational age and condition of the pregnancy. Some cases go to term with few untoward signs or symptoms (Fig. 9–8A, B). These cases can go undetected until labor fails to occur. There are several reports of failed attempts at induction of labor in such cases.[48] Separation of the placenta or death of the fetus is often the first sign of trouble. Placental separation can be catastrophic and result in fetal demise and rapid exsanguination of the mother.

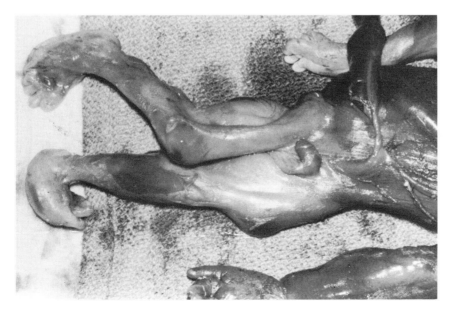

Figure 9–7. Pressure deformities of the lower extremities of the fetus in advanced abdominal pregnancy. (Reprinted with permission from the American College of Obstetricians and Gynecologists. Martin JN Jr, et al.: Abdominal pregnancy: Current concepts of management.)

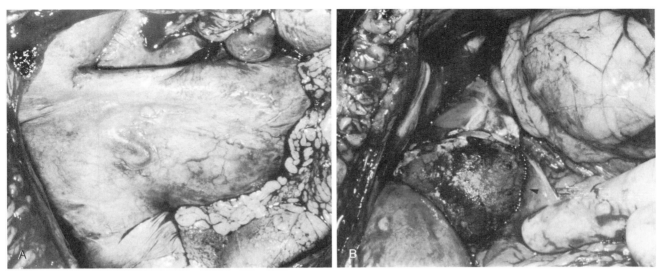

Figure 9–8. Advanced abdominal pregnancy. *A,* Typical appearance of the gestational sac on opening the abdomen. *B,* The fetal head is visible after the gestational sac is opened. (Reprinted with permission from the American College of Obstetricians and Gynecologists. Martin JN Jr et al.: Abdominal pregnancy: Current concepts of management. Obstet Gynecol 71:554, 1988.)

The clinical triad of an extrauterine mass, a positive pregnancy test, and an empty endometrial cavity is the clue to diagnosis of early extrauterine pregnancy. Tubal ectopic gestations and early abdominal gestations display similar clinical pictures. Patients with abdominal pregnancies often have vague gastrointestinal complaints early in gestation, and most report some type of abdominal pain.[47]

As gestation progresses, the patient notes abnormal fetal movement patterns and unusual positions of the fetus. More alarming symptoms that lead to extensive work-up develop by the late second or early third trimester. The average gestational age at diagnosis in the University of Mississippi Medical Center series reported by Martin and colleagues was 26.5 weeks.[48]

Physical examination confirms an unusual transverse or oblique lie in many cases. There is usually no presenting part in the pelvis. The cervix is often displaced far anterior to its normal position. Fetal parts feel very superficial when palpated without intervening uterine muscle wall. Martin and colleagues[47] reported absent fetal heart tones in five of nine patients first seen after 16 weeks' gestation. Four of these patients also reported cessation of fetal movements.

The presence of pre-eclampsia was once thought to rule out the possibility of abdominal pregnancy. This is patently untrue, since pre-eclampsia or eclampsia complicated 32 cases of advanced abdominal pregnancy reviewed by Moodley and coworkers.[51]

Ultrasonography identifies some suspected abdominal pregnancies but is not uniformly accurate in surgically confirmed cases. Magnetic resonance imaging holds promise in diagnosis and preoperative evaluation of placental anatomic relationships.[16, 52] These techniques also provide very useful information about placental involution when the placenta is left in place at surgery (see Figs. 9–5*A, B*).

An abdominal surgical emergency is the presenting problem for a large percentage of abdominal pregnancy patients. Hemoperitoneum is caused by disturbance of the placental bed and partial placental separation. Peritoneal irritation signs may also signal intestinal obstruction or perforation.

SURGICAL MANAGEMENT OF ABDOMINAL PREGNANCY

Most authors suggest prompt operation for abdominal pregnancy as soon as the diagnosis is made.[10, 47] Should management be different when a symptom-free patient is first diagnosed with a live fetus near viability?

Several factors mitigate against a prolonged period of expectant observation. Many fetuses of abdominal pregnancies develop serious pressure and positional deformities of the extremities and head. Separation of a portion of the placental bed can occur at any time. The internal bleeding this causes can result in rapid maternal exsanguination. Unexpected fetal demise is common.

Prompt operation on discovery of the problem is the prudent course in most cases. A short wait for viability when the fetus appears to be normal is not unreasonable when the patient understands and agrees to the risks.

Abdominal pregnancies found very early in gestation are superficial and can sometimes be removed without dangerous bleeding. The depth of implantation quickly increases as gestation progresses. One must then remove the organs on which the placenta implanted, when possible, or allow involution of the placenta at its chosen site.

Advanced abdominal gestations are very dangerous. The natural tendency of the surgeon is to attempt removal of the entire pregnancy. Removal of the placenta is unwise unless it has implanted only on organs one can excise with impunity.

Do not attempt removal or even the gentlest exploration of the placental site unless all blood supply to the placenta can be safely ligated. Leave it alone and leave it in place.[10, 43, 53]

An effective approach for advanced cases is to open the abdomen very carefully. Incise the amniotic sac if it is still present and remove the fetus. Clamp, ligate, and divide the umbilical cord close to its insertion on the placental surface. Make no attempt to disturb the placental site. To do so risks brisk, uncontrollable bleeding. Close the abdomen with the placenta in place. Follow the patient during the period of placental involution with serial ultrasonography or other imaging procedures. Resorption of the placenta is a slow process. The placental mass persists for many months or even years.

Uncontrollable hemorrhage from the placental bed in abdominal pregnancy seldom responds to packing or attempts to ligate visible vessels. Angiographic arterial embolization can selectively occlude the placental blood supply. Kivikoski and colleagues[53] reported success with this procedure in a patient who was exsanguinating despite multiple vessel ligations and packing of the pelvis (Fig. 9–9). Clamping or compressing the aorta for temporary hemostasis can help clear the operating field. Chervenak and colleagues[54] reported application of an aortic clamp for 40 minutes, during which time removal of the abdominal pregnancy and control of bleeding were possible.

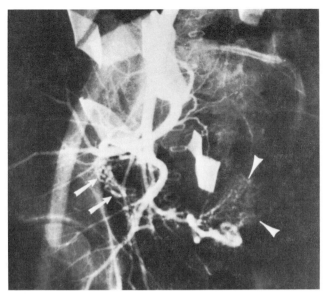

Figure 9–9. Arterial angiography prior to embolization of placental blood supply in abdominal pregnancy. Right internal iliac artery injection. Arrows indicate the placental bed circulation on the right pelvic side wall. Arrowheads indicate the uterus. The coiled tapes are markers for surgical sponges. (Reprinted with permission from the American College of Obstetricians and Gynecologists. Kivikoski AI, et al.: Angiographic arterial embolization to control hemorrhage in abdominal pregnancy: A case report. Obstet Gynecol 71:457, 1988.)

ADJUNCTIVE THERAPY

Methotrexate destroys trophoblastic tissue and accelerates the involution of the placenta.[55] Chemically accelerated placental involution after operation for advanced abdominal gestations creates large amounts of fluid and detritus within the abdomen.[27] These conditions favor colonization by gut bacteria and increase the chance of suppuration at the placental site.

Lathrop and Bowles[56] used a 5-day course of 12.5 mg of intramuscular methotrexate daily. Their patient experienced both stomatitis and leukopenia. The placental mass actually expanded and required reoperation and drainage. Despite these complications, as well as delayed closure of the drain site, this group recommended judicious use of methotrexate therapy.

Rahman and colleagues[27] found the complications of methotrexate to outweigh its advantages in the management of retained abdominal placentas. They recommended limitation or abandonment of methotrexate for this purpose. The Louisiana State University service at Charity Hospital has not used methotrexate adjunctive therapy for abdominal pregnancies.

Bright and Maser[57] recommended in 1961 that patients have a second laparotomy for removal of the placenta. They felt that at least 9 weeks should elapse to reduce placental vascularity. Current majority opinion favors nonintervention and resorption without reoperation unless complications ensue.

Rudimentary Horn Pregnancy

Mauriceau described the first case of pregnancy in a rudimentary uterine horn in 1669. A comprehensive review of this subject by O'Leary and O'Leary in 1963 discovered only 328 reported cases (Fig. 9–10A, B).[56] Pregnancy in a rudimentary uterine horn is ten times less common than abdominal pregnancy.

Ninety per cent or more of rudimentary uterine horns do not communicate with the principal uterine cavity. The mode of fertilization involves migration of sperm or the fertilized ovum.[58] The former is apparently much more common, since 90 to 95% of corpora lutea associated with pregnancies in rudimentary horns are in the ipsilateral ovary.[58, 59]

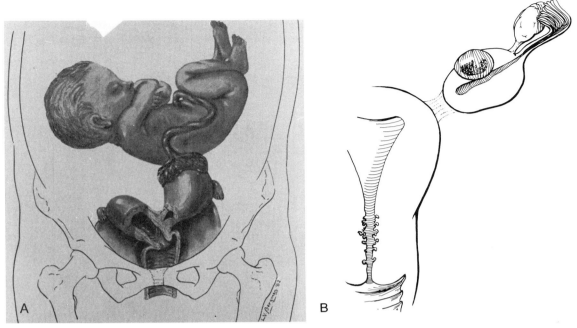

Figure 9–10. *A, B,* Rudimentary horn pregnancy. The rudimentary uterine horn usually does not connect with the principal uterine cavity. In this case, the pregnancy is seen free in the abdominal cavity with placental attachment solely to the rudimentary uterine horn. (*A* is reprinted with permission from the American College of Obstetricians and Gynecologists. O'Leary JL, O'Leary JA: Rudimentary horn pregnancy. Obstet Gynecol 22:374, 1963.)

MORBIDITY AND MORTALITY

The O'Leary review[58] revealed a somber prognosis for implantation in a rudimentary horn. The pregnancy ruptured in 89% of cases. Rupture occurred in the first trimester in 33% and in the second trimester in 61%. Fetal death occurred in 98% of cases when rupture complicated pregnancy in a rudimentary horn. Fifteen per cent of fetuses in rudimentary horns undergo mummification and develop into lithopedions.[59] The few pregnancies that advanced to term had a fetal mortality rate of 80%. A small percentage of cases become secondary abdominal pregnancies. Only 2 of 240 cases suitable for review of fetal outcome had a live birth at term.[58] Table 9–11 summarizes the prognosis for implantations in a uterine horn.

Table 9–11. PROGNOSIS FOR IMPLANTATION IN A RUDIMENTARY UTERINE HORN

Outcome	%
Rupture	89
First trimester	33
Second trimester	61
Third trimester	6
Fetal mummification	15
Proceed to term	<5
Fetal mortality at term	80+
Overall live births (2/240)	0.83

From O'Leary JL, O'Leary JA: Rudimentary horn pregnancy. Obstet Gynecol 22:371, 1963.

CLINICAL FINDINGS IN RUDIMENTARY HORN PREGNANCY

Eastman[60] wisely said that often the only complaint of the patient with extrauterine pregnancy is that "things are not quite right." There are often no specific symptoms or signs. Diagnosis of rudimentary horn pregnancy before operation occurred in only 5% of reported cases.

The passing of a decidual cast raises the physician's suspicions in a few instances. The presence of other maternal congenital anomalies, such as septate vagina or absent kidney, cues the possible existence of a rudimentary uterine horn.

Pregnancy progresses longer in the thick, muscular sac of the rudimentary horn than in the fallopian tube. The crisis of rupture of the horn usually occurs in the middle or early third trimester.

Close examination may disclose a small uterus lateral to the enlarging uterine horn pregnancy mass. The round ligament on the side of the pregnancy uniformly goes into the lateral portion of the mass. The round ligament is not stretched over the pregnancy, as in an intraligamentous gestation. The opposite round ligament goes to the principal uterine horn. Palpation of a round ligament leading into the ectopic gestation identifies pregnancy in a uterine horn. This physical finding is most difficult to elicit.

Ultrasonography in the early stages of pregnancy in a uterine horn reveals a complex adnexal mass. The uterus is displaced and contains no gestational sac. The fetus is only occasionally recognized in a separate uterine horn early in pregnancy. The wall of the rudimentary horn becomes thinned beyond recognition in advanced gestations.

SURGICAL MANAGEMENT OF UTERINE HORN PREGNANCY

Management of pregnancy in a uterine horn is surgical. The logical operation removes the pregnancy and the offending uterine anomaly as soon as the diagnosis is certain, early in gestation. Unfortunately, diagnosis before rupture is rare.

These cases mimic midpregnancy cornual or other spontaneous uterine rupture. Authorities advise special care in securing the ovarian vessels supplying the bulk of the blood flow to the pregnancy mass. Distortion of the course of the ureter or duplication of the ureter is likely. Dissect the ureter and ensure its safety before ligating the adnexal pedicle. Simply clamp, cut, and ligate the fibrous ligament that connects the rudimentary horn with the principal horn.

Careful two-layer closure is wise in the rare instance of communication between the cavity of the anomalous uterine horn and that of the principal uterine cavity. There is no need to resect the unaffected uterine horn.

Advanced cases and those that rupture and become secondary abdominal pregnancies present much more difficult surgical problems. The exact location of the pregnancy and placenta is often not clear. Authorities advise removal of the fetus and leaving the placenta in situ with or without subsequent reoperation. Total excision risks the massive hemorrhage that characterizes disturbance of the placental site in abdominal pregnancy.

Intraligamentous Pregnancy

Intraligamentous or broad ligament pregnancies grow between the anterior and posterior leaves of the broad ligament (Fig. 9–11). These are extraperitoneal abdominal pregnancies.[61] Most develop after rupture of tubal pregnancies on the mesosalpingeal border of the fallopian tube. A few cases follow lateral rupture of intramural pregnancies. Loschge first described broad ligament pregnancy in 1816.[62]

INCIDENCE

Champion and Tessitore[62] estimated broad ligament pregnancy to constitute one in 613 ectopic gestations and approximately one in 184,000 pregnancies. It is difficult to establish the exact incidence of such an unusual disorder.

CLINICAL FINDINGS IN INTRALIGAMENTOUS PREGNANCY

The following descriptions developed from several reports of single cases and small groups of cases. There are no large series of cases to draw on.

Patients have the signs and symptoms of tubal pregnancy early in the course. Many cases oper-

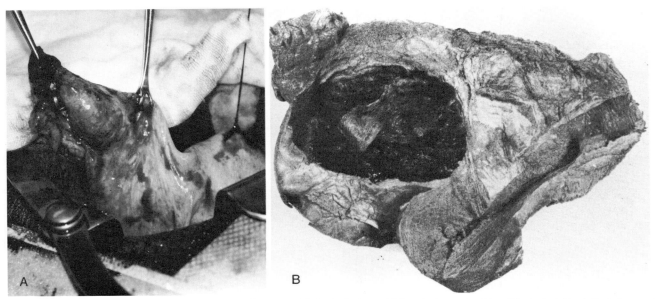

Figure 9–11. *A*, Early intraligamentous gestation. (Courtesy Michael Graham, M.D.; photographed by Rita L. Letellier.) *B*, Advanced intraligamentous pregnancy, right broad ligament. (From Wolfe SA, Neigus I: Broad ligament pregnancy with reports of 3 early cases. Am J Obstet Gynecol 66:106, 1953, Fig. 1, p. 114.)

ated on at this stage are indistinguishable from tubal ectopic pregnancies with broad ligament hematomas. Figure 9–11 shows an early intraligamentous pregnancy in a patient who had a previous tubal ligation.

In a small percentage of such cases, the tubal rupture event is minor and does not trigger investigation or exploration. The patient's signs and symptoms subside. The pregnancy begins its growth in a secondary gestational sac formed by the leaves of the broad ligament.[62] Patients with advanced intraligamentous pregnancies report few symptoms other than local pressure unless rupture or hemorrhage occurs.

The gestation follows one of two courses. The pregnancy may progress to near term when pseudolabor occurs and the fetus expires. When fetal demise occurs earlier in pregnancy, the result is either resorption of the fetus or the formation of an intraligamentous lithopedion.

Physical examination of an advanced case reveals upward and lateral displacement of the uterus. The cervix is neither dilated nor effaced. The pregnancy seems fixed in the pelvis. Palpation reveals no space lateral to the gestation on one side. The pregnancy feels fused to the lateral pelvic side wall. The upper vaginal fornix is often obliterated. Previous authors report that the palpation of the hypertrophied round ligament stretched tightly over the surface of the pregnancy is pathognomonic for intraligamentous pregnancy. Similar findings occur, however, with advanced abdominal pregnancy in the posterior pelvis.

Advanced intraligamentous pregnancies develop as either anterior or posterior forms.[63] Anterior types grow principally by stretching the anterior leaf of the broad ligament. The uterovesical fold may reach the level of the umbilicus. Fetal parts are easily palpable. Posterior forms grow into the cul-de-sac of Douglas. The pregnancy displaces the mesocecum and the mesosigmoid. Fetal parts are

difficult to outline on abdominal examination. The placenta lies anterior and high in both types.

Hysterography or other imaging means occasionally confirm a suspected case, but the diagnosis is rarely clear before operation.

MORBIDITY AND MORTALITY

Wolfe and Niegus[63] offer a maternal mortality rate of 16% for intraligamentous pregnancies. This estimate is an extrapolation from data on more common abdominal pregnancies.[9] Intraligamentous pregnancies produce few liveborn infants.

SURGICAL MANAGEMENT OF INTRALIGAMENTOUS PREGNANCY

Management of intraligamentous pregnancy is surgical. Symptoms of hemorrhage and peritoneal irritation require prompt exploratory surgery. Recall that the placenta is always high and anterior in these cases.

Make the incision into the gestational sac low on the implantation to avoid dislodging the placenta. Extract the fetus, then ligate and divide the umbilical cord near the placenta. Leave the placenta in place, as in an abdominal pregnancy. Bleeding occurs if there is separation of even a small portion of the placenta. When packs do not control this bleeding, hysterectomy is indicated. Anatomic distortion is such that this surgery is formidable. The surgeon must carefully trace the course of the ureter before any deep clamping and ligation. The patient often loses a lot of blood and almost always requires transfusion.

Pregnancies Within the Uterine Wall

Nidation of the developing pregnancy normally takes place in the endometrial cavity. Occasionally, the ovum implants within the uterus but not in the uterine cavity (Fig. 9–12). The result is

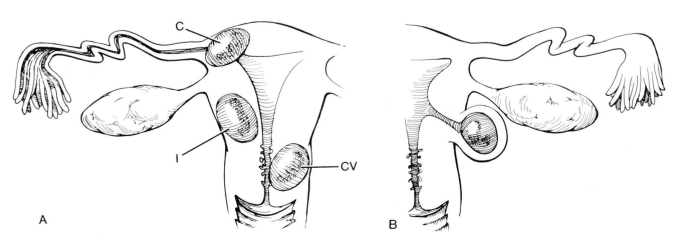

Figure 9–12. *A,* Pregnancies within the uterus but outside the uterine cavity. C—cornual pregnancy; I—intramural pregnancy; CV—cervical pregnancy. *B,* Pregnancy within a sacculation of the uterine wall.

Table 9–12. UTERINE PREGNANCIES OUTSIDE THE ENDOMETRIAL CAVITY

Cornual pregnancy
   Angular
   Interstitial
Intramural pregnancy
Pregnancy in a uterine sacculation
Cervical pregnancy

cornual gestation, intramural pregnancy, pregnancy in a uterine sacculation, or cervical pregnancy (Table 9–12). These rare ectopic gestations constitute 3 to 11% of ectopic pregnancies.[7]

Cornual Pregnancy

It is impossible to distinguish, on clinical findings, pregnancies in the cornual portion of the uterus from those in the interstitial portion of the tube. These are the most frequent pregnancies within the uterine wall. Pregnancies at these sites grow normally for several months, then rupture through the cornual portion of the uterus with disastrous effects (Fig. 9–13).

Cornual and interstitial pregnancies constitute about 2.5% of all ectopic gestations.[64] Cornual pregnancies are nidations that take place in the thinned portion of the uterus near the ostia of the fallopian tubes. These are properly labeled angular or cornual gestations and are excluded from the numbers of tubal gestations.

Previous tubal surgery is the factor most commonly associated with cornual pregnancy. Ron-El and colleagues[65] illustrate this with a patient who had a previous tubal resection for ectopic preg-

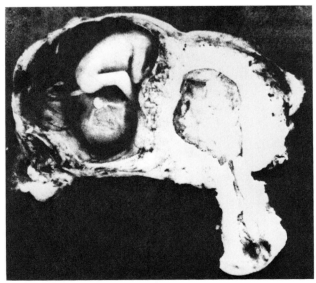

Figure 9–13. Interstitial (cornual) pregnancy. (Reprinted by permission from the Southern Medical Journal. Gray CL: Interstitial pregnancy. South Med J 73:1278, 1980.)

nancy. She later developed a combined midtrimester ruptured cornual gestation with an intrauterine pregnancy that carried to 37 weeks.

Repeated ipsilateral ectopic gestations after tubal resection must be the result of recanalization of the cornual resection site. The resulting uteroperitoneal fistula permits passage of sperm and entry of a fertilized ovum. Wechstein[66] proposes that the voyage of the ovum slows because of scarring or distortion at the fistula site; therefore implantation of the ovum occurs in the uterine cornu. Current practice abandons cornual resection of tubal pregnancy for more conservative tubal surgical procedures (see Chapter 8).[64]

CLINICAL FINDINGS IN CORNUAL PREGNANCY

Cornual pregnancies give few warnings of their presence before catastrophic rupture in the middle trimester. The uterus may feel asymmetric in early pregnancy. The examiner often reports the presence of a fundal leiomyoma. Ultrasonography may show the gestational sac to be in an unusual location high in one corner of the endometrial cavity. The condition mimics pregnancy in one horn of a double uterus. The examiner cannot distinguish the two without prior knowledge of the anatomy.

The true nature of the disorder becomes overt when the patient develops sudden severe pain, shock, and signs of intraperitoneal hemorrhage. An occasional case advances to near term without rupture.

The Louisiana State University Obstetrics Service at Charity Hospital of New Orleans recently had such a case. The patient's nonprogressive labor pattern necessitated cesarean delivery. The fetus was in an opaque but thin sac. We entered this sac immediately on opening the abdomen. After removal of the fetus, it was obvious that the pregnancy had occupied the right cornu of the uterus. The gestation did not occupy the general endometrial cavity. We resected the sac that had held the gestation. The pathologist reported an interstitial pregnancy, based on the finding of smooth muscle in multiple samples from the gestational sac. Debate continues as to whether this represented a term pregnancy in the interstitial portion of the tube or a cornual pregnancy at term.

SURGICAL MANAGEMENT OF CORNUAL PREGNANCY

The management of cornual pregnancy is surgical. In early, unruptured cases, resect the cornu around the implantation. Close the defect in two or three layers as you would close a classic cesarean incision.

Surgical exploration of an advanced ruptured cornual pregnancy reveals one side of the upper uterus violently blown outward. The fetus is usually free in the abdominal cavity. The cavity in the wall of the uterus has a ragged wall of torn myometrium and placental tissue. Bleeding is brisk, and a large amount of blood collects in the pelvis and abdominal cavity.

Surgical options are cornual suture reconstruction, cornual resection and repair, and hysterectomy. Hysterectomy is often necessary to gain control of blood loss and to remedy extensive damage to the uterus. Previous ectopic gestations have already threatened the health and lives of many of these patients.

It is sometimes possible to perform a more conservative cornual repair. Every effort is made to repair the uterus when the patient has expressed a wish to become pregnant again. Freshen the edges of the rupture and close the defect with two or three layers of 00 or 000 polyglycolic/polyglactan absorbable suture.

Long-term follow-ups of repaired cases are too few to predict reliably the course of later pregnancy. Ron-El and colleagues[65] and Beckmann and colleagues[67] reported cases of coexistent normal implantations and cornual gestations. They resected the cornual gestations early in pregnancy. The normally implanted pregnancies continued until cesarean delivery near term without further complication.

Brandes and colleagues[68] reported successful treatment of a cornual pregnancy with systemic methotrexate. The presumed diagnosis was gestational trophoblastic disease, for which the patient received an 8-day course of methotrexate. A cornual gestation suspected on later hysterosalpingogram was confirmed by laparoscopy. The cornual pregnancy resolved without further surgery. The authors commented on the possible utility of this method when surgery is contraindicated or for patients who wish future pregnancies.

Methotrexate management depends on reliable prerupture diagnosis. Diagnosis of cornual pregnancy before rupture is, unfortunately, quite unusual. Biochemical assessment of very early gestation is increasingly accurate. Early, reliable detection of extratubal ectopic gestation would make nonsurgical management feasible.

Ling and co-workers at the University of Tennessee in Memphis are evaluating a protocol for all patients of childbearing age who appear in the emergency department, regardless of diagnosis. They are screened for pregnancy with a sensitive test for human chorionic gonadotropin. A serum progesterone concentration is checked on human chorionic gonadotropin-positive patients. If serum progesterone is below 6.5 ng per mL the pregnancy is deemed to be nonviable. Curettage is performed to look for villi. If none are seen, a gestational sac is searched for, using vaginal ultrasonic imaging.

Gestational sacs over 3 cm in diameter or those containing cardiac activity are managed by traditional laparotomy or laparoscopy. Patients whose gestational sac is less than 3 cm and who show no cardiac activity are treated with methotrexate. If this or similar management plans become standard, many extratubal ectopic gestations will be managed very early in gestation. Many surgical emergencies could be avoided.

Intramural Pregnancy

Intramural pregnancies develop within the uterine wall (see Fig. 9–12A). They must be separate from the uterine cavity and fallopian tube and surrounded by myometrium to support this diagnosis. There must be no congenital sacculation, diverticulum, or congenital anomaly of the uterus.[7] We found only 19 reported cases in literature searches from 1924 to the present.

Two possible scenarios could explain this rare phenomenon. Nidation could take place in a deep endometrial gland that is later sequestered within the wall of the uterus. Implantation could occur on the serosal surface of the uterus and burrow inward.

It is difficult to point out etiologic or clinical features of so rare a phenomenon. The most consistently reported associated pathologic finding is deficient decidua in the endometrial cavity. Previous uterine trauma and infection are common cohorts. Cava and Russell[7] suggested an etiologic pattern similar to that of placenta accreta.

Intramural pregnancy is an operating table diagnosis in most cases. Intramural pregnancies give few signs before they rupture in the second trimester. The patient has severe pain in the lower abdomen and signs of peritoneal irritation and hypovolemia.

Treatment includes exploratory laparotomy and blood transfusion. Damage to the uterus is usually extensive enough to necessitate hysterectomy. Hysterectomy in the presence of widespread trauma and hematoma formation is always challenging. Hemostasis and a clear operating field are difficult to obtain. The ureters and large pelvic vessels are at risk during dissection. Ligation of the internal iliac arteries or aortic compression provides temporary hemostasis and allows the surgeon to identify anatomic landmarks.

Maternal and fetal morbidity and mortality are similar to those for spontaneous rupture of normally implanted gestations (see Chapter 13).

Cervical Pregnancy

Cervical pregnancy is a most unusual manifestation of ectopic gestation and a dangerous one. Jauchler and Baker,[69] in 1970, found 37 reported cases in their broad search of the literature. In 22 of these, the diagnosis was unconfirmed by surgical pathologic specimens. Various studies estimate the incidence at one in 2400 to one in 18,000 pregnancies. Our estimated incidence is ten times lower than the latter. It is difficult to ascertain the true incidence of so rare a condition. Shinagawa and Nagayama[70] reported an unusually large series of 19 cases of cervical pregnancy among several thousand therapeutic abortion cases in Japan.

Studdiford[71] defined cervical pregnancy as nidation and development of the fertilized ovum within the structure of the cervix, with the uterine corpus remaining uninvolved. Surgical pathologic specimens must show cervical glands adjacent to the placenta. The placenta must intimately attach to the cervix below the entrance of the uterine vessels. There must be no fetal elements in the corpus uteri. Figures 9–14 and 9–15 show examples of early and advanced cervical pregnancies.

ETIOLOGIC FACTORS IN CERVICAL PREGNANCY

Schneider[72] proposed an attractive theory about the etiology of certain ectopic pregnancies that may explain cervical pregnancies. He examined the time span of ovum transit through the tube and the endometrial cavity and out of the cervix. At some time during this transit, the fertilized ovum develops the capability for implantation. Schneider proposed that slowing of transit or acceleration of implantation capability produces tubal or cornual gestations. Similar logic indicates that speeding of transit or delayed nidation capability would occasionally produce placenta previa and cervical pregnancy.

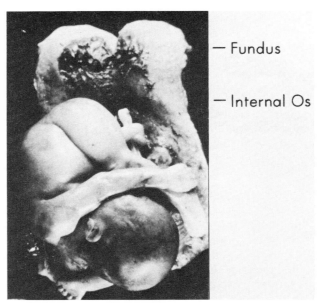

Figure 9–15. Advanced cervical pregnancy—20 weeks' gestation. Fetus in situ. (Reprinted with permission from the American College of Obstetricians and Gynecologists. Parente JT: Cervical pregnancy. Obstet Gynecol 62:81, 1983.)

Uterine trauma or infectious injury to the endometrium plays a role in development of cervical as well as other uterine ectopic gestations. In the 19 patients in Shinagawa and Nagayama's series, all but one had previous elective abortions. Each of the five cases in the report by Parente and colleagues[74] had had previous curettages. This group found that 25 of 31 patients in literature review cases of cervical pregnancy had previous uterine curettages.

Thomasen and Johansen[73] reported two women with cases of cervical pregnancy, both of whom had had previous therapeutic abortions. One also had had a previous cesarean delivery. Four of the eight most recently reported patients with cervical pregnancy had had previous cesarean deliveries.[69, 73] Uterine scarring may speed the passage of the fertilized egg or slow its implantation. This usually results in undetected abortion, but cervical gestation can occur if the fertilized ovum implants in cervical glands.

There are two possible clinical courses for cervical pregnancies. They may grow and eventually rupture the cervix, or they may abort. The latter course is much more common. Advanced cervical pregnancy is very rare.

CLINICAL FINDINGS IN CERVICAL PREGNANCY

Cervical pregnancies mimic threatened abortions early in their course. The patient displays signs and tests positive for pregnancy. There is a varying period of amenorrhea, usually of 6 to 12 weeks. Vaginal bleeding without cramping pain

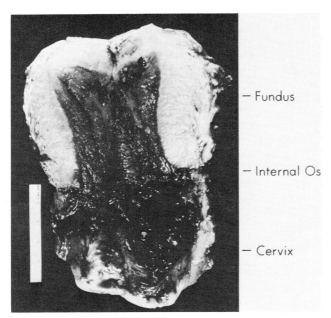

Figure 9–14. Early cervical pregnancy—10 weeks' gestation. (Reprinted with permission from the American College of Obstetricians and Gynecologists. Parente JT: Cervical pregnancy. Obstet Gynecol 62:81, 1983.)

brings the patient to the physician. The cervix is discolored and enlarged. The external os is usually open. It may be possible to palpate the uterus as a mass separate from and above the cervical mass.

SURGICAL MANAGEMENT OF CERVICAL PREGNANCY

Incomplete or inevitable abortion is the usual presumptive diagnosis. There is little indication of the extent of the problem until attempts at evacuation begin. Bleeding that does not respond to oxytocic agents quickly becomes profuse. Packing of the evacuated cavity may temporarily slow or stop the hemorrhage, but bleeding frequently recurs after packing. New hemostatic materials, such as Avitene or fibrin glue, can be helpful in such situations. Transfemoral embolization of branches of the internal iliac arteries can also be attempted.

Hysterectomy is necessary when packing and other efforts at hemostasis fail to control bleeding. Enlargement of the cervix and pericervical hemorrhage distort anatomic relationships. Dissection must be attempted with caution.

Pelosi[75] described and illustrated an inventive cervicotomy approach to cervical pregnancy evacuation. He ascribed the method to Dubrovici of Romania. He placed hemostatic sutures at 3 and 9 o'clock at the lateral edges of the cervix. Incision of the vaginal mucosa permits reflection of the bladder from the cervix and isthmus. Anterior cervicotomy opens the cervical canal, permitting digital removal and curettage of the gestation. Sutures are used to close the cervix and vagina.

The currently recommended management sequence for cervical pregnancy is evacuation and application of pressure by cervical packing with hemostatic agents and gauze. Perform embolization or hysterectomy if hemostasis is not secure.

Pregnancy in Uterine Sacculations

Defects in the muscle layers of the uterine wall that resemble diverticula of the bowel are rare developmental anomalies. Nidation in these sites can enfold and grow as though within the uterine wall. The clinical presentation, signs, symptoms, and management of these cases are the same as in intramural gestations. Some pregnancies in sacculations carry to near term, whereas others rupture in the middle or last trimester.

A case from the Louisiana State University-Charity Hospital service offers an example of a sacculated pregnancy. The patient had no complications with her first pregnancy except that she had Marfan syndrome. She complained of pelvic discomfort and back pain early in her second pregnancy. Two manipulations early in her second pregnancy repositioned what was thought to be a symptomatic retroflexed uterus. On the second attempt, the uterus was manually elevated from the hollow of the sacrum at 16 weeks' gestation with the patient under spinal anesthesia. The patient continued to be uncomfortable throughout pregnancy but otherwise had no difficulties.

Cesarean delivery was performed at 37 weeks' gestation because of oligohydramnios, an undergrown fetus, and a nonreactive nonstress test. The normal fetus and placenta were in a thin-walled fibromuscular sac that replaced the normal posterior uterine wall. The remainder of the uterus appeared normal. The endometrial cavity was hardly distorted by the pregnancy. We excised the anomalous sac and repaired the uterus in two layers, as in classic cesarean incision repair, but on the posterior surface of the uterus. Tubal ligation was done at the patient's previous request. She recovered without incident.

SUMMARY

Ectopic gestations occur throughout the abdominal cavity and at aberrant sites within the fallopian tubes and uterine wall. Early diagnosis is enhanced by technologic improvements in imaging and biochemical detection and evaluation of pregnancies. It is now possible to manage some very early ectopic gestations without surgical intervention. This capability doubtless will expand in the future.

Advanced ectopic gestations at any site pose formidable surgical problems for the obstetrician. Birth of a living baby from an extratubal ectopic gestation is a rare and reportable event. The later stages of extrauterine pregnancy also threaten the life of the mother. Rupture of the uterus and separation of the abnormally implanted placenta are difficult surgical adversaries.

Surgical management decisions reflect concern for the preservation of the life of the mother, her health, and her reproductive capacity. Moral and ethical concerns about the baby modify these decisions, particularly when the fetus approaches viability.

Emergencies arising from extratubal ectopic gestations challenge the anatomic knowledge, operative skills, and ingenuity of the obstetric surgeon. Final decisions in nonemergency cases develop from multiple consultations and open discussion with colleagues, the patient, and her family.

References

1. Iffy L: Ectopic pregnancy. In Iffy L, Kaminetsky HA (eds.): Principles and Practice of Obstetrics and Perinatology, Vol. 1. New York: John Wiley and Sons, pp. 609–633, 1981.
2. Studdiford WD: Primary peritoneal pregnancy. Am J Obstet Gynecol 44:487, 1942.
3. Niebyl JR: Pregnancy following total hysterectomy. Am J Obstet Gynecol 119:512, 1974.

4. Nehra PC, Loginsky SJ: Pregnancy after vaginal hysterectomy. Obstet Gynecol 64:735, 1984.
5. Milosevic M, Toth JR: Intrafollicular ovarian gestation. In Kaminetsky HA, Iffy L (eds.): New Techniques and Concepts in Maternal and Fetal Medicine. New York: Van Nostrand Reinhold, 1979, Figure 16a.
6. Nicholas JS: Experiment on developing rats. Anat Rec 53:387, 1934.
7. Cava EF, Russell WM: Intramural pregnancy with uterine rupture: A case report. Am J Obstet Gynecol 131:214, 1978.
8. Broomes ELC: Full term abdominal pregnancy with delivery of a living child. JAMA 145:399, 1951.
9. Ware HH: Observations on 13 cases of late extrauterine pregnancy. Am J Obstet Gynecol 55:561, 1948.
10. Beacham WD, Hernquist WC, Beacham DW, et al.: Abdominal pregnancy at Charity Hospital of New Orleans. Am J Obstet Gynecol 84:1257, 1962.
11. Badawy AH: Abdominal pregnancy in a previously ruptured uterus. Lancet 2:510, 1962.
12. Makinen JI: Increase of ectopic pregnancy in Finland: Combination of time and cohort effects. Obstet Gynecol 73:21, 1989.
13. Gray C: Interstitial pregnancy. South Med J 73:1278, 1980.
14. Thomsen M, Johansen F: Two cases of cervical pregnancy. Acta Obstet Gynecol Scand 40:99, 1961.
15. Quilligan EJ, Zuspan FP: Ectopic pregnancy. In Douglas-Stromme Operative Obstetrics, Fourth Edition. New York: Appleton-Century-Crofts, pp. 219–252.
16. Harris GJ, Al-Jurf AS, Yuh WTC, et al.: Intrahepatic pregnancy. A unique opportunity for evaluation with sonography, computed tomography, and magnetic resonance imaging. JAMA 261:902, 1989.
17. Yackel DB, Panaton ONM, Martin D, et al.: Splenic pregnancy: A case report. Obstet Gynecol 71:471, 1988.
18. Friedrich MA: Primary omental pregnancy. Obstet Gynecol 31:104, 1967.
19. Hallatt JG: Primary ovarian pregnancy: A report of 25 cases. Am J Obstet Gynecol 132:134, 1978.
20. Malkasian GD, Pratt JA, Dockerty MB: Primary ovarian pregnancy: Report of two cases. Obstet Gynecol 21:632, 1963.
21. Boronow RC, McElin TW, West RH, et al.: Ovarian pregnancy: Report of 4 cases and 13 year review of English literature. Am J Obstet Gynecol 91:1095, 1965.
22. McBride WA, Weed JC: Pregnancy of the broad ligament. South Med J 51:1544, 1958.
23. Kobak AF, Fields C, Pollack SL: Intraligamentous pregnancy. Am J Obstet Gynecol 70:175, 1955.
24. Schaefer G: Extrauterine pregnancy with concomitant term uterine pregnancy. Clin Obstet Gynecol 5:875, 1962.
25. Westerhout FC Jr: Ruptured tubal hydatidiform mole. Obstet Gynecol 23:138, 1963.
26. Stafford JC, Ragan WD: Abdominal Pregnancy: Review of current management. Obstet Gynecol 50:548, 1983.
27. Rahman MS, Al-Suleiman SA, Rahman J, et al.: Advanced abdominal pregnancy: Observations in 10 cases. Obstet Gynecol 59:366, 1982.
28. Delke I, Veridiano NP, Tancer ML: Abdominal pregnancy: Review of current management and addition of 10 cases. Obstet Gynecol 60:200, 1982.
29. Dixon HG, Stewart DB: Advanced extrauterine pregnancy. Br Med J 2:1103, 1960.
30. Tan KL, Goon SM, Wee JH: The pediatric aspects of advanced abdominal pregnancy. Br J Obstet Gynaecol 76:1021, 1969.
31. Pelosi MA, Apuzzio JJ: Abdominal pregnancy. In Iffy L, Charles D (eds.): Operative Perinatology. New York: Macmillan Publishing Co., pp. 515–536.
32. Clark SFJ, Jones SH: Advanced ectopic pregnancy. J Reprod Med 14:30, 1975.
33. Grimes HG, Nosal RA: Ovarian pregnancy. In Iffy L, Charles D (eds.): Operative Perinatology. New York: Macmillan Publishing Co., pp. 368–375.
34. Hertig AT: Discussion of Gerin-Lajoie L. Am J Obstet Gynec 62:920, 1951.
35. Bercovici B, Pfau A, Liban E: Primary ovarian pregnancy: Report of three cases, one with implantation in an endometrial cyst of the ovary. Obstet Gynecol 12:596, 1958.
36. Bacile VA, Nagler W: Unruptured ovarian pregnancy. Am J Obstet Gynecol 81:320, 1961.
37. Dowling EA, Collier FC, Bretschneider A: Primary ovarian pregnancy. Obstet Gynecol 15:58, 1960.
38. Lehfeldt H, Tietze C, Gorstein F: Ovarian pregnancy and the intrauterine device. Am J Obstet Gynecol 108:1005, 1970.
39. Ellis RW: Ovarian pregnancy. Obstet Gynecol 14:54, 1978.
40. Gray CL, Ruffolo EH: Ovarian pregnancy associated with intrauterine contraceptive devices. Am J Obstet Gynecol 132:134, 1978.
41. Williams PC, Malvar TC, Kraft JR: Term ovarian pregnancy with delivery of a live female infant. Am J Obstet Gynecol 142:589, 1982.
42. Spiegelberg O: Zur casuistik der Ovarialschwangerschaft. Arch Gynaekol 13:73, 1878.
43. Rubin IC: Discussion. Am J Obstet Gynecol 62:929, 1951.
44. Baden WF, Heins OH: Ovarian pregnancy. Am J Obstet Gynecol 64:353, 1952.
45. McCullough AM: Abdominal pregnancy case report and review of the literature. J R Army Med Corps 132:16, 1986.
46. Kellett RJ: Primary abdominal (peritoneal) pregnancy. J Obstet Gynaecol Br Commonwealth 80:1102, 1973.
47. Atrash HK, Friede A, Hogue CJR: Abdominal pregnancy in the United States: Frequency and maternal mortality. Obstet Gynecol 69:333, 1987.
48. Martin JN Jr., Sessums JK, Martin RW, et al.: Abdominal pregnancy: Current concepts of management. Obstet Gynecol 71:549, 1988.
49. Norenberg DD, Gunderson JH, Janis JF, et al.: Early pregnancy on the diaphragm with endometriosis. Obstet Gynecol 49:620, 1977.
50. Novak E: Gynecological and Obstetrical Pathology. Philadelphia: W. B. Saunders Co., 1940, p. 397.
51. Moodley J, Subrayen KT, Sankar D, et al.: Advanced extrauterine pregnancy associated with eclampsia: A report of 2 cases. S Afr Med J 71:460, 1987.
52. Mattison DR, Angtuaco T: Magnetic resonance imaging in prenatal diagnosis. Clin Obstet Gynecol 31:353, 1988.
53. Kivikoski AI, Martin C, Weyman P, et al.: Angiographic arterial embolization to control hemorrhage in abdominal pregnancy: A case report. Obstet Gynecol 71:456, 1988.
54. Chervenak FA, Adams J, Reyniak JV: An emergency in abdominal pregnancy. The Female Patient 6:38, 1981.
55. Hreshchyshyn MM, Bogen B, Loughran LH: What is the actual present-day management of the placenta in late abdominal pregnancy? Analysis of 101 cases. Am J Obstet Gynecol 81:302, 1961.
56. Lathrop JC, Bowles GE: Methotrexate in abdominal pregnancy: Report of a case. Obstet Gynecol 32:81, 1968.
57. Bright AS, Maser AH: Advanced abdominal pregnancy. Obstet Gynecol 17:316, 1961.
58. O'Leary JL, O'Leary JA: Rudimentary horn pregnancy. Obstet Gynecol 22:371, 1963.
59. Speert H, Nash W, Kaplan A: Tubal pregnancy. Obstet Gynecol 7:322, 1956.
60. Eastman N: Williams Obstetrics, 11th Edition. New York: Appleton-Century-Crofts, 1956.
61. Eden TW, Lockyer C: Gynecology. New York: Macmillan Publishing Co., 1928, p. 210.
62. Champion PM, Tessitore NJL: Broad ligament pregnancy. Am J Obstet Gynecol 36:281, 1938.
63. Wolfe SA, Neigus I: Broad-ligament pregnancy with report of three early cases. Am J Obstet Gynecol 66:106, 1953.
64. Pritchard JA, MacDonald PC, Gant NF: Ectopic pregnancy. In Williams Obstetrics, 17th Edition. Norwalk, Connecticut: Appleton-Century-Crofts, p. 426.
65. Ron-El R, Langer R, Herman A, et al.: Term delivery following mid-trimester ruptured cornual pregnancy with combined intrauterine pregnancy. Case report. Br J Obstet Gynaecol 95:619, 1987.

66. Wechstein LN: Current perspectives on ectopic pregnancy. Obstet Gynecol Surv 40:259, 1985.
67. Beckmann CRB, Tomasi AM, Thomason JL: Combined interstitial and intrauterine pregnancy: Cornual resection in early pregnancy and cesarean delivery at term. Am J Obstet Gynecol 149:83, 1984.
68. Brandes MC, Youngs DD, Goldstein DP, et al.: Treatment of cornual pregnancy with methotrexate: Case report. Am J Obstet Gynecol 155:655, 1986.
69. Jauchler GW, Baker RL: Cervical pregnancy: Review of the literature and a case report. Obstet Gynecol 35:870, 1970.
70. Shinagawa S, Nagayama M: Cervical pregnancy as a possible sequel of induced abortion. Report of 19 cases. Am J Obstet Gynecol 105:282, 1969.
71. Studdiford WE: Cervical pregnancy: A partial review of the literature and a report of two probable cases. Am J Obstet Gynecol 49:160, 1945.
72. Schneider P: Distal ectopic pregnancy. Am J Surg 12:526, 1946.
73. Thomsen M, Johansen F: Two cases of cervical pregnancy. Acta Obstet Gynec Scand 40:99, 1961.
74. Parente JT, Chau-Su OU, Levy J, et al.: Cervical pregnancy analysis: A review and report of 5 cases. Obstet Gynecol 62:79, 1983.
75. Pelosi MA: Cervical pregnancy. In Iffy L, Charles D (eds.): Operative Perinatology. New York: Macmillan Publishing Co., pp. 344–352, 1981.

10

Surgical Correction of Uterine Anomalies

David N. Jackson
Thomas J. Garite

Pregnancy in a patient with uterine or cervical anomaly has two potential sequelae. First, the uterus may function normally, leading to a successful delivery and no opportunity for diagnosis or therapy. Conversely, the gestation may be severely compromised, with consequences of recurrent pregnancy loss, preterm delivery, placental abruption, fetal growth abnormalities, or malpresentation alerting the physician to intrauterine pathology. The purpose of this chapter is to familiarize the reader with uterine anomalies that cause adverse obstetric outcome and to detail the current diagnostic and therapeutic modalities used to address these complications.

HISTORICAL PERSPECTIVES

The history of uterine pathophysiology is a fascinating mixture of myth and enlightened science. Cultural superstitions, religious dictums, and the infrequent opportunity to pursue authorized human dissection hindered the development of the concepts of modern gynecology well into the fourteenth century.[1] The earliest teachings regarding uterine development were based almost entirely on the study of animals. In the fourth century BC, prominent physicians and philosophers, such as Hippocrates and Aristotle, regarded the uterus as being composed of several cavities and horns, with an endometrial surface of cotyledons, similar to that of cattle.[2] In regard to the function of these horns, the *Aphorisms of Hippocrates* state that "the male fetus is usually seated in the right and the female fetus in the left side."[2] An ongoing concept was that of a multichambered uterus containing seven cells, allowing for male embryo development in three cells on the right, female development in the three cells on the left, and hermaphrodites to develop in the middle cell.[3]

It was not until the sixteenth century that the statements and drawings of Berengario da Carpi and Vesalius unequivocally supported that the uterus had only a single cavity. Vesalius (the Latin name of Andreas Wesel, 1514–1564) was the first to use the term "uterus" in a treatise dated 1543, but he still diagrammed the uterine cavity as having a partial septum at the fundus.[2, 4]

With the increased availability of human studies, Gabriel Fallopio (1523–1562), William Harvey (1578–1657), and Regnier de Graaf (1641–1673) helped differentiate human function from corresponding structures in lower animals.[2] Cervical incompetence was recognized in 1658, although the term was not applied until 1865.[5, 6] In the eighteenth century, detailed placental anatomy and the relationships of the fetus to the gravid uterus were documented in preparations by William Hunter.[7, 7a]

With refinements in microscopic and endocrinologic study, the nineteenth and twentieth centuries have seen an explosion of understanding regarding human conception and early fetal organogenesis. Embryology of the reproductive organs has evolved into an expansive subject, and the timing of events leading to the development of the adnexae, uterus, and vagina has become known. Understanding the embryology of uterine development allows for classification of anomalies and forms the basis for the following discussion.

EMBRYOLOGY

By 6 weeks' gestation, the multipotential germ cells appear in the endoderm of the yolk sac and migrate along the dorsal mesentery to invade the gonadal ridge. In the absence of a Y chromosome, the fallopian tubes form as extensions of the paramesonephric (müllerian) ducts. Fusion of these ducts is completed by approximately 8 weeks' gestation, and the midline portion is destined to become the uterine body. Resorption of the fused

medial walls is generally complete by 10.5 weeks, creating a single uterine cavity. The caudal tip of the fused ducts projects into the posterior wall of the urogenital sinus by 11 to 12 weeks and forms the vaginal fornices, as well as the upper one third of the vagina. The process of vaginal canalization is completed by 20 weeks.

Defects in female organ development prior to 5 weeks' gestation lead to absence of the paramesonephric ducts, with no formation of the uterus, fallopian tubes, or upper vagina (müllerian agenesis). Because ovarian germ cell migration and lower vaginal development are still possible, the patient has a blind vaginal pouch with hormonally active gonads but no active end organ. Menses and reproductive potential are absent, but heterosexual intercourse can be initiated following successful vaginoplasty procedures.

Defects at 5 to 9 weeks' gestation allow for paramesonephric duct formation without proper midline uterine fusion. Ovaries, fallopian tubes, and the lower vagina are present without the uterus, cervix, or upper vagina. The remnant fallopian tubes may be unilateral or bilateral.

Defects at 10 to 12 weeks' gestation lead to a variety of fusion and resorption disorders. Ovaries, fallopian tubes, and a lower vagina should be present, with mild to severe uterine malformation. Variations in uterine form may be accompanied

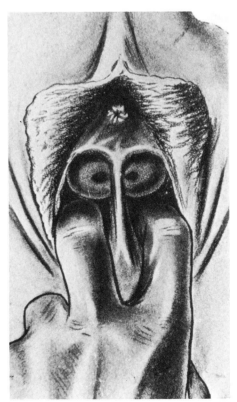

Figure 10–1. Uterus didelphys (Class III). Duplicated cervix and vagina. (From DeLee JB: The Principles and Practice of Obstetrics. Philadelphia: W.B. Saunders Co., 1924, p. 546.)

by a double cervix and possibly a double upper vagina (Figs. 10–1, 10–2). Using the standards of the American Fertility Society,[8] the most severe anomaly leads to uterine and cervical duplication (uterus didelphys) with a double upper vagina. The least severe anomaly leads to an arcuate uterus (Fig. 10–3).

As a terminal product of aberrant uterine fusion, sagittal or transverse septa of the upper vagina may exist in conjunction with other müllerian defects. The identification of a vaginal defect should prompt physicians to suspect coexistent uterine anomalies. Although not directly associated with increased fetal wastage, they impact on reproductive function through dyspareunia, obstruction of menses, and dystocia during labor. Transverse septa are possible anywhere along the vaginal canal but are most common at the junction between the middle and upper thirds of the vagina.[9, 10] There is some evidence that complete transverse septa may be inherited as an autosomal recessive disorder, but this form is rare.[11] An obstructive transverse vaginal septum may be encountered during childhood and necessitates incision to avoid destructive hydromucocolpos.[9–13] A patient with an incomplete transverse vaginal septum that does not impair menstruation or intercourse is likely to conceive and deliver without obstruction. A longitudinal or transverse septum can be incised just prior to descent of the fetal head if dystocia from the septum is obvious. Following delivery, the labor anesthesia can be extended to allow for adequate repair of the vaginal epithelium. If the septum is complex and dystocia occurs, cesarean delivery is an option.

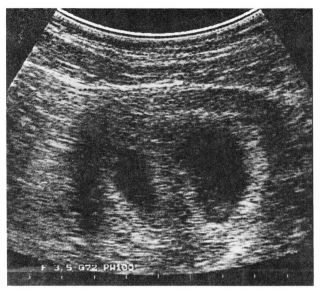

Figure 10–2. Ultrasound study of a double uterine pregnancy. A single uterus shows a thick septum and has a single cervix and vagina (Class V—septate uterus). A gestational sac with a fetal pole appears in each of the two uterine cavities. (Courtesy John Freeman, M.D.)

MÜLLERIAN ANOMALIES

Incidence

The frequency of uterine anomalies is reported at 0.1% to 3.3% of pregnancies, with most authors agreeing on an incidence approximating 0.25%.[13–18] At Long Beach Memorial Hospital, there were 36 müllerian anomalies in 35,303 de-

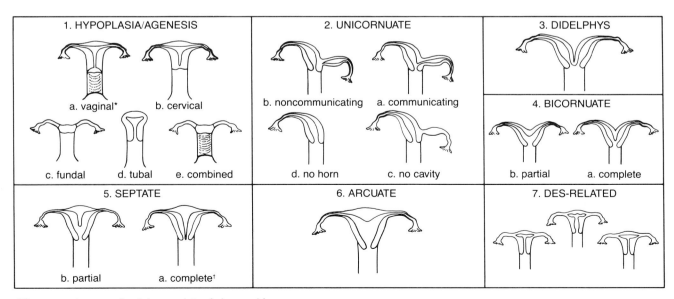

*Uterus may be normal or take a variety of abnormal forms.
†May have two distinct cervices.

Figure 10–3. American Fertility Society classification of müllerian anomalies. (Redrawn from Fertil Steril 49:944, 1988).

liveries between 1982 and 1988 (bicornuate, 64%, septate, 33%, and uterus didelphys, 3%). This incidence of 0.1% at our center is similar to the 0.13% incidence recently reported in 164 patients identified with müllerian anomalies in 124,598 deliveries at Los Angeles County University of Southern California Medical Center from 1979 to 1986 (bicornuate, 39%, septate, 30%, didelphys, 17%, unicornuate, 8%, and arcuate, 6%).[19] The populations at these two centers represent private, high-risk referral and public patients but do not include patients in whom pregnancy loss occurred prior to viability or in whom normal outcome failed to stimulate diagnosis. Until a large prospective study evaluates consecutive patients for uterine anomaly, its true incidence in pregnancy may never be determined.

Classification and Repair

Class I is composed of müllerian agenesis or hypoplasia and has five subdivisions. Vaginal agenesis (Class IA or IE) occurs in 1 of 5000 phenotypic females (see Fig. 10–3).[20] The presence of a transverse vaginal septum prevents an adequate outflow tract for menstruation and is diagnosed when menarche does not follow thelarche and adrenarche. Diagnosis is confirmed by physical examination, karyotype (to discriminate between androgen insensitivity syndrome or chromosomal anomalies), and laparoscopy (to identify associated genital tract anomalies). Because the prevalence of associated renal anomalies is high (50%), intravenous pyelography is recommended. The vagina may be corrected by surgical or nonsurgical means.[14, 21, 22] For patients with a normal, functioning uterus, pregnancy is possible, with a 36% liveborn rate reported.[9, 20, 23] Elective cesarean section is recommended to avoid destruction of the artificial vagina.

Cervical agenesis (Class IB) prevents appropriate passage of sperm, and pregnancy is unlikely. In 35 patients reported by Farber and colleagues,[24, 25] 25 had surgical anastomosis of the vagina to the uterus, with two becoming pregnant and giving birth to term neonates. The rarity of this syndrome makes generalizations difficult, but it appears that once pregnancy is achieved, term delivery is possible. Cesarean section is recommended to avoid damage to the surgical anastomosis.[26]

Uterine agenesis (Class IC) is rarely reported, and treatment to allow conception is lacking. Tubal agenesis (Class ID) is usually seen in conjunction with a unicornuate uterus without a rudimentary horn. Successful gestation is determined by the extent of the associated unicornuate malformation.

Class II malformations involve the unicornuate uterus and have several forms (see Fig. 10–3). Over 100 pregnancies in unicornuate uteri have been reported, with a spontaneous abortion rate of 33 to 48% (range 15 to 75%), a preterm birth rate of 17 to 29%, and a live birth rate of 40 to 66%.[20, 27] Diagnosis may be suspected from the presence of a firm, solid pelvic mass (representing the rudimentary horn) contralateral to a deviated uterine fundus. If the horn is noncommunicating, dysmenorrhea may be a predominant feature of the gynecologic history. Diagnosis is confirmed by hysterosalpingogram (Fig. 10–4), laparoscopy, or laparotomy.

If the pregnancy is implanted in the rudimentary horn, it is a potential surgical emergency. Over 89% are diagnosed after uterine rupture, usually occurring at approximately 20 weeks' gestation.[28, 29] Rarely, successful pregnancy in a rudimentary horn has been reported.[30, 31] Another rare complication is the obstruction and abscess of a rudimentary horn during pregnancy.[32]

Pregnancy in a unicornuate uterus is at risk for intrauterine growth retardation, preterm labor, and abnormal presentation of the fetus.[33–35] There is a high incidence of dysfunctional labor (50%) and an overall cesarean section rate of 70%. In separate reports, Fedele and colleagues[34] and Maneschi and colleagues[35] evaluated 67 pregnancies in 31 women with unicornuate uteri. There were 38 abortions (57%), one rupture of a rudimentary horn (1.5%), and 28 viable births (42%). Of the 28 births there were 22 term deliveries (78%) and 20 cesarean sections (71%).

Uterus didelphys is the third category (Class III) (Fig. 10–5). Surgical resection of the intervening septum is not routinely advocated unless pregnancy loss has occurred. In a report by Musich and Behrman,[36] eight of 14 women with uterus didelphys had viable gestations without surgery. In Stein and March's[19] report of 27 pregnancies delivered by women with uterus didelphys, 75% of the

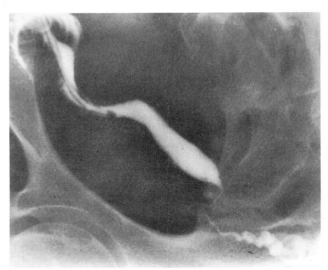

Figure 10–4. Hysterosalpingogram of unicornuate uterus (Class II müllerian anomaly). (Courtesy Greg Rosen, M.D.)

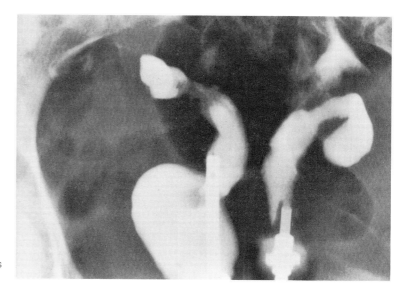

Figure 10–5. Hysterosalpingogram of uterus didelphys (Class III müllerian anomaly).

women had term births with an average birth weight of 2731 ± 131 g. Compared with bicornate or unicornuate anomalies, there is a lower incidence of breech or transverse presentations (33%); however, cesarean delivery is still required in up to 80% of patients because of the high incidence of dysfunctional labor.[19] Surgical intervention at delivery for uterus didelphys often involves removal of symptomatic vaginal septa. If the septum is thick, blood vessels must be secured after incision.

The bicornuate uterus (Class IV) has the widest variation of morphology, with complete and partial forms designated as Class IVA and Class IVB, respectively (see Fig. 10–3). The uterus is characterized by two separate fundal bodies (Fig. 10–6). Outcome is variable, with spontaneous abortion

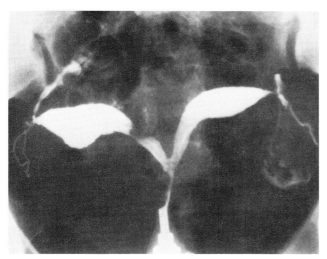

Figure 10–6. Hysterosalpingogram of a bicornuate uterus (Class IV müllerian anomaly). Note the two separate uterine bodies. The hysterosalpingogram cannot always distinguish bicornuate from septate uteri.

reported in 35% of patients, early delivery in 23%, and cesarean birth in 70 to 90%. Viable birth rates range from 40% for complete lesions to 90% for the milder partial forms.[9, 12, 20, 27] Overall mean birth weights of 2982 to 3117 g indicate good potential for neonatal survival.[19] If recurrent midtrimester loss occurs, repairs by procedures such as the Strassman unification are associated with improved reproductive outcome.[36, 37] Strassman unification is recommended for the bicornuate uterus; it involves unification of the cavities with minimal tissue removal (Fig. 10–7). The patient is placed in the supine position. The approach to the uterus is through a transverse or midline incision. To help exposure, traction sutures may be placed at the uterine fundus. Pitressin solutions (10 U/20 mL saline) may decrease bleeding when injected into the myometrium but have known cardiovascular effects on the mother and may inhibit healing. As suggested by Mattingly and Thompson, the use of hypotensive anesthetic agents and the use of a 0.5-inch Penrose drain as a tourniquet assist hemostasis when the drain is passed through an avascular space in the broad ligament and tied anterior to the uterus around the lower uterine segment. A similar occlusion around the infundibulopelvic ligament decreases blood loss further.[51] Care must be taken to occlude both the arterial and venous flows for maximal hemostasis. After exposure, a fundal incision is made transversely between the round ligaments (see Fig. 10–7). This incision opens the two uterine cornua to expose the cavities. Care must be taken superiorly to avoid damaging the interstitial portion of the fallopian tubes and inferiorly to avoid expanding the incision into the cervix. After incision, the exposed sides generally evert and approximate well. A three-layered vertical myometrial closure then completes the unification (see Fig. 10–7).

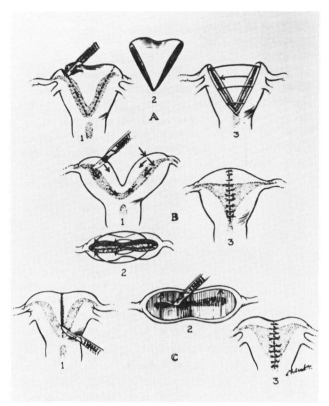

Figure 10–7. Transabdominal repair of müllerian anomalies. A—Jones wedge excision of a small uterine septum. B—Strassman reunification operation for a bicornuate uterus. C—Tompkin's repair of a septate uterus. (From Jones HW: Reproductive impairment and the malformed uterus. Fertil Steril 36:137, 1981.)

The septate uterus (Class V) may be complete or partial and in older reports has been quoted as the most common uterine anomaly unrelated to drug exposure (Fig. 10–8). It is hard to distinguish a septate from a bicornuate uterus by hysterosalpingogram alone (Fig. 10–9). In one report, 38 of 39 patients with septate uteri were incorrectly labeled through radiographic study as having bicornuate uteri.[20, 28] The distinction of the septate from the bicornuate uterus is important for predicting perinatal complications. In a septate uterus, spontaneous abortion occurs in up to 67% of cases (bicornuate 35%), the overall live birth rate is 28% (bicornuate 40 to 90%), and the chance of preterm delivery is 33%, compared with a 24% chance of preterm birth in patients with bicornuate uteri.[19, 20, 38] Counseling as to outcome may be aided by sonography. Placental implantation away from the septum is associated with lower rates of abortion and preterm birth.[39] Proposed etiologies for the higher reproductive wastage in the septate uterus include disorders of placental implantation on the septum, a poor blood supply to the septum, and a thin uterine musculature, leading to increased irritability and preterm labor. Without surgery, 25 to 33% of pregnancies in a septate

uterus can be expected to achieve viability, with an average birth weight of 2839 ± 102 g and a cesarean section rate of 76%.[19] In patients with a septate uterus and a history of reproductive loss, unification procedures have been successful in improving pregnancy outcome.[36, 40–50] When surgery for septate uterus is deemed appropriate, therapy by hysteroscopy should initially be considered (Fig. 10–10).[40–45] Advantages of hysteroscopic resection as opposed to laparotomy include low operative morbidity, decreased hospitalization time, earlier time to conception, and increased chance for subsequent vaginal delivery.[45] The procedure is usually completed in less than 20 minutes and is rarely associated with significant hemorrhage. Impressive results have been obtained by this approach, with 95% pretreatment reproductive wastage reduced to approximately 10% after surgery. Over 50% of patients deliver at term.[40–45] Although transcervical division of uterine septa without hysteroscopic visualization has been reported, this technique is improved by hysteroscopic guidance.[46, 47]

For patients treated by laparotomy, Jones[49] describes the technique of wedge resection as an alternative operation (see Fig. 10–7).[51] The patient is positioned in the supine position. The approach to the uterus is through a transverse or midline incision. To help exposure, traction sutures may

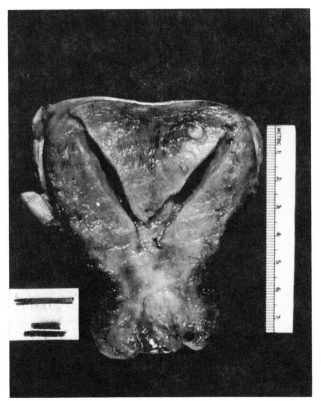

Figure 10–8. Gross pathologic specimen of a bicornuate uterus. Note the single cervix, two uterine cavities, and single uterine fundus with indentation on the superior surface.

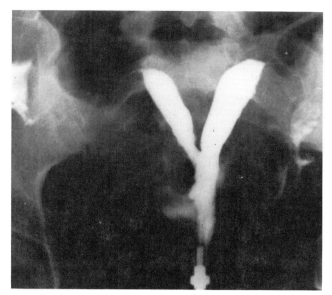

Figure 10–9. Hysterosalpingogram of a septate uterus (Class V müllerian anomaly). (Courtesy Greg Rosen, M.D.)

be placed at the uterine fundus. Because the exterior of the uterus often appears normal, the incision is guided by the hysterosalpingographic findings. Hemostasis is obtained through the use of hypotensive anesthetics, vasopressin (Pitressin) solutions, or tourniquet applications around the lower uterine segment and infundibulopelvic ligaments.[51] A small wedge is removed approximately 1 to 2 cm from the insertion of the fallopian tubes. The apex of the wedge is directed to encompass the defect, with care to limit removal of normal endometrial and myometrial tissues. If septal tissue remains after the initial wedge, it is removed with a subsequent wedge. Closure of the uterus is accomplished with interrupted sutures of delayed absorbable material. The uterus is closed in three layers. The inner layer approximates the endometrium and the myometrium. The intermediate layer approximates the myometrium. The superficial layer approximates the serosa. In order to allow the incision to heal, effective barrier contraception for 3 to 6 months should be stressed.

Good reproductive performance after wedge metroplasty is reported, with a 96% pregnancy rate. A 76% term delivery rate is reported following wedge resection of a septate uterus.[52]

In the Thompkins metroplasty, a single midline incision rather than a wedge exposes the septum. Each half of the septum is incised, with no septal tissue removed. It is a simple technique, with good results reported. Thompkins metroplasty is recommended for patients in whom hysteroscopic repair of a septate uterus would be considered difficult (see Fig. 10–7). After a vertical midline uterine incision is made, the septum is dissected, and the uterus is closed in three layers.

Class VI lesions include the arcuate form of the uterine cavity (Fig. 10–11). The "partial septum" at the fundus causes few obstetric problems.[8] The risk of preterm delivery is low (10%), but the incidence of malpresentation and cesarean section remains high (70–80%).[19]

Drug-induced uterine anomalies (Class VII) have been the most commonly detected uterine anomalies (see Fig. 9–3).[53-59] The synthetic estrogen diethylstilbestrol (DES) is the main agent of reproductive tract anomalies. A uterine abnormality following DES exposure presents as a T-shaped, constricted, or small uterine cavity (Fig. 10–12).[53] Cervicovaginal abnormalities include adenosis, clear-cell adenocarcinoma, cervical hoods, collars, and a "cockscomb" appearance.[53-58] There is no increased incidence of renal anomalies, and thus pyelograms are not routinely recommended. In 579 pregnancies of women who had in utero exposure to DES, as summarized by Buttram and Gibbons,[20, 38] 5.4% were ectopic, 27% ended in spontaneous abortion, 28% delivered early, and 63% had viable gestations. Diethylstilbestrol-exposed pregnancies have a high incidence of late first and

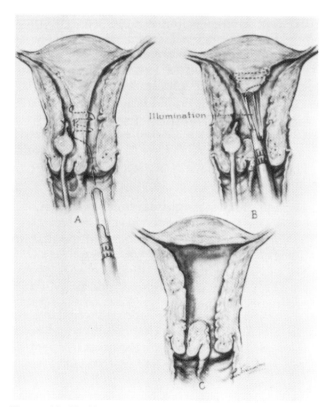

Figure 10–10. Hysteroscopic resection of a complete uterine septum. A—Foley bulb is inserted into the right uterine cavity, and the septum is progressively excised until the bulb is seen. B—Electrosurgical excision of a thick upper septum. C—Remaining single uterine cavity. (From Rock JA: Resectoscopic techniques for the lysis of a class V: Complete uterine septum. Fertil Steril 48:495, 1987.)

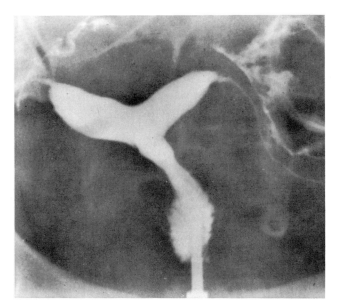

Figure 10–11. Hysterosalpingogram of an arcuate uterus (Class VI müllerian anomaly). (Courtesy Greg Rosen, M.D.)

early second trimester losses. Improved outcome has been demonstrated by utilizing cervical cerclage.[57–59] Because DES was not used after the early 1970s, the adverse consequences should be historic after the next decade. Until that time, reproductive history should include questions regarding possible in utero exposure to DES, especially in the setting of repeated pregnancy loss or a documented uterine cavity anomaly.

Cervical Incompetence and Uterine Anomalies

The overall incidence of incompetent cervix in patients with uterine anomalies is reported to be 17 to 30%.[12, 60] Serial ultrasonography may be useful in determining the appropriate patient for cerclage, with 80 to 97% of patients having had prior pregnancy loss and confirmed müllerian anomaly and demonstrating reduction in cervical length on serial ultrasonography.[60] When treated with cerclage, these patients have a 97% term delivery rate.[60] Unfortunately, controlled studies are lacking. A complete discussion of cerclage technique is found later in this chapter.

Genetic Considerations and Fetal Concerns

Patients with uterine anomalies invariably are concerned about the risk of a female fetus' having a similar uterine defect. Benirschke and colleagues[61] summarized the topic in 1973, reporting seven instances of neonatal uterine anomalies in mothers with similar anomalies.[61] Since that summary, Elias reported that transmission of uter-

ine anomalies among female relatives is unlikely, with congenital uterine anomalies found in only 2.7% of first-degree relatives and no anomalies found in second- or third-degree relatives.[62] There are reports of twin- and sibling-related anomalies with an autosomal pattern of inheritance, but the majority of defects undoubtedly represent polygenic or multifactorial occurrence.[11, 63, 64] For multifactorial anomalies, recurrence risk can be quoted at 2 to 3%.

Many women with uterine anomalies have concomitant infertility, increasing the chance that advanced maternal age necessitates genetic screening. There are no reports of increased complications of ultrasonically directed amniocentesis for genetic studies in women with uterine anomalies. Transabdominal chorionic villus sampling in women with a bicornuate uterus has been reported.[65, 66]

Constriction of the fetus because of an abnormal uterine cavity may lead to limb reduction and other defects. In four cases reported by Graham and colleagues,[67] a bicornuate uterus was associated with fetal distal arm and leg reduction, leading to absence of fingers, hand, or forearm.[67] Brachial plexus injury, phrenic nerve palsy, a small left arm, and deformed ribs in a neonate carried in a bicornuate uterus has also been documented.[68] Although the risk is small, there is an increasing number of reports of fetal defects associated with uterine malformation.[69, 70] Ultrasonography can be utilized to document intact and freely moving limbs before delivery.

Urinary Tract Anomalies

Eleven to 31% of women with genital malformations have associated urinary tract anomalies.[14,

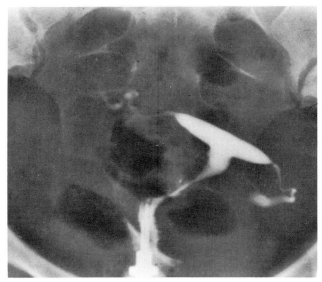

Figure 10–12. Hysterosalpingogram of T-shaped uterus from exposure to diethylstilbestrol (DES) in utero (Class VII müllerian anomaly).

[19, 20] Those with a unicornuate uterus have the highest incidence of associated renal lesions (70%), usually renal agenesis (Fig. 10–13).[27] Conversely, patients with unilateral renal agenesis have a 20% incidence of major genital malformation, usually unicornuate uterus. Other forms of uterine anomalies have a 10% risk of associated urinary tract abnormalities.[71] Intravenous pyelography is recommended in all patients with Class I through Class V anomalies but is not routinely advocated for patients with anomalies secondary to DES exposure (Class VII) or with arcuate uteri (Class VI).

Postpartum Hemorrhage

Postpartum hemorrhage in patients with müllerian anomalies is often secondary to incomplete placental extrusion or uterine atony. Manual placental extraction for retained placenta followed by curettage with a large curette should be available. Eobolic agents, such as oxytocin, ergonovine maleate, and prostaglandin derivations can be used to treat uterine atony. The patient should be prepared for these possibilities during prenatal counseling, especially if malpresentation, preterm labor, abruption, or recurrent pregnancy loss alerts the physician to the possibility of a uterine malformation. Ultrasonographic confirmation of septal implantation alerts the physician to increased potential for retained placenta.

Diagnosis at Cesarean Section

When a uterine anomaly is diagnosed at cesarean section, repair depends on classification. Class V (septate) lesions warrant removal at the time of cesarean section. Small, thin septal lesions are usually avascular and seldom bleed on incision. Check the uterine cavity by hysteroscopy before the next conception to be certain that the septa was adequately removed and healed. Extensive repairs of thick septae, bicornuate, or didelphic lesions are best managed post partum, prior to the next conception. For patients with a communicating rudimentary uterine horn (Class II), the horn should be removed prior to the next conception to avoid the risk of uterine rupture from implantation in the horn.

Conclusions

Uterine anomalies may be encountered in 1 in 300 women and in 1 in 1000 deliveries. Abortion, preterm delivery, abruptio placentae, fetal malpresentation, dysfunctional labor, and postpartum hemorrhage are the most common obstetric manifestations of uterine anomalies. Overall, there is a 28% abortion rate for women with anomalies and a 10 to 15% incidence of müllerian anomalies in women with two or more consecutive pregnancy losses.[72, 73] For ongoing pregnancies beyond 20 weeks' gestation, there is a 25% incidence of preterm delivery and a cesarean section rate of 70 to 90%. Breech and transverse lie complicate up to 70% of pregnancies, and unsuccessful external version should open the consideration of a possible anomaly, especially if the uterine fundus is found to be abnormal on palpation.[74]

Individual patient counseling necessitates a knowledge of defect classification, relative cavity size, prior pregnancy history, and location of placental implantation. Monitoring for appropriate fetal growth and normal fetal limb development should be pursued with serial ultrasonographic examination.

Cervical incompetence may be associated with a uterine anomaly in up to 30% of patients.[12] Cerclage in a previous or current pregnancy should prompt uterine exploration to rule out uterine defect. Cerclage should be utilized if cervical incompetence is documented by ultrasonography or physical examination, especially for the patient with two or more early midtrimester losses.

At delivery, retained placentae and postpartum hemorrhage should be anticipated in patients with

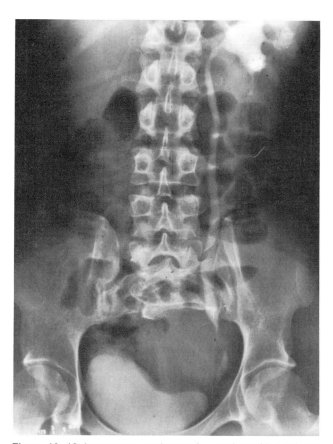

Figure 10–13. Intravenous pyelogram in a patient with a unicornuate uterus (Class II). Note agenesis of left kidney and ureter. (Courtesy Greg Rosen, M.D.)

uterine malformations. The maternal urinary system should be evaluated by intravenous pyelogram in all but Class VII lesions (DES exposure) and Class VI lesions (arcuate uterus). Referral for metroplasty depends on defect classification and history of reproductive wastage. Hysteroscopic approach to septal repair appears to offer the least morbidity without sacrificing efficacy. In general, pregnancy after metroplasty has up to a 95% success rate for viable gestation.

CERVICAL INCOMPETENCE AND CERCLAGE

The first description of recurrent early pregnancy loss related to an inability of the "inner orifice of the womb" to retain the "seed" can be traced to 1658.[75] It was another 200 years before the term "cervical incompetence" was first used by Gream[5] in 1865; it was not until the 1950s that surgical repair of the pregnant and nonpregnant cervix for patients who had habitual spontaneous abortions became popular. Perhaps the most influential article was V.N. Shirodkar's landmark report on cervical cerclage in 1955, describing cervical incompetence in this way:

> There are some unfortunate women who abort repeatedly between the fourth and seventh months; no amount of rest and treatment with hormones seems to help them in retaining the products of conception. . . . The attempts of obstetricians all over the world to solve this problem have met with very little success.[76]

As reflected in the above paragraph, women had to suffer repeated spontaneous abortions prior to resorting to surgical repair. The minimum number of prior miscarriages in Shirodkar's series was four per patient, and one patient had experienced 11 consecutive losses prior to cerclage placement.[76] Forty years later, the modern-day obstetrician faces the same syndrome but is often forced to define and treat cervical incompetence after a single pregnancy loss.[77] The following section deals with the frequency, definition, and treatment of cervical incompetence, with an emphasis on differentiating prophylactic from therapeutic cerclage procedures.

The term "cervical incompetence" implies a lack of lower uterine integrity in retaining the expanding pregnancy. The cervix is primarily composed of fibrous components, with only 10 to 30% smooth muscle.[78] At the junction of the fibrous cervix to the muscular uterine body, there is a functional transition, which is termed the internal cervical os. The integrity of this transition area is responsible for maintaining the patency of the cervix as gestation progresses. In the early second trimester, elongation of the uterine isthmus begins, and patients with cervical incompetence manifest dilatation of the cervix without uterine contractions. This dilatation of the internal os is visible on ultrasonography and is palpable on vaginal examination. Differential diagnosis of recurrent midtrimester pregnancy loss includes parental balanced translocations, uterine leiomyomata, müllerian anomalies, inadequate luteal phase, parental sharing of human leukocyte antigens, maternal systemic illness (such as systemic lupus erythematosus or diabetes mellitus), infectious disorders of the lower genital tract, and chromosomal anomalies of the fetus.[79–36] This differential diagnosis for midtrimester loss should be considered before making a diagnosis of incompetent cervix and proceeding to therapeutic alternatives.[87, 88]

The patient with cervical incompetence often gives a history of in utero exposure to DES, cervical trauma from prior deliveries, or cervical surgery.[89–95] Diethylstilbestrol-exposed patients have a high incidence of late first and early second trimester losses. Improved outcome has been demonstrated by utilizing cervical cerclage.[89, 90] Traumatic delivery may initiate subsequent weakness of the internal os, and a history of normal term delivery does not rule out incompetent cervix.[87, 88] Dilatation and curettage is implicated in incompetent cervix, especially if the internal os was dilated more than 10 mm.[91–93] Operative reports detailing prior cervical conization should be investigated to assess whether an excessive amount of tissue was removed or if the procedure was exceptionally difficult. Congenital cervical weakness is suspected when primary cervical incompetence is found in primigravidas without cervical trauma.[96]

It has been suggested that biochemical and hormonal influences play a major role in the development of incompetent cervix.[96, 97] Rechberger and associates[97] postulated that a high turnover of collagen in cervices of patients with incompetent cervix leads to decreased cervical integrity. Premature release of cervical prostaglandin may promote passive dilatation by lowering the normal cervical collagen content.[98, 99]

Diagnosis

The frequency of cervical incompetence has been reported in between 1 in 54 and 1 in 1000 deliveries.[87, 88, 100–102] The classic history is two consecutive midtrimester pregnancy losses, characterized by painless cervical dilatation in the absence of labor.

Symptoms include a watery vaginal discharge (sometimes bleeding) prior to an atypical mild cramping or pressure in the lower pelvis. At examination, the cervix is found to be significantly dilated. After passive progression to 5 to 6 cm, there is active labor, with monitored uterine activity. Without intervention, the patient rapidly delivers a fetus with a normal appearance, sometimes with membranes intact.

To aid the obstetrician in diagnosing such a diverse and multifactorial entity, several tools are available to identify the patient at risk for cervical incompetence. In patients with a history of pregnancy loss resulting from painless cervical dilatation, a vaginal examination should be performed. Preconceptual findings suggestive of cervical incompetence include (1) the ability to easily pass a No. 8 Hegar dilator through the nonpregnant internal os; (2) withdrawal of a 2-mL (6-mm diameter) Foley balloon catheter through the cervical canal with minimal resistance; (3) hysterosalpingogram demonstrating cervical funneling; (4) clinical evidence of cervical anomalies secondary to DES exposure; and (5) clinical evidence of extensive obstetric trauma to the cervix.[103-105]

If the patient is pregnant and at risk for cervical incompetence, serial vaginal examination to assess dilation of the cervix is aided by sonographic evidence of cervical funneling or shortening.[106-110] An internal os transverse diameter of less than 2 cm on ultrasonographic examination has low correlation with cervical incompetence.[109] A decrease in sagittal cervical length to less than 4 cm and funneling of the amniotic membranes into the cervical canal are suggestive of incompetence.[110] The ultrasonographic examination should be performed by experienced sonographers, and transvaginal study is useful when abdominal findings are equivocal. If necessary, the cervix should be viewed with the bladder full and empty and with the patient standing and supine.

A documented change in cervical length or dilation in a patient at risk is suggestive of cervical incompetence and the need for therapy. The American College of Obstetrics and Gynecology Task Force on Quality Assurance has promulgated useful guidelines for evaluating the patient at risk and has quantified treatment with cerclage as prophylactic or therapeutic (Table 10–1).[103] These recommendations include that fetal gestational age assessment and sonographic status of the pregnancy be determined prior to cerclage placement. Contraindications to cerclage are preterm labor, active uterine bleeding, chorioamnionitis, premature rupture of membranes, fetal anomaly incompatible with life, and fetal demise.[103]

Treatment

Once the diagnosis of incompetent cervix is determined, therapeutic alternatives consist of surgery (cerclage, Lash, or Mann procedures) or nonsurgical modalities (bed rest, tocolytic agents, hormonal therapy). Preconceptual procedures, such as the Mann or Lash cervical repairs, reported fetal salvage rates of 78 to 85%.[99, 104] The procedures involve exposing the anterior cervix by cephalad reflection of the bladder by anterior colporrhaphy in the same manner as for preparation for vaginal hysterectomy. A wedge of tissue at the cervicouterine junction is excised, and plication of the exposed anatomic defect within the cervical body completes the repair. A high incidence of postoperative infertility as a result of cervical scarring makes this a less desirable surgical modality than postconceptual cerclage.

CERCLAGE

Reinforcement of the junction between fibrous cervix and muscular uterine isthmus (internal cervical os) is the basis for cerclage repair. Case-controlled series utilizing this approach show fetal survival improved from 0 to 20% before surgery to 75 to 100% after surgery. Over 80% deliver after 36 weeks' gestation.[87, 88, 99-102, 111, 112] Although these are optimistic statistics, control patients in these reports are historical, and randomization is lacking. Three randomized reports have shown no benefit from cerclage for patients at low to moderate risk for preterm delivery from cervical incompetence. These included patients with twin[113] and singleton gestations.[114, 115] In these reports, the incidence of birth prior to 33 weeks in cerclage patients compared with control subjects was not reduced. Unfortunately, selection bias for low-risk patients places the significance of these studies in question. The largest and most recent prospective report has obtained different results.[116] Pregnant women at risk for incompetent cervix were randomized to cerclage or to control groups. The cerclage patients showed improvement in delivery

---

Table 10–1. INDICATIONS FOR CERVICAL CERCLAGE: OBSTETRIC CRITERIA OF THE AMERICAN COLLEGE OF OBSTETRICIANS AND GYNECOLOGISTS

Prophylactic Cerclage
1. History of prior pregnancy in which patient has had classic signs of incompetent cervix
2. Prepregnancy physical findings suggesting possible cervical incompetence in a patient with history of a prior spontaneous midtrimester abortion. At least one of the following should be present:
   a. Ability to introduce a No. 8 Hegar dilator through the internal os when the patient is not pregnant
   b. Withdrawal of a Foley balloon catheter with 2 to 3 mL of water through the cervical canal with minimal resistance
   c. Hysterosalpingogram demonstrating cervical funneling
   d. Clinical evidence of significant cervical anomalies suggestive of in utero exposure to DES
   e. Clinical evidence of extensive obstetric trauma to the cervix

Therapeutic Cerclage
1. Premature effacement or dilation or both of the cervix in the absence of labor prior to 28 weeks of gestation
2. Sonographic evidence of cervical funneling, especially in a patient with prior history of midtrimester delivery

prior to 33 weeks (13% cerclage compared with 18% control; p = 0.03) and had fewer stillbirths, spontaneous abortions, or neonatal deaths (8% cerclage compared with 12% control; p = 0.06). The procedure was felt to be beneficial in 1 of 20 patients, with 5% fewer deliveries occurring in cerclage patients between 20 and 32 weeks' gestation. The authors point out that the statistical differences were small, and the trial is currently ongoing.

In summary, patients who have had two or more painless midtrimester pregnancy losses (or physical evidence of a passively dilating internal os on serial ultrasonography or physical examination) are most likely to benefit from cerclage placement. Patients with an atypical history who are at low to moderate risk for cervical incompetence may not benefit from cerclage.

CERCLAGE TECHNIQUES. There is no demonstrated advantage of one cerclage technique over another.[117] The surgeon should be familiar with four main categories (Shirodkar, McDonald, emergent, and transabdominal). Each has advantages for specific patients. The choice of anesthetic is based on physician and patient preference. Because studies have shown an increase in prostaglandin metabolites for up to 24 hours after cerclage,[118-121] the use of prostaglandin synthetase inhibitors prior to surgery may be useful. The most experience in pregnancy has been with indomethacin (Indocin R).[122, 123] The initial dose of indomethacin is 50 mg by rectal suppository. A repeat dose at 2 to 4 hours may be necessary, based on patient symptoms.[124] Maintenance dosage is 25 mg orally every 4 to 6 hours or rectal suppository 25 mg every 8 hours. The medication is not used for more than 48 hours and is rarely required past 24 hours. Uterine contractions more than 24 hours after cerclage should alert the obstetrician to infection, uterine anomaly, or unsuspected premature ruptured membranes. Alternative tocolytic agents include β-mimetics (terbutaline, ritodrine) or magnesium sulfate. Unfortunately, controlled studies on the efficacy of these agents with cerclage are lacking.

Shirodkhar Cerclage. The Shirodkar cerclage places a submucosal suture at the level of the cervicovaginal junction.[76, 125] The original description utilized a 1/4-inch wide strip of maternal fascia lata introduced with an aneurysm needle. Most surgeons now use a flat, wide suture, such as 5-mm Mersilene. The needle tip should be blunt in order to avoid perforation of the cervical-vaginal mucosa (Fig. 10–14A). The perineum is prepared by operating room staff, but the surgeon and his or her assistant should gently clean the vagina under direct visualization to avoid trauma to the cervix or membranes.

Grasp the cervix on the posterior lip with relatively atraumatic instruments (Babcock or ring forceps, preferably nonserrated). The cervix is pulled forward and then elevated toward the symphysis to allow for a vertical incision in the posterior vaginal wall at the level of the internal os (Fig. 10–14B). The incision should extend only through the vaginal mucosa. The anterior cervix is then grasped, and the cervix is pulled downward. A 1- to 2-cm transverse incision is made in the midline similar to that used in an anterior colporrhaphy (Fig. 10–14C). If necessary, the bladder is gently pushed above the level of the internal os by midline blunt dissection. The needle is advanced under the mucosa toward the opposite incision (Fig. 10–14D). Direct the needle posteriorly to anteriorly, allowing for easier exposure of the needle tip after insertion. The rotation is a gentle procedure, with little resistance felt when the needle is submucosal and not within the body of the cervix. After the procedure is performed bilaterally, the suture is tied to achieve an internal cervical diameter of approximately 5 mm (Fig. 10–14E). Usually most bleeding will cease after the suture is tied, and hemostasis is rarely a problem (Fig. 10–14F). If necessary, the mucosal incisions can be reapproximated with fine, absorbable sutures.

Modifications involve placement of the knot posteriorly, various degrees of burying the knot submucosally, and securing the cerclage to the cervix with interrupted suture to avoid displacement. Novy[99] recommends the use of a 1:1000 solution of epinephrine in 20 mL of saline in the anterior vaginal fornix and posteriorly at the level of the uterosacral ligaments to aid hemostasis. If an aneurysm needle technique is utilized, Druzin and Berkeley[126] recommend the use of a curved tonsil clamp to retract the mucosa laterally for improved submucosal suture placement.

Theoretical advantages of the Shirodkar technique include a high cervical suture placement and an absence of directing the needle toward the amniotic membranes. With proper placement, the Shirodkar technique may provide stronger circumferential support of the internal os, with less risk of erosion into the cervical canal.[99] There are data to suggest that the rate of preterm births is lower after elective Shirodkar cerclage when compared with elective McDonald cerclage.[87, 99, 101] Fetal survival is reported at 87% after elective Shirodkar procedures and 68% after emergent procedures.[87, 96, 99, 101]

McDonald Cerclage. Modifications of a purse string cerclage can be traced to the original series of 70 patients reported by McDonald.[112] McDonald originally recommended placing a No. 4 silk suture at 20 to 24 weeks' gestation. Modifications involve placing the cerclage at 14 to 16 weeks' gestation and using an alternative suture, such as Mersilene (No. 2 or 5 mm), Prolene, or silk (No. 2).[125]

After preparation of the perineum and the vagina, the cervix is grasped and the junction of the cervix to the vagina is identified. The suture place-

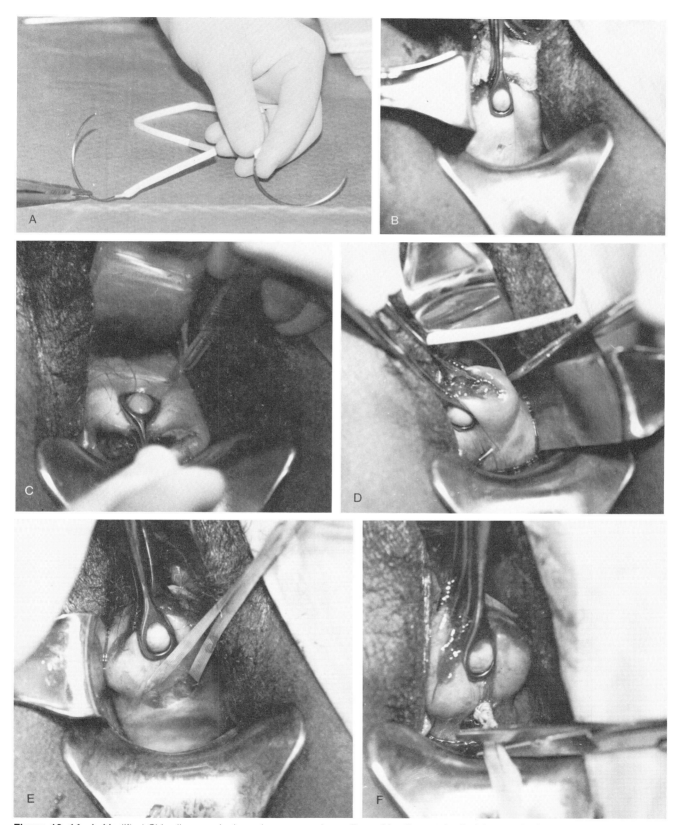

Figure 10–14. *A,* Modified Shirodkar cervical cerclage: preparing a 5-mm Mersilene strip doubly armed with large, blunt needles; *B,* posterior incision in the vaginal epithelium; *C,* anterior incision in the vaginal epithelium; *D,* passing the needle beneath the vaginal epithelium on the left side of the cervix; *E,* a Mersilene suture has been passed on both sides and encircles the cervix, ready to tie; *F,* the suture is tied posterior to the cervix to achieve an internal cervical diameter of approximately 5 mm. (Courtesy Duane E. Neumann, M.D.; photographed by Rita L. Letellier.)

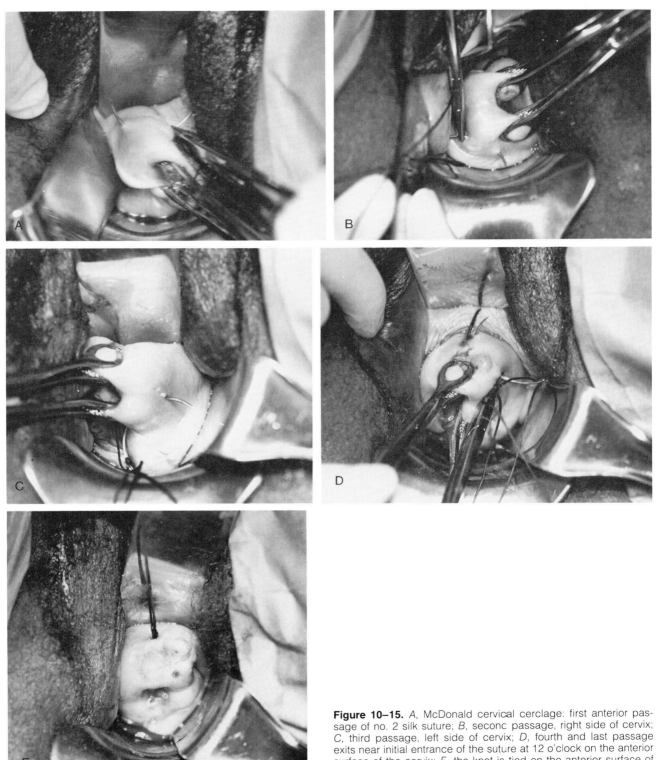

Figure 10–15. A, McDonald cervical cerclage: first anterior passage of no. 2 silk suture; B, second passage, right side of cervix; C, third passage, left side of cervix; D, fourth and last passage exits near initial entrance of the suture at 12 o'clock on the anterior surface of the cervix; E, the knot is tied on the anterior surface of the cervix.

ment is begun anteriorly and directed downward with rotation of the wrist (Fig. 10–15A). Because the needle tip curves toward (then away from) the internal os, the surgeon must be alert to the location of the cervical canal to avoid membrane rupture.

Circumferential placement of the suture in four sequential bites completes the purse string. It is usually tied anteriorly (Figs. 10–15B–E). A second purse string is sometimes required for optimal internal os support. Caution should be exercised in placing multiple sutures because of the risk of cervical damage from devascularization. Because displacement of the suture most often occurs posteriorly, secure placement in the posterior cervix is stressed.[125] The advantages of this procedure are its technical simplicity and usefulness in emergent procedures. Fetal survival following McDonald cerclage is reported at 78 to 86%.[87, 101]

Abdominal Cerclage. An abdominal approach to the reinforcement of the internal os has been practiced since 1965.[127] The technique is advocated in the second trimester, when viable gestation is confirmed.[127–132] Because of the added morbidity of laparotomy, it is generally reserved for those patients in whom cervical defect precludes transvaginal cerclage placement. The patient should be made aware of a higher potential blood loss (an average of 150 mL) and the need for cesarean section at delivery.

A laparotomy is performed through a transverse or vertical skin incision. After 15 weeks' gestation, the vertical incision is advocated. The vesicouterine junction is identified, and the peritoneal reflection of the bladder is incised transversely. The bladder is reflected off the lower uterine segment with midline blunt or sharp dissection. Care must be taken to avoid the lateral vascular plexus. The uterus is gently elevated with cephalic traction, and the level of the internal cervical os is identified at the junction of the development of the uterine isthmus.

The avascular space between the ascending and descending branches of one uterine artery is found lateral to the cervicoisthmic junction (Fig. 10–16). Blunt dissection medial to the vessels and lateral to the uterine isthmus dissects this space. Using right-angled forceps, the avascular space between the ascending and descending branches is bluntly dissected to allow passage of a 5-mm Mersilene suture. This may require a 1 to 2-cm tunnel. If parametrial veins are disrupted, hemostatic clips are useful in controlling bleeding. The dissection is repeated on the contralateral side. The posterior leaf of the broad ligament is then punctured, and a 15-cm segment of 5-mm Mersilene suture is passed around the posterior peritoneum and tied anteriorly with a single knot. The suture should lie flat and fit snugly. The peritoneum is reapproximated after securing the ends of the knot to the main band with nonabsorbable suture. Presurgical

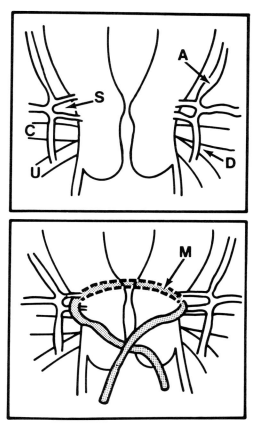

Figure 10–16. Transabdominal cervical cerclage: A—ascending branch of uterine artery; D—descending branch of uterine artery; C—cardinal ligament; U—uterosacral ligament; S—avascular space; M—Mersilene band suture is placed through the avascular spaces and around the cervix. (From Marx PD: Transabdominal cervicoisthmic cerclage: A review. Obstet Gynecol Surv 44:518, 1989.)

salvage rates of 16 to 20% are reported to be improved to 85 to 95% with this procedure.[127–132]

Emergent Cerclage. Emergent cerclage is performed in the setting of advanced cervical dilatation (usually beyond 3 cm), and such cases are usually complicated by herniation of intact amniotic membranes through the cervical os.[133] The criteria for cerclage placement must be rigidly adhered to. There must be no evidence of chorioamnionitis, preterm labor, or fetal anomaly. The patient should be counseled that the chance for success is low, with a 24% fetal survival rate reported when cerclage is placed at 5-cm or greater dilatation.[134] A retrospective review by Whitehead and colleagues[135] showed a live birth rate of only 12% when emergent cerclage was placed at greater than 3-cm dilatation. Recent reports are more optimistic. In a report by Barth and colleagues,[133] 11 of 15 patients had an average gestational prolongation of 63 days following emergent cerclage. Olatunbosun and Dyck[136] reported success with emergent cerclage in 10 of 12 patients treated with cervical dilatation greater than 4 cm and no bleeding. Their technique consisted of placing the patient under general anesthesia with halothane and endotracheal intubation, followed by placing the patient in a deep Trendelenburg position supported by shoulder harnesses. The vagina is irrigated carefully with an antiseptic solution to avoid injuring the exposed membranes. Grasping of a thin, effaced cervix may lead to trauma and bleeding, as well as membrane rupture. To avoid this, six to ten stay sutures of 2–0 silk are placed circumferentially around the cervix and used to pull the cervix over the protruding membranes. A moist

swab can be used to aid in replacement of the membranes (Fig. 10–17A–C). Two purse string sutures of Mersilene or nylon are placed around the cervix as high as possible toward the internal os. All but four of the stay sutures are then removed, and the remainder are tied across the cervix. Prophylactic tocolysis, antibiotic therapy, and an indwelling catheter are recommended and should be maintained for 24 hours after the procedure. Failure occurs as a result of intractable labor or rupture of membranes.

Several technical problems are specific to emer-

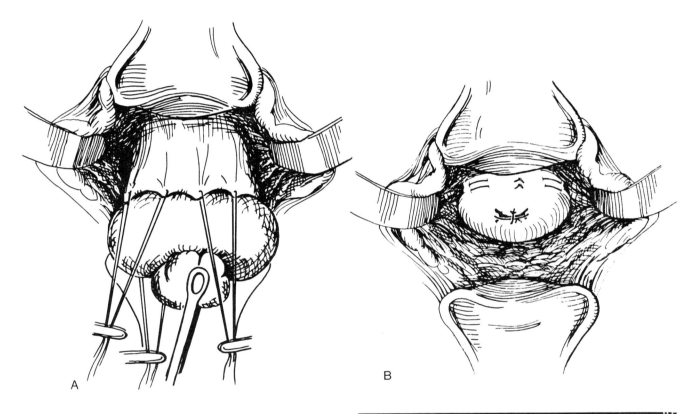

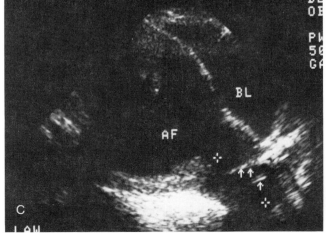

Figure 10–17. Emergent cerclage: *A,* traction sutures pull the dilated cervix downward. A moist sponge gently assists in reduction of bulging membranes; *B,* appearance of the cervix after suture placement. (From Olatunbosun OA, Dyck F: Cervical cerclage operation for a dilated cervix. Obstet Gynecol 57:166, 1981); *C,* ultrasound study after placement of emergent cerclage at 24 weeks' gestation with the cervix dilated 5 cm. Cervix appears closed and membranes retracted. BL—the bladder, AF—the amniotic fluid, two cerclage sutures *(arrows).*

gent cerclage, the most important being the ability to reduce the herniated membranes before suture placement. To assist in membrane reduction, deep Trendelenburg positioning and manual replacement of the membranes are needed. One technique is to remove the tip of a No. 16 Foley catheter and gently insert the catheter through the cervical os. The 30-mL balloon is then inflated to elevate the membranes before suture placement.[137, 138] Similar results may be obtained by having an assistant elevate the uterine fundus by cephalic abdominal retraction. This raises the lower uterine segment and allows for retraction of the amniotic membranes. Overdistending the bladder with up to 1000 mL of saline has also been reported as useful in elevating the lower uterine segment and reducing the herniated membranes.[139, 140] If noninvasive maneuvers are unsuccessful, transabdominal amniocentesis has been employed to decrease intra-amniotic fluid volume and facilitate membrane retraction. This may increase the risk of membrane rupture associated with cerclage placement.[141]

Progesterone (hydroxyprogesterone caproate),[142] pessaries,[143, 144] and tocolytic agents have been used along with bed rest as alternatives to cerclage for patients with incompetent cervices. Success using pessaries and tocolytics is most likely for patients experiencing early uterine irritability rather than passive cervical incompetence. The efficacy of progesterone use was reported by Sherman.[142] Fetal survival rates improved from 25% pretreatment to 92% survival after treatment with high doses of 17 α-hydroxyprogesterone caproate weekly in patients with presumed cervical incompetence. Additional noninvasive techniques include cervical scarring by electrocauterization[145] or a mechanical cervical "collar" made of a silicone-plastic cuff.[146] The cuff is inflated to provide support to the internal os from external compression. Electrocautery scars the cervix and is potentially associated with cervical stenosis. These modalities have not been accepted as substitutes for cerclage.

PLACENTA PREVIA AND CERVICAL PREGNANCY. Transvaginal cerclage has also been used to avert bleeding complications in placenta previa.[147] A prospective randomized trial by Arias[147] in 25 patients with placenta previa had 13 patients receiving cerclage, compared with 12 control subjects. The patients with cerclages achieved a more advanced gestational age at delivery (34.9 ± 3.0 compared with 31.6 ± 2.9 wks; p = 0.02) and had less maternal bleeding. Although the numbers are small, they provide an interesting series from which to consider the use of cerclage in patients with symptomatic placenta previa early in gestation. Other reports on the efficacy of cerclage in placenta previa are needed for corroboration.

Cerclage is reported to decrease blood loss in evacuation of a distal cervical pregnancy.[148, 149] The rarity of this condition precludes detailed study, but case reports relate successful evacuation of cervical ectopic pregnancy aided by McDonald-type cerclage.[148, 149]

Complications

Complications of cerclage placement include premature rupture of amniotic membranes (1 to 9%), chorioamnionitis (1 to 8%), displaced cervical suture (3 to 13%), cervical laceration at delivery (1 to 13%), and increased incidence of emergent cesarean section (10%).[111, 115–117, 150–153] Perioperative membrane rupture, chorioamnionitis, and cerclage failure are all increased when the suture is placed in a cervix dilated more than 3 cm.[153, 154] Cervical bacterial colonization in patients with cerclage occurs at the same rate found among control subjects without cerclages.[154, 155] The incidence of positive cultures is not decreased significantly by administration of prophylactic antibiotics.[154, 155] If preterm premature rupture of membranes occurs, the cerclage should be removed, and the patient should be managed expectantly.[156] If the cerclage fails for other reasons (bleeding, dilatation), the opportunity may exist for repeat cerclage placement.[157]

Rare complications include excessive bleeding, which necessitates blood transfusion. The average blood loss during vaginal cerclage is only 30 to 50 mL, and during abdominal cerclage, 150 mL.[87, 128, 130] Uterine rupture is reported from labor prior to cerclage removal.[158, 159] Bladder injuries may occur during cerclage placement or from suture erosion.[160, 161] One reported case of bladder trigone ulceration occurred 22 years after cerclage placement, reinforcing the need for cerclage removal after delivery.[162]

There is no universal protocol for postoperative care after cerclage. Outpatient cerclage placement is shown to be cost-effective and efficacious but must be individualized.[163] Bed rest, tocolysis, and prophylactic antibiotics become less justifiable after 24 to 48 hours. After cerclage placement, the patient is advised to avoid intercourse or cervical stimulation. The patient should be educated as to the signs and symptoms of preterm uterine activity, infection, and rupture of the amniotic membranes. Bed rest, oral tocolysis, and home uterine activity monitoring are individualized, based on patient symptoms. Vaginal examinations and serial ultrasonography are used to identify recurrent cervical dilation (see Fig. 10–9).[164] If cervical dilation is noted, aggressive tocolysis and strict bed rest may improve outcome.[164]

Conclusion

Cervical incompetence occurs in 1 in 54 to 1 in 1000 deliveries. Painless cervical dilatation is the hallmark of this condition, but clinical presentations vary. The obstetrician should advise prophylactic cerclage placement, based on preconceptual findings as outlined in the guidelines of the American College of Obstetricians and Gynecologists. Therapeutic cerclage for progressive cervical dilatation shown on physical examination or ultrasonography can be accomplished with either McDonald or Shirodkar techniques. Emergent cerclage at greater than 4 to 5 cm of dilation requires additional technical modifications and should be considered on an individual basis. When transvaginal cerclage is not possible because of cervical dysmorphology, the transabdominal approach can be utilized. Although randomized studies of cerclage placement in patients at low to moderate risk for cervical incompetence are contradictory as to efficacy, the patient with cervical incompetence and prior fetal survival of 10 to 25% can be expected to have a 70 to 90% success rate following cerclage placement.

UTERINE LEIOMYOMATA IN PREGNANCY

Prospective study of uterine leiomyomata in pregnancy has been hindered by the limitations of noninvasive diagnosis. Only 10 to 40% of ultrasonically detected leiomyomata in pregnancy are also diagnosed by physical exam.[165] A recent retrospective study discovered a 2% incidence of leiomyomata in 6005 consecutive pregnancies referred for ultrasonography.[166] The authors estimated that 10% of pregnant patients with leiomyomata would be expected to have complications. In a separate report, 93 of 6706 pregnancies between 1981 and 1985 had leiomyomas by ultrasonography (1.4%). Of these 93 patients, 9% developed placental abruption, 15% had significant pain, and 21.5% suffered preterm labor.[167] This is in contrast to the historical 50 to 70% complication rate quoted when leiomyomata during pregnancy were discovered without the aid of ultrasonography.[168] Recent studies indicate that 10 to 20% of patients with early, ultrasonically detected leiomyomata will have complications.[166–168, 169, 170] This figure increases when leiomyomata are diagnosed by palpation.

Complications related to leiomyomata in pregnancy include preterm labor and delivery, spontaneous abortion, and premature rupture of the membranes. In one series of 28 patients with significant leiomyomata, 14% delivered before 25 weeks, 18% delivered between 28 and 36 weeks, and 68% delivered after 37 weeks.[166]

Hospital admission is often related to pain, which occurs most commonly in the second or early third trimester. The pain is caused by degeneration and may be noted with or without signs of peritoneal irritation. On questioning, the patient can usually outline a specific uterine focus rather than diffuse abdominal tenderness. If uterine irritability accompanies the pain, differentiation among placental abruption, intrauterine infection, and adnexal torsion may be difficult. In the report by Katz and colleagues,[166] ibuprofen was suggested to be an efficacious analgesic. This may relate to its prostaglandin-inhibiting effects on uterine irritability as well as its analgesic properties.

Vaginal bleeding in patients with uterine leiomyomata is usually found early in gestation and is often a prelude to spontaneous abortion. The risks of bleeding, premature rupture of membranes, and abortion are increased when the myoma is located in close proximity to the placental implantation site.[165] Complications are also expected to increase when the myomata are noted to enlarge on serial ultrasonographic examinations.[166–170]

Diagnosis

When a patient is identified as having a pelvic mass consistent with leiomyomata during pregnancy, the differential diagnosis includes other solid tumors of the uterus and adnexae. Until direct observation (usually at delivery) excludes ovarian or abdominal pathology, scrutiny for malignant changes, such as cyst formation, rapid growth, maternal ascites, and unusual abdominal symptoms, must be maintained. Any suspicious mass should be investigated by detailed radiologic studies or by laparotomy.

When the diagnosis of benign myoma is fairly certain, patient counseling includes the anticipation of painful crises related to degeneration, infarction, or (if pedunculated) torsion. Parasitic omental and bowel adhesions may be suggested by colicky gastrointestinal pain. If the myomata are close to the lower uterine segment, their expansion may cause bowel tenesmus posteriorly or urinary obstruction anteriorly.[171, 172] Enlargement of the myoma occurs in approximately 30% of cases. Small myomata (less than 6 cm in diameter) are more likely to expand than large myomata (greater than 10 cm in diameter).[169] When growth of the myoma is less than 25% of initial volume, the 6-week postpartum size generally equals prepregnancy size.[173]

Management

Individual treatment depends on the gestational age at the time of complications, associated bleeding, and preterm labor. Development of cystic, anechoic spaces in the myoma on serial ultrasonographic examinations heralds degenerative changes associated with abdominal pain and uterine irritability (perhaps from prostaglandin release).[166–169, 173]

At delivery, myomata in the lower uterine segment are often associated with fetal malpresentation, dysfunctional labor, and the need for cesarean section (see Fig. 10–18). Because a classic uterine incision may be required in a uterus with a distorted lower uterine segment and a malrotated fundus, adequate skin incision for exposure should be utilized. Although uterine healing in a noninfected uterus should be excellent, when patients have had extensive fundal myomectomy prior to pregnancy, elective cesarean delivery at 37 to 38 weeks with documented fetal pulmonary maturity is currently practiced. Vaginal delivery in patients with leiomyomata is often complicated by postpartum hemorrhage from placental retention. When the placenta is implanted over the myoma, the patient is reported to be at higher risk for postpartum complications.[170] Rarely, a submucous myoma is spontaneously expelled post partum.[174]

Surgical excision of the myoma in the first or second trimester is rarely advocated because of the highly vascularized myometrium and poor results for pregnancy continuation. If pregnancy loss occurs related to leiomyomata, then removal by hysteroscopy, laparoscopy, or laparotomy should be considered before the next conception. Pregnancy following gonadotropin-releasing hormone agonist (or analogue) is reported, but further studies are needed to document the safety and efficacy of this treatment.[175, 176] When the leiomyomata are associated with infertility, laser myomectomy shows promise, with conception rates of 69% and a viable term delivery rate of 59%.[177, 178]

Complications

Patients frequently ask about the effect of myomata on fetal development. Reports have documented submucosal leiomyomata that impinge on the fetus, causing limb or cranial deformation.[179, 180] Serial ultrasonographic studies should assist in reassuring the patient of uncompromised fetal growth.

Conclusion

Leiomyomata in pregnancy are diagnosed with greater frequency with the use of obstetric ultrasonography. Approximately 1 to 2% of pregnancies have ultrasonically detected leiomyomata, and 10 to 20% of these have complications. If the leiomyomata are palpable, then 50 to 70% are expected to have complications. Any lesions that are suspected of malignant change should be investigated. Enlargement of the leiomyoma occurs in approximately 30% of patients, and leiomyomata close to the placental implantation site have a higher correlation with bleeding, premature ruptured membranes, abortion, and pain. The majority of patients (68%) deliver at term, but fetal malposition or dystocia during labor from leiomyomata in the lower uterine segment increases the incidence of cesarean section.

RETROVERSION AND UTERINE SACCULATION

Pregnancy in a uterus with the fundus displaced toward the cul-de-sac (e.g., retroverted, retroflexed) occurs in 11 to 19% of obstetric patients.[181] Although fertility is not impaired, vaginal bleeding and spontaneous abortion are reportedly increased.[182, 183] In prior reviews, one per 3000 pregnancies was reported to have incarceration of a retroverted gestation.[184, 185] In a recent review by Hess, "incarceration of a retroverted uterus occurred in one per 10,384 live births."[186] The four patients in his review had successful replacement followed by term delivery. Retroversion rarely persists past 14 to 16 weeks' gestation, when the expanding uterus elevates above the fixed boundaries of the pelvic side walls. If displacement does not occur, the expanding uterus potentially compresses the bowel, bladder, and urethra. Fetal wastage may approach 33% from spontaneous labor and forced evacuation of the uterus. The highest success is achieved by manual replacement before 16 weeks' gestation.

Diagnosis

Symptoms of abdominal pain, bleeding from the vagina, urinary retention, paradoxic incontinence, tenesmus, and constipation may occur.[181, 186] Retroversion persisting up to the third trimester is infrequent and produces confusion as to fetal

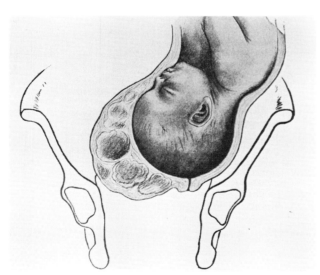

Figure 10–18. Cervical myoma obstructing labor. (From DeLee JB: The Principles and Practice of Obstetrics. Philadelphia: W.B. Saunders Co., 1924, p. 558.)

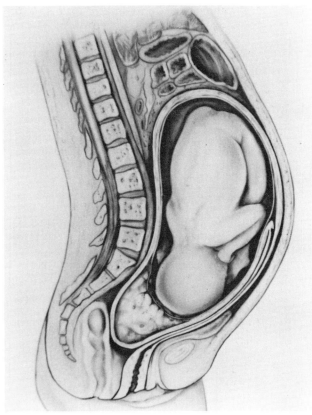

Figure 10–19. Persistent retroversion of the uterus at 36 weeks' gestation is seen. There is a false impression of fetal cephalic presentation and of placenta previa, which is actually a breech presentation with a fundal placenta at cesarean delivery. (From Jackson DN: Gestational retroversion at term. Obstet Gynecol 71(3):466, 1988.)

presentation and uterine orientation (Fig. 10–19).[181, 187] Physical examination in these patients reveals the cervix to be malrotated beneath the symphysis pubis. A posterior mass is felt through the cul-de-sac and has a soft consistency. Ultrasonographic and radiographic findings are not conclusive, and the practitioner needs a high degree of suspicion for correct diagnosis.

Management

After bowel and bladder are emptied, pressure through the vagina or rectum is applied to the retroverted fundus in an effort to displace it up out of the pelvis. Epidural anesthesia or intravenous analgesia may be necessary to reduce patient discomfort during a difficult replacement, especially if tenaculum traction on the cervix is required. If no movement is achieved, the patient should be positioned on her knees with her head and shoulders lowered.[188] When retroversion is diagnosed near term, the delivery is best managed by cesarean section. Care must be exercised to

identify the proper surgical orientation of the lower uterine segment during abdominal delivery, and the incision to access the gestation is often through the malrotated uterine fundus.[181]

UTERINE SACCULATION

Sacculation of a pregnant uterus unrelated to müllerian malformation has been infrequently reported.[189, 190] The uterine wall is thin and ballooning, with the defect size ranging from 2 to 10 cm. The location of the defect may be in the body or the fundus of the uterus and may contain the placental implantation site. Dysfunctional labor, cesarean section, and placental retention are all increased with uterine sacculation. If the defect is discovered during cesarean section, the sacculated uterus should be differentiated from müllerian anomalies by careful inspection of the intrauterine cavity for septa and of the fundus for bicornuate notching.[191]

Management

Laparotomy with excision and repair of the sacculation may be necessary to effect removal of an adherent placenta. If the sacculation is discovered after uncomplicated vaginal delivery, hysteroscopy or hysterosalpingogram as an interval procedure can direct repair before the next conception.

References

1. Ramsey, EM: The history of the uterus. In Norris HJ, Hartig AT, Abell MR (eds): The Uterus. Baltimore: Williams & Wilkins, 1973, pp 1–16.
2. Radcliff W: Milestones in Midwifery and the Secret Instrument. San Francisco: Norman Publishing, 1989.
3. Kudlien, F: The seven cells of the uterus: The doctrine and its roots. Bull Hist Med 39:415, 1965.
4. Vesalius A: De Humani Corporis Fabrica. Basilae, 1543 (Facsimile, Brussels, 1964). In Ramsey EM: The History of the Uterus (see ref. no. 1).
5. Gream GT: Dilation or division of the cervix uteri. Lancet 1:381, 1865.
6. Harger JH: Cervical cerclage: Patient selection, morbidity, and success rates. Clin Perinatol 10:321, 1983.
7. Hunter W: The Gravid Uterus. Birmingham, 1774.
7a. Hunter W: An anatomical description of the human gravid uterus and its contents. London: J. Johnson. 1794.
8. The American Fertility Society: Classification of adnexal adhesions, distal tubal occlusion, tubal occlusion secondary to tubal ligation, tubal pregnancies, müllerian anomalies and intrauterine adhesions. Fertil Steril 49:944, 1988.
9. Jones HW: Reproductive impairment and the malformed uterus. Fertil Steril 36:137, 1981.
10. Bowman JA Jr, Scott RB: Transverse vaginal septum: Report of four cases. Obstet Gynecol 3:441, 1954.
11. McKusick VA, Baver RL, Koop CE, Scott RB: Hydrome-

trocolpos as a simply inherited malformation. JAMA 189:813, 1964.

12. Biair RG: Pregnancy associated with congenital malformations of the reproductive tract. Br J Obstet Gynaecol 67:36, 1989.

13. Pinsonneault O, Goldstein DP: Obstructing malformations of the uterus and vagina. Fertil Steril 44:241, 1985.

14. Golan A, Langer R, Bukovsky I, Caspi E: Congenital anomalies of the müllerian system. Fertil Steril 51:747, 1989.

15. Geiss FC, Mauzy FH: Genital anomalies in women. Am J Obstet Gynecol 82:330, 1961.

16. Zabrieski JR: Pregnancy and the malformed uterus: Report of 92 cases. West J Surg Obstet Gynecol 70:293, 1962.

17. Green LK, Harris RE: Uterine anomalies: Frequency of diagnosis and associated obstetrical complications. Obstet Gynecol 47:427, 1976.

18. Holmes JA: Congenital abnormalities of the uterus and pregnancy. Br Med J 1:1144, 1956.

19. Stein AL, March CM: The outcome of pregnancy in women with müllerian duct anomalies. J Reprod Med 35:411, 1990.

20. Buttram VC: Müllerian anomalies and their management. Fertil Steril 40:159, 1983.

21. Rock JA, Reeves LA, Retto H, et al.: Success following vaginal creation for müllerian agenesis. Fertil Steril 339:809, 1983.

22. Garcia J, Jones HW Jr: The split thickness graft technic for vaginal agenesis. Obstet Gynecol 49:328, 1977.

23. Jeffcoate TNA: Advancement of the upper vagina in the treatment of hematocolpos and hematometria caused by vaginal aplasia: Pregnancy following the construction of an artificial vagina. J Obstet Gynecol Br Comm 76:961, 1969.

24. Farber M, Mitchell GW Jr, Marchant DJ: Congenital atresia of the uterine cervix: Long term results. Trans Am Gynecol Obstet Soc 1:113, 1982.

25. Farber M, Noumoff J, Freedman M, Oberkotter L: Understanding and correcting genital anomalies. Contemp Ob Gyn 24:113, 1984.

26. Zarou GS, Esposito JM, Zarou DM: Pregnancy following the surgical correction of congenital atresia of the cervix. Int J Gynaecol Obstet 11:143, 1973.

27. Ansbacher R: Uterine anomalies and future pregnancies. Clin Perinatol 10:295, 1983.

28. O'Leary JL, O'Leary JA: A rudimentary horn pregnancy. Obstet Gynecol 27:806, 1966.

29. Andolf E, Helm G, Svalenius E, Westrom L: Seventeen week pregnancy in a rudimentary uterine horn revealed at routine ultrasonography. Acta Obstet Gynecol Scand 67:379, 1988.

30. Jarrell J, Effer SB, Mohide PT: Pregnancy in a rudimentary horn with fetal salvage. Am J Obstet Gynecol 127:676, 1977.

31. Akhtar AZ: Term pregnancy in a rudimentary horn of a bicornuate uterus with foetal salvage: a case report. Asia-Oceania J Obstet Gynaecol 14:143, 1988.

32. Orr JW, Bull J, Younger JB: Infected müllerian anomaly: An unusual cause of pelvic abscess during pregnancy. Am J Obstet Gynecol 155:368, 1986.

33. Andrews MC, Jones HW Jr: Impaired reproductive performance of the unicornuate uterus: Intrauterine growth retardation, infertility, and recurrent abortion in five cases. Am J Obstet Gynecol 144:173, 1982.

34. Fedele L, Zamberletti D, Vercellini P, et al: Reproductive performance of women with unicornuate uterus. Fertil Steril 47:416, 1987.

35. Maneschi M, Maneschi F, Fuca G: Reproductive impairment of women with unicornuate uterus. Acta Eur Fertil 19:273, 1988.

36. Musich JR, Behrman SJ: Obstetric outcome before and after metroplasty in women with uterine anomalies. Obstet Gynecol 52:63, 1978.

37. Strassman EL: Fertility and unification of double uterus. Fertil Steril 17:165, 1966.

38. Buttram VC Jr, Gibbons WE: Müllerian anomalies: A proposed classification (an analysis of 144 cases). Fertil Steril 32:40, 1979.

39. Fedele L, Dorta M, Brioschi D, et al.: Pregnancies in septate uteri: Outcome in relation to site of uterine implantation as determined by sonography. AJR 152:781, 1989.

40. Rock JA, Murphy A, Cooper WH: Resectoscopic techniques for the lysis of a Class V: Complete uterine septum. Fertil Steril 48:495, 1987.

41. March CM, Israel R: Hysteroscopic management of recurrent abortion caused by septate uterus. Am J Obstet Gynecol 156:834, 1987.

42. Valle RF, Sciarra JJ: Hysteroscopic treatment of the septate uterus. Obstet Gynecol 67:253, 1986.

43. Perino A, Mencaglia L, Hamou J, Cittadini E: Hysteroscopy for metroplasty of uterine septa: Report of 24 cases. Fertil Steril 48:321, 1987.

44. DeCherney AH, Russell JB, Graebe RA, Polan ML: Resectoscopic management of müllerian fusion defects. Fertil Steril 45:726, 1986.

45. Hassiakos DK, Zourlas PA: Transcervical division of uterine septa. Obstet Gynecol Surv 45:165, 1990.

46. Records JW: Vaginal approach in repair of uterine septal defect. Obstet Gynecol 25:387, 1965.

47. Mossop RT: Pervaginal correction of the septate uterus. Cent Afr J Med 15:284, 1969.

48. Carapetyan H: Metroplasty: Unification of a bicornuate or septate uterus. Clin Obstet Gynecol 17:5, 1974.

49. Jones HW Jr: Operations for congenital anomalies of the uterus and vagina. Clin Obstet Gynecol 17:5, 1974.

50. Mahgoub SE: Unification of a septate uterus: Mahgoub's operation. Int J Gynecol Obstet 15:400, 1978.

51. Surgery for anomalies of the müllerian ducts. In Mattingly, RF, Thompson, JD (eds.): Telinde's Operative Gynecology. Philadelphia: J.B. Lippincott Co., 6th Edition, 1985, p. 369.

52. Jones HW Jr, Rock JA (eds.): Reparative and Constructive Surgery of the Female Generative Tract. Baltimore: Williams & Wilkins, 1983, p. 185.

53. Stilman RJ: In utero exposure to diethylstilbestrol: Adverse effects on the reproductive tract and reproductive performance in male and female offspring. Am J Obstet Gynecol 142:905, 1982.

54. Kaufman RH, Adam E, Binder GL, Gerthoffer E: Upper genital tract changes and pregnancy outcome in offspring exposed in utero to diethylstilbestrol. Am J Obstet Gynecol 137:299, 1980.

55. Herbst AL, Scully RE: Adenocarcinoma of the vagina in adolescence: A report of seven cases, including six clear cell carcinomas (so-called mesonephromas). Cancer 25:745, 1970.

56. Sandberg EC: Benign cervical and vaginal changes associated with exposure to stilbestrol in utero. Am J Obstet Gynecol 125:777, 1976.

57. Goldstein DP: Incompetent cervix in offspring exposed to diethylstilbestrol in utero. Obstet Gynecol 52(suppl):735, 1978.

58. Ben-Baruch G, Menczer J, Mashiach S, Serr DM: Uterine anomalies in diethylstilbestrol exposed women with fertility disorders. Acta Obstet Gynecol Scand 60:395, 1981.

59. Ludmir J, Landon MB, Gabbe SG, et al.: Management of the diethylstilbestrol-exposed pregnant patient: A prospective study. Am J Obstet Gynecol 157:665, 1987.

60. Ayers JWT, DeGrood RM, Compton AA, et al.: Sonographic evaluation of cervical length in pregnancy: Diagnosis and management of preterm cervical effacement in patients at risk for premature delivery. Obstet Gynecol 71:939, 1988.

61. Benirschke K: Survey of pathologic anatomy. In Norris HJ, Hartig AT, Abell MR (eds.): The Uterus. Baltimore: Williams & Wilkins, 1973.

62. Elias S, Simpson JL, Carson SA, et al.: Genetic studies in incomplete müllerian fusion. Obstet Gynecol 63:276, 1984.

63. Daw E, Toon P: Identical twins with uterus didelphys and duplex kidneys. Postgrad Med J 61:269, 1985.
64. Sarto GE, Simpson JL: Abnormalities of the müllerian and Wolffian duct systems. Birth Defects 14:37, 1978.
65. Johnson JM, Elias S, Simpson JL, et al.: Transabdominal chorionic villus sampling in a patient with a bicornuate uterus. Am J Perinatol 6:292, 1989.
66. Bagnasco JF, Trabin JR, Manko GF: Prenatal sampling and bicornuate uterus [letter]. Prenat Diagn 9:447, 1989.
67. Graham JM, Miller ME, Stephan MJ, Smith DW: Limb reduction anomalies and early in utero limb compression. J Pediatr 96:1052, 1980.
68. Dunn DW, Engle WA: Brachial plexus palsy: Intrauterine onset. Pediatr Neurol 1:367, 1985.
69. Matsunaga E, Shiota K: Ectopic pregnancy and myoma uteri: Teratogenic effects and maternal characteristics. Teratology reported in Graham. J Pediatr 96:1052, 1980.
70. Miller ME, Dunn PM, Smith DW: Uterine malformation and fetal deformation. J Pediatr 94:387, 1979.
71. Rock JA, Jones HW Jr: The clinical management of the double uterus. Fertil Steril 28:798, 1977.
72. Harger JH, Archer DF, Marchese SG, et al.: Etiology of recurrent pregnancy losses and outcome of subsequent pregnancies. Obstet Gynecol 62:574, 1983.
73. Tho PT, Byrd JR, McDonough PG: Etiologies and subsequent reproductive performance of 100 couples with recurrent abortion. Fertil Steril 32:389, 1979.
74. Semmens JP: Abdominal contour in the third trimester: An aid to diagnosis of uterine anomalies. Obstet Gynecol 25:779, 1965.
75. Parisi VM: Cervical Incompetence. In Creasy RK, Resnick R (eds.): Maternal Fetal Medicine: Principles and Practice. Philadelphia: W.B. Saunders Co., 1989.
76. Shirodkar VN: A new method of operative treatment for habitual abortions in the second trimester of pregnancy. Antiseptic 52:299, 1955.
77. Crombleholme WR, Minkoff HL, Delke I, Schwarz RH: Cervical cerclage: An aggressive approach to threatened or recurrent pregnancy wastage. Am J Obstet Gynecol 146:168, 1983.
78. Rorie DK, Newton M: Histological and chemical studies of the smooth muscle in human cervix and uterus. Am J Obstet Gynecol 99:466, 1967.
79. McIntyre JA, McConnachie PR, Taylor CG, Faulk WP: Clinical immunologic and genetic definitions of primary and secondary recurrent spontaneous abortions. Fertil Steril 42:849, 1984.
80. Byrd JR, Askew DE, McDonough PG: Cytogenetic findings in fifty-five couples with recurrent fetal wastage. Fertil Steril 28:246, 1977.
81. Coechock S, Smith BJ, Gocial B: Antibodies to phospholipids and nuclear antigens in patients with repeated abortions. Am J Obstet Gynecol 155:1002, 1986.
82. Hensleigh PA, Fainstst T: Corpus luteum dysfunction: Serum progesterone levels in diagnoses and assessment of therapy for recurrent and threatened abortion. Fertil Steril 32:396, 1979.
83. Stray-Pedersen B, Stray-Pedersen S: Etiologic factors and subsequent reproductive performance in 195 couples with a prior history of habitual abortion. Am J Obstet Gynecol 148:140, 1984.
84. Adno J: The "incompetent cervix" associated with bicornuate uterus. S Afr Med J 36:1015, 1962.
85. Craig CJ: Congenital abnormalities of the uterus and fetal wastage. S Afr Med J 47:2000, 1973.
86. Waintraub G, Milwidsky A, Weiss D: Prevention of premature delivery in a unicornuate uterus by cervical cerclage. Acta Obstet Gynaecol Scand 54:497, 1975.
87. Harger JH: Cervical cerclage: Patient selection, morbidity, and success rates. Clin Perinatol 10:321, 1983.
88. Cousins L: Cervical incompetence, 1980: A time for reappraisal. Clin Obstet Gynecol 23:467, 1980.
89. Schmidt G, Fowler WC Jr, Talbert LM, et al.: Reproductive history of women exposed to diethylstilbestrol in utero. Fertil Steril 33:21, 1980.
90. Nunley WC, Kitchin JD: Successful management of incompetent cervix in a primigravida exposed to diethylstilbestrol in utero. Fertil Steril 31:217, 1979.
91. Johnstone FD, Beard RJ, Boyd IE, McCarthy TH: Cervical diameter after suction termination of pregnancy. Br Med J 1:68, 1976.
92. Caspi E, Schneider D, Sadovsky G, et al.: Diameter of cervical internal os after induction of early abortion by laminaria or rigid digitation. Am J Obstet Gynecol 146:106, 1983.
93. Embrey MP: Prostaglandin induced abortion and cervical incompetence [letter]. Br Med J 2:497, 1975.
94. Leiman G, Harrison NA, Robin A: Pregnancy following conization of the cervix. Complications related to cone size. Am J Obstet Gynecol 136:14, 1980.
95. Larsson G, Grundsell H, Gullberg B, et al.: Outcome of pregnancy after conization. Acta Obstet Gynecol Scand 61:461, 1982.
96. Shortle B, Jewelewicz R: Cervical incompetence. Fertil Steril 52:181, 1989.
97. Rechberger T, Uldbjerg N, Oxlund H: Connective tissue changes in the cervix during normal pregnancy and pregnancy complicated by cervical incompetence. Obstet Gynecol 71:563, 1988.
98. Blum M: Prevention of spontaneous abortion by cervical suture of the malformed uterus. Int Surg 62:213, 1977.
99. Novy MJ: Combatting recurrent abortion and premature delivery with cervical cerclage. Contemp Obstet Gynecol 25:113, 1985.
100. Wright EA: Fetal salvage with cervical cerclage. Int J Gynaecol Obstet 25:13, 1987.
101. Harger JH: Comparison of success and morbidity in cervical cerclage procedures. Obstet Gynecol 56:543, 1980.
102. Toaff R, Toaff ME, Ballas S, et al.: Cervical incompetence: Diagnosis and therapeutic aspects. Isr J Med Sci 13:39, 1977.
103. Meeker CI, Carey WB, Freedman WL, et al.: Quality Assurance in Obstetrics and Gynecology. American College of OB Gyn Task Force on Quality Assurance. Am Coll Ob Gyn, May 1989.
104. Lash AF, Lash SR: Habitual abortion: The incompetent internal os of the cervix. Am J Obstet Gynecol 59:68, 1950.
105. Bergman R, Svennerud S: Traction test of demonstrating incompetence of the internal os of the cervix. Int J Fertil 2:163, 1957.
106. Sarti DA, Sample WF, Hobel CJ, Staisch KJ: Ultrasonic visualization of a dilated cervix during pregnancy. Radiology 130:417, 1979.
107. Jackson G, Pendleton HJ, Nichol B, Wittmann BK: Diagnostic ultrasound in the assessment of patients with incompetent cervix. Br J Obstet Gynecol 91:232, 1984.
108. Varma TR, Patel RH, Pillai U: Ultrasonic assessment of the cervix in "at risk" patients. Acta Obstet Gynaecol Scand 65:147, 1986.
109. Feingold M, Brook I, Zakut H: Detection of cervical incompetence by ultrasound. Acta Obstet Gynecol Scand 63:407, 1984.
110. Costantini S, Valenzano M, Venturini PL, et al.: Ultrasonic evaluation of cervical incompetence. Biol Res Pregnancy Perinatol 7:11, 1986
111. Seppala M, Vara P: Cervical cerclage in the treatment of incompetent cervix. Acta Obstet Gynecol Scand 49:343, 1970.
112. McDonald IA: Suture of the cervix for inevitable miscarriage. J Obstet Gynaecol Br Comm 64:346, 1957.
113. Dor J, Shalev J, Mashiach G, et al.: Elective cervical suture of twin pregnancies diagnosed ultrasonically in the first trimester following induced ovulation. Gynecol Obstet Invest 13:55, 1982.
114. Lazar P, Gueguen S: Multicentered controlled trial of cervical cerclage in women at moderate risk of preterm delivery. Br J Obstet Gynaecol 91:731, 1984.
115. Rush RW, Isaacs S, McPherson K, et al.: A randomized

controlled trial of cervical cerclage in women at high risk of spontaneous delivery. Br J Obstet Gynecol 91:724, 1984.

116. Macnaughton MC, Chalmers IG, Chamberlain GVP, et al.: Interim report of the Medical Research Council/Royal College of Obstetricians and Gynaecologists multicentre randomized trial of cervical cerclage. Br J Obstet Gynaecol 95:437, 1988.

117. Cardwell MS: Cervical cerclage: A ten-year review in a large hospital. South Med J 81:15, 1988.

118. Reptke JT, Niebyl JR: Role of prostaglandin synthetase inhibitors in the treatment of preterm labor. Semin Reprod Endocrinol 3:259, 1985.

119. Novy MJ, Ducsay CA, Stanczyk FZ: Plasma concentrations of prostaglandin $F_{2\alpha}$ and prostaglandin E_2 metabolites after transabdominal and transvaginal cervical cerclage. Am J Obstet Gynecol 156:1543, 1987.

120. Toplis PJ, Shephard JH, Youssefniejadian E, et al.: Plasma prostaglandin concentrations after cerclage in early pregnancy. Br J Obstet Gynaecol 87:669, 1980.

121. Bibby JG, Brunt J, Mitchell MD, Turnbull AC: The effect of cervical encerclage on plasma prostaglandin levels during early human pregnancy. Br J Obstet Gynaecol 86:19, 1979.

122. Niebyl JR, Blake DA, White RD, et al.: The inhibition of preterm labor with indomethacin. Am J Obstet Gynecol 136:1014, 1980.

123. Zuckerman H, Shalev E, Gilad G, et al.: Further study of the inhibition of premature labor by indomethacin. Double blind study. J Perinat Med 12:25, 1984.

124. Knight A: Prostaglandin synthesis inhibitors as tocolytic agents. In Petrie RH (ed.): Perinatal Pharmacology, New Jersey: Med Ec Books, 1989, p. 276.

125. Branch W: Operations for cervical incompetence. Clin Obstet Gynecol 29:240, 1986.

126. Druzin ML, Berkeley AS: A simplified approach to Shirodkar cerclage procedure. Surg Gynecol Obstet 162:375, 1986.

127. Bensen RC, Durfee RB: Transabdominal cervicouterine cerclage during pregnancy for the treatment of cervical incompetency. Obstet Gynecol 25:145, 1965.

128. Novy MJ: Transabdominal cervicoisthmic cerclage for the management of repetitive abortion and premature delivery. Am J Obstet Gynecol 143:44, 1982.

129. Herron MA, Parer JT: Transabdominal cerclage for fetal wastage due to cervical incompetence. Obstet Gynecol 71:865, 1988.

130. Marx PD: Transabdominal cervicoisthmic cerclage: A review. Obstet Gynecol Surv 44:518, 1989.

131. Wallenburg HC, Lotgering FK: Transabdominal cerclage for closure of the incompetent cervix. Eur J Obstet Gynecol Reprod Biol 25:121, 1987.

132. Anthony GS, Price JL: Successful use of transabdominal isthmic cerclage in the management of cervical incompetence. Eur J Obstet Gynecol Reprod Biol 22:379, 1986.

133. Barth WH Jr, Yeomans ER, Hankins GDV: Emergent cerclage. Surg Gynecol Obstet 170:323, 1990.

134. Forster FMC: Abortion and the incompetent cervix. Med J Aust 2:807, 1967.

135. Whitehead KD, Wise RB, Dunnihoo DR, Otterson WN: Retrospective analysis of cervical cerclage procedures at the Louisiana State University, Shreveport (1980 to 1987). South Med J 83:159, 1990.

136. Olatunbosun OA, Dyck F: Cervical cerclage operation for a dilated cervix. Obstet Gynecol 57:166, 1981.

137. Orr C: An aid to cervical cerclage. Aust NZ J Obstet Gynaecol 13:114, 1973.

138. Holman MR: An aid for cervical cerclage. Obstet Gynecol 42:478, 1973.

139. Scheerer LJ, Lam F, Bartolucci L, Katz M: A new technique for reduction of prolapsed fetal membranes for emergency cervical cerclage. Obstet Gynecol 74:408, 1989.

140. Pelosi MA: A new technique for reduction of fetal membranes for emergency cervical cerclage [letter]. Obstet Gynecol 75:143, 1990.

141. Goodlin RC: Cervical incompetence, hourglass membranes and amniocentesis. Obstet Gynecol 54:748, 1979.

142. Sherman AI: Hormonal therapy for control of the incompetent os of pregnancy. Obstet Gynecol 28:198, 1966.

143. Oster S, Javert CT: Treatment of the incompetent cervix with the Hodge pessary. Obstet Gynecol 28:206, 1966.

144. Vitsky M: The incompetent cervical os and the pessary. Am J Obstet Gynecol 87:144, 1963.

145. Barnes A: Conization and scarification as a treatment for cervical incompetence. Am J Obstet Gynecol 82:920, 1961.

146. Yosowitz EE, Haufrect F, Kaufman RH, et al.: Siliconeplastic cuff for the treatment of the incompetent cervix in pregnancy. Am J Obstet Gynecol 113:233, 1972.

147. Arias F: Cervical cerclage for the temporary treatment of patients with placenta previa. Obstet Gynecol 71:545, 1988.

148. Wharton KR, Gore B: Cervical pregnancy managed by placement of a Shirodkar cerclage before evacuation. A case report. J Reprod Med 33:227, 1988.

149. Wharton KR: [Letter] J Reprod Med 34:69, 1989.

150. Peters WA, Thiagarajah S, Harbert GM: Cervical cerclage: Twenty years experience. South Med J 72:933, 1979.

151. Kuhn RJP, Pepperel RJ: Cervical ligation: A review of 242 pregnancies. Aust N Z J Obstet Gynaecol 17:79, 1977.

152. Hofmeister FJ, Schwartz WR, Vondrak BF, et al.: Suture reinforcement of the incompetent cervix. Am J Obstet Gynecol 101:58, 1968.

153. Aarnoudse JG, Huisjes HJ: Complications of cerclage. Acta Obstet Gynaecol Scand 58:255, 1979.

154. Charles D, Edwards WR: Infectious complications of cervical cerclage. Am J Obstet Gynecol 141:1065, 1981.

155. Kessler I, Shoham Z, Lancet M, et al.: Complications associated with genital colonization in pregnancies with and without cerclage. Int J Gynaecol Obstet 27:359, 1988.

156. Yeast JD, Garite TR: The role of cervical cerclage in the management of preterm premature rupture of the membranes. Am J Obstet Gynecol 158:106, 1988.

157. Schulman H, Farmakides G: Surgical approach to failed cervical cerclage: A report of three cases. J Reprod Med 30:626, 1985.

158. Lindberg BS: Maternal sepsis, uterine rupture, and coagulopathy complicating cervical cerclage. Acta Obstet Gynaecol Scand 58:317, 1979.

159. Thurston JC: Rupture of uterus following Shirodkar suture. Br Med J 2:1293, 1963.

160. Bates JL, Cropley T: Complications of cervical cerclage. Lancet 2:1035, 1977.

161. Ulmsten U: Complication of cervical cerclage. Lancet 2:1350, 1977.

162. Hortenstine JS, Witherington R: Ulcer of the trigone: A late complication of cervical cerclage. J Urol 137:109, 1987.

163. Wetchler BV, Brick J: Safety of outpatient cerclage. J Reprod Med 35:243, 1990.

164. Rana J, Davis SE, Harrigan JT: Improving the outcome of cervical cerclage by sonographic follow-up. J Ultrasound Med 9:275, 1990.

165. Muram D, Gillieson M, Walters JH: Myomas of the uterus in pregnancy: Ultrasonographic follow-up. Am J Obstet Gynecol 138:16, 1980.

166. Katz VL, Dotters DJ, Droegemueller W: Complications of uterine leiomyomas in pregnancy. Obstet Gynecol 73:593, 1989.

167. Rice JP, Kay HH, Mahony BS: The clinical significance of uterine leiomyomas in pregnancy. Am J Obstet Gynecol 160:1212, 1989.

168. Grandin DJ: A review of 445 pregnancies complicated by fibromyomas. Am J Obstet Gynecol 58:727, 1949.

169. Lev-Toaff AJ, Coleman BG, Aryer PH, et al.: Leiomyomas in pregnancy: Sonographic study. Radiology 164:375, 1987.

170. Winer-Muram HT, Muram D, Gillieson MS: Uterine myoma in pregnancy. J Assoc Can Radiol 35:168, 1984.

171. Goldberg KA, Kwart AM: Intermittent urinary retention in the first trimester of pregnancy. Urology 17:270, 1981.

172. Schwartz Z, Dgani R, Katz Z, Lancet M: Urinary retention caused by impaction of leiomyoma in pregnancy. Acta Obstet Gynecol Scand 65:525, 1986.

173. Aharoni A, Reiter A, Golan D, et al.: Patterns of growth of uterine leiomyomas during pregnancy. A prospective, longitudinal study. Br J Obstet Gynaecol 95:510, 1988.

174. Honore LH, Reid DW: Uncomplicated, spontaneous expulsion of a uterine leiomyoma post partum: A case report. J Reprod Med 30:358, 1985.

175. Kessel B, Liu J, Mortola J, et al.: Treatment of uterine fibroids with agonist analogs of gonadotropin-releasing hormone. Fertil Steril 49:538, 1988.

176. Gardner RL, Shaw RW: Cornual fibroids: A conservative approach to restoring tubal patency using a gonadotropin-releasing hormone agonist (goserlin) with successful pregnancy. Fertil Steril 52:332, 1989.

177. Starks GC: CO_2 laser myomectomy in an infertile population. J Reprod Med 33:184, 1988.

178. Reyniak JV, Corenthal L: Microsurgical laser technique for abdominal myomectomy. Microsurgery 8:92, 1987.

179. Graham JM, Miller ME, Stephan MJ, Smith DW: Limb reduction anomalies and early in utero limb compression. J Pediatr 96:1052, 1980.

180. Romero R, Chervenak FA, DeVane G, et al.: Fetal head deformation and congenital torticollis associated with a uterine tumor. Am J Obstet Gynecol 141:839, 1981.

181. Jackson D, Elliot J, Pearson M: Asymptomatic uterine retroversion at 36 weeks gestation. Obstet Gynecol 71:466, 1988.

182. Weekes AL, Atley RD, Brown VA, et al.: The retroverted gravid uterus and its effect on the outcome of pregnancy. Br Med J Clin Res 1:622, 1976.

183. Barr SJ, Barr KJ: Retroversion and infertility. Am J Obstet Gynecol 146:990, 1933.

184. Gibbons JM, Paley WB: The incarcerated gravid uterus. Obstet Gynecol 33:842, 1969.

185. Fudel HE, Misenheimer RH: Incarceration of the retroverted gravid uterus with sacculation. Obstet Gynecol 43:46, 1974.

186. Hess LW, Nolan TE, Martin RW, et al.: Incarceration of the retroverted gravid uterus: Report of four patients managed with uterine reduction. South Med J 82:310, 1989.

187. Vleugels MP, Meuwissen JH: Confusing presentation in a retroflexed septate uterus at term. Eur J Obstet Gynecol Reprod Biol 24:237, 1987.

188. Terry RB: Incarcerated retroflexed gravid uterus: Simple maneuver for its correction. Obstet Gynecol 13:630, 1959.

189. Becker SM, Kant E, Carlson L: Sacculation of the pregnant uterus: A potential complication of tuboplasty. Fertil Steril 21:521, 1970.

190. Rubovits WH: True sacculation of the contractile portion of the pregnant uterus. Am J Obstet Gynecol 62:1044, 1951.

191. Rudolph L: Pseudouterus arcuatus and functional malformations of the uterus. Am J Obstet Gynecol 39:975, 1940.

11

Surgical Management of Trophoblastic Disease

John C. Weed, Jr.
Verda J. Hunter

The incidence of molar gestations varies considerably with geography. Moles occur as frequently as 1 in 125 pregnancies in Southeast Asia and 1 in 1200 pregnancies in industrialized nations.[1] Molar gestations associated with gross or microscopic evidence of fetal development are reported in 1 in 10,000 to 1 in 100,000 pregnancies. The incidence of malignant gestational trophoblastic disease (GTD) is difficult to determine. It is reported as "other" in statistics of the American Cancer Society. The reported incidence of malignant GTD after evacuation of hydatidiform mole varies from 6 to 25%.[2] Approximately half of the incidences of malignant GTD arise directly from nonmolar gestation.

Gestational trophoblastic disease is the term used to describe a spectrum of pathologic entities associated with abnormal placentation. These abnormalities are conveniently grouped into the following:

● Benign GTD (syndromes of molar pregnancies),
● Malignant GTD,

• Placental site trophoblastic tumor.

This group of diseases shares the characteristics of (1) being associated with an event of conception, (2) having the presence of human chorionic gonadotropin (hCG) as a tumor marker, and (3) having a remarkable rate of successful therapy even in the face of metastatic disease. Of equal importance is the ability to preserve reproductive capacity in the population at risk for these neoplasms, which is the younger range of the reproductive age group.

Surgical intervention plays a critical role in both the diagnosis and treatment of trophoblastic disease. We shall discuss the role of surgery as a diagnostic procedure as well as the indication for aggressive extirpation. A vigorous attack on the neoplasm must be weighed against the patient's desire to retain reproductive function.

BENIGN TROPHOBLASTIC DISEASE (SYNDROMES OF MOLAR PREGNANCY)

Benign GTD encompasses the syndromes of complete hydatidiform mole (classic mole), incomplete hydatidiform mole (partial mole), and hydatidiform degeneration of spontaneous abortion due to genetic or other abnormalities of the first trimester.

Clinical Findings

Complete moles are characterized by the absence of fetal parts. The vast majority lack maternal chromosomes. Histopathology shows trophoblastic hyperplasia accompanied by edematous villi with scant cellularity. These villi contain a "villous lake" of acellular material. Partial moles are distinguished by the presence of triploidy and fetal vascular structures. The villous lake is absent, and trophoblastic hyperplasia is much less marked. The majority of patients present with the clinical picture of early spontaneous abortion. Often the patient has passed the grape-like vesicles by the time she arrives at the hospital. The increasing use of ultrasonography to evaluate early pregnancy has led to the diagnosis of molar syndromes before the onset of bleeding. In either case, evacuation is necessary.

Surgical Management

Suction curettage is the procedure of choice for evacuation of molar pregnancies. This is true even for the 50% of patients with uterine enlargement that is greater than expected for gestational age. Before the availability of suction curettage, patients with markedly enlarged uteri were subjected to evacuation via hysterotomy. Hysterotomy reportedly was required for better control of extensive bleeding. Curry and co-workers[3] reviewed the experience of molar evacuation at the Southeastern Trophoblastic Disease Center (SETDC). Evacuation by hysterotomy was associated with the persistence of molar pregnancy in 46% of patients. This finding was believed to be related to the volume of molar tissue rather than the technique of evacuation.

The evacuation of molar pregnancies should not be taken lightly. The degree of risk of perforation or other complications increases with the size of the uterus. The corpus is enlarged and hypervascular, as seen in the arteriogram shown in Figure 11–1. Bleeding is always a potential problem. Other risks include complications associated with the use of general anesthetics, such as drug reaction, aspiration, the development of acute respiratory distress secondary to trophoblastic embolization, or the precipitation of acute thyroid storm in patients presenting with signs and symptoms of hyperthyroidism.

Caution dictates the evacuation of molar pregnancies as an inpatient procedure under appropriate (usually general) anesthesia. Before surgery, hematologic and serum chemistry studies must be performed, the operating room must be equipped for suction curettage as well as pelvic laparotomy, blood must be immediately available for transfusion, and appropriate consent of the patient for evacuation and emergency laparotomy must be obtained. A preoperative chest radiograph is highly desirable. Arterial blood gas determination and hemodynamic monitoring via pulmonary artery catheterization are advocated by Twiggs and colleagues[4] for patients with the clinical picture of toxemia.

Evacuation should proceed after surgical preparation of the perineum, vulva, and vagina. Shaving the labia is unnecessary and unkind. Evacuation of the bladder by straight catheter is routine. Prior placement of cervical laminaria 12 to 24 hours before surgery may be very helpful for those patients who have not begun to dilate spontaneously.

The evacuation should begin by using the largest suction curette that can be inserted easily without mechanical dilation of the cervix. Once suction has been applied and evacuation is noted by the aspiration of tissue and blood and the palpable reduction in size of the uterine corpus, one may begin the infusion of oxytocin (usually 30 units of oxytocin in 1000 ml of 5% dextrose in normal saline or 5% dextrose in Ringer's lactate running rapidly). To decrease the possibility of trophoblastic embolization, one should not begin oxytocin infusion before active evacuation. The addition of methergine for uterine contraction without infusion of large volumes of fluid or highly concen-

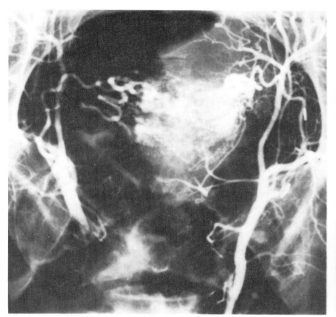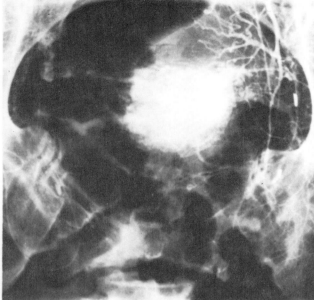

Figure 11–1. Pelvic arteriogram demonstrates uterine hypervascularity and tumor blush.

trated oxytocin is helpful. Sharp curettage is not necessary after thorough suction curettage, and it does nothing but add to the risk of uterine perforation. Post-evacuation observation for 12 to 18 hours is recommended.

Evacuation of molar pregnancy by hysterectomy is the treatment of choice for those women who have completed childbearing or who have associated pelvic pathology for which hysterectomy is indicated. Although Curry and co-workers[3] reported a dramatic decrease in trophoblastic sequelae after evacuation of primary moles by hysterectomy (3.5% versus 20%), hysterectomy does not obviate the necessity for close follow-up by serial serum β-hCG determination. Ovarian preservation is recommended for young women. Theca lutein cysts of the ovary should not constitute a reason for oophorectomy because they will regress spontaneously after molar evacuation. Torsion and other ovarian complications are rare.

PERSISTENT TROPHOBLASTIC NEOPLASIA

Persistent molar pregnancy is considered malignant by definition. Patients require extensive evaluation for the presence of metastatic disease.

Staging

There are two staging systems currently in use for GTD. One is the World Health Organization (WHO) system, which combines anatomic and prognostic scoring,[5] and the other is the clinical classification[6] (Tables 11–1 and 11–2). Staging studies to provide information include a history, physical examination, chest radiograph, chest computed tomography (CT) scan, head CT or brain

Table 11–1. THE PROGNOSTIC SCORE FOR MALIGNANT GESTATIONAL TROPHOBLASTIC DISEASE*

	0	1	2	4
Age (years)	<39	>39		
Antecedent pregnancy	Mole	Abortion	Term pregnancy	
Interval (months)	4	4–6	7–12	>12
Pretreatment hCG (log)	<3	<4	<5	>5
ABO group: female × male		0 × A	B	
		A × 0	AB	
Largest tumor (cm)		3–5	5	
Site of metastasis		Spleen, kidney	Gastrointestinal tract, liver	Brain
Number of metastases identified		1–4	4–8	>8
Previous chemotherapy failed			Single drug	Two or more drugs

*A total score of <4 indicates low risk; a total score of 5–7 indicates medium risk; a total score of >7 indicates high risk.

Table 11–2. THE SOUTHEASTERN TROPHOBLASTIC DISEASE CENTER'S CLINICAL CLASSIFICATION OF MALIGNANT GESTATIONAL TROPHOBLASTIC DISEASE (GTD)

I. Nonmetastatic GTD
II. Metastatic GTD
   A. Good prognosis
      1. <40,000 mIU/ml of serum hCG
      2. Symptoms present for less than 4 months
      3. No brain or liver metastases
      4. No prior chemotherapy
      5. Pregnancy event is not term delivery (i.e., mole, ectopic, or spontaneous abortion)
   B. Poor prognosis
      1. >40,000 mIU/ml of serum hCG
      2. Symptoms present for more than 4 months
      3. Brain or liver metastases
      4. Prior chemotherapeutic failure
      5. Antecedent term pregnancy

scan, electroencephalogram, pelvic and abdominal ultrasound or CT, serum hCG, and ABO blood group determination. All studies may not be necessary for every patient.[7] There is no role for surgery for the confirmation of lesions in staging of GTD today. Histologic diagnosis of choriocarcinoma is desirable but not necessary for initiation of therapy.

Once staging studies are completed, patients are assigned to risk categories. In the WHO staging system, patients are considered to be at low risk if the total value of risk factors is less than or equal to 4, medium risk if the total value of risk factors is 5 to 7, and high risk if the total value of risk factors is greater than 7.[5] The New England Trophoblastic Disease Center uses a similar prognostic scoring system to place patients in low- versus high-risk categories.

The SETDC uses the clinical classification. The patient is considered to have nonmetastatic choriocarcinoma if there is no evidence of extrauterine metastases after staging studies are completed.

Nonmetastatic choriocarcinoma is not divided into "good" and "poor" prognostic categories because these patients achieve 100% remission at the SETDC.[6] Any of the following factors place a patient with metastatic disease in the "poor-prognosis" group: a pretreatment hCG titer of greater than 40,000 mIU/ml, duration of more than 4 months since the onset of symptoms, antecedent term pregnancy, or brain and/or liver metastases.

Nonmetastatic Gestational Trophoblastic Disease

In nonmetastatic GTD, the patient's desire to bear children is an important factor in the determination of treatment. Young patients who have not completed their families should receive intensive chemotherapy. The SETDC has shown excellent success for both remission and fertility using this approach for patients with nonmetastatic disease.[5] Eighty percent of patients with nonmetastatic disease are able to retain reproductive function, and 47 of 109 patients had 57 pregnancies. Among young patients who still wish to bear children, surgery is reserved for salvage when cure is not achieved by drug therapy alone. Most often small-volume residual disease is found deep in the myometrium, confirming the impressions of pelvic arteriography (Fig. 11–2). Salvage hysterectomy contributed to the cure of 17 patients with nonmetastatic, persistent disease refractory to drugs.

Primary hysterectomy for patients with nonmetastatic disease is an adjuvant to therapy. Hammond and colleagues[6] documented the advantages of early surgery and concomitant chemotherapy. A shorter treatment course was possible with few chemotherapy side effects. There was no increase in postoperative complications secondary to chemotherapy. The approach of tumor debulking is accepted in other gynecologic malignancies.

Low-risk, nonmetastatic GTD is treated with single-agent chemotherapy using methotrexate or actinomycin D. Both agents are highly effective, and there is usually no cross resistance. We prefer

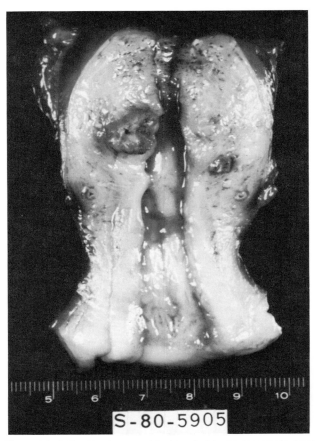

Figure 11–2. Small-volume residual trophoblastic disease is deep within the myometrium.

to initiate treatment with methotrexate, the reason being that the possibility of viral or toxic hepatitis may require change from methotrexate and the availability of actinomycin D offers a nonhepatotoxic, effective alternative. Single-agent regimens are listed in Table 11–3. Methotrexate may be given orally or parenterally. The addition of leukovorin rescue has decreased toxicity without decreasing response.[8] All regimens are adaptable to outpatient administration. Actinomycin D is a highly effective single agent. Table 11–3 gives the doses of two current regimens. The conventional 5-day course is difficult to administer on an outpatient basis because it causes considerable nausea, which is refractory to antiemetics. The higher dose, biweekly regimen is better tolerated.[9] The use of actinomycin D in therapeutic doses carries the side effect of extensive alopecia. Cosmetic considerations, such as the possibility of alopecia, are significant in this patient population, but they should not interfere with effective therapy.

Metastatic Gestational Trophoblastic Disease

Similar principles of age, hCG titer, and fertility status govern the surgical approach to metastatic GTD. Hammond and colleagues[6] suggested that there is benefit from early hysterectomy combined with vigorous drug therapy. The reduction in morbidity (measured by shortened hospital stay) did not reach statistical significance, however. Nonetheless, the concept is similar to that of cytoreduction in ovarian cancer. Tumor debulking in chemosensitive tumors appears to be advantageous, especially when distant tumor burden is small. When the uterus and adnexae harbor bulky disease and there is severe damage to normal architecture (as shown in Fig. 11–3), we believe primary hysterectomy is a benefit to the patient. Patients with "good-prognosis" metastatic disease required fewer courses of therapy for cure with primary hysterectomy and chemotherapy (3.8 courses) than with chemotherapy alone (5.9 courses) and chemotherapy plus salvage hysterectomy (8.4

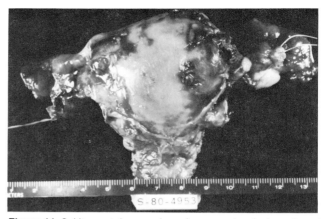

Figure 11–3. Uterus, tubes, and ovaries are extensively replaced by choriocarcinoma with impending uterine rupture and hemoperitoneum.

courses), although these figures only approached statistical significance.[6]

GOOD PROGNOSIS

There is a role for surgery in the treatment of metastatic lesions. Common sites for metastases are vagina, lung, liver, kidney, and brain. Each patient's site requires individual surgical planning interfaced with chemotherapy. Vaginal metastases of choriocarcinoma are among the most frequently encountered. Lesions may be found from the fornices to the perineum. Although confirmation of malignancy by biopsy is a sound principle in other tumors, one should not biopsy vaginal metastases of choriocarcinoma. Such biopsies are very dangerous because of the vascularity of choriocarcinoma and the proximity of the bladder, ureter, urethra, and rectum. Surgery for removal of vaginal metastases is not indicated. Hemostasis may be extremely difficult to achieve in friable areas of tumor. However, spontaneous bleeding from these lesions usually responds to packing, transfusion, and chemotherapy.

Pulmonary metastases are also common in choriocarcinoma.[10] Smith and co-workers[8] demonstrated the presence of multiple lung nodules if CT scan of the chest is used. These lesions usually respond well to systemic therapy. However, resection should be considered when resistant disease is encountered. Pulmonary metastases are characterized by slow resolution. Resection of solitary nodules may be therapeutic if no other site of protected resistance (e.g., uterus) remains. Careful restaging should be performed with careful repeat CT scans of the head, chest, abdomen, and pelvis. Repeat radioimmunoassays of serum and cerebrospinal fluid for hCG are recommended. Figure 11–4 shows a large pulmonary metastasis resected as the only demonstrable site of residual neoplasia. Despite the lesion's size, only microscopic foci of

Table 11–3. SINGLE-AGENT CHEMOTHERAPY

Agent	Regimen*	Reference
Methotrexate	15–25 mg IM† or p.o. daily × 5	6
Methotrexate	1 mg/kg IM days 1, 3, 5, 7 0.1 mg/kg IM leukovorin days 2, 4, 6, 8	6
Actinomycin D	12–15 μg/kg IVP‡ daily × 5	6
Actinomycin D	40 μg/kg IV§	20

*Repeat courses every other week provided granulocyte level is >1500/mm³, level of platelets is >150,000/mm³, and other toxicity has cleared.
†Intramuscularly.
‡Intravenous, push.
§Intravenously.

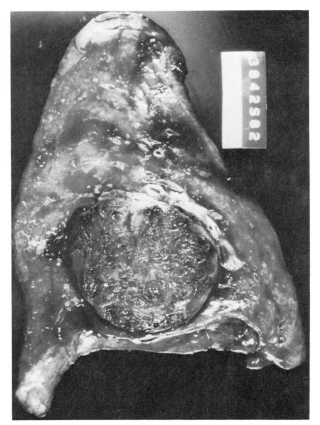

Figure 11–4. Isolated 8-cm lesion in the left lung. Histologically, the lesion was mostly clot and scar, with a few viable areas of trophoblast at the perimeter.

Table 11–4. MULTIAGENT CHEMOTHERAPY

Acronym	Agents
MAC	Methotrexate, actinomycin D, and chlorambucil
VBP	Velban, bleomycin, and platin
EMA-Co	Etoposide, methotrexate, actinomycin D, folinic acid, vincristine, and cyclophosphamide

From Surwit EA: Management of high-risk gestational trophoblastic disease. J Repro Med 32:657, 1987.

presumably viable trophoblast could be demonstrated at the periphery of the lesion. Such resections should be performed while the patient is on chemotherapy.

POOR PROGNOSIS

High-risk, metastatic disease is best managed by aggressive multiagent chemotherapy. Table 11–4 outlines the regimens in current use. Chemotherapy with the methotrexate/actinomycin D/chlorambucil combination has been the "gold standard"; however, the newer agents such as platinol and VP-16-213 (etoposide) have been shown to be effective as primary and salvage therapies. These combinations are quite toxic, and they should be administered only by physicians who are thoroughly familiar with the compounds as well as the disease entity.

Optimal management for patients with central nervous system metastasis remains a matter for discussion. The salvage rate for patients with central nervous system metastasis approaches 45%, which is amazing compared with that for patients with brain metastasis from any other malignancies.[11–13] Surgical intervention for the sole purpose

of diagnosis is to be condemned. The presence of a brain lesion by imaging techniques in a woman with elevated hCG is diagnostic. There is a consensus that surgical decompression of acute intracerebral bleeding is productive.[13] However, Weed and colleagues[11] suggested that this complication is prevented by prompt institution of whole-brain irradiation concomitant with multiagent chemotherapy.

The surgical extirpation of persistent lesions should be strictly individualized. Rustin and co-workers[12] reported that early craniotomy was of benefit to two of five patients who presented with brain lesions as the first sign of recurrence.

Soper and co-workers[14] reported experience with renal metastases of GTD in eight patients. The three surviving patients presented with "limited" systemic tumor load, in that metastatic disease was limited to lungs and one kidney only. Those patients treated successfully had prompt nephrectomy under cover of multiagent chemotherapy. There were no survivors if bilateral renal or other "poor-prognosis" sites of metastases were present.

Liver metastases carry a significantly poor prognosis, as reported by Barnard and colleagues.[15] Resection of liver lesions is of little benefit. Operative intervention is required for hemoperitoneum from bleeding lesions. Anecdotal experiences with selective hepatic infusion have been equally unsuccessful.[16] Surgical intervention at other areas of metastatic choriocarcinoma should be individualized. Emergent control of intra-abdominal bleeding may be required for invasion of bowel or omentum, uterine perforation, or lesions of liver or spleen. There appears to be no therapeutic advantage to aggressive cytoreduction during operation for complications of overwhelming disease.

PLACENTAL SITE TROPHOBLASTIC TUMOR

Placental site trophoblastic tumor is a rare form of trophoblastic disease that was described by Kurman and co-workers[17] in 1976. Clinical experience has been accumulated by Finkler and colleagues[18] and others.[19] These tumors may follow spontaneous abortion, therapeutic abortion, molar pregnancy, or delivery. The characteristic pathology of the tumor shows trophoblast cells that infiltrate the myometrium and vasculature. Hemorrhage and necrosis are minimal, and villi are rare. The mitotic index is a fairly reliable measure of tumor aggressiveness. Placental site tumors are associated with low levels of serum hCG, and they are reported to be resistant to chemotherapy. Hysterectomy is recommended;[18] however, curettage alone may be curative. Metastases and fatalities have been reported.

SUMMARY

Centers for the treatment of GTD have demonstrated extremely high cure rates for this group of chemosensitive malignancies when appropriate aggressive therapy is based on careful staging.[20] For women who have completed childbearing, early hysterectomy with chemotherapy shortens the length of treatment required for remission. This approach reduces expense and complications of chemotherapy for patients with nonmetastatic or good-prognosis metastatic disease. In selected patients with poor-prognosis metastatic disease, surgery in conjunction with chemotherapy results in a 40 to 50% cure rate. Tumor debulking for extensive metastatic disease may confer a similar advantage. Surgical salvage by resection of resistant foci of disease can be life saving.

References

1. Atrash HK, Hogue CJ, Grimes DA: Epidemiology of hydatidiform mole during early gestation. Am J Obstet Gynecol 154:906, 1986.
2. Soper JT, Hammond CB: Gestational trophoblastic disease and gestational choriocarcinoma. In Gusberg SB, Hugh M, Shingleton HM, Deppe G: Female Genital Cancer. New York: Churchill-Livingstone, 1988, p. 440.
3. Curry SH, Hammond CB, Tyrey L, et al.: Hydatidiform mole: Diagnosis, management, and long-term follow-up of 347 patients. Obstet Gynecol 45:1, 1975.
4. Twiggs LB, Morrow CP, Schlaerth JB: Acute pulmonary complications of molar pregnancy. Am J Obstet Gynecol 135:189, 1979.
5. World Health Organization: Gestational Trophoblastic Disease: WHO Technical Report Series 692. Geneva, Switzerland: World Health Organization, 1983.
6. Hammond CB, Weed JC Jr, Currie JL: The role of operation in the current therapy of gestational trophoblastic disease. Am J Obstet Gynecol 136:844, 1980.
7. Hunter VJ, Raymond E, Christensen C, et al.: Efficacy of the metastatic survey in the staging of gestational trophoblastic disease. Cancer 65:1647, 1990.
8. Smith EB, Weed JC Jr, Tyrey L, et al.: Treatment of nonmetastatic gestational trophoblastic disease: Results of methotrexate alone versus methotrexate-folinic acid. Am J Obstet Gynecol 144:88, 1982.
9. Twiggs LB: Pulse actinomycin D scheduling in non-metastatic gestational trophoblastic neoplasia: Cost-effective chemotherapy. Gynecol Oncol 16:190, 1983.
10. Libshitz HI, Barber CE, Hammond CB: The pulmonary metastases of choriocarcinoma. Obstet Gynecol 49:412, 1977.
11. Weed JC Jr, Woodward KT, Hammond CB: Choriocarcinoma metastatic to the brain: Therapy and prognosis. Semin Oncol 9:208, 1982.
12. Rustin GJ, Newlands ES, Begent RH, et al.: Weekly alternating etoposide, methotrexate, and actinomycin/vincristine and cyclophosphamide chemotherapy for the treatment of CNS metastases of choriocarcinoma. J Clin Oncol 7:900, 1989.
13. Yordon EL, Schlaerth J, Gaddis O, et al.: Radiation therapy in the management of gestational choriocarcinoma metastatic to the central nervous system. Obstet Gynecol 69:627, 1987.
14. Soper JT, Mutch DG, Chin M, et al.: Renal metastases of gestational trophoblastic disease: A report of 8 cases. Obstet Gynecol 72:796, 1988.
15. Barnard DE, Woodward KT, Young SG, et al.: Hepatic metastasis of choriocarcinoma. Gynecol Oncol 25:73, 1986.
16. Maroulis GB, Hammond CB, Johusrude IS, et al.: Arteriography and infusional chemotherapy in localized trophoblastic disease. Obstet Gynecol 45:397, 1975.
17. Kurman RJ, Scully RE, Norris HJ: Trophoblastic pseudotumor of the uterus. An exaggerated form of "syncytial endometritis": Simulating a malignant tumor. Cancer 38:1214, 1976.
18. Finker NJ, Berkowitz RS, Driscoll SG, et al.: Clinical experience with placental site trophoblastic tumors at the New England Trophoblastic Disease Center. Obstet Gynecol 71:854, 1988.
19. Lathrop J, Lauchlan S, Lathrop R, et al.: Placental site trophoblastic tumor (PSTT): A clinical and therapeutic assessment. Gynecol Oncol 32:113, 1989 [abstract].
20. Weed JC Jr, Jelovsek FR, Tyrey L, et al.: Intensive inpatient therapy and survival in gestational trophoblastic disease. Gynecol Oncol 16:315–363, 1983.

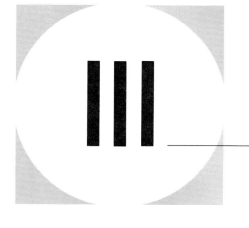

III

Surgical Problems
of Late Pregnancy

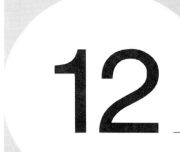

12

Placental Abnormalities:
Previa, Abruption, and Accreta

Susan M. Ramin
Larry C. Gilstrap III

Abnormalities of the placenta may result in significant complications that can potentially be life threatening to the mother, the fetus, or both. This chapter focuses on three serious "placental" complications—placenta previa, abruption, and accreta.

PLACENTA PREVIA

Definition

Placenta previa, a potentially life-threatening complication of pregnancy, can be classified into three types according to the relationship between the placenta and the internal cervical os before the onset of labor.[1, 2] In a low-lying or marginal placenta, the placental edge implants in the lower uterine segment but does not reach the internal cervical os. A partial placenta previa covers a portion of the internal cervical os, whereas in a total placenta previa the internal cervical os is completely covered. This classification is relatively unimportant in terms of predicting the clinical course or serving as a guideline for decisions regarding management.

Incidence

Placenta previa is a relatively common sonographic finding in the second trimester, with a reported incidence of 5.3 to 45%.[2–5] At term it is significantly less common (one in 150 to one in 400 births).[5–8] It has been hypothesized that this change in incidence as gestation progresses is due to "placental migration" secondary to a relative growth of the lower uterine segment.[9]

Etiology

The etiology of placenta previa remains unknown. Several associated factors include increasing maternal age, multiparity, multiple fetuses, cigarette smoking, a prior abortion, a previous previa, and prior cesarean births (Table 12–1).[6, 10] In a retrospective study, 3.8% of patients had placenta previa following an induced first-trimester abortion.[6] The relationship between prior cesarean delivery and subsequent development of placenta previa was first proposed by Bender.[11] Singh and co-workers[12] reported a 3.9% incidence of placenta previa in such women compared with 1.9% in those without prior abdominal births. Nielsen and associates[13] found placenta previa in 1.22% of women with a scarred uterus compared with 0.25% of women with an unscarred uterus. Women with scarred uteri also had an increased incidence of unexplained antepartum hemorrhage

Table 12–1. FACTORS REPORTED TO BE ASSOCIATED WITH PLACENTA PREVIA

Increasing maternal age
Multiparity
Multiple fetuses
Cigarette smoking
Prior abortion
Prior placenta previa
Prior cesarean section
Male fetus

Data from Barrett JM, Boehm FH, Killam AP: Induced abortion: A risk factor for placenta previa. Am J Obstet Gynecol 141:769, 1981; and Brenner WE, Edelman DA, Hendricks CH: Characteristics of patients with placenta previa and results of "expectant management." Am J Obstet Gynecol 132:180, 1978.

(3.81% vs. 0.40% of controls). There also appears to be a linear relationship between the number of previous cesarean sections and the risk of placenta previa. Women with four or more prior cesarean sections have up to a 10% risk of placenta previa.[14]

Several authors have reported that an increased number of women with placenta previa had a male fetus. The significance of this finding remains unknown.[1, 10] Brenner and associates[10] reported an increased risk of congenital anomalies in pregnancies complicated by placenta previa (6.7% vs. 3.2% of controls). The major congenital malformations involved the cardiovascular system, central nervous system, gastrointestinal tract, and respiratory system.

Women with placenta previa that "migrates" in the second trimester to a normal position may be at risk for other complications. Newton and colleagues[15] found that 45% of these women had one or more of the following perinatal complications: antepartum hemorrhage, abruptio placentae, intrauterine growth retardation, and cesarean delivery. Moreover, there was a significant increase in prematurity, low birth weight, and perinatal mortality among these patients.

Diagnosis

SIGNS AND SYMPTOMS

The diagnosis of placenta previa is suggested by the sudden onset of painless vaginal bleeding in the second or third trimester of pregnancy. An important distinction between placenta previa and abruptio placentae is the lack of uterine contractions and abdominal pain in most cases. There may be a coexisting abruption in up to 10% of cases of placenta previa. Furthermore, approximately 10% of cases are diagnosed when women report uterine contractions. Also, the lack of vaginal bleeding does not necessarily exclude placenta previa.

The bleeding most often begins without any obvious precipitating event. The initial episode of bleeding is rarely catastrophic and will usually abate spontaneously. The bleeding is related to the physiologic development of the lower uterine segment with subsequent partial separation of the placenta. As the lower uterine segment continues to "thin," the bleeding will recur. The initial episode of bleeding was found to occur before 30 weeks' gestation in 35%, between 30 and 35 weeks' gestation in 33%, and after 36 weeks' gestation in 32% of cases.[7] There was a relationship between the degree of placenta previa and the initial bleeding episode. Total and partial placenta previas initially bleed earlier in pregnancy (35 weeks or earlier), whereas bleeding from marginal or low-lying previas was first noted after 36 weeks' gestation, often occurring with the onset of labor.

Furthermore, maternal hemorrhage tended to be more severe, requiring blood transfusion if total or partial previas were noted to bleed earlier in gestation.

A careful physical examination of the abdomen may be helpful in differentiating a placenta previa from an abruptio placentae. Suggestive findings include a soft uterus, no palpable contractions, and an abnormal fetal lie. In a recent report of 173 cases of placenta previa by Cotton and co-workers,[1] abnormal fetal presentation (breech or transverse lie) was present in 34%. Often, the presenting fetal part will be high above the pelvic brim and the placental souffle heard best over the symphysis.

ULTRASONOGRAPHY

Although a gentle speculum examination of the vagina and cervix can be performed to rule out local pathologic causes of the bleeding without inciting hemorrhage,[16] it is probably safer to defer this until localization of the placenta has been accomplished and a placenta previa has been ruled out. The most accurate, noninvasive technique available today for localization of the placenta is transabdominal ultrasonography, which has essentially replaced soft-tissue placentography and radioisotopic placental localization (Figs. 12–1 to 12–4). Real-time sonography should be routinely used in patients who are bleeding to precisely visualize the placenta and its location in relation to the internal cervical os. Recently, transvaginal sonographic examination has been employed for the

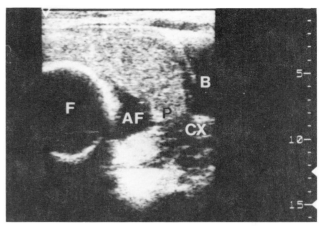

Figure 12–2. Sonogram of anterior total placenta previa at 32 weeks' gestation. AF—Amniotic fluid; B—bladder; CX—cervix; F—fetal head; P—placenta. (Courtesy Rigoberto Santos, M.D.)

diagnosis of placenta previa and appears to have improved the accuracy rate (Fig. 12–5).[17]

In 1965, Donald first introduced the concept of placental localization via abdominal ultrasound, and in 1966 Gottesfeld and co-workers published the first report of this method in 112 pregnant cases, with an accuracy of 97%.[18] The placental location was confirmed by cesarean delivery, manual extraction, or amniocentesis. In a series of 613 cases, Donald and Abdulla[19] reported a diagnostic accuracy of 94% for previa using ultrasound for placental localization. A similar accuracy rate for ultrasound was reported by Campbell and Kohorn.[20] Finally, Bowie and associates[21] examined the accuracy, sensitivity, and specificity of ultrasound diagnosis in a retrospective study of 164 patients. They found ultrasound diagnosis to be 93% accurate, 93% sensitive, and 92% specific. Placenta previa was proved in 13 cases; however, there was one false-negative in this group.

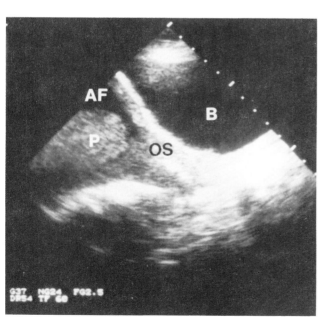

Figure 12–1. Sonogram of marginal placenta previa at 26 weeks' gestation. Placenta (P) borders on the internal cervical os (OS). AF—Amniotic fluid; B—maternal bladder. (Courtesy Rigoberto Santos, M.D.)

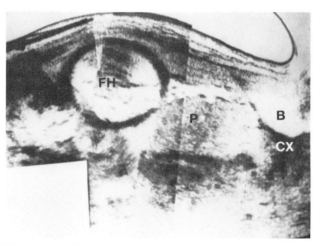

Figure 12–3. Sonogram of posterior total placenta previa. B—Bladder; CX—cervix; FH—fetal head; P—placenta. (Courtesy Rigoberto Santos, M.D.)

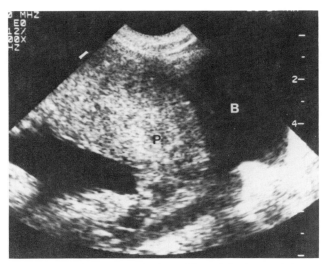

Figure 12–4. Sector scan in the midline of the lower abdomen shows an anterior total placenta previa. B—Bladder; P—placenta. (Courtesy Rigoberto Santos, M.D.)

Because there are no specific markers to accurately identify the internal cervical os by ultrasound, both false-positive and false-negative results have been reported. The majority of errors are due to false-positive diagnoses. Bladder distention and absence of fetal parts in the lower uterus contribute to this false-positive error.[21] Repeat ultrasonography with an empty bladder should be performed to minimize false-positive results. The false-negative rate for ultrasonographic diagnosis

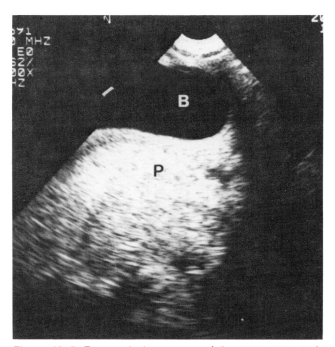

Figure 12–5. Transvaginal sonogram of the same case as in Figure 12–4. B—Bladder; P— placenta. (Courtesy Rigoberto Santos, M.D.)

of placenta previa has been reported to be as low as 2% and as high as 7.3%.[1, 21, 22] According to Laing,[22] the inability to visualize a posterior placenta previa (fetal head position), failure to recognize a laterally positioned previa, and difficulty in differentiating between amniotic fluid and blood near the internal cervical os are the most common reasons for a false-negative result. Clinically, a false-negative diagnosis of placenta previa is more important than a false-positive diagnosis.

MAGNETIC RESONANCE IMAGING

Another recent modality employed in the diagnosis of placenta previa is magnetic resonance imaging (MRI), which uses nonionizing radiation and has no known biologic hazard when properly used.[23–25] The major advantages of MRI over ultrasound include better definition of maternal soft-tissue anatomy, more accurate definition of the cervix and placenta, and the absence of the need for a full bladder.[25] The value of MRI in obstetric patients is currently being examined in several centers.

DOUBLE SET-UP EXAMINATION

In the recent past the "double set-up examination" was considered the main diagnostic step for placenta previa; however, given the present accuracy of sonographic placental localization, it is seldom used. This examination may be considered when a woman presents in labor at term with continued bleeding that is not life threatening. An operating room is the appropriate place for a double set-up, with blood available for transfusion and the capacity for prompt delivery if severe hemorrhage occurs. A scrub nurse, anesthesiologist, and surgeons other than the examining obstetrician should be present. Once all preparations have been made, a digital examination is performed by gently sweeping the vaginal fornices. If the fetal head can be precisely palpated in all quadrants through the lower uterine segment and the cervix is sufficiently dilated, an amniotomy can be done and vaginal delivery allowed. On the other hand, if digital examination reveals the suspected placenta (a "boggy" sensation) or incites hemorrhage, immediate cesarean delivery is indicated. A double set-up examination is rarely indicated in the preterm gestation.

Management

In the past, active management with vaginal delivery of placenta previa was associated with a maternal mortality rate of 10% and a perinatal mortality rate of 70%.[10] Because the approach has changed to one of expectant management with liberal use of cesarean section, there has been a dramatic reduction in the maternal mortality rate to less than 1% and in the perinatal mortality rate to 10%.

A pregnant woman with continued bleeding requires prompt evaluation in the hospital. The examiner inserts a large-bore intravenous catheter and draws blood for crossmatch and hematocrit determination. If the woman is hemodynamically unstable, adequate fluid and blood replacement is a priority. Uterine activity and fetal condition can be assessed by external electronic monitoring. Ultrasonography can be employed to localize the placenta after the mother is stabilized. If sonography confirms placenta previa, the obstetrician must then formulate a plan for the timing and method of delivery, which will depend on the gestational age of the fetus and the severity of hemorrhage. The ultimate goal is to achieve fetal maturation with minimal risk to the mother and fetus.

Absence of bleeding allows expectant management when the fetus is premature. Ideally, the patient should remain hospitalized at bedrest until fetal maturation is documented, labor ensues, or recurrence of hemorrhage is severe enough to necessitate delivery. Once the diagnosis of placenta previa is made, it is of utmost importance to avoid any intravaginal manipulation. If it is not possible for the patient to remain hospitalized, she may be managed on an ambulatory basis. The patient and her family must understand the risks associated with placenta previa, the necessity for the patient to maintain a sedentary life-style, and the need for the availability of a support person who can promptly transport the patient to the hospital.

In a study by Cotton and co-workers,[1] expectant management was practiced in 66% of the patients and included the aggressive use of antepartum blood transfusions and selective use of tocolytic agents. Despite a loss of more than 500 mL of blood at the initial bleeding episode in 20% of the patients, the gestation was extended by a mean of 16.8 days in 50% of the patients. Unfortunately, even with this approach 20% of the patients were delivered before 32 weeks' gestation, which accounted for 73% of all perinatal deaths. Ultimately, an elective termination of the pregnancy by cesarean section is preferred to an emergency cesarean section. Approximately 28% of the newborns delivered under emergency situations were anemic, compared with 3% of those delivered electively.[1]

Another potential advantage of expectant management is migration of the placenta away from the internal cervical os. Recently, Arias[26] reported excellent results in patients with placenta previa who were bleeding by placing cervical cerclages between 24 and 30 weeks' gestation. Further studies are required before this procedure can be routinely recommended for patients with placenta previa.

Cesarean section is the accepted method of delivery in virtually all patients with placenta previa. This is true from both the maternal and fetal standpoints. A rare exception might be with a previable fetus. The choice of uterine incision depends on the fetal lie and placental location. The transverse uterine incision is preferable with a cephalic presentation, a well-formed lower uterine segment, and a posteriorly located placenta previa. Otherwise, a vertical uterine incision should be performed, especially with an anteriorly located placenta previa, to minimize the bleeding.

Myometrial contractions occlude the blood vessels and control bleeding after delivery of a normally implanted placenta. However, significant blood loss may occur after delivery of a placenta that is implanted in the lower uterine segment because this area does not contract well. Blood loss can be controlled with sutures if specific bleeding sites can be identified. If this approach is unsuccessful, ligation of the hypogastric and uterine arteries or even hysterectomy may be necessary. The techniques for these procedures are discussed in Chapters 21 and 26.

PLACENTAL ABRUPTION

Placental abruption is potentially one of the most serious complications that can occur during pregnancy. It may be associated with life-threatening hemorrhage and is a significant cause of maternal and fetal morbidity, as well as perinatal mortality. Hemorrhage associated with placental abruption remains one of the major obstetric causes of maternal mortality.

Definition

Placental abruption is the premature separation of the placenta from the maternal surface of the uterus secondary to hemorrhage into the decidua basalis (Figs. 12–6 and 12–7). *Placental abruption* is the most commonly used term. Other terms that have been used to describe this condition include *abruptio placentae, ablatio placentae,* and *accidental hemorrhage.*[27] Placental abruption may be classified as acute or chronic, although the majority of cases are associated with acute hemorrhage and require intervention and delivery. The abruption may present with vaginal bleeding, or the clot may remain sequestered behind the placenta (concealed abruption).

Incidence

Like many other complications of pregnancy, the exact incidence of placental abruption remains unknown. It depends on the criteria used for mak-

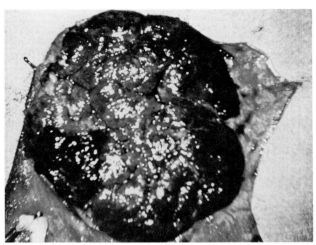

Figure 12–6. Placental abruption. Note the blood clot on the left lower margin.

ing the diagnosis, especially in the case of chronic abruptions. In several studies the incidence has varied from a low of 0.44% to a high of 1.3%.[28–30] The Swedish nationwide birth registry of 894,619 births from 1973 to 1981[30] reported an abruption rate of 0.44%. The rate of 1.3% was based on 4545 deliveries in a single American institution.[29] Pritchard and Brekken[31] reported that the incidence of abruption severe enough to kill the fetus was approximately 0.2% (one in 443 deliveries).

Etiology

Although several conditions have been reported to be associated with placental abruption, the etiology is unknown in the majority of cases. Some of the reported factors are summarized in Table 12–2.[32–42] In one study of 201 women with placental abruption severe enough to kill the fetus, Pritchard and colleagues[32] reported that approximately

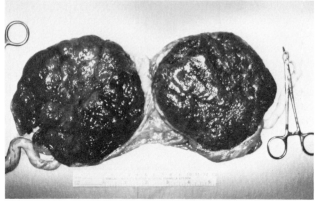

Figure 12–7. Placental abruption in twin gestation. Note the large blood clot on the right lower margin of the left placenta. (Courtesy Cristela Hernandez, M.D.)

Table 12–2. FACTORS REPORTED TO BE ASSOCIATED WITH PLACENTAL ABRUPTION

Hypertension
Trauma
Short umbilical cord
Folate deficiency
Multiparity
Compression of vena cava
Uterine anomaly
Previous abruption
Premature rupture of membranes
Chorioamnionitis
Cigarette smoking
Cocaine abuse

half of the women were hypertensive. This figure was 5 times the incidence of hypertension in their population. In contrast, Paterson,[30] in a review of 193 cases of placental abruption, reported only a 14% incidence of associated hypertension, which was similar to the 13% incidence of hypertension in the total population. Population differences, severity of abruption, or volume replacement could cause this discrepancy.

Trauma causes only a few placental abruptions. In a series of severe abruptions, trauma could be implicated in only 2 (1%) patients.[32] Higgins and Garite[33] reviewed 1542 abruptions (five series) and noted that only 15 (1%) were associated with trauma. However, pregnant patients who experience trauma do have a significant risk for placental abruption. Placental abruption occurred in 47 (27%) of 176 women (seven series) who experienced severe trauma, with a frequency of abruption ranging from 7 to 66%.[33] Significant placental abruption may occur even if the mother is not significantly injured.[34] Placental abruption following maternal trauma may also be occult with no obvious vaginal bleeding or abdominal pain, and the diagnosis may be suspected only because of an abnormal fetal heart rate pattern.[35]

It seems logical that a short umbilical cord might cause placental abruption, but this association is rarely confirmed. Pritchard and associates[32] were unable to identify an association between a short umbilical cord and placental abruption in a large series of severe placental abruption. It has been postulated that maternal dietary deficiencies, such as folate deficiency, may be associated with placental abruption.[36] However, Whalley and co-workers,[37] using plasma folate determinations and marrow cytomorphology to detect folate deficiency, could find no association between folate deficiency and placental abruption. The history of previous placental abruption is a significant risk factor for the development of placental abruption in subsequent pregnancies.[28, 30, 31] Pritchard and co-workers[33] reported a 10% recurrence rate for placental abruption. The recurrence rate increases to 25% after two consecutive abruptions.[36]

Inferior vena caval occlusion, uterine anomalies, and sudden uterine decompression have also been associated with placental abruption.[32] However, Pritchard and co-workers[32] were able to attribute placental abruption to either uterine decompression or a uterine anomaly in only one case each, and in no case was abruption associated with occlusion of the vena cava. In fact, placental abruption did not occur in three women who had inferior vena caval ligation. Other conditions reported to be associated with placental abruption include premature rupture of the membranes,[38] chorioamnionitis,[39] and cigarette smoking.[40] The association between cocaine abuse and placental abruption is becoming a serious problem. Chasnoff and colleagues[41] observed that the onset of labor with placental abruption occurred in 4 of 23 cocaine abusers immediately following intravenous self-injection. In another report of 50 women who abused cocaine during pregnancy, there were eight stillbirths secondary to placental abruption.[42]

Diagnosis

CLINICAL FINDINGS

The classic signs and symptoms of placental abruption include vaginal bleeding, hypertonic contractions, and uterine tenderness and irritability. Central retroplacental bleeding may be concealed. In cases secondary to maternal trauma, uterine contractions and tenderness and abdominal pain may be absent or minimal.[35] An abnormal fetal heart rate may be the most significant finding. Common signs and symptoms of placental abruption are summarized in Table 12–3.[29] Hurd and associates[29] found that the most common signs and symptoms were vaginal bleeding (78%), uterine tenderness (66%), fetal distress (60%), and hypertonic uterine contractions (34%).

ULTRASOUND FINDINGS

Although ultrasound is extremely accurate in the diagnosis or exclusion of placenta previa, it is unreliable in excluding placental abruption. Sonographic findings of placental abruption are quite variable (Figs. 12–8 and 12–9). A retroplacental hematoma is the most commonly documented sonographic finding with abruptio placentae. In a

Table 12–3. SIGNS AND SYMPTOMS OF PLACENTAL ABRUPTION

Vaginal bleeding
Uterine tenderness
Back pain
Hypertonic uterine contractions
Fetal distress
Dead fetus

Adapted from Hurd WW, Miodovnik M, Hertzberg V, Lavin JP: Selective management of abruptio placentae: A prospective study. Obstet Gynecol 61:467, 1983.

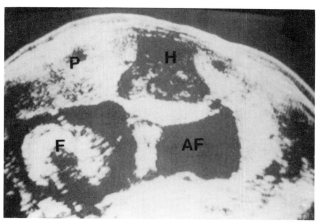

Figure 12–8. Sonogram of abruptio placentae at 25 weeks' gestation. AF—Amniotic fluid; F—fetal parts; H—retroplacental hematoma; P—placenta. (Courtesy Rigoberto Santos, M.D.)

retrospective study of 57 cases of placental abruption, Nyberg and associates[43] found the hematoma location to be subchorionic in 81%, retroplacental in 16%, and preplacental in 4%. The echogenicity of hemorrhage changes with time and may be difficult to differentiate from the placenta initially. When compared with the sonographic appearance of the placenta, the sonographic appearance of acute hemorrhage was hyperechoic to isoechoic and gradually became sonolucent within 14 days.[43] Negative sonographic findings do not rule out placental abruption.

LABORATORY FINDINGS

When the diagnosis of placental abruption is suspected, an evaluation of hematologic and clotting studies should be performed, including hematocrit with platelets, prothrombin time (PT), partial thromboplastin time (PTT), fibrinogen, fibrin degradation products, and urinalysis. Additional laboratory work that should be examined includes serum creatinine, aspartate aminotransferase, and total bilirubin. Unfortunately, the laboratory results are quite variable in cases of placental abruption and may not be helpful especially with milder degrees of this complication.

The initial hematocrit value may not be representative of the severity of the abruption, especially if the symptoms are of recent onset. Because there will be a delay time in obtaining results from the laboratory, one can quickly identify the presence of disseminated intravascular coagulation by the clot observation test, which can be performed at the bedside. If this test reveals a small or absent clot, the coagulation studies will be abnormal, with prolongation of the prothrombin and partial thromboplastin times, elevated fibrin degradation products, and hypofibrinogenemia. Thrombocytopenia may or may not be initially present with overt hypofibrinogenemia; however,

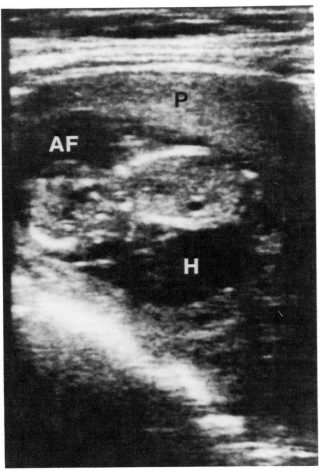

Figure 12–9. Transverse scan of placental abruption at 13 weeks' gestation with dead fetus. Placenta separated at left margin. AF—Amniotic fluid; H—hematoma; P—placenta. (Courtesy Rigoberto Santos, M.D.)

Table 12–4. MANAGEMENT OF PLACENTAL ABRUPTION AND A LIVE FETUS

Complete blood count, platelet count, and urinalysis
Clotting studies
Clot observation test
Four units of crossmatched blood
Intravenous hydration with large-bore catheter
Foley catheter to monitor urinary output
Monitoring of maternal vital signs and fetal status
Consideration of cesarean section if indicated

Adapted, in part, from Hurd WW, Miodovnik M, Hertzberg V, Lavin JP: Selective management of abruptio placentae: A prospective study. Obstet Gynecol 61:467, 1983.

Laboratory work that should be performed includes hematocrit, platelets, urinalysis, and clotting studies (PT, PTT, fibrinogen, and fibrin degradation products). The patient should also be crossmatched for 4 units of blood, and a large-bore intravenous line should be inserted promptly and fluid administration started. A Foley catheter should be placed to monitor urinary output. Maternal vital signs and fetal status must be monitored closely. If both mother and fetus remain stable, expectant management can be employed remote from term in carefully selected patients. The obstetrician must maintain close observation and plan prompt intervention if necessary. Delivery is indicated near term or if serious hemorrhage or fetal distress is present. Cesarean section should be performed when there is evidence of a compromised fetus, massive hemorrhage, failure to progress, or any situation that is a contraindication to labor.

In a recent retrospective study by Sholl[44] of 130 patients with placental abruption, 72 pregnancies were preterm (between 26 and 37 weeks). Almost half were delivered within 3 days of admission for either significant hemorrhage or fetal distress. There was a 57% cesarean delivery rate for those women who required delivery promptly after admission and also for those in whom delivery was delayed for 3 or more days. Metzger and associates[45] employed expectant management in two previable pregnancies with partial placental abruptions and achieved favorable outcomes. One patient was admitted at 24 weeks' gestation with vaginal bleeding and was managed expectantly until 27 weeks, when delivered by cesarean section because of recurrent bleeding and labor. The second patient was admitted at 26 1/2 weeks' gestation with vaginal bleeding and placed at bedrest with expectant care until 32 weeks, when she labored and delivered vaginally.

Significantly more complications occur in patients who have placental abruption severe enough to kill the fetus. Consumptive coagulopathy is present in almost one third of the patients and is usually evident at the time of admission or shortly thereafter.[31] Blood loss averages almost one half of the patient's blood volume.[31] Significant blood

with repeated blood transfusions low platelet counts are common. Clinically significant hypofibrinogenemia is defined as a plasma fibrinogen level below 150 mg/dl. Of 141 cases of severe abruption with a dead fetus reported by Pritchard and Brekken,[31] the fibrinogen concentration was below 150 mg/dl in 38% and below 100 mg/dl in 28%. They observed that severe hypofibrinogenemia developed within 8 hours after onset of initial symptoms.

Management

Once the diagnosis of placental abruption has been made, management depends on the status of the mother and fetus. If the fetus is alive, the abruption is thought to be mild. However, it is impossible to determine the extent of placental separation and whether the fetus is capable of tolerating additional insult. Treatment of women who have placental abruption and a live fetus is summarized in Table 12–4.[29]

loss can lead to hypovolemic shock with subsequent maternal death or renal failure. Krupp and co-workers[46] identified renal failure in 6 of 10 fatal cases, with most being related to renal cortical necrosis. Acute tubular necrosis, however, is the most common form of renal failure seen in association with severe placental abruption. Proteinuria is quite common, occurring in 48%.[31] Uteroplacental apoplexy (Couvelaire uterus) may occur in severe abruptions with blood infiltrating the myometrium beneath the serosa. Rarely, this condition interferes with uterine contractility and results in postpartum hemorrhage.

Management of severe placental abruption with a dead fetus is outlined in Table 12–5.[29, 47] Because potentially serious complications can occur with massive hemorrhage, the patient should receive prompt volume replacement, including both electrolyte solution (lactated Ringer's solution) and blood, to maintain the hematocrit at least 30% and urine output at least 30 mL/hr.[47] If vigorous fluid therapy does not correct oliguria, the central venous pressure must be monitored. An amniotomy with insertion of an intrauterine pressure catheter should be performed promptly. The preferable route of delivery is vaginal. A cesarean section should be performed for obstetric indications. Although it once was advocated that delivery occur within 8 hours or so from the time of diagnosis,[31] the most important determinant in a favorable outcome is vigorous and adequate fluid administration.

Treatment of consumptive coagulopathy is controversial. If management is aimed toward adequate fluid replacement and delivery, it is rarely necessary to treat the coagulopathy. Improvement of the coagulopathy usually does not occur until after delivery.[47] Therapy is indicated when there is significant alteration of coagulation with uncontrolled bleeding from multiple sites (intravenous lines, catheter, gums, vagina). In the past, fibrinogen was used in cases of coagulopathy resulting from placental abruption, but it is no longer available because of the substantial risk of hepatitis B. Other therapeutic agents have been advocated in such cases, including cryoprecipitate, platelets, and fresh frozen plasma. Fifteen to 20 units of cryoprecipitate supply 4 g of fibrinogen.[27] Platelets should be given if the platelet count is lower than 50,000/μL and there is oozing from trauma sites. Ten platelet packs will increase the platelet count to greater than 50,000/μL.[27] Only a portion of these platelets are viable.

Patients with both consumptive coagulopathy and renal failure present a special therapeutic dilemma. The clinician must walk a thin line between blood and volume replacement and fluid overload. Indications for dialysis in these patients include fluid overload and electrolyte imbalance such as hyperkalemia.

PLACENTA ACCRETA

Definition

Placenta accreta may be defined as an "abnormal" adherence of the placenta to the uterus. The abnormal adherence is secondary to the attachment of placental villi directly to the myometrium without evidence of intervening decidua.[48] The decidua basalis is partly or entirely absent. The pathogenesis of this absence or paucity of intervening decidua is unclear. Khong and Robertson[49] have suggested that placenta accreta results from a defective interaction between maternal tissue and migrating trophoblast, with development of an abnormal uteroplacental vasculature.

Placenta accreta can generally be classified into three major types: accreta, increta, and percreta.[48, 50] Accreta refers to the condition in which the placental villi are attached to, but do not invade, the myometrium. Increta refers to the condition in which the villi actually invade the myometrium, and percreta refers to the condition in which the villi invade or penetrate the full thickness of the uterine wall.[50] The placenta may actually invade the urinary bladder.[51, 52] The three major types of placenta accreta are summarized in Figure 12–10. In a study of 40 patients by Breen and co-workers,[48] 78% had an accreta, 17% an increta, and 5% a percreta.

Incidence

The exact prevalence of placenta accreta varies widely, with reports ranging from 1 in 500 deliveries to 1 in 70,000 deliveries (average of 1/7000 deliveries).[48] Read and colleagues,[53] in a review of 22 cases, reported an incidence of 1 in 2562 deliveries and postulated better case reporting in recent times.

Table 12–5. MANAGEMENT OF SEVERE PLACENTAL ABRUPTION WITH A DEAD FETUS

Hematocrit, platelet count, and urinalysis
Prothrombin time, partial thromboplastin time, fibrinogen, fibrin degradation products
Clot observation test
Six units of crossmatched blood
Two large-bore intravenous catheters and Foley catheter
Infusion of intravenous fluids
Infusion of at least 2 units of blood immediately
Maintenance of hematocrit at ≥30 and urine output at ≥30 mL/ hr (check hourly)
Amniotomy with intrauterine pressure monitoring
Goal of vaginal delivery; however, cesarean section if indicated

Adapted, in part, from Hurd WW, Miodovnik M, Hertzberg V, Lavin JP: Selective management of abruptio placentae: A prospective study. Obstet Gynecol 61:467,1983; Pritchard JA: Haematological problems associated with delivery, placental abruption, retained dead fetus, and amniotic fluid embolism. Clin Haematol 2:563, 1973.

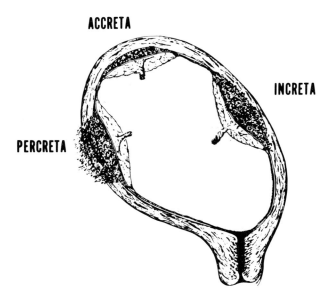

ACCRETA

INCRETA

PERCRETA

Figure 12–10. The three major types of placenta accreta. (From Breen, et al.: Placenta accreta, increta, and percreta: A survey of 40 cases. Obstet Gynecol 49:43 1977.)

Etiology

The precise etiology of placenta accreta is not known. Accreta appears to be associated with conditions that predispose the invasion of myometrium by placental villi. These conditions include previous cesarean section, uterine curettage, myomectomy, and treatment of Asherman's syndrome.[14, 48, 50, 53–55] Other associated factors include multiparity, implantation of the placenta in the lower uterine segment, placenta previa, and previous uterine infection (Table 12–6).[14, 50, 53]

Two of the most important associated factors are previous cesarean section and placenta previa.[14, 48, 50, 53] Clark and associates[14] reported a 5% incidence of placenta accreta when placenta previa was associated with an unscarred uterus, compared with 24% when placenta previa was associated with one previous cesarean section. As the number of cesarean sections increased, the risk of accreta increased, to a high of 67% when placenta previa was associated with four or more cesarean births.

Diagnosis

It is very difficult to make the diagnosis of placenta accreta during the antepartum period. The diagnosis is almost always made after birth

(Fig. 12–11). Cox and associates[54] did, however, report the diagnosis of placenta percreta made at 26 weeks' gestation by ultrasonography. MRI may also prove useful for diagnosing this extreme form of placenta accreta.

The majority of women with placenta accreta have an uncomplicated antepartum course.[50] Although 30% of the patients reported by Fox[50] did experience some antepartum bleeding, the majority of these (86%) had placenta previa. Breen and associates[48] reported similar findings with regard to antepartum bleeding (six of nine such cases were in women with placenta previa). The possibility of accreta should be considered when the diagnosis of placenta previa is made. Patients with placenta percreta may also rarely present with sudden gross hematuria.[52, 56] Litwin and associates[52] recently reported three such cases, one of which was diagnosed preoperatively by ultrasonography.

With the exception of vaginal bleeding associated with placenta previa, there are few signs and symptoms of placenta accreta that are manifested during labor.[48, 50] Fox[50] reported that 12 cases (2%) of intrapartum uterine rupture were associated with placenta accreta. Placenta accreta was associated with uterine rupture in a patient with a 23-week gestation.[57]

The two most common findings of placenta ac-

Table 12–6. FACTORS ASSOCIATED WITH PLACENTA ACCRETA

Factor	Fox[50] (1972)	Breen and co-workers[48] (1977)	Read and co-workers[53] (1980)
Placenta previa	34%	17%	64%
Post-cesarean section	25%	30%	27%
Prior dilation and curettage	30%	18%	27%
Previous manual removal of placenta	10%	10%	9%*
Multiparity (≥5)	40%	—	23%

*Prior postpartum hemorrhage with retained placenta.

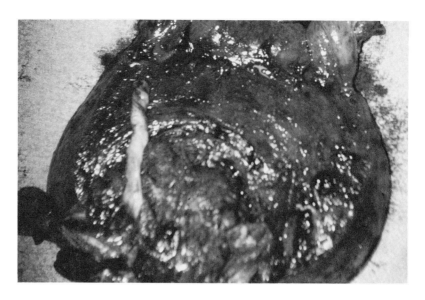

Figure 12–11. Placenta accreta.

creta during the third stage of labor are postpartum hemorrhage and a retained placenta.[50] The two most serious complications that also occur during this time are uterine inversion and uterine rupture. Fox[50] reported that uterine inversion occurred in 2% and uterine rupture in 3% of patients during the third stage of labor. Krysiewicz and associates[56] reported a very unusual complication of placenta percreta, a vesicouterine fistula, occurring during the postpartum period.

Management

Hysterectomy, either at the time of cesarean section or in the immediate postpartum period, is often required because of complications of placenta accreta such as hemorrhage or uterine rupture. Hysterectomy is the therapy of choice in the multiparous patient who wishes sterilization. However, the young nulliparous woman with placenta accreta presents a somewhat more difficult therapeutic dilemma, especially if the infant is too immature to survive. Unfortunately, hysterectomy may also be the treatment of choice in the management of these patients.

In the review by Fox,[50] 309 (68%) had an immediate hysterectomy, whereas conservative therapy was attempted in 143 (32%). Of this latter group, 61 had a delayed hysterectomy. The maternal mortality was 6.1% for the group who underwent immediate hysterectomy, compared with 26% for those treated conservatively.[50]

Breen and associates[48] reported 40 patients with placenta accreta. Thirty-eight (95%) had a hysterectomy, one patient was treated conservatively, and one patient died before surgery could be performed. Read and associates[53] reported that hysterectomy was required in 14 (67%) of 22 cases. One patient died intraoperatively from hemor-

rhage. Eight patients were managed successfully with a conservative approach consisting of uterine curettage or suturing of bleeding sites and uterine artery ligation.[53] Others have reported successful conservative management of placenta accreta.[54, 58] Hysterectomy, uterine artery ligation, and hypogastric artery ligation are described and illustrated in this textbook. Chapter 26 describes peripartal hysterectomy. Chapter 21 contains the illustrations and techniques of uterine artery ligation. Hypogastric artery ligation is discussed in both Chapters 21 and 26.

Although conservative therapy as described above may be a reasonable consideration for the individual patient, this approach should not be carried to the extreme because it may jeopardize the life of the mother. It may indeed be tragic for the young nulliparous patient to undergo hysterectomy, especially if the newborn did not survive, but it is even more tragic for her to die from hemorrhage. Hysterectomy remains the primary mode of therapy in the majority of patients with placenta accreta.

MISCELLANEOUS PLACENTAL CONDITIONS

Vasa Previa

Vasa previa occurs in one in 2000 to 3000 deliveries.[59] It is frequently misdiagnosed as placenta previa or abruptio placentae. Vasa previa is associated with an extremely high fetal mortality rate (50 to 75%) because it involves the loss of fetal blood. By definition, vasa previa exists when there is a velamentous insertion of the cord in the lower uterine segment with the fetal vessels coursing through the membranes, often across the internal cervical os in advance of the presenting fetal part

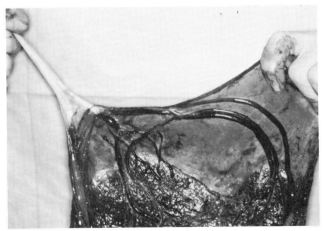

Figure 12–12. Vasa previa. Note the velamentous cord insert on and the fetal vessels coursing through the membrane. (Courtesy Gary Hankins, M.D.)

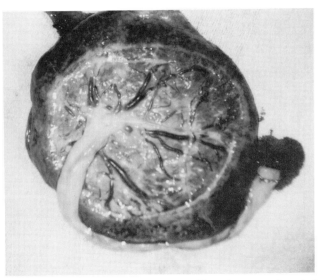

Figure 12–13. Circumvallate placenta. Note the area of central depression on the fetal surface encircled by a thickened, grayish-white ring.

(Fig. 12–12).[59] The fetal vessels are prone to lacerations, especially at the time of ruptured membranes, with subsequent fetal exsanguination being the rule. With significant vaginal bleeding an immediate cesarean delivery is mandatory to save the fetus.

The diagnosis of vasa previa is most often made during the postpartum period via examination of the placenta, although the diagnosis can be made antepartum by confirming the presence of fetal cells in the vaginal blood with the Apt test, hemoglobin electrophoresis, or Kleihauer-Bethke techniques. The fetus may also exhibit a sinusoidal heart rate pattern. The finding of this fetal heart rate pattern in association with bleeding on rupture of the membranes should raise the suspicion of vasa previa. Vasa previa occurs more commonly with multiple gestation and is associated with velamentous insertion of the cord.

Circumvallate Placenta

Circumvallate placenta refers to an extrachorial placenta where the fetal chorionic plate is smaller in size than the maternal basal plate. The placenta has an area of central depression on the fetal surface encircled by a thickened, grayish-white ring representing folded amnionic and chorionic membranes (Fig. 12–13).[60] The etiology for this placental condition is unknown. Antepartum bleeding, prematurity, and fetal malformations have been reported to be associated with this placental condition. The diagnosis is made by examination of the placenta after delivery.

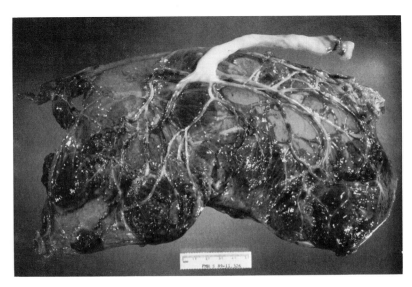

Figure 12–14. Membranaceous placenta. (Courtesy Cristela Hernandez M.D.)

Membranaceous Placenta

Severe hemorrhage secondary to a membranaceous placenta can resemble that of a total placenta previa. This rare placental anomaly has functioning villi completely covering the fetal membranes with the chorion's periphery occupied by a thin membranous placental structure (Fig. 12–14).[60] There may be an associated prolonged third stage of labor that often requires a difficult manual extraction of the placenta. This complication has been diagnosed during the antepartum period with high-resolution ultrasonography.[60] It is not associated with adverse fetal effects.

References

1. Cotton DB, Read JA, Paul RH, Quilligan EJ: The conservative aggressive management of placenta previa. Am J Obstet Gynecol 137:687, 1980.
2. Wexler P, Gottesfeld KR: Second trimester placenta previa: An apparently normal placentation. Obstet Gynecol 50:706, 1977.
3. Artis III AA, Bowie JD, Rosenberg ER, Rauch RF: The fallacy of placental migration: Effect of sonographic techniques. Am J Radiol 144:79, 1985.
4. Rizos N, Doran TA, Miskin M, et al.: Natural history of placenta previa ascertained by diagnostic ultrasound. Am J Obstet Gynecol 133:287, 1979.
5. Wexler P, Gottesfeld KR: Early diagnosis of placenta previa. Obstet Gynecol 54:231, 1979.
6. Barrett JM, Boehm FH, Killam AP: Induced abortion: A risk factor for placenta previa. Am J Obstet Gynecol 141:769, 1981.
7. Crenshaw C Jr, Jones DED, Parker RT: Placenta previa: A survey of twenty years experience with improved perinatal survival by expectant therapy and cesarean delivery. Obstet Gynecol Surv 28:461, 1973.
8. Naeye RL: Placenta previa. Predisposing factors and effects on the fetus and surviving infants. Obstet Gynecol 52:521, 1978.
9. King DL: Placental migration demonstrated by ultrasonography. Radiology 109:167, 1973.
10. Brenner WE, Edelman DA, Hendricks CH: Characteristics of patients with placenta previa and results of "expectant management." Am J Obstet Gynecol 132:180, 1978.
11. Bender S: Placenta praevia and previous lower segment cesarean section. Surg Gynecol Obstet 98:625, 1954.
12. Singh PM, Rodrigues C, Gupta AN: Placenta previa and previous cesarean section. Acta Obstet Gynecol Scand 60:367, 1981.
13. Nielsen TF, Hagberg H, Ljungblad ULF: Placenta previa and antepartum hemorrhage after previous cesarean section. Obstet Gynecol Surv 45:181, 1990.
14. Clark SL, Koonings PP, Phelan JP: Placenta previa/accreta and prior cesarean section. Obstet Gynecol 66:89, 1985.
15. Newton ER, Barss V, Cetrulo CL: The epidemiology and clinical history of asymptomatic midtrimester placenta previa. Am J Obstet Gynecol 148:743, 1984.
16. Hibbard LT: Placenta previa. Am J Obstet Gynecol 104:172, 1969.
17. Farine D, Fox HE, Jakobson S, Timor-Tritsch IE: Vaginal ultrasound for diagnosis of placenta previa. Am J Obstet Gynecol 159:566, 1988.
18. Gottesfeld KR, Thompson HE, Holmes JH, Taylor ES: Ultrasonic placentography—a new method for placental localization. Am J Obstet Gynecol 96:538, 1966.
19. Donald I, Abdulla U: Placentography by sonar. J Obstet Gynaecol Br Commonw 75:993, 1968.
20. Campbell S, Kohorn EI: Placental localization by ultrasonic compound scanning. J Obstet Gynaecol Br Commonw 75:1007, 1968.
21. Bowie JD, Rochester D, Cadkin AV, et al.: Accuracy of placental localization by ultrasound. Radiology 128:177, 1978.
22. Laing FC: Placenta previa: Avoiding false-negative diagnoses. J Clin Ultrasound 9:109, 1981.
23. Johnson IR, Symonds EM, Kean DM, et al.: Imaging the pregnant human uterus with nuclear magnetic resonance. Am J Obstet Gynecol 148:1136, 1984.
24. McCarthy SM, Stark DD, Filly RA, et al.: Obstetrical magnetic resonance imaging: Maternal anatomy. Radiology 154:421, 1985.
25. Powell MC, Buckley J, Price H, et al.: Magnetic resonance imaging and placenta previa. Am J Obstet Gynecol 154:565, 1986.
26. Arias F: Cervical cerclage for the temporary treatment of patients with placenta previa. Obstet Gynecol 71:545, 1988.
27. Cunningham FG, MacDonald PC, Gant NF: Williams Obstetrics, 18th Edition. Norwalk, CT: Appleton & Lange, 1989, pp. 701.
28. Karegard M, Gennser G: Incidence and recurrence rate of abruptio placentae in Sweden. Obstet Gynecol 67:523, 1986.
29. Hurd WW, Miodovnik M, Hertzberg V, Lavin JP: Selective management of abruptio placentae: A prospective study. Obstet Gynecol 61:467, 1983.
30. Paterson MEL: The aetiology and outcome of abruptio placentae. Acta Obstet Gynecol Scand 58:31, 1979.
31. Pritchard JA, Brekken AL: Clinical and laboratory studies on severe abruptio placentae. Am J Obstet Gynecol 97:681, 1967.
32. Pritchard JA, Mason R, Corley M, Pritchard S: Genesis of severe placental abruption. Am J Obstet Gynecol 108:22, 1970.
33. Higgins SD, Garite TJ: Late abruptio placenta in trauma patients: Implications for monitoring. Obstet Gynecol 63:10S, 1984.
34. Stafford PA, Biddinger PW, Zumwalt RE: Lethal intrauterine fetal trauma. Am J Obstet Gynecol 159:485, 1988.
35. Kettel LM, Branch DW, Scott JR: Occult placental abruption after maternal trauma. Obstet Gynecol 71:449, 1988.
36. Hibbard BM, Jeffcoate TNA: Abruptio placentae. Obstet Gynecol 27:155, 1966.
37. Whalley PJ, Scott DE, Pritchard JA: Maternal folate deficiency and pregnancy wastage: I. Placental abruption. Am J Obstet Gynecol 105:670, 1969.
38. Gonen R, Hannah ME, Milligan JE: Does prolonged preterm premature rupture of the membranes predispose to abruptio placentae? Obstet Gynecol 74:347, 1989.
39. Darby MJ, Caritis SN, Shen-Schwartz S: Placental abruption in the preterm gestation: An association with chorioamnionitis. Obstet Gynecol 74:88, 1989.
40. Naeye RL, Harkness WL, Utts J: Abruptio placentae and perinatal death: A prospective study. Am J Obstet Gynecol 128:740, 1977.
41. Chasnoff IJ, Burns WJ, Schnoll SH, Burns KA: Cocaine use in pregnancy. N Engl J Med 313:666, 1985.
42. Bingol N, Fuchs M, Diaz V, et al.: Teratogenicity of cocaine in humans. J Pediatr 110:93, 1987.
43. Nyberg DA, Cyr DR, Mack LA, et al.: Sonographic spectrum of placental abruption. Am J Radiol 148:161, 1987.
44. Sholl JS: Abruptio placentae: Clinical management in nonacute cases. Am J Obstet Gynecol 156:40, 1987.
45. Metzger DA, Bowie JD, Killam AP: Expectant management of partial placental abruption in previable pregnancies. A report of two cases. J Reprod Med 32:789, 1987.
46. Krupp PJ Jr, Barclay DL, Roeling WM, Wegener G: Maternal mortality: A 20-year study of Tulane Department of Obstetrics and Gynecology at Charity Hospital. Obstet Gynecol 35:823, 1970.
47. Pritchard JA: Haematological problems associated with delivery, placental abruption, retained dead fetus and amniotic fluid embolism. Clin Haematol 2:563, 1973.

48. Breen JL, Neubecker R, Gregori CA, Franklin JE Jr: Placenta accreta, increta, and percreta. A survey of 40 cases. Obstet Gynecol 49:43, 1977.

49. Khong TY, Robertson WB: Placenta creta and placenta praevia creta. Placenta 8:399, 1987.

50. Fox H: Placenta accreta, 1945–69. Obstet Gynecol Surv 27:475, 1972.

51. Ochshorn A, David MP, Soferman N: Placenta previa accreta: A report of nine cases. Obstet Gynecol 33:677, 1969.

52. Litwin MS, Loughlin KR, Benson CB, et al.: Placenta percreta invading the urinary bladder. Br J Urol 64:283, 1989.

53. Read JA, Cotton DB, Miller FC: Placenta accreta: Changing clinical aspects and outcome. Obstet Gynecol 56:31, 1980.

54. Cox SM, Carpenter RJ, Cotton DB: Placenta percreta: Ultrasound diagnosis and conservative surgical management. Obstet Gynecol 71:454, 1988.

55. Friedman A, DeFazio J, DeCherney A: Severe obstetric complications after aggressive treatment of Asherman syndrome. Obstet Gynecol 67:864, 1986.

56. Krysiewicz S, Auh YH, Kazam E: Vesicouterine fistula associated with placenta percreta. Urol Radiol 10:213, 1988.

57. Nagy PS: Placenta percreta induced uterine rupture and resulted in intraabdominal abortion. Am J Obstet Gynecol 161:1185, 1989.

58. Hollander DI, Pupkin MJ, Crenshaw MC, Nagey DA: Conservative management of placenta accreta. A case report. J Reprod Med 33:74, 1988.

59. Pent D: Vasa previa. Am J Obstet Gynecol 134:151, 1979.

60. Cunningham FG, MacDonald PC, Gant NF: Williams Obstetrics, 18th Edition. Norwalk, CT: Appleton & Lange, 1989, p. 533.

13

Surgical Problems Involving the Pregnant Uterus:

Uterine Inversion, Uterine Rupture, and Leiomyomas

Warren C. Plauché

UTERINE INVERSION

Uterine inversion is simply the turning of the uterus inside out. This usually happens in the third stage of labor but can occur even in the nonpregnant uterus in relation to the expulsion of an intrauterine tumor. Table 13-1 outlines the types of uterine inversions encountered in the practice of obstetrics and gynecology. This chapter deals only with puerperal inversions.

Puerperal uterine inversion is divided into acute, subacute, and chronic forms.[1] Because most uterine inversions are immediately treated by replacement of the uterus, the subacute and chronic forms have become rare and isolated events. Subacute inversion implies that the uterus has been extruded long enough for a contraction ring to form in the lower uterine segment. Occasionally a case may be encountered that has been neglected or misdiagnosed long enough to be termed chronic. There is some variation in the literature concerning the interval of time that denotes chronic inversion. Watson and co-workers[2] suggested 4 days, whereas others require a remarkable 4 weeks.[1,3]

Prevalence and Morbidity

Uterine inversion is a rare complication of obstetric delivery. A literature survey by Watson and co-workers[2] in 1980 found the incidence of uterine inversion to vary from a high of 1 in 2000 deliveries to a low of 1 in 20,000 deliveries. In 1940 Das[4] described the incidence of uterine inversion in the United States to be 1 in 23,000 deliveries. He found the incidence in the United Kingdom to be 1 in 28,000 deliveries. In recent studies from individual hospital services, a prevalence near the 1 in 10,000 range has been reported.[5-8]

Rodriguez and colleagues[7] first reported puerperal uterine inversion at vaginal delivery in patients who had previous cesarean births. The prevalence of uterine inversion among 854 vaginal deliveries of previous section patients was 1 inversion per 427 cases. This compared with 1 inversion per 5797 vaginal deliveries of patients without previous cesarean birth. More studies are required to confirm this difference in risk.

The mortality rate for uterine inversion has been reported to vary from 0 to 41%.[2,8] Earlier reports showed 13 to 41% mortality.[8] Death from this complication is quite rare in modern obstetrics. Effective management now exists for the principal causes of death in uterine inversion, that is, blood loss, shock, and infection. Uterine inversion has caused no deaths among the 55,000 confinements at Charity Hospital of New Orleans in the last 10 years.

Causes of Uterine Inversion

Typically, a case of acute puerperal uterine inversion develops when a fundal placenta fails to separate promptly from the wall of an atonic uterus after obstetric delivery. The attendant succumbs to the temptation to pull vigorously on the umbilical cord. He or she may attempt to express the placenta with fundal pressure.

Uterine inversion begins when a dimple develops in the fundus of the uterus as the uterine wall is drawn or pushed into the uterine cavity. At this point the inversion is partial or incomplete (Fig. 13-1A). Progression of the forces that draw the uterus downward will eventually result in complete inversion (Fig. 13-1B). The uterus then presents as a mass in the vagina. The placenta usually remains attached, and it is sometimes difficult to recognize that an inverted uterus is present with the placenta. In some cases the uterus is extruded through the introitus, adding prolapse to the diagnosis of complete inversion (Fig. 13-1C).

Table 13-2 lists some of the factors said to contribute to the development of uterine inversion. The placenta is most commonly, but not always, implanted in the uppermost fundus. Acute inversion can occur with any placental location and can develop even though the placenta has separated and been expelled.

The uterus is usually atonic in inversion cases and fails to contract tightly after delivery of the infant. The usual mechanism for separation of the placenta requires contraction of the uterus to reduce the area of implantation. The placenta is normally attached to the uterine wall by a few anchoring villi. Sharply reduced uterine volume

Table 13-1. UTERINE INVERSION—A CLASSIFICATION

Puerperal
By duration
Acute
Subacute
Chronic
By extent
Partial
Complete
Complete with prolapse
Nonpuerperal

Table 13-2. UTERINE INVERSION—CONTRIBUTING CAUSES

Common causes
Umbilical cord traction
Uterine atony
Placenta accreta—focal or general
Fundal pressure before placental separation
Unusual causes
Short umbilical cord
Uterine anomalies
Tumors—submucous myomas
Cervical incompetence
Cervical anomalies

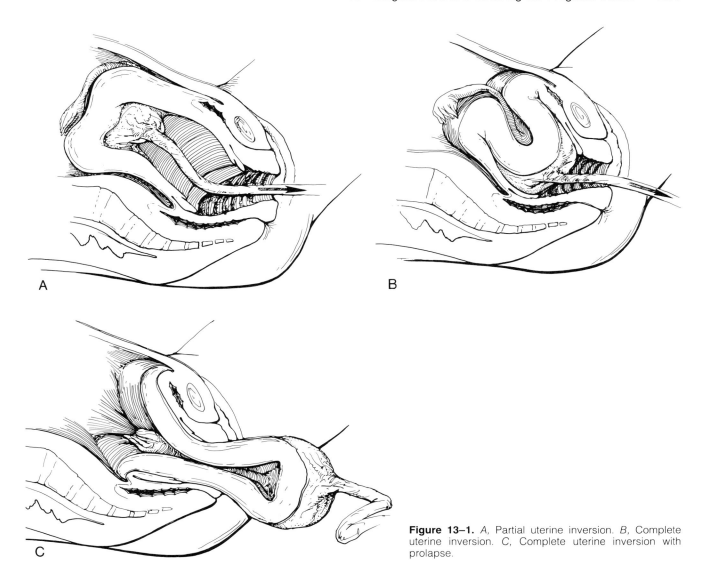

Figure 13–1. *A*, Partial uterine inversion. *B*, Complete uterine inversion. *C*, Complete uterine inversion with prolapse.

shears off the placenta at the decidual plate, and the placenta is expelled from the uterine cavity. When the uterus is atonic, the placenta will not quickly separate. Traction on the umbilical cord may result in inversion of the atonic uterus.

Placenta accreta attaches firmly to the myometrium. Villi grow directly into the myometrial wall, and no plane for decidual separation exists. The absence of the decidual plate is usually focal but can involve the entire placental surface. Persistent efforts to deliver such a placenta may result in uterine inversion.

The myometrial wall is thin and easily inverted when congenital sacculation of the uterine fundus exists. A shortened or incompetent cervix offers an unusually accommodating opening for inversion. A short umbilical cord combined with fundal implantation of the placenta may also contribute to inversion of the puerperal uterus. Uterine, cervical, and cord anomalies actually are rare contributors to uterine inversion.

Diagnosis of Uterine Inversion

The diagnosis of uterine inversion should be considered in all cases of postpartum shock or hemorrhage (Table 13–3). The diagnosis is obvious when the uterus inverts and prolapses during attempts to expel the placenta. Cases of partial inversion may display minimal symptoms and signs.

Ultrasonography can be an aid to the diagnosis of occult partial uterine inversion.[9] In more subtle

Table 13–3. UTERINE INVERSION—DIAGNOSIS

Maternal anxiety and shock
Postpartum hemorrhage
Bimanual pelvic examination
  Partial inversion—dimple in fundus
  Complete inversion—uterine mass in vagina or outside
    introitus
Ultrasound evidence of occult inversion

cases, the patient may initially exhibit only discomfort, pressure, and anxiety after delivery of her baby. Bleeding is often profuse and unrelenting because of the uterine atony that commonly accompanies inversion.

As blood loss increases, the patient becomes diaphoretic, her blood pressure falls, and her pulse rises. Prompt investigation of the cause of postpartum hemorrhage should always include inspection, bimanual pelvic examination, and intrauterine exploration.

In cases of partial uterine inversion, the attendant will feel the infolding of the fundus and a restricted uterine cavity. Complete inversion presents a large, velvety, purple-red, bloody mass either within the vagina or prolapsed outside the introitus.

The anatomic region just above the cervix should be promptly assessed because a contraction ring could constrict the opening available for replacement of the uterus. Management is much more difficult when this constricting ring is fully developed.

Chronic inversion is recognized by the presence of the involuting inverted uterus, either within the vagina or prolapsed through the introitus, for a prolonged period of time. A constriction ring at the level of the lower uterine segment may become tight enough to cause ischemic necrosis of the uterus. The earlier obstetric literature remarkably recommended that the uterus be allowed to complete the process of post-partal involution before treatment was attempted.[10]

Management

The modern obstetrician is wise to pursue an aggressive management program consisting of supportive therapy and prompt uterine replacement in cases of acute puerperal uterine inversion. Supportive treatment should begin immediately. An anesthetist should be available and prepared for the possibility of general anesthesia, using a uterine-relaxing agent such as halothane if necessary. The anesthetist should comfort the anxious patient, explain the situation to her, and provide pain relief.

Two intravenous access lines should be available if possible. The patient's hematologic and coagulation status should be assessed and a sample of her blood sent for crossmatching. Large quantities of blood products are often required in this unusual emergency. A common request of the blood bank on our service is "Give me four units of packed cells and stay two ahead of me." Prepare for immediate replacement of the uterus.

Uterine Replacement Technique

Several procedures have been recommended for the immediate replacement of the uterus in cases of acute inversion. Attempts at replacement of the uterus should be made immediately. The only reasons to delay uterine replacement are to stabilize the patient or to get a consultant with skill and experience in replacement procedures. A trained attendant, even one without experience in uterine replacement, should make the first attempt if there will be considerable delay in consultation. Prompt replacement can often be quite a simple matter.

The placenta is usually still attached to the leading edge of the inverted uterus. The placenta can be removed before replacement of the uterus is attempted. The operator can peel the placenta away from the uterine wall by developing a decidual cleavage plane at one edge of the placenta as though performing manual extraction of the placenta. First attempts at uterine replacement should begin as soon as the placenta is removed.

Foci of placenta accreta can be manually separated in most cases, and residual fragments can be curetted away under direct vision. Bleeding is usually brisk during removal of the placenta. Replacement of the uterus should be performed without delay. Total placenta accreta or percreta defies manual removal. In these rare cases, the uterus should be replaced with the placenta in situ, and prompt peripartal hysterectomy should be performed.

Next the operator forms his or her hand into a fist and presses upward against the leading edge of the inverted fundus. This may suffice for replacement if the uterus is very lax and no constriction ring has formed. This maneuver is remarkably easy if recognition of the problem has been prompt and replacement immediate. The operator's internal hand remains within the uterus as the abdominal hand massages the uterus and oxytocics are administered to ensure tight uterine contraction.

A maneuver described by Johnson[11] is very effective when a constriction ring has begun to form but manual replacement is still possible. The open hand is introduced into the vagina under appropriate anesthesia. The fundus rests in the palm, and the fingers and thumb fit around the cervix, within the developing contraction ring. Simultaneously, the ring is dilated with the fingers and the reversion of the uppermost portion of the inverted fundus is encouraged. The last part to invert is replaced first, progressing up the fundal wall by pressing upward with the palm of the hand. Tocolytic agents help in these difficult cases. Halothane anesthesia was used in the past to accomplish relaxation of the contraction ring, but this agent has been largely replaced by parenteral tocolytic drugs.

Kovacs and DeVore[12] in 1984 described the successful use of a bolus dose of 0.25 mg of terbutaline sulfate before attempting to replace the uterus in two cases of subacute uterine inversion. Although the drug caused transient exacerbation of maternal tachycardia, the replacement procedure was dramatically facilitated. The uterus was found to relax within 2 minutes, at which time it was easily replaced. Oxytocin was administered after replacement to ensure contraction.

Fenoterol and ritodrine were the β-mimetic tocolytic agents used in the uterine inversion cases reported by Thiery and Delbeke in 1985.[13] This group from Belgium added intramyometrial prostaglandin $F_{2\alpha}$ in a dose of 250 μg after replacement of the inverted uterus. The uterus and contraction ring were first relaxed with the β-mimetic agent. The uterus was then effortlessly replaced and held in place until it became firm 15 minutes after administration of prostaglandin $F_{2\alpha}$. Attempts at replacement under ketamine and halothane anesthesia had failed in one of the cases in this series.

Magnesium sulfate assisted uterine replacement in four of six cases of subacute puerperal uterine inversion reported by Catanzarite and colleagues[5] in 1986. Intravenous magnesium sulfate, 4 g over 5 minutes, was found to relax the contraction ring in two of the cases. The tocolytic agent obviated the need for general anesthesia for uterine replacement. Intramyometrial Prostin-15M was administered in several of these cases with improvement of uterine tone and no side effects.

We currently recommend tocolysis, replacement of the uterus, and prostaglandin administration for inversion cases when immediate simple replacement fails (Table 13–4). Broad-spectrum antibiotics should be administered after these extensive manipulations to prevent endomyometritis.

SURGICAL MANAGEMENT OF CHRONIC INVERSION

When the uterus has been inverted for a long time, the supracervical contraction ring becomes firmly developed and fixed. Manual replacement by the vaginal route may be very difficult despite attempts using anesthetics and tocolytic agents. Several surgical procedures have been described to address this problem.

Operative vaginal approaches were described by Spinelli[14] and Kustner.[3] The former involves an anterior culpotomy and incision of the cervix ex-

Table 13–4. UTERINE INVERSION—MANAGEMENT

Acute and subacute inversion
  Supportive measures
    Fluids and electrolytes
    Blood replacement
    Pain relief
  Prompt manual replacement of uterus
    Tocolysis—β-mimetic agents
        magnesium sulfate
    Oxytocics—oxytocin
        prostaglandin
Chronic inversion
  Surgical replacement operations
    Vaginal approach
    Abdominal approach

tending into the fundus. The latter takes a posterior approach to a similar end.

Huntington and co-workers[15] in 1928 described an abdominal procedure for chronic uterine inversion (Fig. 13–2A–C). The inversion funnel is visualized from above. The round ligaments and adnexal structures course into a depression in the base of the cul-de-sac of Douglas. Although there are no published cases, administration of tocolytic agents might be a helpful adjunct preceding Huntington's maneuvers. In 1989 Shah-Hosseini and Evrard[8] reported the modern use of the Huntington procedure.

The uterine wall and round ligament are grasped with Allis or similar clamps an inch or so down each side of the funnel. Slow, patient, gentle traction gradually everts the uterine wall. Successive clamping sites down the uterine wall progressively replace the uterus. The hand of an assistant pressing upward from below helps in this process. Prostaglandins administered into either cornu of the replaced uterus ensure tight myometrial contraction, guarding against recurrent inversion. Antibiotics should be administered before and after surgery.

Occasionally, the constriction ring in the lower uterine segment will not relax, and the uterus cannot be surgically replaced by simple traction. The contraction ring in the posterior lower uterine segment can be incised to allow uterine replacement. This procedure was described by Haultain[10] in 1901 (Fig. 13–2D). After replacement of the uterus, the incision in the posterior uterine segment is repaired with two layers of 00 or 000 absorbable sutures.

In rare instances, ischemic changes in the uterus make it necessary to remove the uterus in cases of chronic inversion. Extirpation of the uterus is a routine matter if the uterus can be repositioned. If the uterus cannot be replaced, the operation becomes very complex and dangerous because of gross distortion of anatomic relationships.

UTERINE RUPTURE

Rupture of the pregnant uterus can be the most difficult of surgical obstetric complications. Careful study of uterine rupture, however, reveals that nearly half of the cases are not dramatic or life threatening.[16] Many separations of previous uterine scars, although technically classified as uterine ruptures, occur with few symptoms or signs. These separations are discovered incidentally at the time of repeat cesarean operations or uterine exploration after vaginal delivery. Asymptomatic dehiscences should be considered separately from major, life-threatening uterine ruptures.

The obstetric literature contains many articles on uterine rupture that do not identify the severity of all cases. Their results combine simple dehis-

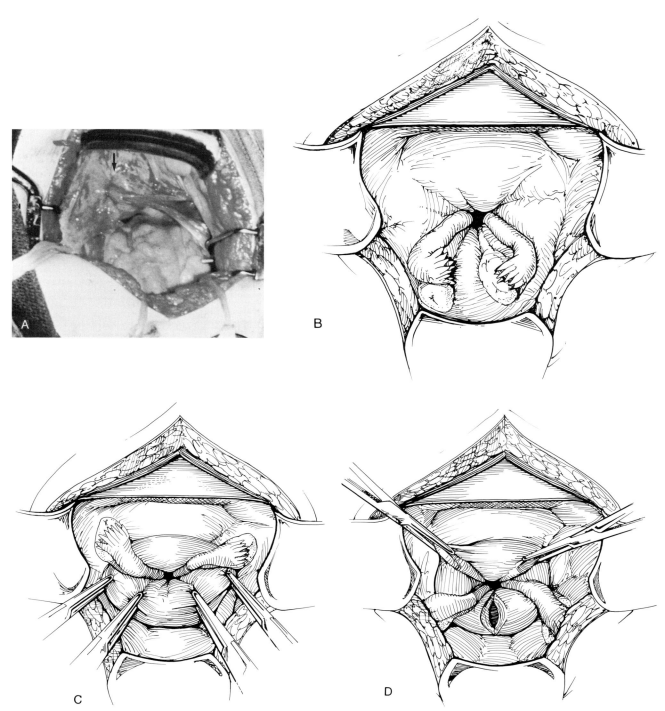

Figure 13–2. *A*, Complete uterine inversion. View of the pelvis at laparotomy. Round ligaments drawn into inversion site in midpelvis *(arrow)* (courtesy Clarence E. Ehrlich, M.D.). *B*, Complete uterine inversion viewed from above. Round ligaments and fallopian tubes disappear into a depression in the cul-de-sac of Douglas. *C*, Huntington procedure: traction to restore the inverted uterus to normal position. *D*, Haultain procedure: traction after incision of the posterior lower uterine segment to replace an inverted uterus.

cences and major ruptures. The resulting morbidity and outcome statistics and management suggestions do not apply well to either separate group.

Studies of uterine rupture from major university referral centers often focus on catastrophic ruptures. Their conclusions cannot be held to apply to minor uterine wound dehiscence events.[16] Conversely, studies of minimal cesarean wound separations do not prepare us for massive spontaneous uterine rupture cases. The student of this subject must read widely and critically to reach valid conclusions.

The controversy regarding rupture of previous cesarean scars during trial of labor is an example of the clinical problems in this field. After 50 years of "once a cesarean, always a cesarean" thinking, the winds of change currently blow in the direction of allowing vaginal birth after cesarean section (VBAC).

There were supporters of VBAC as far back as the 1930s. They believed that the uterus healed by regeneration of smooth muscle without scar tissue. This theory was disproved by the definitive work of Schwartz and co-workers.[17] The early VBAC advocates gave over to the "once a cesarean" group, who recruited two generations of obstetricians to their banner.

Careful clinical studies of VBACs in the past decade document the rarity of serious uterine rupture during these labors.[18–22] Recent researchers brave unknown previous scars, multiple scars, and oxytocin augmentation of labor. They report few untoward events.[22]

Half or more of all cases of major uterine rupture are related to disruption of previous cesarean scars.[16, 23] The implications for maternal and fetal risk must be carefully considered. Several authors have expressed fear of an increase in uterine rupture as the incidence of cesarean birth increases.[16, 24–26] Most study groups, including the Committee on Obstetrics of the American College of Obstetricians and Gynecologists, interpret the available data positively and support VBAC as national policy.[27]

Table 13–5 lists some of the variables to consider when classifying the spectrum of obstetric problems associated with rupture of the pregnant uterus.

Incidence

Keifer[28] in 1964 published a survey of reports of 9300 cases of uterine rupture that appeared in a 30-year span of the world's English-language literature beginning in 1932. These reports estimated the incidence of rupture of the gravid uterus from a high of 1 in 800 deliveries to a low of 1 in 3000.

Eden and colleagues[29] examined 53 years of Duke University Medical Center records begin-

Table 13–5. UTERINE RUPTURE—CLASSIFICATION AND MANAGEMENT ISSUES

Prepartal vs. intrapartal
Spontaneous vs. traumatic
Partial vs. complete
Minimal vs. life threatening
Scarred uterus vs. no scar

ning in 1931. This group found an incidence of 1 rupture in 1424 deliveries. Separate analysis of the last decade of the Duke experience revealed an incidence of only 1 rupture in 2251 deliveries. There was a fivefold rise in the cesarean delivery rate over that of the preceding decade and a tenfold increase over that of the first two decades of the study. The Duke group was convinced that uterine rupture was rare among patients with previous cesarean scars.

Shrinsky and Benson[30] in 1978 reported a 25-year survey in which 1 uterine rupture in 2695 deliveries occurred on their service at the University of Oregon. Their survey of the world literature is difficult to interpret because some researchers reported only complete major ruptures, whereas others recorded all uterine wound separations. The incidence of all uterine ruptures in 33 articles published between 1945 and 1975 varied from 1 in 93 deliveries to 1 in 4900 deliveries.

In 1984 I and my colleagues reported an incidence of 1 in 2174 deliveries during the preceding decade of catastrophic, life-threatening uterine rupture at Louisiana State University obstetric service at Charity Hospital.[16] The mean incidence of complete rupture of the uterus from our English literature survey was 1 in 1148 deliveries.[16]

Causes of Obstetric Uterine Rupture

Figure 13–3 and Table 13–6 outline the interrelationships and some of the principal causes of rupture of the pregnant uterus. The leading cause, responsible for 50 to 70% of all cases and 30% of major complete ruptures, is a previous uterine scar. The large majority of scars that result in uterine rupture are those from previous cesarean births.

Nielsen and co-workers,[31] in 1989, reported a large prospective study from Sweden on the incidence of rupture and dehiscence of previous cesarean scars. This 10-year study followed 2036 women who had had previous cesarean delivery. Trial of labor was attempted in 1008 patients and was successful in 92.2%. Nielsen and co-workers defined uterine scar dehiscence as separation of the scar without rupture of the membranes. Uterine rupture implied open rupture into the peritoneal cavity of both the uterine wall and amniotic membranes (Table 13–6).

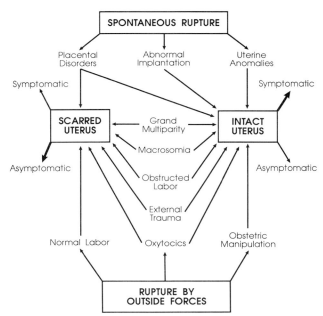

Figure 13–3. Causes of obstetric uterine rupture and their interrelationships.

Nielsen and colleagues found uterine dehiscence in 4% of cases and uterine rupture in 0.6%. Two of the ruptures occurred before labor, both in T incision scars. The true incidence of dehiscence in this study is uncertain because the authors did not routinely examine the interior of the uterus after vaginal delivery. This group concluded that there were no serious complications in either the mothers or the offspring in the trial of labor group.

I and my colleagues have reported 23 catastrophic uterine ruptures from the hospitals of the Louisiana State University (LSU) School of Medi-

cine-New Orleans Department of Obstetrics and Gynecology. Fourteen (61.3%) of these life-threatening cases occurred in uteri that bore scars of previous cesarean deliveries.[16] Trials of labor in 307 patients with previous cesarean scars of all types, including unknown scars, were examined by the University Medical Center branch of the same LSU Department of Obstetrics and Gynecology in 1987. Two major uterine ruptures required emergency hysterectomies, and seven dehiscences of uterine scars required repair (2.9%).[32]

Meehan and Magani[33] reviewed 1350 patients with trials of labor after previous cesarean delivery from University Hospital in Galway between 1972 and 1987. There were six true scar ruptures in the group (0.44%, or 1 in 225).

The method of closure of cesarean incisions may affect subsequent scar strength and therefore the incidence of subsequent rupture. I have long taught that cesarean closure techniques that turn endometrial glandular tissue into the wound create surgical endometriosis that could weaken the eventual scar.

Dunihoo and co-workers[34] investigated the effect of closure method on scar integrity in rabbits. Two wounds were made in each uterine horn. Continuous everted, continuous inverted, interrupted everted, and interrupted inverted closure methods were used. No difference was found in the tensile strength of the scars formed after 28 to 30 days of healing time.

Uterine scars from hysterotomies, myomectomies, perforations from curettage, and even laparoscopy trochar punctures have been related to uterine rupture. These events make up less than 20% of the cases.[35, 36] The widely held notion that myometrial incisions that do not enter the endometrial cavity will not subsequently rupture appears to be an unsubstantiated myth.

The uterus may be more prone to rupture in women who were exposed to diethylstilbestrol (DES) in utero. Adams and colleagues[37] described a spontaneous intrapartum uterine rupture in a DES-exposed patient. Review of the case reveals a preconceptual Shirodkar cerclage that was removed because of erosion through the cervical mucosa. The subsequent massive rupture from the upper cervix through the left corpus into the broad ligament could have been related to complications of either cerclage or DES, or to a combination of these factors. The course of the tear is suspicious for a defect in müllerian duct fusion related to early intrauterine DES exposure.

Post-cesarean endomyometritis was formerly thought to be an important factor in uterine rupture in later pregnancies. Studies on the LSU obstetric service indicate that the relationship between postpartum infection and wound rupture is inconstant. Post-delivery infection is not an absolute indicator of defective cesarean wound strength.

Table 13–6. UTERINE RUPTURE—CONTRIBUTING CAUSES

Uterine scar dehiscence
Trauma
  Indirect
    Blunt trauma—blows, seat belt injury
    Excessive manual fundal pressure
    Extension of cervical tears
  Direct
    Penetrating wounds
    Intrauterine manipulations
    Forceps application and rotation
    Postpartum curettage
    Manual placental extraction
    Version and extraction
    External version
Inappropriate use of oxytocin
Grandmultiparity
Uterine anomalies
Placenta percreta
Tumors—trophoblastic disease, cervical carcinoma
Fetal problems—macrosomia, malposition, anomalies,
  destructive procedures

Uteri involved in severe postpartum infections occasionally develop early postpartum dehiscence of the cesarean wound. These dehiscence sites are localized and sealed off by adherence of the omentum and bladder and attachment of the wound site to the anterior abdominal wall. There may be little or no myometrium remaining between the abdominal wall and the chorioamniotic sac with the next pregnancy. Trial of labor in such a situation might be inappropriate. Obstetricians cannot always detect this condition or other examples of abnormal healing of cesarean incisions.

Trauma is responsible for approximately 20% of obstetric uterine ruptures (Fig. 13–4). Trauma may be related to obstetric maneuvers or outside forces. The majority of traumatic ruptures due to obstetric manipulations are associated with forceps delivery. Reviews of uterine rupture from 1930 to 1970 usually cited Kielland forceps and rotation maneuvers as the most frequent forceps operations causing uterine injury.[30] Forceps delivery also increases the number of extensions of cervical tears into the lower uterine segment.

Obstetric manipulations of the fetus contribute the next largest share of uterine injuries. Older studies found internal podalic version of transverse lies and breech extractions to be involved in 4 to 6% of uterine ruptures.[30] External version has been only an occasional visitor to the lists of uterine rupture since the advent of effective tocolytic agents and ultrasound monitoring of the process.

Parity of five or more has been associated with uterine rupture.[16, 30] Multiparity, oxytocin misuse, fetal macrosomia, and excessive fundal pressure for delivery contributed to many older cases of obstetric uterine rupture. These factors are quite rare in modern case collections. Unsuspected macrosomia, malpositions, anomalies, and cephalopelvic disproportion remain important considerations as we enter an era of more universal trial of labor for patients with scars from previous cesarean sections.

Rupture of the gravid uterus has repeatedly been reported in relation to oxytocin administration.[38] Present methods demand supervised administration of carefully measured, minute quantities of dilute oxytocin by mechanisms that can immediately stop administration of the drug if hyperstimulation occurs. Uterine contractions can be monitored by internal pressure transducers so that both timing and intensity of contractions are known. Under these circumstances, hyperstimulation of the uterus should be rare. If the forces of normal labor are considered acceptable for uterine and fetal safety, similar oxytocin-induced contractions should be equally safe.

Prostaglandin agents for uterine stimulation raise the question of safety of oxytocics once again. McCarthy and McQueen[39] in 1980 reported uterine rupture complicating intra-amniotic injection of prostaglandin E_2 for second-trimester abortion when contractions were augmented with synthetic oxytocin. Valenzuela and co-workers,[40] Sawyer and co-workers,[41] and others have recorded cases of rupture of the uterus after intravaginal suppositories of prostaglandin E_2 were used to ripen the cervix at term.

Prostaglandins are very powerful oxytocic agents. Their physiologic action seems to closely mimic the normal process of labor. Their pharma-

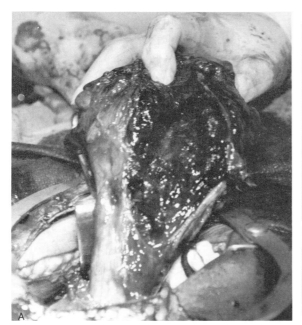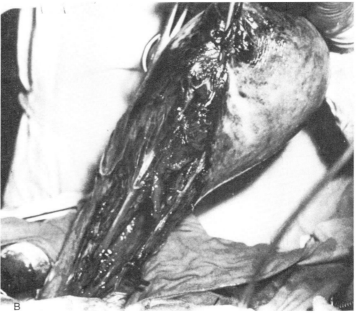

Figure 13–4. *A,* Massive rupture of a classic cesarean scar near term. *B,* Massive traumatic rupture of the pregnant uterus. Lateral rupture caused by head-on auto accident at 32 weeks' gestation. (Courtesy Duane E. Neumann, M.D.; photographed by Rita L. Letellier.)

cologic instability has made it difficult to develop a delivery system that approaches the safety of carefully metered dilute oxytocin. Prostaglandins are not, at the time of this writing, approved by the Food and Drug Administration for induction of labor or other use in late pregnancy.

Automobile accidents, stab wounds, and gunshot wounds are the principal causes of uterine rupture from outside forces. These cases constitute no more than 10% of ruptures.[16] The English-language obstetric literature contains only 22 cases of stab wounds of the pregnant uterus.[42] A small number of researchers have described gunshot and other penetrating wounds of the pregnant uterus. Franger and co-workers[43] found reports of only nine cases of self-inflicted gunshot wounds to the pregnant uterus.

A more extensive literature discusses seat belt and other motor vehicle injuries to mothers and fetuses.[44] These cases of traumatic uterine rupture are often severe and frequently involve injury to the bowel, bladder, spleen, kidney, liver, soft tissues, and pelvic bones.

Spontaneous rupture of the intact pregnant uterus is usually unanticipated and among the most vivid examples of this pregnancy complication.[45] Ruptures of the intact uterus made up 38% of our Charity Hospital series of catastrophic ruptures and 70% of our literature survey of complete uterine rupture. Many spontaneous uterine ruptures defy explanation. Small subgroups are related to congenitally weak areas of the myometrial wall, fetal macrosomia, or polyhydramnios. Makar and colleagues[46] reported a case of spontaneous perforation of the pregnant uterus by a leiomyoma undergoing red degeneration and necrosis.

Deaton and co-workers[47] reported a rare case of spontaneous uterine rupture in pregnancy after hysteroscopic lysis of intrauterine adhesions in a case of Asherman's syndrome.

Other rare instances of spontaneous uterine rupture are associated with placenta percreta or invasive moles in which the placental villi grow entirely through the uterine wall. Ruptures of abnormal pregnancy implantations such as cornual pregnancies and cervical pregnancies are rare but devastating events (see also Chapter 9). Aggressive malignant tumors rarely complicate pregnancy. The most aggressive of all tumors, choriocarcinoma, may cause hemoperitoneum from uterine perforation (Fig. 13–5).

Infections occasionally play a role in spontaneous rupture of the pregnant uterus. Jones and Mitler[48] reported rupture of the uterus in a gravid bicornuate uterus infected with *Bacteroides* and *Clostridial* organisms. Lindberg[49] recorded a case of uterine rupture from a β-hemolytic streptococcal infection after cervical cerclage.

Morbidity and Mortality

An examination of morbidity and mortality from rupture of the pregnant uterus must consider several confounding variables. The threat to mother and baby varies with the length of gestation at the time of rupture and with placental implantation in relation to the rupture site. Additional factors include the presence or absence of previous uterine scars, the extent of the rupture, and the inciting event, whether spontaneous or traumatic. The variables are so confounding that estimations of morbidity and mortality rates should be directed at specific segments of the spectrum of uterine rupture.

Dehiscence of a scar from a previous cesarean section is the most frequent type of uterine rupture encountered in the practice of obstetrics and gynecology. All obstetric surgeons have encountered these openings in thin, white, relatively avascular scars through which amniotic membranes are visible or extruded. Problems occur when the membranes rupture, the placenta is directly under the dehiscence, or the dehiscence extends into the uterine vessels. The strength of the healed scar and the location of the placenta in relation to the scar are important considerations when contemplating vaginal deliveries after a previous cesarean birth. Both factors are particularly difficult to assess.

Rupture of the scarred uterus causes less blood

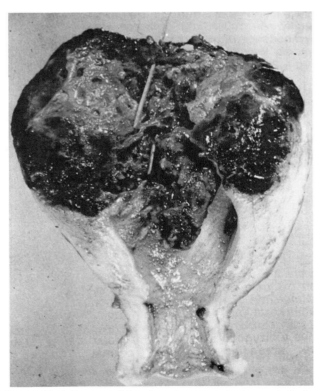

Figure 13–5. Rupture of the uterus because of advanced choriocarcinoma.

loss and threat to the life of the baby and mother than does rupture of the intact organ.[16] Our literature survey from 1978 to 1983 indicated a maternal mortality rate of 13.5% for 162 complete ruptures of the intact uterus. All mothers survived the 38 complete ruptures of the scarred uterus. Fetal mortality was 76.1% in complete ruptures of the intact uterus, compared with 32.4% in complete ruptures of the scarred uterus. Ruptures of the scarred uterus clearly present only a small threat to the life of the mother when operating facilities, surgical skills, blood transfusions, and potent antibiotics are rapidly available. The threat to the baby, despite dramatic improvement in neonatal intensive care, remains considerable.

Extensive ruptures of uterine scars before term occur most often in uteri that bear vertical scars extending into the fundal portion of the uterus. Incisions were involved in 68% of the ruptures of vertical scars and 12% of catastrophic ruptures in our review.[16] The number of classic sections in the risk pool was unknown. Separation of a classic scar opens a large portion of the anterior uterine wall. This disrupts large uterine vascular channels and is likely to expose a portion of the placental implantation site. Both of these factors provoke brisk bleeding. Rupture of classic scars is often a dramatic event accompanied by intraperitoneal and vaginal bleeding, abdominal pain, and fetal distress or death.

Rupture of a transverse scar is less explosive than rupture of a classical scar but should not be dismissed as an insignificant event. Sixty percent of uterine scar disruptions occur in transverse scars. Transverse scar ruptures during labor tend to be relatively innocuous dehiscences. They are much less vascular and less likely to involve the placental implantation site than are vertical scars. The threat to mother and baby is therefore greatly reduced. Many dehiscences of transverse cesarean scars are partial, small, and asymptomatic.

The descriptions of typical vertical and transverse scar dehiscences do not hold true for every case. I and my colleagues have performed a repeat cesarean on a symptom-free patient and found complete bivalving of a classic scar. There was little bleeding, despite total extrusion of a live baby into the free peritoneal cavity. We have also seen extensive transverse scar dehiscences extend into the major uterine vessels and broad ligament with devastating consequences.

Traumatic ruptures are among the most difficult cases of obstetric uterine rupture. Automobile accidents, gunshot wounds, and stab wounds to the abdomen of pregnant patients carry high risk of morbidity and mortality for the mother and especially for the fetus. Franger and co-workers[43] reported a 47 to 71% perinatal mortality from gunshot wounds of the uterus. Such cases are seldom simple and often require the skills of a multidisciplinary team of surgeons.

Spontaneous rupture of the intact pregnant uterus is a rare but catastrophic event that poses great risk to mother and baby. Spontaneous rupture of the intact uterus before labor is much more devastating than most scar separations that occur during labor. These ruptures may occur at any time during pregnancy but are most common in the last trimester.

Spontaneous ruptures of aberrant implantations in the cornual portion of the uterus, in anomalous uterine horns, or in the cervix usually occur in the middle trimester of gestation. These ruptures may be life threatening for the mother and are usually fatal to the fetus. Cornual, cervical, and other extratubal ectopic pregnancies are discussed fully in Chapter 9.

Diagnosis

Spontaneous occult dehiscence of the central portion of transverse uterine scars often occurs without symptoms or signs. It is encountered as an incidental finding at the time of repeat cesarean delivery or at the time of uterine exploration after delivery.

Table 13–7 outlines features of diagnostic value in cases of overt uterine rupture. The classic signs are vaginal hemorrhage, shock, cessation of labor, and recession of the presenting part. This tetrad is easily recognized but seldom seen. The physician hopes to recognize early signs of the disorder in order to intervene effectively. Premonitory signs seldom appear before the actual rupture.

There have been instances of fortuitous recognition of asymptomatic uterine dehiscence by ultrasonic imaging.[50] Fetal stress occasionally is detected during routine electronic monitoring. The mother may complain of unusual suprapubic discomfort or tenderness. These signs appear immediately preceding or during the rupture event.

Loss of pressure in an intrauterine pressure transducer system occurs in some cases of uterine rupture. Loss of catheter pressure is not a rare

Table 13–7. UTERINE RUPTURE—INTRAPARTAL DIAGNOSIS*

Maternal anxiety
Vascular instability and shock
Vaginal bleeding
Fetal distress or demise
Pain not associated with contractions
Cessation of labor
Recession of presenting part
Easily palpable fetal parts through abdominal wall
Point tenderness of uterus
Ultrasound evidence of rupture or extrusion of uterine contents
Decompression of intrauterine pressure catheter
Signs of peritoneal irritation

*All diagnostic signs and symptoms may be present in varying degrees or may be entirely absent.

event in normal labor monitoring. This sign is not reliable. Rodriguez and colleagues[51] reviewed 76 cases of uterine rupture, 39 of which had intra-uterine pressure catheters. Loss of pressure was not observed in any of the patients.

Interval hysterograms or ultrasound imaging before labor may identify some distorted uterine scars. This does not always presage rupture. Visual perfection of a scar similarly does not guarantee its tensile strength. There are, at present, no reliable signs, symptoms, or tests that allow the physician to predict which scars or uteri will re-main intact or rupture before or during labor.

CONFIRMATION OF SUSPECTED UTERINE RUPTURE

Massive spontaneous or traumatic prepartal uterine ruptures are suspected from the history and signs of shock, vaginal bleeding, fetal death or distress, and an acute abdominal emergency. Confirmation of diagnosis is by laparotomy.

Intrapartal, major, complete ruptures of the uterus are usually found among cases of severe postpartum hemorrhage after difficult labor or instrumental delivery. Confirmation of the diag-nosis in these cases depends on careful examina-tion of the pelvic organs and genitalia to rule out other causes of postpartum bleeding and rule out a rent in the wall of the uterus.

POSTPARTUM MANUAL EXPLORATION OF THE UTERINE CAVITY

The obstetrician carefully introduces his or her dominant hand into the uterus and palpates the endometrial cavity in a systematic fashion, feeling for a gap in the wall of the uterus. The lower uterine segment after vaginal delivery is normally thin and buttery soft. The uterus may be intact yet feel almost as though no uterine wall exists. It is very difficult to be certain of the presence or absence of a lower segment tear under these cir-cumstances.

Anterior isthmic or upper cervical ruptures are identified when the fingers pass through a rent and are felt by the abdominal hand. The inside fingers feel as though they are just beneath the anterior abdominal wall. Palpation of bowel or other organs is certain confirmation of major rup-ture but is seldom detected in ruptures of the lower uterus.

Ruptures of the posterior uterus are not rare. They are difficult to detect and are often not considered by the inexperienced examiner.

Massive bleeding often signals a lateral tear into the major uterine vessels. The lateral portion of the isthmus of the uterus and the upper cervix must be carefully assessed. The fingers may enter a full-thickness tear in the uterine wall and pass right into the broad ligament. The diagnosis is then sufficiently confirmed to warrant laparotomy.

Complete ruptures that extend into the anterior fundal portion of the uterus are easier to detect than lower segment ruptures. The uterine muscle at the junction of the upper cervix and myome-trium normally forms a firm ring that can be palpated around its entire circumference. A gap in this ring signals a rupture of the uterus until proved otherwise. Major ruptures may allow the examiner's fingers or entire hand to pass into the peritoneal cavity. Palpation of extrauterine organs may be possible. There can even be extrusion of bowel or omentum into the uterine cavity. The diagnosis is then obvious, and immediate laparot-omy is indicated.

Obstetricians are often insecure about their as-sessment of uterine integrity after delivery. Anx-iety increases with an unexplained postpartum hemorrhage. The uterine cavity should be exam-ined frequently after normal delivery, with close attention paid to the feel of the normal organ. This will increase an obstetrician's confidence in his or her ability to reliably detect an abnormality.

Given a massive postpartum hemorrhage and no other obvious cause, uterine rupture must be sus-pected. Laparotomy is the appropriate confirma-tory step as soon as proper preparations are com-plete. The patient should be stabilized while operating facilities, anesthesia, and blood replace-ment are prepared. The patient often cannot be stabilized in the presence of massive uterine rup-ture until bleeding is surgically secured. Prolonged attempts at stabilization before exploration can waste precious time.

Management of Asymptomatic Uterine Scar Dehiscence

Previous uterine scars should be carefully eval-uated after every subsequent delivery. The integ-rity of the previous scar determines current man-agement and influences advice to the patient about future pregnancies.

Small asymptomatic dehiscences that are en-countered at the time of repeat cesarean operation are simply debrided and closed with the uterine incision.

When small, asymptomatic dehiscences are de-tected after VBAC, current management practice favors observation of the patient and spontaneous healing. Wound dehiscence complicated by post-partum hemorrhage demands exploratory surgery.

What do we tell the patient with dehiscence of a previous cesarean scar about further pregnancies and surgical sterilization? If the patient wants another pregnancy, I recommend repeat cesarean birth near term without labor. The cesarean op-eration includes surgical sterilization by tubal ligation or hysterectomy, depending on coexisting problems. If the patient is certain she wants no more pregnancies, peripartal hysterectomy at the time the dehiscence is discovered is preferred.

Management of Major Uterine Rupture (Fig. 13–6)

Catastrophic obstetric uterine rupture is among the most dramatic and difficult obstetric problems. Such uterine ruptures challenge the skills and ingenuity of the most meticulously trained obstetric surgical team. Table 13–8 outlines the limited choices available to an obstetric surgeon addressing the problem of major uterine rupture.

UTERINE PACKING

Packing the uterus for postpartum hemorrhage was commonplace in the era preceding safe obstetric surgery. Packing a uterus when uterine rupture is diagnosed or suspected is only a stopgap measure, not a definitive treatment.

An incomplete rupture without major arterial bleeding may occasionally be controlled with packing. Blood loss can be reduced while preparations are made for definitive surgical treatment. Successful packing dramatically reduces blood loss from the uterus. The obstetrician who chooses to use an intrauterine pack must introduce fold after fold of gauze packing into the uterine cavity (see Chapter 22 for details).

Uterine packs do not always control uterine bleeding; indeed, some surgeons feel that the packs

Table 13–8. UTERINE RUPTURE—MANAGEMENT OPTIONS

Uterine packing*
Débridement and repair
Peripartal hysterectomy
Subtotal (supracervical)
Complete
Internal iliac artery ligation*

*Auxiliary procedure; seldom definitive therapy.

never control it. Packs have several possible complications. Among the most common are perforation of the uterus and endomyometritis. Placing a uterine pack can extend a previous laceration of the uterus. Uterine packing requires repeated entries into the uterine cavity with an instrument that can perforate the uterus. Bacteria are introduced into the uterus with each transit of the cervix.

The pack that successfully controls bleeding should be left in no longer than 12 to 24 hours. It is then removed slowly and gently while oxytocics are administered to ensure tight uterine contraction. Pack removal requires only analgesia, not general anesthesia.

Packing and expectant management do not allow assessment of retroperitoneal or intraperitoneal bleeding. The extent of the injury to the uterus or other abdominal organs cannot be evaluated. Uterine packing is therefore seldom the wisest management choice for uterine rupture in modern obstetrics.[52] Extensive ruptures of the uterus are now commonly managed by exploratory surgery with either repair of the defect or removal of the uterus.

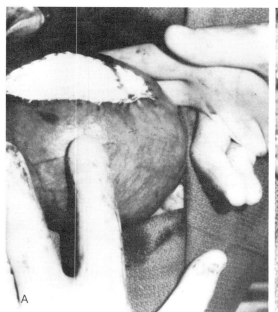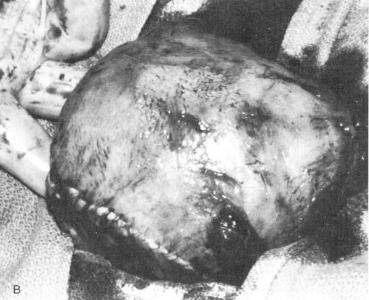

Figure 13–6. *A,* Repair of a spontaneous midtrimester uterine rupture using a synthetic fiber textile patch (Gore-Tex). Pregnancy continued to near term when cesarean delivery was performed. *B,* Gore-Tex soft tissue patch repair of uterine rupture. The appearance of the repair site at cesarean delivery near term. (From Martin JN Jr, Brown DW, Rush LV Jr, et al: Successful pregnancy outcome following mid-gestational uterine rupture and repair utilizing Gore-Tex soft tissue patch. Obstet Gynecol 75:518–521, 1990. Courtesy James N. Martin, Jr., M.D.)

In addressing major uterine rupture, the surgeon must decide whether or not to remove the uterus. If the patient's condition is unstable and the surgeon is not comfortable with the concept of peripartal hysterectomy, hemostatic repair of the rupture may be the safest course. The obstetric surgeon who is trained and capable of rapid, safe peripartal hysterectomy has a choice. He or she may attempt to repair the rent in the uterus or remove the uterus.

The uterus that has explosive damage and is beyond safe repair should be removed. Removal of the uterus may also be suggested when the patient is a multipara with previous cesarean deliveries who does not want more children. The presence of other gynecologic disorders such as uterine leiomyomata may influence this decision. This subject is discussed fully in Chapter 27 on peripartal hysterectomy.

SUTURE REPAIR OF UTERINE RUPTURE

Repair rather than removal of the ruptured uterus has found favor in the recent obstetric literature. Aguero and Kizer,[53] from Caracas, reported a large series of suture repairs in 462 (67.5%) of 684 uterine ruptures and dehiscences. Their survey of the literature revealed that 41.3% of uterine ruptures were managed by suture repair.

Sheth,[54] from Bombay, reported a series of 110 uterine ruptures, 66 (63%) of which were managed by suture repair. In Mexico, Reyes-Ceja and co-workers[55] reported 100 uterine ruptures, 65% of which were managed by hysterorrhaphy rather than hysterectomy. These investigators believed that, in their environments, repair was safer than hysterectomy.

TECHNIQUE OF UTERINE REPAIR AFTER RUPTURE

Repair of minor uterine ruptures and wound dehiscences discovered at the time of repeat cesarean entails no more than simple débridement and resuturing of the wound. Old scar tissue is removed and the dehiscence is closed with the current cesarean incision.

Repair of major uterine ruptures is much like the layered closure of a classical cesarean incision. Blood loss must first be rapidly controlled to stabilize the patient and clear the operative field. Control of blood loss may require uterine artery ligation, internal iliac artery ligation, or transient aortic compression. The full extent of the injury must be inspected before the decision is made whether to repair or remove the uterus.

The repair site must be débrided of all necrotic and ragged tissues. What remains should be a smooth although perhaps irregular wound in the myometrial wall. This wound can be closed with two or three layers of continuous absorbable suture such as 0 chromic or 00 polyglactin/polyglycolic suture. The first row of sutures approximates the deep myometrium, inverting the endometrium into the uterine cavity. A second layer closes the bulk of the myometrial wall. A third layer is often necessary for neat closure of the subserosal myometrium and visceral peritoneum.

What is the fate of the repaired uterine rupture in subsequent pregnancy? A body of literature is building on this subject. Sheth[54] reported 21 pregnancies in 13 patients who had suture repairs of previous uterine ruptures. Seventeen pregnancies occurred in 11 patients after repair of a lower segment rupture, with only one repeat rupture. Four pregnancies were recorded in two patients after suture repair of a rupture in the fundal portion of the uterus. Three of these reruptured, and only one child survived.

Reyes-Ceja and co-workers[55] recorded 22 pregnancies in 19 patients with previous uterine rupture. It was the policy of these authors to deliver subsequent pregnancies by cesarean operation at 38 weeks' gestation. Eight pregnancies culminated in vaginal delivery, however. Only one (4.5%) repeat uterine rupture was encountered. This was an incomplete rupture discovered on examination of the uterus after a vaginal delivery. The Reyes-Ceja group felt that pregnancy after repaired uterine rupture was appropriate. They suggested that international consensus favors cesarean delivery for patients with pregnancies after repair of uterine rupture.

In 1971 Ritchie[56] reported a series of 36 pregnancies in 28 patients after uterine rupture. There were two reruptures (5.5%) in his group, both of classical scars. Ritchie's survey of the literature of the classical cesarean era before 1932 revealed 86 pregnancies after uterine rupture with 52 (61%) repeat ruptures. Ritchie's data from 1932 to 1971 are summarized in Table 13–9. There were a total of 253 pregnancies in 194 patients with previous uterine rupture. Rerupture occurred in 10% of cases and resulted in 2 maternal deaths (0.8%) and 11 perinatal deaths (5.9%) (Table 13–10). Ruptures of classical scars dominated these statistics and were responsible for the most severe cases.

Table 13–9. PREGNANCIES AFTER SUTURE REPAIR OF UTERINE RUPTURE BY TYPES OF PREVIOUS SCARS

	Number	% of Cases
Patients	194	
Pregnancies	253	
Site of original scar		
Classical	94	48
Lower segment	28	15
Not recorded	72	37

Adapted from Ritchie EH: Pregnancy after rupture of the pregnant uterus. J Obstet Gynaecol Br Commonw 78:642, 1971.

The patient's wish for future pregnancies influences the choice to repair rather than remove a uterus that has ruptured. The risk of rerupture must be considered and communicated clearly to the patient and her family. More long-term follow-up of such cases is needed for certain prognosis. The body of literature currently available indicates that subsequent pregnancy imposes a modest risk of rerupture of the repaired uterus and a small risk of maternal death.

Most of the risk of rerupture accrues to cases of repaired fundal ruptures. A tubal sterilization procedure with rupture repair or hysterectomy should be considered for patients who experience major fundal ruptures unless they insist on future pregnancies. Repaired ruptures of the lower segment appear safer for another pregnancy.

INTERNAL ILIAC (HYPOGASTRIC) ARTERY LIGATION

Ligation of the anterior division of the internal iliac (hypogastric) arteries reduces blood flow and pulse pressure to the site of a major uterine rupture and clears the operating field for safe dissection (Fig. 13–7*A* and *B*). Ligation usually must be performed on both sides because of extensive collateral circulation. Internal iliac ligation is an auxiliary operation to control blood loss and is not sufficient treatment for most cases of rupture of the gravid uterus. The utility of transient aortic compression should be recalled when nothing else will stem the hemorrhagic tide. Internal iliac artery ligation is discussed in detail in Chapter 22.

Table 13–10. OUTCOME OF PREGNANCIES AFTER SUTURE REPAIR OF UTERINE RUPTURE (1932–1971)

	Number	Rate
Pregnancies	253	
Outcome		
Rerupture	25	10%
Maternal death	2	0.8%
Perinatal death	11*	5.9%

*Thirty-nine abortions not included; 174 surviving infants.
Adapted from Ritchie EH: Pregnancy after rupture of the pregnant uterus. J Obstet Gynaecol Br Commonw 78:642, 1971.

HYSTERECTOMY FOR UTERINE RUPTURE

Removal of the ruptured uterus is a proper choice when the uterus is damaged beyond safe repair. Hysterectomy in these cases may be a life-saving procedure. The procedure for peripartal hysterectomy is described in detail in Chapter 27.

The surgeon must remember to examine the entire abdomen for injuries and to repair other injured organs. The bowel, bladder, ureters, and adnexal structures are at greatest risk. Organs as distant as the liver and spleen may be involved in blunt trauma cases or penetrating injuries to the pregnant abdomen.

Whether to perform a complete or subtotal peripartal hysterectomy has been argued for years. At the Department of Obstetrics and Gynecology at LSU, we have consistently recommended total hysterectomy whenever this procedure is feasible.

A uterine rupture confined to the fundus of the uterus in an unstable patient can be addressed by subtotal (supracervical) hysterectomy. This oper-

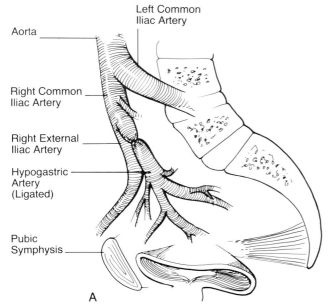
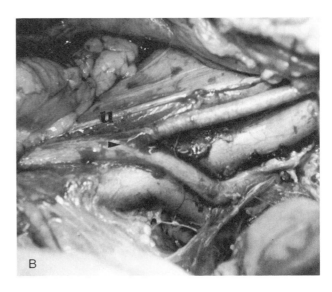

Aorta
Left Common Iliac Artery
Right Common Iliac Artery
Right External Iliac Artery
Hypogastric Artery (Ligated)
Pubic Symphysis
A
B

Figure 13–7. *A.* Blood vessels of the right lateral pelvic wall. *B,* The vessels of the left lateral pelvic wall. The common iliac artery (at the 9 o'clock position) bifurcates into the external iliac artery (anterior) and the internal iliac (hypogastric) artery (posterior). Note the intimate relationships with the accompanying iliac veins and the ureter (U). (Courtesy Ruth Higdon, M.D.; photographed by Rita L. Letellier.)

ation is certainly faster and easier than complete hysterectomy. It is difficult to be certain of the lower extent of a uterine tear at the time of operation. If the rupture extends into the lower segment and cervix, subtotal hysterectomy will not suffice. It is a major tragedy to perform laparotomy and partial hysterectomy on a patient with postpartum hemorrhage only to have bleeding continue unabated after surgery because of uterine rupture that extends into the cervix.

Regular screening for pelvic cancer must be emphasized to patients after subtotal hysterectomy. Many of these patients may not return for long-term follow-up examinations. The insidious development of cancer in a cervical stump is often not discovered until late in the disease. Complete hysterectomy is recommended as the definitive treatment whenever feasible.

LEIOMYOMAS IN PREGNANCY

Leiomyomas (fibroids) of the uterus complicate approximately 1.5% of pregnancies.[57] They influence pregnancy adversely in several ways. Rice and colleagues[57] indicated that 15% of 93 patients with leiomyomas complicating pregnancy required narcotic analgesia at some time during pregnancy. Twenty percent of their patients experienced premature labor.

Submucous fibroids cause some abortions. A 57% incidence of abruptio placentae is reported when myomas underlie the placental implantation site.[57] Intramural leiomyomas can distort the uterine cavity and cause abnormal fetal positions and presentations. Large fibroids can distort the birth canal and obstruct descent of the fetus during labor (Fig. 13–8).[58]

Torsion

Torsion of a pedunculated leiomyoma presents much the same clinical picture as torsion of an adnexal mass. The patient has acute abdominal pain, peritoneal irritation, and an exquisitely tender pelvic or abdominal mass. The mass may be confirmed and described by imaging techniques. The presence of a surgical abdomen mandates exploratory laparotomy at any stage of gestation.

Management at the time of exploratory surgery is usually simple. In most cases a vertical low abdominal incision will allow adequate exposure and extended exploration of the abdomen if necessary. The involved leiomyoma may be cyanotic or completely infarcted. The surgeon doubly clamps the twisted pedicle with Kelly or Ochsner (Kocher) clamps. Care must be taken to ensure that the ureter or other structures have not become involved in the mass or its pedicle. The surgeon divides the pedicle between clamps and removes the mass.

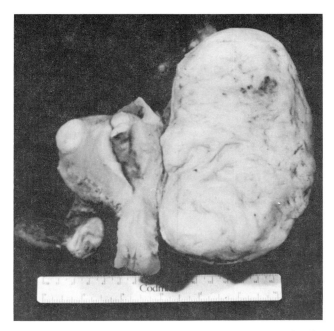

Figure 13–8. Uterine leiomyomas may cause recurrent abortion (submucous) or obstruction of labor (intramural or subserous), or may undergo degeneration during pregnancy. (Courtesy Michael Graham, M.D.; photographed by Rita L. Letellier.)

Degeneration

Leiomyomas are subject to a unique form of "red degeneration" during pregnancy. Red degeneration usually occurs in the second trimester of pregnancy.[57] It starts with acute edema of the tumor. The tumor capsule and its peritoneal covering are stretched, causing severe pain. The leiomyoma develops liquefaction necrosis accompanied by some interstitial hemorrhage. These events give the tumor its characteristic red color and soft consistency. Makar and colleagues[46] reported a rare case of uterine perforation that resulted from rupture of a leiomyoma undergoing red degeneration.

Pregnant patients who present with acute abdominal pain are always a difficult problem in differential diagnosis.[59] Degeneration of leiomyomas causes the acute onset of abdominal pain that is localized to the offending fibroid and often quite severe. There are often signs of localized peritoneal irritation. There is usually an area of exquisite tenderness on the pregnant uterus that may contain one or more fibroids.

The patient is obviously uncomfortable. She may exhibit mild fever and leukocytosis. There is difficulty in differentiating the symptom complex from appendicitis when the pain is in the right lower abdomen. Serum levels of smooth muscle enzyme markers, glutamic-oxaloacetic transaminase, and lactate dehydrogenase may be elevated.[58]

Ultrasound imaging can confirm the presence of leiomyomas. Ultrasound follows the progress of necrosis by the appearance and changes in sono-lucent areas within the tumor. Laparoscopy is occasionally necessary for definitive diagnosis. Laparoscopy is particularly useful in early pregnancy when ectopic gestation is a major differential diagnostic consideration.

Management of degenerating leiomyomas in pregnancy usually consists of support, rest, and analgesia. The course may be prolonged for several weeks. The intensity and duration of discomfort challenge the tolerance of the patient and physician.

Surgical excision is rarely necessary or indicated. The tumor site is very vascular and does not hold sutures well. Attempts to excise the tumor risk uncontrollable hemorrhage, premature labor, and loss of the pregnancy.

Hysterectomy may be required to control hemorrhage from dissection at the site of a necrotic leiomyoma in pregnancy. If it becomes necessary to excise a degenerating fibroid, these risks must be made clear to the patient. Permission should be obtained before laparotomy for both hysterectomy and pregnancy termination as well as myomectomy.

References

1. Kellogg FS: Puerperal inversion of the uterus: Classification for treatment. Am J Obstet Gynecol 18:815, 1929.
2. Watson P, Besch N, Bowes WA: Management of acute and subacute puerperal inversion of the uterus. Obstet Gynecol 55:12, 1980.
3. Quilligan EJ, Zuspan F (eds.): Douglas-Stromme Operative Obstetrics, 4th Edition. New York: Appleton-Century-Crofts, 1982, pp. 764.
4. Das P: Inversion of the uterus. J Obstet Gynaecol Br Emp 47:525, 1940.
5. Catanzarite VA, Moffitt KD, Baker ML, et al.: New approaches to the management of acute puerperal uterine inversion. Obstet Gynecol 68:7S, 1986.
6. Townsend HH: Acute puerperal uterine inversion: Report of a case and review of management. JAOA 84:282, 1984.
7. Rodriguez MH, Wang R, Clark SL, et al.: Previous cesarean birth: Management considerations in the patient with acute puerperal uterine inversion. Am J Obstet Gynecol 150:433, 1984.
8. Shah-Hosseini R, Evrard JR: Puerperal uterine inversion. Obstet Gynecol 73:567, 1989.
9. Gross RC, McGahan JP: Sonographic detection of partial uterine inversion. Am J Radiol 144:761, 1985.
10. Haultain FWN: The treatment of chronic uterine inversion by abdominal hysterotomy, with a successful case. Br Med J 2:974, 1901.
11. Johnson AB: A new concept in the replacement of the inverted uterus and a report of nine cases. Am J Obstet Gynecol 57:557, 1949.
12. Kovacs BW, DeVore GR: Management of acute and subacute puerperal uterine inversion with terbutaline sulfate. Am J Obstet Gynecol 150:784, 1984.
13. Thiery M, Delbeke L: Acute puerperal uterine inversion: Two-step management with a β-mimetic and a prostaglandin. Am J Obstet Gynecol 153:891, 1985.
14. Spinelli PG: Inversion of the uterus. Riv Ginec Contemp 1:1, 1897.
15. Huntington JL, Irving FC, Kellog FS: Abdominal reposition in acute inversion of the puerperal uterus. Am J Obstet Gynecol 15:34, 1928.
16. Plauché WC, Von Almen W, Muller R: Catastrophic uterine rupture. Obstet Gynecol 64:792, 1984.
17. Schwartz OH, Paddock R, Bortnick AR: The cesarean scar: An experimental study. Am J Obstet Gynecol 25:962, 1938.
18. Morrison J: Vaginal delivery after cesarean section. Am J Obstet Gynecol 146:262, 1983.
19. Merrill BS, Gibbs CE: Planned vaginal delivery following cesarean section. Obstet Gynecol 52:50, 1978.
20. Meier P, Porreco R: Trial of labor following cesarean section: A two year experience. Am J Obstet Gynecol 144:671, 1982.
21. Lavin J, Stephens R, Miodovnik M, et al.: Vaginal delivery in patients with a prior cesarean section. Am J Obstet Gynecol 59:135, 1982.
22. Graham AR: Trial of labor following previous cesarean section. Am J Obstet Gynecol 149:35, 1984.
23. Chestnut D, Eden RD, Gall SA, et al.: Peripartum hysterectomy. Obstet Gynecol 65:365, 1985.
24. Pruett KM, Kirshon B, Cotton DB: Unknown uterine scar and trial of labor. Am J Obstet Gynecol 159:807, 1988.
25. Garnett JD: Uterine rupture during pregnancy: An analysis of 133 patients. Obstet Gynecol 23:898, 1964.
26. Palerme GR, Friedman EA: Rupture of the gravid uterus in the third trimester. Am J Obstet Gynecol 94:571, 1966.
27. American College of Obstetricians and Gynecologists: Guidelines for Vaginal Delivery after a Cesarean Birth. Statements of the Committee on Obstetrics: Maternal and Fetal Medicine. Washington, DC: American College of Obstetricians and Gynecologists, 1989.
28. Keifer WS: Rupture of the uterus. Am J Obstet Gynecol 89:335, 1964.
29. Eden RD, Parker RT, Gall SA: Rupture of the pregnant uterus: A 53-year review. Obstet Gynecol 68:671, 1986.
30. Shrinsky DC, Benson RC: Rupture of the pregnant uterus: A review. Obstet Gynecol Surv 33:217, 1978.
31. Nielsen TF, Ljungblad U, Hagberg H: Rupture and dehiscence of cesarean section scar during pregnancy and delivery. Am J Obstet Gynecol 160:569, 1989.
32. Woodbridge A, Gonsoulin W: Trial of Labor after Cesarean Birth: The UMC Lafayette Experience. LSU resident research day presentation, New Orleans, October 1988.
33. Meehan FP, Magani IM: True rupture of the cesarean section scar (a 15 year review, 1972–1987). Br J Obstet Gynecol Reprod Biol 30:129, 1989.
34. Dunnihoo DR, Otterson WN, Mailhes JB, et al.: An evaluation of uterine scar integrity after cesarean section in rabbits. Obstet Gynecol 73:390, 1989.
35. Golan A, Sanbank O, Tear AJ: Trauma in late pregnancy. S Afr Med J 547:161, 1980.
36. McNabey W, Smith EI: Penetrating wound of the gravid uterus. J Trauma 12:1024, 1972.
37. Adams DM, Druzin ML, Cederqvist LL: Intrapartum uterine rupture. Obstet Gynecol 73:471, 1989.
38. Awais GM, Lebherz TB: Ruptured uterus: A complication of oxytocin induction and high parity. Obstet Gynecol 36:465, 1970.
39. McCarthy T, McQueen J: Uterine rupture as a complication of second trimester abortion using intraamniotic prostaglandin E2 and augmentation with other oxytocic agents. Prostaglandins 19:849, 1980.
40. Valenzuela G, Hayashi RH, Lackritz RM, et al.: Uterine rupture at term with vaginal prostaglandin E2. Am J Obstet Gynecol 138:1223, 1980.
41. Sawyer MM, Lipshitz J, Anderson GD, et al.: Third-trimester uterine rupture associated with vaginal prostaglandin E2. Am J Obstet Gynecol 140:710, 1981.
42. Degefu S, O'Quinn AG, Pernoll M, et al.: Stab wound of the gravid uterus: A case report and literature update. Journal of the Louisiana State Med Society 140:39, 1988.
43. Franger AL, Buchsbaum HJ, Peaceman AM: Abdominal gunshot wounds in pregnancy. Am J Obstet Gynecol 160:1124, 1989.
44. Dyer I, Barclay DL: Accidental trauma complicating pregnancy. Am J Obstet Gynecol 83:907, 1962.

45. Taylor PJ, Cumming DC: Spontaneous rupture of a primigravid uterus. J Reprod Med 22:168, 1979.
46. Makar APh, Meulyzer PR, Vergote IB, et al.: A case report of unusual complication of myomatous uterus in pregnancy: Spontaneous perforation of myoma after red degeneration. Eur J Obstet Gynecol Reprod Biol 31:289, 1989.
47. Deaton JL, Maier D, Andreoli J Jr: Spontaneous uterine rupture during pregnancy after treatment of Asherman's syndrome. Am J Obstet Gynecol 160:1053, 1989.
48. Jones DE, Mitler LK: Rupture of a gravid bicornuate uterus in a primigravida associated with *Clostridial* and *Bacteroides* infection. J Reprod Med 21:185, 1978.
49. Lindberg BS: Maternal sepsis, uterine rupture and coagulopathy complicating cervical cerclage. Acta Obstet Gynecol Scand 58:317, 1979.
50. Acton CM: The ultrasonic appearance of a ruptured uterus. Aust Radiol 22:254, 1978.
51. Rodriguez MH, Masaki DI, Phelan JP, et al.: Uterine rupture: Are intrauterine pressure catheters useful in the diagnosis? Obstet Gynecol 161:666, 1989.
52. Weingold AB, Sall S, Sherman DH, et al.: Rupture of the gravid uterus. Surg Gynecol Obstet 21:1233, 1966.
53. Aguero O, Kizer S: Suture of the uterine rupture. Obstet Gynecol 31:806, 1968.
54. Sheth SS: Results of treatment of rupture of the uterus by suturing. J Obstet Gynaecol Br Commonw 75:55, 1968.
55. Reyes-Ceja L, Cabrera R, Insfran E, et al.: Pregnancy following previous uterine rupture. Study of 19 patients. Obstet Gynecol 34:387, 1969.
56. Ritchie EH: Pregnancy after rupture of the pregnant uterus. J Obstet Gynaecol Br Commonw 78:642, 1971.
57. Rice JP, Kay HH, Mahony BS: The clinical significance of uterine leiomyomas in pregnancy. Am J Obstet Gynecol 160:1212, 1989.
58. Barter RH, Parks J: Myomas in pregnancy. Clin Obstet Gynecol 1:519, 1958.
59. Abramovici H, Factor JH: Uterine myomas during pregnancy. Am J Obstet Gynecol 140:484, 1981 [Letter].

14

Nonobstetric Abdominal Surgery During Pregnancy

James N. Martin, Jr.

Pregnancy and abdominal surgical disease of non-reproductive organs frequently occur simultaneously, either as independent or associated events.[1–5] The diagnosis and management of these conditions present many challenges to the obstetrician and his or her consultants. Not only are there myriad diagnostic possibilities to consider, but pregnancy alters the symptoms and signs normally associated with individual conditions and the normal ranges for many laboratory values. Thus, definitive diagnosis of a surgical condition often eludes the clinician, and procrastination leads to dangerous delays in the decision to operate. Reluctance to utilize indicated diagnostic irradiation or related techniques because of an irrational fear of fetal safety frequently and needlessly postpones diagnosis and ultimately worsens maternal and perinatal prognosis. The interests of the mother and child are best served by truly collaborative and sustained management of these patients by obstetrician-gynecologists, general surgeons, and anesthesiologists until complete disease resolution is achieved.

APPENDICITIS

The most common acute general surgical condition in nonpregnant or pregnant patients is acute appendicitis, with a peak occurrence during the second and third decades of life.[6, 7] It is the most common extrauterine complication of pregnancy for which a laparotomy is performed.[2, 4, 8–15] Appendicitis accounts for nearly two-thirds of all conditions in which laparotomy is performed during pregnancy. Its incidence is reported to range from 1 to 28 per 10,000 deliveries, with an average of 7 per 10,000.[4, 8, 16–25] Despite the progesterone-induced hypomotility of the intestinal tract, appendicitis does not appear to occur with greater frequency during gestation. It also appears to be unrelated to maternal age and parity. Although appendicitis can occur at any time during the antepartum, intrapartum, or postpartum period, the highest percentage of cases (about 50%) cluster in the second trimester.[4, 8, 12, 17, 18, 20, 22, 26–28]

Acute appendicitis almost always occurs following luminal obstruction.[6] Lymphoid tissue, fecalith, parasites (schistosomiasis),[29] foreign bodies, and benign or malignant tumors[30] can obstruct the appendiceal lumen. Distension, venous engorgement, arterial ischemia, bacterial overgrowth, suppuration, arterial ischemia, venous thrombosis, and, ultimately, perforation distal to the blocked lumen ensue. Inflammation surrounding the appendix and cellulitis or abscess may produce a palpable mass. With appendiceal perforation comes the release into the peritoneal cavity and surrounding tissues of bacteria-laden exudate and fecal material. The omentum and tissues proximate to the appendiceal rupture usually contain the spread of exudate and prevent its wider dissemination. Retroplacental appendiceal perforation may cause the formation of a large phlegmon.

Approximately 24 to 48 hours may pass from the time of initial appendiceal obstruction to perforation. For embryologic reasons, the visceral component of the pain is perceived in the periumbilical or epigastric areas, irrespective of actual appendiceal location. Pain localized to the appendiceal site occurs when the overlying parietal peritoneum is irritated.

Acute appendicitis during pregnancy is difficult to diagnose in spite of modern diagnostic and therapeutic techniques. Diversity of clinical presentation characterizes appendicitis, even in nonpregnant patients. The diagnosis is a frustrating challenge for those physicians with the welfare of two patients at stake. Diagnosis becomes progressively more difficult as the patient approaches term.[2, 18, 19, 22, 26–28] This is primarily because of upward displacement of the appendix during pregnancy, altered physiologic responses to the inflamed appendix, and the confusion of normal pregnancy symptoms with that of appendiceal inflammation.

Progressive displacement of the appendix by the enlarging uterus and the counterclockwise rotation of the tip of the uterus into the right upper quadrant have been described for almost 50 years (Fig. 14–1). In Baer's studies, 93% of appendices by the eighth month of gestation were above the iliac crest as opposed to the normal nonpregnant location below that line in the right lower quadrant in 65% of the cases, the pelvis in 30%, and retrocecal in 5%.[31] The abdominal wall is lifted away from the appendix by the enlarging uterus. Muscular laxity occurs, and the guarding, tenderness, and rebound generally associated with irritation of the parietal peritoneum may be diminished or absent.

Symptoms and signs unreliably distinguish the gravid patient with appendicitis from women with other disorders.[32] The most consistent clinical symptom encountered in acute appendicitis associated with pregnancy is vague right-sided abdom-

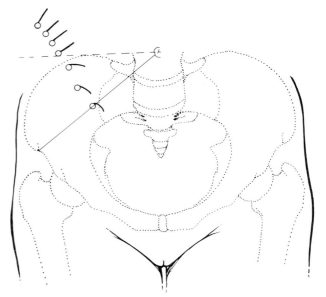

Figure 14–1. During pregnancy, the appendix is progressively displaced upward and outward by the enlarging uterus as the tip rotates counterclockwise. By midgestation, the appendix is usually at the level of the umbilicus.

inal pain. With the progression of pregnancy, pain associated with appendicitis may be located in the right upper quadrant, right side, or right flank. This pain, produced by inflammation and distension of the unruptured appendix, often is perceived in the periumbilical or epigastric areas without regard to the exact location of the appendix. In later stages of the disease, however, acute suppuration, gangrene, or perforation of the appendix produces a point of maximal tenderness resulting from contact of the inflamed appendix with the overlying peritoneum. A small number of patients may have little or no pain, particularly if the appendix is retrocecal and far removed from the abdominal wall.[8, 11, 24, 27, 33] The enlarging uterus late in gestation tends to keep the appendix away from the abdominal wall, leading to milder and less well localized symptoms that can confuse the clinician into a delay in diagnosis and a higher incidence of gangrene and perforation.

Although nausea is so common in the first trimester that it loses its significance as an early symptom of appendicitis, vomiting beyond the first trimester may be particularly significant. Approximately three of four gravid patients with appendicitis suffer from vomiting.[8, 12, 23] In contrast to almost universal occurrence in the nonpregnant patient, anorexia occurs in only 25 to 71% of all pregnant patients with appendicitis.[2, 12, 16, 23, 24, 27, 28]

Several aids to the physical diagnosis of appendicitis are available but none has been rigorously tested in the pregnant patient. Blumberg's sign describes the finding of rebound tenderness in the area of the appendix itself. A useful maneuver to differentiate uterine from appendiceal pain is to turn the patient on her left side while pressing on the point of maximal tenderness (Alder's sign).[34, 35] If the pain shifts to the left side after patient turning, pain is assumed to be of uterine or adnexal origin. If the pain remains in the right lower quadrant, appendicitis is suspected. If pain is elicited when the gravid uterus is shifted back to the right side when the patient is moved in that direction, then appendicitis is considered to be more likely (Bryant's sign).[13]

Rovsing's sign describes the production of right lower quadrant pain following pressure and release of the abdominal wall over the left lower quadrant and uterus.[17, 19, 22, 24] Markle's "heel-drop-jarring" test, involving striking or having the patient drop down abruptly on her heels, is alleged to elicit pain in the site of the inflamed appendix in 75% of cases.[36, 37] Closely related is "bump tenderness," elicited with jarring movements of the patient while she is being transported on a stretcher or a positive fanny-drop test, which is discomfort elicited by lifting up the patient's midsection and dropping it back onto the stretcher. Collected series reveal that guarding is present in slightly more than 50% of pregnant patients with appendicitis, rebound pain in about 75%, and less of both in later gestations.[8, 12, 22, 23, 27, 28]

At least half of all patients with acute appendicitis in pregnancy remain afebrile.[2, 12] An elevated temperature, however, may help make the diagnosis of appendiceal perforation. The highest pulse rates are also found in cases with perforation but may be less than 100 beats per minute even in the presence of significant disease.[22, 23, 27, 28] Because leukocytosis is physiologic in pregnancy, interpretation of white blood cell counts of up to 16,000/mm^3 and left shifts approaching 80% are problematic.[2, 8, 22, 27] If the white blood cell count is very high or progressively rising, it is a cause for concern relative to appendiceal perforation.[38] A minimum of 25% of patients with appendicitis have neither an elevated white blood cell count nor a left shift. A large number of white blood cells or bacteria in a catheterized specimen of urine suggests urinary tract infection or acute pyelonephritis with or without a stone as a cause for pain and elevated temperature. Close proximity of the urinary collecting system to an inflamed appendix late in pregnancy may result in pyuria, but usually there are less than 10 white blood cells and few red blood cells per high power field. Pyuria and hematuria may occur in 10 to 29% of pregnant patients with appendicitis.[8]

The differential diagnosis of acute gestational appendicitis is extensive. Horowitz's compilation of data from 545 patients found that 73% of patients had acute appendicitis, 21% had nothing detectable, and 6% had a variety of conditions, including pyelonephritis, cholecystitis, twisted ovarian cysts, salpingitis, degenerating myomas, and infarcted or torsed adnexal tumors.[24] The correct diagnosis of appendicitis during pregnancy in published accounts ranges from 28 to 80%.[4, 8, 22, 26, 28, 39] Between 5 and 60% of pregnant patients have perforated appendices at surgery, a risk of almost 1 in 4.* The risk of perforation increases throughout gestation.

The use of graded compression ultrasonography in nonpregnant individuals has been reported to be helpful in the diagnosis of 75% of patients later shown to have appendicitis.[40, 41] Puylaert's group reported that ultrasonography used in this manner was specific in excluding the diagnosis in 100% of 31 patients without acute nonperforated appendicitis.[41] Similar investigations have not been performed in pregnant patients. The presence of an appendiceal abscess or appendolith (Fig. 14–2) may be apparent on ultrasonographic examination and thereby facilitate timely therapy.[42]

Thus, the diagnosis of appendicitis in pregnancy depends primarily on clinical acumen. Often history is more important than examination; pain migrating from the upper abdomen to the lower right quadrant is more likely appendicitis than

---

*See references 8, 9, 12, 17, 18, 20–24, 27, 28, and 35.

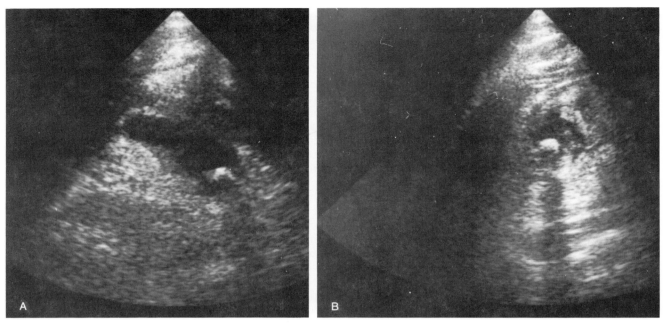

Figure 14–2. A, A large, tubular retrocecal appendix with an appendolith is seen in longitudinal and B, transverse ultrasonographic views (courtesy John Gibson, M.D.).

the upward migrating pain of pelvic inflammatory disease. Because physical findings and laboratory tests are often not sensitive or specific, the obstetrician and his or her consultants usually lack confidence in the diagnosis. The price of avoiding treatment delay is a degree of overdiagnosis, something that is expected in the nonpregnant patient in at least 30% of cases. The price of delay is underdiagnosis and probably higher maternal and perinatal morbidity and mortality. Surgical removal of the inflamed appendix more than 24 hours after the onset of symptoms is associated with an approximate increase in risk of perforation from one in three to 50%.[18, 28]

Prompt presumptive diagnosis and operative treatment, in addition to better fluid nutritional support, antibiotic availability, better anesthesia, and improved surgical technique, have resulted in a significant reduction from the 40% maternal mortality rate quoted by Babler in 1908.[43] When maternal deaths secondary to appendicitis have occurred in recent years, they have involved women with advanced, perforated appendices.[16] Perinatal loss is more a function of disease severity as a reflection of delayed diagnosis than of surgical intervention itself (3%). Fetal loss rates associated with unruptured, nonperforated appendicitis and disease with perforation in a total of 680 reported cases collected by McGee[25] were 29 and 187 in 1000, respectively.

The optimal management of appendicitis is always surgical. The best interests of the patient and progeny are served if the operation is undertaken immediately on making a reasonably certain diagnosis. After the first trimester of pregnancy, a 30-degree left tilt should be maintained during

surgery to improve uteroplacental blood flow, prevent supine hypotension, minimize uterine handling with the attendant risk of preterm labor, and finally, to improve access to the appendix. The majority of patients undergo general anesthesia, although spinal and epidural anesthesias have been utilized successfully.[32]

Pregnant patients with presumed appendicitis are prepared for surgery with intravenous fluid therapy using lactated Ringer's solution at a rate sufficient to establish adequate diuresis. Nasogastric intubation is undertaken with a sump-type tube to prevent vomiting with aspiration or acute gastric dilatation. Prior to surgery, broad-spectrum intravenous antibiotics are administered. These usually include an aminoglycoside, ampicillin, and clindamycin. Prophylactic antibiotics are utilized, presumably to reduce the incidence of postoperative intraperitoneal and wound complications. Although arguable, utilization of triple-drug therapy is particularly recommended for the patient with suspected perforation. Antibiotics are not continued postoperatively for more than two doses in nonperforated cases.[44]

The operative approach to a patient with appendicitis depends on the presumed location of the infected appendix, the trimester of pregnancy, and the body habitus of the patient.[6] The traditional approach to the first-trimester patient with suspected acute unruptured appendicitis is a McBurney (gridiron) or lower midline incision, or less frequently, a paramedian or Pfannenstiel incision (Fig. 14–3A). In the first trimester, when appendicitis is suspected the McBurney incision is preferred by many.[6, 16, 20, 22, 25, 26, 35] It affords adequate operative exposure and is stronger than other

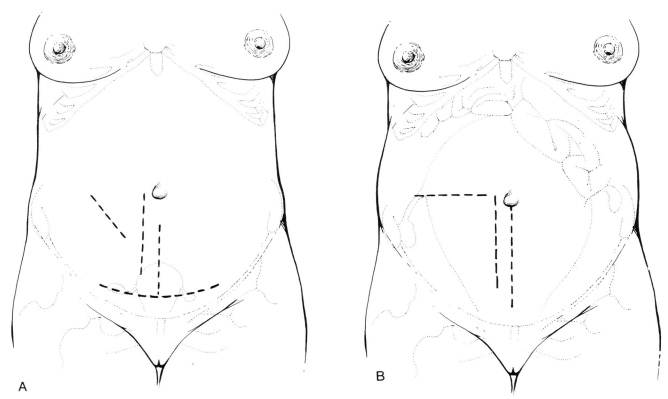

Figure 14–3. Surgical incisions are illustrated for use with appendectomy or other abdominal operations in *A*, first trimester gravidas, and *B*, those in the second or third trimesters.

types of incisions during the early postoperative period. The best rule is to make the midpoint of the incision over the area of maximal tenderness. Otherwise, the midpoint of the incision is placed over the McBurney point, which is at the junction of the lateral and middle thirds of a line drawn from the anterior superior spine to the umbilicus. The incisional direction is made parallel with the inguinal ligament.

The incision is carried sharply through the skin and subcutaneous tissue down to the fascia of the external oblique muscle. The thin fascial covering over this muscle is incised, and the muscle is split bluntly in the direction of its fibers. Using large hemostat forceps, the internal oblique muscle beneath the external oblique muscle is split again in the direction of its fibers to reveal the transverse muscle beneath it. It is split similarly to expose the preperitoneal fat and the peritoneum. The latter is grasped with forceps and incised in order to enter the peritoneal cavity. Enlargement of this wound can be undertaken by incision of the anterior rectus sheath, retraction of the rectus muscle medially, and incision of the posterior rectus sheath and peritoneum. The inferior epigastric vessels traversing posterior to the rectus muscle on the posterior rectus sheath are identified prior to incision and ligated.

The appendix and cecum are delivered into the incision. Babcock clamps are used to atraumatically grasp the appendix at its tip and near its base (Fig. 14–4). A 3–0 delayed absorbable suture is utilized to ligate en masse the mesoappendix, including the appendiceal artery. Otherwise, successive clamping of the mesosalpinx with Kelly clamps is undertaken with small bites and suture ligatures. Moistened packs are placed around the appendix to isolate it from the operative field. The appendix is crushed at its base with a Kelly or Halstead clamp, followed by placement of a medium ligature of absorbable suture at this site. A Kelly clamp is placed on the appendix a short distance distal to the ligature, leaving sufficient space between the ligature and the clamp to permit passage of a scalpel or an electrocautery.

The clamped appendix is amputated with a scalpel. The appendix, attached clamp, and the scalpel are dropped into a small basin and removed from the operative field as contaminated instruments. The ligature about the base of the appendix is now cut short, the distal ends of the stump are lightly cauterized, and the moist packs are removed from the field. The area is generously lavaged with warm saline or antibiotic-containing solution, and the procedure is completed. The ligated appendiceal stump is not buried.

Closure of the McBurney incision is performed with a continuous suture of 2–0 or 3–0 delayed absorbable suture in the fascia. Interrupted or continuous sutures in the fascia over the internal and external oblique muscles may be utilized to eliminate dead space. Skin staples or subcuticular

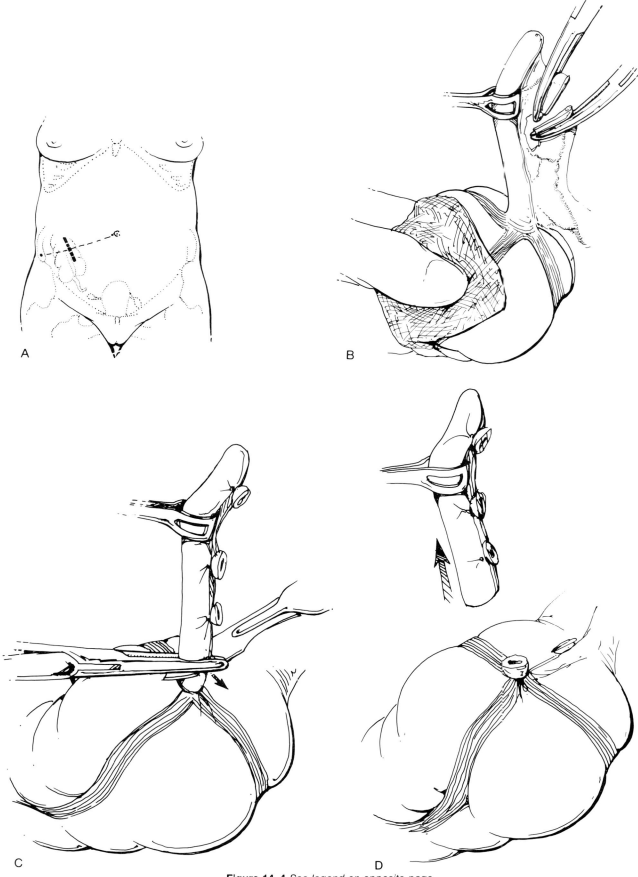

Figure 14–4 *See legend on opposite page*

sutures are then used to approximate the skin over the incised area. Skin staples are removed on the fourth postoperative day with placement of supportive Steri-Strips.

Surgical approach to the patient with suspected appendicitis in pregnancy during the second trimester is similar to the approach during the first trimester, although utilization of operative laparoscopy becomes technically more difficult. Utilization of a muscle-splitting transverse incision (Rocky-Davis or McArthur-McBurney) at a point over the area of maximal tenderness is recommended. Also, a lateral left tilt of the patient is performed in order to provide the best operative exposure and optimal uterine blood flow with the uterus off the inferior vena cava.

In the third trimester, a muscle-splitting incision centered over the point of maximal tenderness usually provides the best exposure to the appendix, especially when the patient is tilted approximately 30 degrees to the left (Fig. 14–3B). Others feel that a high paramedian incision is appropriate, particularly when the fetus is viable, because it allows greater operative flexibility. Although generally cesarean delivery is performed only for valid obstetric indications, cesarean birth in association with appendectomy may decrease fetal mortality in cases with appendiceal perforation close to term. The only other indications for cesarean section at the time of appendectomy include incontrovertible evidence of fetal distress, the presence of septic shock, and when access to the appendix is precluded unless the uterus is emptied of its contents.

A paramedian incision is a vertical skin incision made over the belly or lateral margin of the rectus muscle. It is carried through the fat layer to the anterior rectus fascia. This is incised at its lateral margin, and the muscle is deflected medially to expose the underlying peritoneum, which is opened in the usual fashion. Appendectomy is performed as described earlier, and the right paramedian incision is closed.

Very recently, the traditional approach has been supplanted in some hospitals by diagnostic and operative laparoscopy. Initially, laparoscopy was performed in cases of suspected appendicitis in pregnancy and laparotomy was undertaken immediately thereafter in positive cases.[45–49] Laparoscopy also has been utilized to direct the performance of appendectomy through an abdominal stab wound.[50] Most exciting has been the development by Semm and Schreiber of appendectomy by operative laparoscopy.[51–53]

Laparoscopic removal of the inflamed appendix has been performed up to the twenty-fifth week of gestation.[52] It has been emphasized that macroscopic or optical findings of the appendix do not always correlate with the histopathologic findings. Therefore, removal of the appendix is recommended in all situations in which abdominal pain leads the obstetric surgeon to operate on the pregnant abdomen for possible appendicitis.[1, 2, 8, 22, 52] Advantages of operative laparoscopy in this setting include the avoidance of postoperative adhesions, a reduced incidence of wound infection or abscess formation in the region of the abdominal wall, and more rapid postoperative recovery.

Laparoscopic appendectomy is undertaken in the manner described by Schreiber (Fig. 14–5).[52] After catheterization of the urinary bladder and preparation of the abdomen and umbilical fossa, the anesthetized patient in a 15- to 30-degree left lateral recumbent position undergoes a stab incision in the lower umbilical fossa. A Verres needle is introduced, and a pneumoperitoneum is applied under electronic control. The Verres needle should be introduced in a straight downward direction away from the uterus. By means of a Z-stab technique, the trocar cartridge is put into position to take the 7-mm Hopkins Lens System. Following a scout viewing of the abdomen, two 5-mm working trocar cartridges are introduced suprasymphysially. As the pregnant uterus increases above the pelvic brim, the perforations for the two 5-mm working trocars are placed sequentially higher in the right middle abdomen and not suprasymphysially as for a nonpregnant individual.

The lesser pelvis and pouch of Douglas are inspected, and the ovaries and tubes may be manipulated anteriorly with atraumatic forceps. If pathologic findings are present on the reproductive organs, these are treated first. Location of the vermiform appendix is followed immediately by blunt or sharp separation of adhesions from the immediate area with atraumatic forceps or tenacular scissors. The appendix is then grasped at the tip and sharply dissected from its mesoappendix. Prior thermocoagulation of the resection site is important. Small snips should be taken. If thermocoagulation is inadequate, such as in the case of a very thick mesoappendix with extensive fat deposits, a recoagulation of a bleeding site can

Figure 14–4. *A,* Standard appendectomy location of muscle splitting (Rocky-Davis) incision for uncomplicated appendectomy. The incision may be placed higher in advanced pregnancies, usually over the point of maximum tenderness. *B,* The cecum and the appendix are stabilized. The mesoappendix and accompanying appendiceal vessels are severed between hemostats. *C,* The base of the appendix is crushed and ligated with absorbable suture. The appendix is severed between the ligature and a clamp 1 cm distal to the ligature. *D,* The appendix is handed off the table with all contaminated instruments. The mucosa of the appendix stump is cauterized, and the area is generously layered with saline. The operation is then complete. It is not necessary to invert the appendix stump, although many surgeons do so.

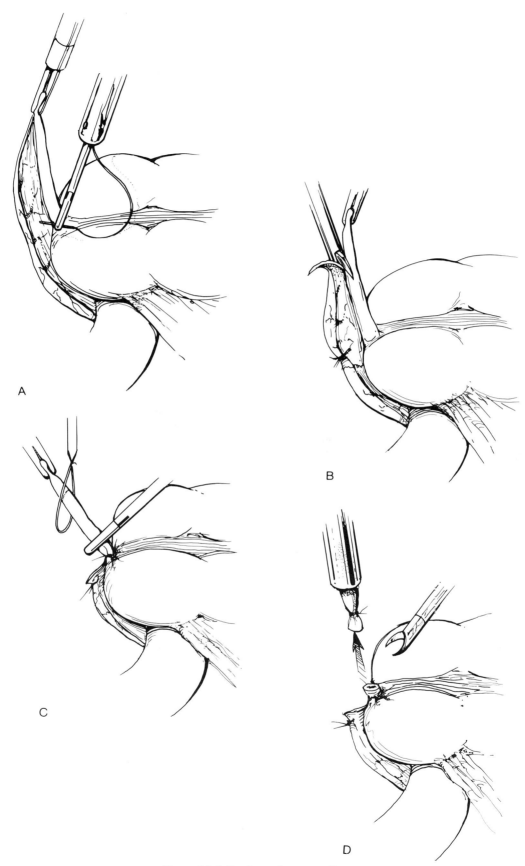

A

B

C

D

Figure 14–5 *See legend on opposite page*

then be performed without difficulty. Thermocoagulation is performed no closer than 5 mm from the cecum for no longer than 30 seconds at 90 to 100°C.

Usually, the appendicular artery can be exposed and ligated if necessary with a Roeder catgut ligature. Following appendiceal skeletonization, thermocoagulation is undertaken at the base for 20 to 30 seconds at 90 to 100°C, with the distance to the cecum corresponding to the length of the stump of 5 mm. These limits are not exceeded, because thermal damage to the cecal wall can evidently occur without the appearance of white discoloration of the serosa. In the region between the endocoagulated area and the orifice of the appendix into the cecum, two Roeder ligatures of 2–0 monofilament polypropylene are applied. The appendix is passed through the preknotted loop, after which the sutures are tightened. Proximal to the end of the endocoagulated area, a catgut ligature is applied in order to prevent peritoneal contamination with appendiceal contents.

The right 5-mm trocar is removed, the incision is extended to 11 mm, and the 11-mm trocar is introduced with the appendix extractor. This is a simple tube 10 mm in diameter and 19 cm in length without a valve but with a 5-mm rubber gasket. The tip of the appendix is pulled through the extractor with a gripping forceps and drawn out of the abdominal cavity after resection. The operation is concluded with stump disinfection with an iodine swab.

At the conclusion of the procedure, the upper abdomen is examined to visualize the liver, spleen, and gallbladder. Approximately 1 m of ileum is examined for a Meckel diverticulum. A skin suture is applied to the 11-mm perforation site, and the operation is concluded. Removal of the gaseous contents is undertaken with interrupted or continuous ligatures placed in the fascial tissue at puncture sites. The skin is reapproximated using Steri-Strips or fine suture. A laxative can be administered 24 hours after the operation, and liquids can be started in the absence of nausea. Hospitalization is continued for at least 24 hours or longer until recovery is clinically apparent.

Ideally, the fetal heart rate should be monitored throughout the operation in any pregnancy in which extrauterine fetal viability is a possibility.[54] However, logistic difficulties and problems with contamination of the operative field often limit such attempts. Under optimal circumstances when practical, gestations at more than or equal to 24 weeks should be monitored either by intermittent external fetal heart rate monitoring or ultrasonography to check fetal heart rates at intervals during the operative procedure. Continuous external electronic fetal heart rate monitoring via the abdominal wall away from the incisional site seems ideal, either by traditional equipment or by telemetry.

The finding of appendiceal perforation or free exudate in the abdomen necessitates suction removal of the fluid and generous irrigation of the abdomen with saline or antibiotic solution until the effluent solution is clear. Intraperitoneal lavage using antibiotic solutions has been recommended to decrease the incidence of wound and abscess complications. An appendiceal abscess site should be drained with a perforated wound hemovac catheter or soft suction drains brought out through a separate stab wound. Wound closure is altered in this circumstance with Smead-Jones or single-layer closure with 0 or 2–0 polyglycolic acid or monofilament, nonabsorbable suture, such as prolene or 28-gauge steel wire. Usually the operator either places a superficial wound drain in the incision with a separate stab exit site and closes the skin over it or leaves in place untied skin sutures, to be tied with secondary wound closure 72 hours after the completion of the operation.

Postoperative care of pregnant patients with appendicitis includes removal of the nasogastric tube and initiation of liquids on the first postoperative day or when peristalsis resumes. When appendiceal abscess, gangrenous appendicitis, or evidence of extensive peritonitis is present at the time of surgery, antibiotic therapy is continued postoperatively until the patient has been afebrile at least 24 hours.[44, 55] Early ambulation is encouraged. Strong bowel stimulants, such as enemas and suppositories, are discouraged for the first 4 postoperative days. Rarely, adult respiratory distress syndrome ensues in the critically ill gravida; termination of pregnancy to accelerate maternal recovery does not appear necessary.[2]

In any pregnancy after midgestation in which there is obvious peritonitis, utilization of prophylactic tocolytic therapy is recommended, although insufficient data are available to identify a threshold gestational age or an obvious benefit.[2] Otherwise, tocolytic therapy is withheld during most appendectomies, but the uterus is monitored for the first 24 to 48 hours postoperatively with electronic tocodynamometry monitoring when the gestation equals or exceeds 20 weeks.

Preterm labor becomes progressively more likely as the pregnancy approaches term (60% incidence

---

Figure 14–5. *A,* The appendix is located and stabilized. A Roeder catgut ligature secures the appendiceal artery. *B,* Tenacular scissors takes small snips of the mesoappendix. Thermocoagulation controls bleeding points. *C,* Thermocoagulation of the appendiceal base (20 to 30 seconds at 90 to 100° C). Two Roeder ligatures are applied to the appendix between the coagulated area and the cecum. *D,* A third ligature occludes the appendix above the coagulated area. The appendix is transected with tenacular scissors. The appendix is drawn out of the abdomen through the appendix extractor tube. The stump may be disinfected with an iodine swab.

in the third trimester),[56] and the appendicitis becomes complicated by perforation, peritonitis, and abscess formation.[4, 12, 23, 27, 28, 57] Most preterm labor associated with appendicitis occurs within 5 days of surgery.[2] However, preterm labor and fetal loss can occur several weeks after an apparently successful operation.[21, 28] There appears to be no objective evidence to encourage the utilization of progestational agents as tocolytic agents or for hormonal support. The use of supplemental progesterone during first trimester surgery for appendicitis has not been investigated. Preterm labor may be the only presenting sign of appendicitis.[28]

If the appendix is perforated or gangrenous at the time of appendectomy, if the uterus is involved in the process with peritonitis, and if the pregnancy is near term, cesarean hysterectomy may be seriously considered; increased maternal morbidity and mortality rates have been seen if the uterus is left in place.[16] The extent of infection, the parity of the patient, the length of gestation, the condition of the patient, and her desires regarding sterilization are all important factors involved in the decision whether to proceed with delivery or hysterectomy or both.

In the unusual occurrence of acute appendicitis during active labor, awaiting vaginal delivery is a safe course to follow if delivery is expected to occur within a reasonable period of 6 to 10 hours.[58] If the progress of labor is slow or desultory or if the maternal and fetal conditions deteriorate, exploration, possibly with cesarean delivery, is indicated. A vertical or right paramedian incision is appropriate in this circumstance. If prodromal labor is occurring, appendectomy can be performed with anticipated subsequent vaginal delivery.

Cesarean delivery is indicated in association with appendicitis only if there is evidence of overt fetal distress, insufficient access to the appendix, or extensive peritonitis with advanced gestational age.[8, 25, 59] Because intrauterine fetal demise has been observed following third-trimester appendectomy with perforation and peritonitis,[20, 21, 23, 57, 59, 60, 61] intensive fetal surveillance, with induction of labor when the fetus is mature, is recommended.

CHOLECYSTITIS AND CHOLECYSTECTOMY

Cholecystectomy is the second most frequent nongynecologic abdominal operation performed in pregnant women, exceeded only in frequency by appendectomy.[15, 62–64] The most common cause of cholecystitis is cholelithiasis. The incidence of cholelithiasis increases with age. For reasons not totally understood, changes in biliary lipid metabolism and gallbladder function because of altered biliary physiology during pregnancy result in an increased incidence of maternal gallstones.[33, 63, 65, 66] Approximately 3.5% of pregnant women harbor

gallstones, and during the second or third trimester of pregnancy, the gallbladder volume increases almost twofold.[67–69] Moreover, the rate and percentage of bile that is discharged from the gallbladder are reduced following stimulation.[70] Eighty-one percent of women who are destined to exhibit symptoms of gallbladder disease encounter their first symptoms within 1 year of pregnancy.[71]

The full range of gallbladder disease is seen in pregnancy, from mild biliary colic to severe gallbladder inflammation and infection. The incidence of gestational cholecystectomy generally has varied between 3 and 8 in 10,000 pregnancies, with higher rates (1 in 1000) reported from selected hospitals and referral medical centers.[5, 62, 63, 72–74]

Acute cholecystitis usually presents with the abrupt onset of epigastric pain that radiates into the right upper quadrant. During the last trimester of pregnancy, the point of maximal tenderness is often displaced to a position over the upper uterine fundus. Although early in this process pain is described frequently as colicky or stabbing, it soon becomes constant. A low-grade fever is a frequent finding. Patients usually have nausea and vomiting.

Right upper quadrant tenderness is the most consistent sign in gravidas with peritonitis contiguous to an inflamed gallbladder. Although tenderness at the tip of the right ninth costal cartilage at the time of inspiration (Murphy's sign) is often seen in the nonpregnant individual, it occurs rarely in pregnant patients.[62, 64] Rebound and rigidity in the right upper quadrant are infrequent signs. If present, they may suggest possible intestinal perforation, pancreatitis, or appendicitis in the right upper quadrant. Practitioners should consider that the patient may have a form of severe pre-eclampsia called HELLP syndrome, with signs and symptoms of Hemolysis, Elevated Liver enzymes, and Low Platelet count.[75–79] Many patients with this atypical form of pre-eclampsia have been mistakenly treated for upper abdominal pathology unassociated with pregnancy-induced hypertension, and the proper diagnosis has been long delayed. Patients with HELLP syndrome require delivery as soon as possible as part of effective treatment. Other considerations in the differential diagnosis include acute appendicitis, acute pancreatitis, severe acute viral hepatitis, acute pyelonephritis, perforated ulcer, pneumonia, and myocardial infarction.

Abnormalities in laboratory profiles are generally nonspecific. Laboratory studies may indicate an increase in white blood cell count, and in some patients an elevation of serum amylase and bilirubin may be present. Elevated serum amylase levels suggest accompanying pancreatitis that usually responds to conservative therapy.[80–82] The diagnosis of cholelithiasis by ultrasonography (Figs. 14–6A, B) is accurate and reliable in more than 90% of cases.[83–85] Early in the course of cholecys-

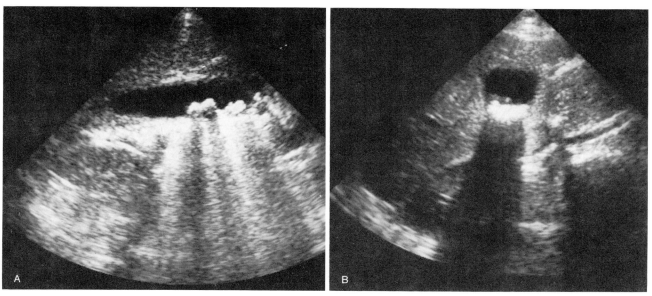

Figure 14–6. *A,* Longitudinal and *B,* cross-sectional sonographic views of gallstones in an enlarged gestational gallbladder (courtesy John Gibson, M.D.).

titis, the patient is found to have gallstones, often in association with a thickened gallbladder wall. Ultrasonography, however, may fail to demonstrate gallstones when a common duct stone is present. In this infrequent circumstance, [99m]TC HIDA (iminodiacetic acid) scanning is recommended. The radiation dose to the fetus with this type of scan is substantially less than 1 rad, even assuming that the technetium conjugate crosses the placenta.[86]

Classic management of acute cholecystitis in pregnancy usually is nonsurgical, with recommended medical treatment including nasogastric suction, intravenous fluids, and modest amounts of narcotic analgesia.[62, 63, 72, 74, 86, 87] Antibiotic administration is undertaken only in those patients who fail to respond to the aforementioned medical management or who are about to undergo surgery. Other investigators recommend routine prophylactic utilization of broad-spectrum β-lactam antibiotics.[80] It is estimated that 70 to 80% of pregnant patients have relief of symptoms with medical therapy alone. Total parenteral nutrition is rarely needed.[86] Currently, medical management is the recommended mode of therapy for all patients with first trimester cholecystitis. Recurrent episodes may occur. Among 26 patients treated conservatively for symptomatic cholelithiasis, 15 (58%) had recurrent episodes of biliary colic during the course of pregnancy.[86] Eight patients were hospitalized once, five twice, and three three times. There is no evidence that pregnancy termination benefits acute cholecystitis; spontaneous abortion may occur following one or more episodes of cholecystitis in pregnancy.

Indications for surgical intervention with cholecystectomy are individualized in the pregnant patient, particularly to exclude first-trimester pa-

tients.[74, 86] Asymptomatic gallstones do not warrant cholecystectomy. However, repeated attacks of biliary colic or failure to respond to medical therapy over a 4-day period, suspected perforation with peritonitis, suspected pancreatitis, severe disease toxicity, significant obstructive jaundice, uncontrolled diabetes mellitus, cases of suspected perforated peptic ulcer, appendicitis, or other intra-abdominal emergencies are indications for immediate surgery.

The advent of laparoscopic cholecystectomy may alter these recommendations for the acute surgical abdomen in the first trimester. The most important advantage of laparoscopic cholecystectomy is the elimination of trauma associated with surgical access, as well as the transient ileus that usually follows open abdominal surgery. Postoperative pain is also minimized, and these patients can be discharged from the hospital fairly soon to resume normal activity and employment. Gallbladder disease in the first trimester appears to be associated with a worse than expected perinatal outcome.[80, 88]

The second trimester of pregnancy appears to be the optimal time for classic cholecystectomy when indicated.[62, 63, 74, 86, 87] Some investigators feel that biliary colic or acute cholecystitis occurring during the second trimester of pregnancy should be treated surgically following medical stabilization.[86] During the third trimester of pregnancy, symptoms should generally be treated medically, as recommended for first-trimester cholecystitis.[74, 80–86] The management objective for the patient with acute cholecystitis is to prepare her for possible cholecystectomy. Prompt abatement of the signs and symptoms of the acute disease process should lead to postponement of operation, except perhaps in the second trimester of pregnancy.

The traditional technique of cholecystectomy involves an upper midline incision or an incision placed obliquely or transversely beneath the right costal margin.[89] A right paramedian incision high above the umbilicus or a transverse muscle-splitting incision over the point of maximal tenderness in the second and third trimesters of pregnancy may offer adequate exposure for performance of cholecystectomy in the event that either cholecystitis or appendicitis is the etiology of the acute abdomen in a second- or third-trimester pregnant patient.

Following manual exploration and determination that the pathologic problem leading to the acute abdomen is an inflamed gallbladder, removal of that organ is begun by depressing the hepatic flexure of the colon inferiorly and retracting the omentum and duodenum medially (Fig. 14–7). Incision of the overlying peritoneum above the cystic duct is undertaken, and the gallbladder is retracted upward, using a Babcock clamp. The junction of the cystic duct and the common bile duct is carefully identified. Once the cystic duct is isolated, a single tie is placed around it in order to prevent migration of calculi through the cystic duct during the remainder of the cholecystectomy.

Operative cholangiography is performed with the radiation dose to the fetus minimized by a lead shield over the abdomen, either preoperatively if the patient is draped for a subcostal incision or intraoperatively if a midline incision is used. Two upper abdominal views are required. The radiation dose to the fetus may be measured by using a film badge beneath the mother's back.[74] Following operative cholangiography, the gallbladder is dissected free from its bed and the cystic artery is ligated. The operation is concluded by drainage of the area with a single soft Penrose drain brought out through a separate stab incision if the area is associated with any bleeding or bile leakage.

Since the first series of laparoscopic cholecystectomies were reported by Reddick and co-workers in 1989,[90, 91] there has been an explosion in the use of laparoscopic gallbladder surgery.[92–94] It is anticipated that first-trimester and selected second-trimester patients could undergo a cholecystectomy by this newer mode of surgery.

During pregnancy, operations on the gallbladder are best undertaken by a general surgeon working in concert with an obstetrician-gynecologist. There are a number of complications of cholecystectomy that necessitate special surgical expertise. These include the possibility of performing a cholecystostomy for those patients who have such marked inflammation that identification of the structures of the region of the gallbladder is seriously impaired. Rare cases of choledochal cyst (cystic dilatation of the common bile duct) exist that require drainage in association with cholecystectomy.[95] Infectious cholecystitis associated with *Salmonella typhi* or parasites, such as those belonging to the genus *Ascaris,* may be encountered in individuals recently arrived in the country from endemic areas.[65] The optimal treatment remains cholecystectomy with preoperative and postoperative antibiotic therapy as appropriate. Tocolytic therapy with magnesium sulfate is recommended postoperatively if surgery is performed in the third trimester.[86] Only a single case of biliary tract carcinoma has been reported during pregnancy.[96] Gallbladder drainage by percutaneous cholecystostomy may have a place in third-trimester treatment, followed by postpartum cholecystectomy.[97]

Biliary lithotripsy is a non–Food and Drug Administration-approved technology for gallstone treatment during pregnancy. All protocols seeking Food and Drug Administration approval exclude gravid patients because of unknown risks to the mother and fetus.

In summary, prepregnancy cholecystectomy is advised for patients with a history of cholelithiasis. During the first trimester of pregnancy, biliary colic or acute cholecystitis should be treated medically if possible, with elective operations scheduled in the second trimester. Biliary symptoms that occur in the second trimester should be treated operatively at that time, in contrast to medical management of symptoms that occur during the third trimester. Although fetal loss rates up to 15% have been described in association with cholecystectomy and cholecystitis during pregnancy,[98] others have not observed negative effects on perinatal mortality.[5, 73]

PANCREATITIS

Acute pancreatitis is an uncommon but life-threatening illness. Its true incidence in pregnancy is unknown,[99–103] but estimates range from two to ten in 10,000.[73, 102] Usually self-limited, the disease is encountered most commonly in the third trimester of pregnancy and in puerperium.[99–105] Four of five cases occur in multigravid patients.[106] Most cases are associated with biliary tract disease,[100, 107–110] although frequently no identifiable cause can be discerned.[99, 111] Less frequent etiologies include drugs, unrecognized hyperlipidemia, and preeclampsia. Regardless of the inciting agent, the ultimate cause of acute pancreatic injury appears to be autodigestion by activated digestive enzymes within the pancreas. These destroy pancreatic parenchyma and cause progressive edema, coagulation, necrosis, and hemorrhage.[112]

Pain secondary to pancreatitis can range from minimal to severe. Characteristically, it is steady epigastric pain that often radiates to the back.[100, 104, 105] It may develop suddenly or may increase gradually for several hours before achieving maximum severity, with persistence for hours or days. Nausea and vomiting frequently accompany the pain. Importantly, a small percentage of patients may present with vomiting only and no significant

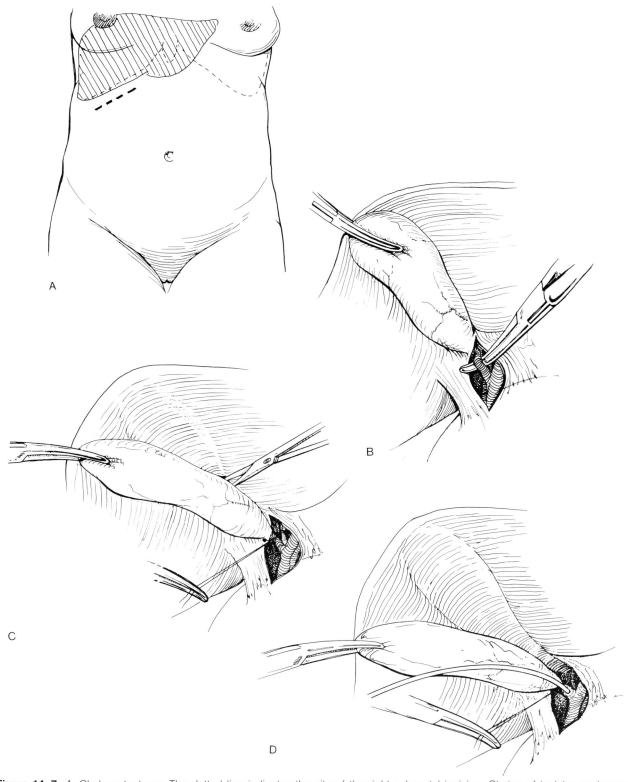

Figure 14–7. *A,* Cholecystectomy. The dotted line indicates the site of the right subcostal incision. Choice of incision and operating team are discussed in the text. (All steps of the operation are not shown.) *B,* The gallbladder is retracted upward. The peritoneum overlying the common bile duct and cystic duct is incised. The cystic duct is identified. *C,* The cystic duct has been ligated. The gallbladder is being dissected from its bed with Metzenbaum scissors. The cystic artery is visualized, ligated, and divided. *D,* Operative cholangiography. A No. 5 polyethylene catheter is passed through a small incision in the cystic duct. Radio-opaque dye is introduced, and radiographic film is exposed to demonstrate the presence or absence of stones in the distal cystic duct or common bile duct. The cystic duct is ligated and divided, and the gallbladder is removed.

abdominal pain. Jaundice may be present in a small percentage of patients.

Other than the elicitation of guarding at the time of upper abdominal examination, the physician usually finds little else that is diagnostic on physical examination.[106] Unusual findings are a faint blue periumbilical discoloration (Cullen's sign) or a bruised discoloration of the flanks (Grey-Turner's sign), usually observed only in association with severe hemorrhagic pancreatitis. A low-grade fever commonly accompanies the disease. Because transudation of fluid into extravascular spaces can be considerable with severe disease, maternal blood volume depletion may be present, with tachycardia and orthostatic hypotension associated with fetal distress. In the most severe cases, maternal hypovolemic shock may be present, with fetal distress or demise.[99] Often, an ileus is present.

Although the cornerstone of diagnosis is elevated serum amylase concentrations, the magnitude of serum amylase elevation does not correlate with disease severity.[106] A normal amylase concentration may be obtained from a patient with acute pancreatitis.[113, 114] Many other intra-abdominal illnesses, including biliary colic, perforated peptic ulcer, and mesenteric infarction, can simulate acute pancreatitis and increase serum amylase concentration. The diagnostic specificity of an increased serum amylase concentration is enhanced by the measurement of serum amylase isoenzymes. Most amylase in the serum of patients with acute pancreatitis is P-type isoamylase.[115] Serum lipase concentrations also are usually increased in patients with acute pancreatitis and remain elevated much longer than serum amylase levels.

Because serum amylase levels usually return to normal within days of an attack of uncomplicated acute pancreatitis, a timed measurement of urinary amylase over a 2-hour span has been recommended to support the clinical diagnosis of pancreatitis.[33] However, normal baseline values for this determination, as well as serum lipase levels during normal gestation, have never been determined. Nies and Dreiss recommend that lipid screening for cholesterol and triglyceride serum concentration be performed to identify the infrequent mother with hyperlipidemic pancreatitis who might respond to therapeutic lowering of lipid concentrations.[116]

Sonography plays an important role in the diagnosis of acute pancreatitis.[108, 117] Although agreement has not been achieved regarding the echo patterns or their intensity in patients with acute pancreatitis, an edematous-appearing gland that appears sonolucent in comparison to the liver supports the diagnosis. Focal or overall pancreatic enlargement may be observed. Imaging of a pseudocyst may also help support the diagnosis, although this is a late finding (Fig. 14–8). Unfortunately, the rate of technically unsatisfactory ultrasonograms of the pancreas is relatively high,

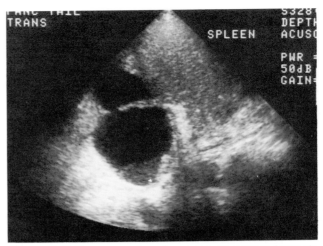

Figure 14–8. Transverse view of a pancreatic septated pseudocyst with dependent debris located beneath the spleen (courtesy John Gibson, M.D.).

particularly in obese patients or those with overlying distended bowel loops. Computed tomography (CAT) and nuclear magnetic resonance imaging offer more promise as diagnostic techniques.[106] The latter technique utilizes intense magnetic fields not likely to be hazardous to the unborn[118] and may be safer than the radiation exposure of almost 1 rad that the fetus can receive with an abdominal CAT scan (0.9 rad).[119, 120]

Medical management of the gravid patient with suspected acute pancreatitis is basically supportive. Because large quantities of extracellular fluid may collect within retroperitoneal spaces with subsequent hypovolemia, intravenous fluid replacement must be aggressive. In order to monitor fluid resuscitation in very ill patients, central monitoring via Swan-Ganz catheter placement has been recommended. To reduce pancreatic secretions, the patient is maintained in a fasting state with nasogastric suction. Meperidine is recommended as the drug of choice for analgesia. Broad-spectrum antibiotics frequently are utilized to treat infection.

Blood glucose levels, complete blood count, liver function tests, lactate dehydrogenase and calcium levels, arterial blood gases, serum electrolytes, and renal function are monitored as clinically indicated. Arterial blood gas measurements should be considered every 12 hours for several days in patients with severe disease. Early in the disease process, total parenteral nutrition for the pregnant patient should be considered.[121–124] Fetal status and well-being are assessed frequently. Plasma exchange has been reported to be an effective therapeutic modality for patients with severe pancreatitis and hyperlipidemia.[125]

Surgical exploration for patients with acute pancreatitis is recommended for three major indications: (1) to rule out surgically correctable disease, (2) to eliminate a disease condition that initiates pancreatic inflammation, and (3) to remove necrotic or infected foci during the septic phase of hemorrhagic necrotizing pancreatitis. Thus, surgery is reserved for patients with pancreatic abscess, ruptured pseudocyst, severe hemorrhagic pancreatitis, and for those patients with pancreatitis secondary to a surgically remediable lesion.[106] The development of a secondary infection in the necrotic debris of residual pancreatitis may not become evident until 7 to 14 days following initial symptoms. Whenever sepsis is encountered after an attack of acute pancreatitis, prompt surgery is required to drain necrotic foci and collections and to irrigate and remove toxic substances from the bed of the pancreas.

Patients with intra-abdominal hemorrhage from necrotic large blood vessels that supply the pancreas are best managed initially by angiographic embolization to control the hemorrhage. Even in the nonpregnant individual, the debate continues as to whether early operative intervention or endoscopic sphincterotomy done within 24 to 36 hours after the onset of symptoms reduces the incidence of hemorrhagic pancreatitis and the mortality rate from gallstone pancreatitis. Removal of the gallbladder and exploration of the common duct appear to be appropriate in this circumstance.

In the woman who responds to medical management, surgery for associated biliary tract disease is best avoided during the acute episode and the first or third trimester of pregnancy. Instead, it is scheduled either for the second trimester or after delivery.[109] Pregnancy termination does not appear to be indicated. However, planned delivery may hasten disease resolution.[126] Most pregnant patients with pancreatitis recover spontaneously within 3 to 7 days with medical management. It is unusual for respiratory insufficiency to develop.[111]

Following hospital discharge, patients are followed closely for the development of a pancreatic pseudocyst. Serum amylase concentrations are monitored every 14 days until they return to normal. Pseudocyst formation usually occurs weeks after the episode of pancreatitis and can be detected reliably by ultrasonography.[106] Their formation usually is attended by recurrent bouts of epigastric pain, fluid collections in the abdomen or pleural spaces, hemorrhage, rupture, or abscess formation. Pseudocysts are usually managed expectantly, as spontaneous resolution occurs unless complications are noted. Most resolve spontaneously within 6 weeks of detection. Percutaneous drainage or laparotomy may be required to excise or drain a pseudocyst.

Although maternal mortality rates of up to 37% have been reported with acute pancreatitis in pregnancy,[100] death is infrequent unless the disease is especially severe.[99, 102, 104, 127] Fetal mortality is a risk in severely ill mothers and in those that have preterm labor. Overall fetal salvage rates have been reported to range between 80 and 89%.[99, 101, 102, 106]

INTESTINAL OBSTRUCTION

Intestinal obstruction is an increasingly common cause for abdominal pain and surgery during pregnancy. It is estimated to occur in approximately 1 to 3 of every 10,000 pregnancies.[5, 128–131] The increasing incidence in recent years is related almost exclusively to more frequent laparotomy in young women, which predisposes to adhesion formation. Adhesions are the most common predisposing factor to intestinal obstruction in either the pregnant or nonpregnant patient.[132] The most frequent antecedent operations are appendectomies and gynecologic surgery.[133, 134] Adhesion formation secondary to pelvic inflammatory disease is considered to be another major etiologic factor in the formation of intra-abdominal adhesions that lead to intestinal obstruction (Fig. 14–9). Acute obstruction occurs most frequently during the third trimester of pregnancy.[129] It can be confused with placental abruption because uterine pain with maternal shock and fetal death can occur in association with bowel strangulation.[135]

Volvulus and intussusception are the second and third most frequent causes of gestational intestinal obstruction, respectively. Volvulus may be responsible for up to one in four cases of obstruction during pregnancy.[136, 137] It has been described ante partum and post partum, particularly following cesarean delivery.[138] Usually it occurs secondary to adhesion formation[139] and is considered to be more common in many African countries than in the Western world.[140, 141] Intestinal volvulus in pregnancy most commonly involves the sigmoid colon, (47%) followed by approximately equal occurrence in the small intestine (28%) and the cecum/large intestine (25%).[137, 142, 143] Harer and

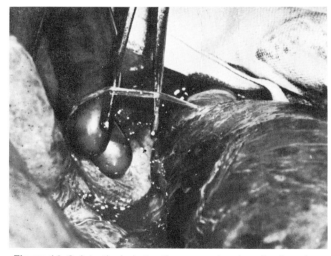

Figure 14–9. Intestinal obstruction secondary to adhesions from previous surgery (courtesy James Hardy, M.D.).

Harer suggest that the mechanism of sigmoid volvulus in pregnancy is displacement, compression, and partial obstruction of an abnormally mobile sigmoid colon by the enlarging uterus.[137] Also, an elongated mesocolon may predispose to volvulus.[144]

Intussusception is somewhat less common but potentially more dangerous for the patient and progeny than is volvulus (Fig. 14–10). It accounts for 4 to 6% of intestinal obstructions during pregnancy.[129, 145–147] In the majority of cases with intussusception, plain abdominal radiographs reveal no abnormality. Thus, the clinician must rely on less exact diagnostic measures, and delay of surgery is a common problem, especially early in pregnancy.[131, 135, 147–150] Although a Meckel diverticulum is the most common cause of intussusception in pregnancy, a precipitating neoplasm, including choriocarcinoma, occurs in 20% of cases.[151] Other etiologies for intestinal obstruction during pregnancy include strangulated hernias, congenital defects, malrotation, recovery from surgery, megacolon, previous weight reduction surgery, primary or metastatic neoplasms, and extrinsic pressure by the gravid or postpartum uterus on the sigmoid colon.[128, 130, 135, 136, 146, 150–164]

In addition to placental abruption, a number of other abdominal conditions can be misdiagnosed when intestinal obstruction is present. These include acute pancreatitis, pyelonephritis, appendicitis, cholecystitis, and gastroenteritis. True mechanical obstruction of the intestinal tract can also be caused by acute adnexal torsion or by degeneration of a fibroid tumor.

The three most likely periods in pregnancy for intestinal obstruction are at midgestation, late in the third trimester, and early in the puerperium as the uterus returns rapidly to normal size, with a consequent alteration in the relationship of intra-abdominal structures.[38, 165, 166] The first pregnancy following abdominal surgery appears to be the one at highest risk for intestinal obstruction.

Abdominal pain, vomiting, and obstipation constitute the classic clinical triad of symptoms in patients with intestinal obstruction. Because all three of these may be seen to some degree with normal pregnancy, the clinician may find it difficult to differentiate physiologic from pathologic symptoms. Abdominal pain, present in the great majority of patients with intestinal obstruction, may be diffuse, constant, or periodic. The varieties of presentation reflect the variability in level of obstruction in the small or large intestine and whether the obstruction is partial or total. Also, the suddenness and time course of the obstruction can influence the severity of pain. Acute upper intestinal obstruction usually produces the most severe pain. In contrast, there can be little or no pain in adults with intussusception or small-gut volvulus. It is emphasized that *the severity of pain cannot be correlated with the seriousness of the disorder.* Symptoms can mimic those of the onset of labor to a great extent.

Bowel sounds are of little value in making an early diagnosis of obstruction. Tenderness on palpation is typically absent with early obstruction. There usually is no guarding or rebound tenderness unless strangulation and gangrene of the bowel are present. Thus, tenderness on palpation is a late finding and usually is generalized. Late in the course of intestinal obstruction, the triad of fever, oliguria, and shock may occur as manifestations of massive fluid loss into the bowel with acidosis and infection.[167] Irreversible damage to the bowel usually has occurred by this time, and surgery is obligatory. Normal bowel sounds may be present until very late in the clinical picture.

Vomiting alone seldom confirms the diagnosis unless the vomitus is feculent. Vomiting, however, is much more likely if strangulation of the intestine has occurred. Although chronic constipation is expected in pregnancy, obstipation (total constipation) is abnormal and most characteristic of low colonic obstruction, such as that associated with sigmoid volvulus. Pulse rate and white cell count are not reliable for diagnostic purposes.

Although a single flat plate and an upright radiograph of the abdomen are nondiagnostic in approximately half of cases early in the course of disease, serial films at 4- to 8-hour intervals usually reveal progressive changes that help to confirm the diagnosis[38, 135, 147, 168] (Fig. 14–11). Concern for the mother and the possibility of intestinal obstruction should outweigh any concern regarding the distant risk and minimal adverse effects of diagnostic radiographs on the fetus. The hazards of undiagnosed intestinal obstruction far exceed the miniscule potential radiation hazard to the fetus.

Simple small bowel obstruction usually produces progressive intestinal dilatation with "stepladder" formation of intestinal loops and air-fluid levels. Large bowel obstruction appears radiologically as dilatation of the bowel with loss of haustration and accumulation of intraluminal fluid. Volvulus

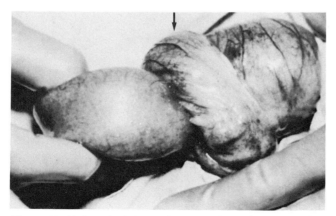

Figure 14–10. Intestinal obstruction secondary to intussusception (*arrow*) (courtesy James Hardy, M.D.).

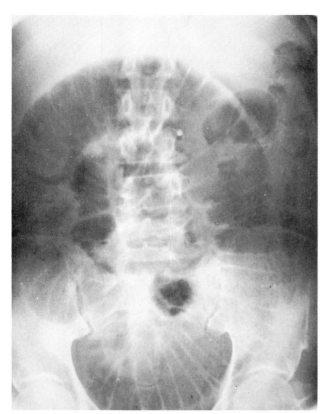

Figure 14–11. Radiographic appearance of small bowel obstruction with "stepladder" formation of intestinal loops and air-fluid levels (courtesy James Hardy, M.D.).

should be suspected whenever there is a single grossly dilated loop of bowel.[38] The radiographic findings associated with intussusception are bizarre, and a correct preoperative diagnosis rarely is made.[145] Repeated enemas that are nonproductive may be helpful in diagnosing a low-level intestinal obstruction. The rectal passage of blood-stained fluid suggests intestinal strangulation. Obstruction also can be inferred if the colon remains distended after an enema. Ultrasonographic findings described as "single or double concentric rings of sonolucency surrounded by a coarse central echogenic focus" have been cited.[169, 170] However, ultrasonographic findings can be misinterpreted and can lead to further treatment delays.[145, 150]

Definitive therapy for intestinal obstruction is surgical. Delay and procrastination with attempted placement of a long tube is ill-advised. It rarely works, can lead to intussusception, and inevitably delays definitive therapy.[147] Any significant delay can be catastrophic to both mother and fetus. Thus, early surgical intervention during pregnancy generally is recommended. Rare case reports have detailed the successful use of a rectal tube inserted through a sigmoidoscope to decompress a sigmoid volvulus and avoid immediate laparotomy.[171–173]

Before surgery, the patient is rapidly stabilized and infused with fluid and electrolytes to correct the metabolic situation, maintain adequate urinary output, and maintain adequate maternal circulating blood volume for uteroplacental sustenance. The patient's vital signs are carefully monitored, and a short nasogastric tube is placed. The patient and her fetus are monitored closely and maintained in a 30-degree left lateral tilt position to prevent supine hypotension. Prophylactic antibiotics are initiated if intestinal perforation or strangulation is anticipated.

Whenever intestinal obstruction is suspected, the abdominal incision must be vertical and ample in order to provide the best operative exposure. Division of adhesive bands is undertaken, and careful assessment for bowel viability is performed. A search is made for multiple sites of obstruction, and the total length of the bowel is examined prior to a decision for resection of any part. In the absence of adhesive bands, volvulus sometimes can be treated simply by detorsion. Resection of nonviable bowel may be necessary, as may a colostomy.[173] Unless delivery by cesarean operation is required for adequate exposure of the bowel or there are obstetric reasons for delivery, usually it is best to leave the pregnant uterus undisturbed. The abdominal incision should maintain its integrity even if vaginal delivery with its expulsive efforts occurs within the first 24 hours postoperatively.[133]

During the postpartum period, intestinal obstruction can develop secondary to compression by the pregnant uterus itself or by an adynamic ileus (pseudo-obstruction). Management of either condition is conservative, with restoration of fluid and electrolyte balance and with nasogastric suction. The uterus is displaced out of the pelvis with the rectal finger. With the patient in the exaggerated knee-chest position, a rectal tube is inserted and serial radiographs are taken to evaluate cecum and colon size. Surgery is indicated only if cecal perforation is expected, if intestinal diameter expands beyond 9 to 12 cm,[174, 175] or if the patient fails to improve within 72 hours of the institution of conservative therapy.

Similar to patient experience with acute appendicitis during pregnancy, maternal mortality (10 to 20%)[128, 137] with intestinal obstruction mostly results from procrastination and postponement of definitive surgical therapy in the hope that the condition will resolve spontaneously. Unfortunately, infection and irreversible shock can develop in the presence of devascularized bowel. In this milieu, perinatal and maternal survival may be compromised. Early diagnosis and aggressive medical-surgical treatment are essential for an optimal maternal-fetal outcome. It is imperative that the physician have a high index of suspicion and a willingness to perform surgery.

The finding of gross feculent material outside the intestinal tract at surgery requires diversionary therapy because the primary anastomosis of unprepared colon is hazardous, particularly in the presence of infection. Postoperatively, intravenous hyperalimentation may be necessary for maintenance of optimal maternal and perinatal nutrition. Prolonged nutritional support is an important issue, particularly in the presence of sepsis. Current thinking emphasizes that, whenever possible, enteral nutrition is better than parenteral nutrition.[164, 165] Enteral feedings maintain the intestinal mucosa and its barrier function to prevent the egress of enteric bacteria or their toxins or both into the peritoneal cavity. Postoperative ileus usually is viewed as a contraindication to enteral feeding. However, ileus is almost always secondary to gastric or colonic dysmotility and the small intestine is rarely involved. Intrajejunal feedings via small catheter can usually be initiated in the early postoperative period to effect optimal nutritional support of the gut and patients. Use of magnesium tocolysis during and immediately following any operation in which peritonitis is identified is recommended.

Patients with inflammatory bowel disease can develop a wide range of complications during pregnancy.[178] These include fistulization from the terminal ileum,[179] intestinal perforation with peritonitis,[145, 180–186] small bowel obstruction,[2, 187, 188] intestinal abscesses,[181, 189–192] and toxic megacolon.[193–199] Fulminating colitis during pregnancy should be treated aggressively in the operating room to remove damaged bowel, re-anastomose vital tissue, perform emergency ileostomy and subtotal colectomy, and form a mucous fistula. Toxic dilatation of the colon is optimally managed with subtotal colectomy and ileostomy formation.[199–201] Patients with a continent ileostomy generally deliver vaginally (75%) and require cesarean delivery only for obstetric reasons.[202]

TRAUMA-RELATED AND OTHER SURGICAL EMERGENCIES

The leading cause of fortuitous injury in pregnancy is motor vehicle accidents.[203–205] These account for at least half of the cases of blunt abdominal trauma encountered during pregnancy.[203, 204] Severe internal injuries in the abdomen are usually accompanied by intraperitoneal bleeding and hypovolemic shock. Fetal compromise and loss are almost always proportional to the severity of maternal injury. Indeed, in association with trauma, the most common cause of fetal death is maternal death[204] and the second most frequent cause of fetal death is premature placental separation.[206] When pelvic fracture occurs, it is often associated with hemorrhage and massive concealed retroperitoneal bleeding, rupture of the uterus, and injury to the bladder, urethra, and portions of the urinary tract.[204, 207–211]

Fetal distress is usually the first sign of maternal distress and shock, involving blunt trauma serious enough to cause extensive intra-abdominal hemorrhage. Steering wheel trauma to the pregnant abdomen may cause immediate or delayed hepatic and splenic rupture. In the presence of fetal distress and a history of significant blunt abdominal trauma, intraperitoneal bleeding is invariably present and immediate laparotomy must be performed. In the absence of fetal distress, ultrasonography, diagnostic peritoneal lavage, or CT scanning of the abdomen may reveal the presence of blood as fluid in the cul-de-sac and abdominal spaces. Trauma to the liver, spleen, and kidneys is best reflected by CT scans; damage to the bowel, mesentery, and gallbladder is more reliably detected by diagnostic peritoneal lavage. Laparotomy should not be delayed if intra-abdominal bleeding is suspected or if a viable fetus is in obvious distress. The diagnosis of intraperitoneal bleeding in the pregnant patient may be hampered because traditional signs of peritoneal irritation are not as pronounced as they are in the nonpregnant state.[210] Kleihauer-Betke testing should be performed to detect fetomaternal transfusion, with its risks of exsanguination and blood group isoimmunization.[212–216]

Because clinical manifestation of internal injuries and placental abruption may be delayed following even seemingly minor trauma,[212, 213, 217, 218] continuous fetal monitoring for gestations of more than or equal to 24 weeks should be performed for at least 24 hours for almost all pregnant patients following all trauma except the most insignificant. Others recommend hospitalization of up to 72 hours.[205] Clinical evidence of a hepatic laceration with hemorrhage and shock may be delayed for several weeks following the event. It may not become apparent until delivery occurs and eliminates the compressive effect of the uterus on a bleeding site.

A conservative nonsurgical approach is often utilized for the pregnant patient with blunt trauma unless signs of fetal distress or internal hemorrhage with major injuries, shock, altered mental status, or neurologic deficit are present.[219] A practice of routine exploration of patients with penetrating injuries is often undertaken. All pregnant patients who suffer penetrating injuries should be considered for exploration by a midline approach.[220] If maternal vital signs and fetal heart rate assessment are stable and there is no evidence of intra-abdominal hemorrhage in a patient with a wound below the uterine fundus, observation of both mother and fetus without immediate surgery is recommended following radiographic evaluation of projectile location.[221] If a bullet is within the uterus, continued observation is recommended. Knife wounds should be probed for peritoneal injury and surgical exploration undertaken for those patients with confirmed peritoneal perforation.[222,223] Exploratory celiotomy should be performed at any time there is fetal or maternal compromise and in all patients in whom the entry wound is above the uterine fundus. Laceration of the diaphragm must be ruled out.

At the time of surgery, the bowel should be thoroughly examined and all injuries should be repaired.[224] Thorough evaluation of bleeding from uterine entry and exit sites must be performed. If uterine injury, including rupture or lacerated uterine vessels with broad ligament or retroperitoneal hematomas, are encountered, delivery is effected immediately, and damage to the vessels is repaired. Removal of the uterus may be needed if damage is extensive.[7] Unless there is lack of exposure or evidence of fetal compromise or injury, cesarean delivery is not undertaken. If there is evidence of fetal injury and the gestation is more than 28 weeks, delivery is encouraged because the risk of fetal death from injury is much greater than the risk of perinatal death from prematurity. If the fetus is dead, conservative measures are followed, with surgery reserved for maternal compromise or entry wounds above the fundus. Spontaneous vaginal delivery thereafter is anticipated or induced. Management is thereafter highly individualized. In the absence of immediate surgery for penetrating abdominal trauma, vigilant observation for maternal or fetal compromise must be maintained for at least 24 hours. Exploration is mandatory if the patient develops any signs of hemodynamic instability or sepsis.

Maternal hemodynamic instability in association with a surgical abdomen may also be caused by spontaneous visceral rupture or aneurysmal rupture. Although infrequent, spontaneous rupture of the liver or spleen has been observed in pregnancy.

The maternal and fetal mortalities associated with splenic rupture are 26 and 63%, respectively.[225] Although the majority of splenic ruptures occur because of trauma, one third occur atraumatically near term without associated health disorders or splenic pathology.[225–232] The diagnosis is often difficult and unsuspected. Splenic rupture can be described as immediate or delayed, spontaneous or traumatic. Blunt abdominal trauma often causes immediate rupture. Delayed rupture may be secondary to trauma, with an intact capsule. When the capsular integrity is overcome by subcapsular pressure, massive peritoneal hemorrhage can occur and be virtually symptom-free. Splenic rupture has been reported in all trimesters, with the predominance of cases occurring late in gestation.[225]

The spleen is the most common visceral organ to undergo rupture following trauma because of its soft consistency, mobility, and tendency to enlarge under a variety of conditions.[233] In addition to external trauma, internal trauma related to torsion and rupture of the splenic pedicle, splenic artery, splenic vein, or splenic capsule can occur.

Lack of ligamentous support for the spleen makes it a very mobile organ predisposed to torsion of the pedicle and to trauma.

Symptoms of splenic rupture reflect massive intra-abdominal hemorrhage. Initially, abdominal pain is localized to the left upper quadrant. The patient often complains of chest, neck, epigastric, or left shoulder pain (Kehr's sign). With progressive hemorrhage, nausea and vomiting may occur, the abdomen may become more rigid, and hemorrhagic shock may develop. Dullness on percussion in the left flank and upper quadrant (Vallance's sign) and tenderness over the posterior edge of the left sternocleidomastoid muscle (Saegusser's sign) may be encountered.[233]

Spontaneous splenic rupture is usually not suspected prior to surgery. Delivery of a mature late third-trimester fetus via cesarean section allows exposure for emergency splenectomy. Recently, the first case of splenic preservation following spontaneous rupture during pregnancy was reported.[231] In this instance, the combination of local pressure and the application of topical thrombin agents was effective, and splenic conservation was possible.

More than 90 cases of pregnancy-related ruptured splenic artery aneurysms have been reported.[234–238] The majority of these have occurred in the third trimester of pregnancy.[235] Portal hypertension is thought to be the cause.[239, 240] Patients usually present with sudden severe upper left quadrant abdominal pain and hypovolemic shock. Once the aneurysm is identified following careful exploration of the abdominal contents, removal of the aneurysm and usually the spleen is undertaken. Usually no palpable mass is found on physical examination prior to surgery. Approximately one of four patients with this surgical disorder in pregnancy undergoes a two-stage rupture in which hemorrhage occurs into the lesser omental sac, accompanied by pain and syncopy.[225, 236] Some recovery occurs in association with partial tamponade of the bleeding vessel. If surgery is not performed promptly thereafter, secondary hemorrhage can occur and lead to death.

Aneurysms in other abdominal sites can also rupture during pregnancy. Ruptured aneurysms of the renal artery, aorta, hypogastric artery, and external iliac, middle colic, and mesenteric arteries have been described.[234, 241–243] A similar sudden shock syndrome is encountered with concealed rupture of any major blood vessel.

Shock, diffuse abdominal pain, nausea, and vomiting usually follow spontaneous rupture of the liver.[224, 244–247] Hepatic rupture usually follows severe pre-eclampsia/eclampsia or trauma.[63, 248–253] Other etiologies include acute fatty liver of pregnancy,[254, 255] hepatic amebic abscesses,[256–259] adenomas,[260–262] hemangiomas,[245] metastatic choriocarcinoma,[263] and hepatocellular carcinoma.[264]

Maternal outcome usually is poor with hepatic rupture because shock develops rapidly and diagnosis is often difficult. A broad spectrum of presentation is associated with hepatic rupture, ranging from minor subcapsular hematomas to exsanguination from a major disruption of the liver parenchyma.

Ultrasonography and CT scans are helpful adjuncts in diagnosing and following suspected liver hematomas. However, signs and symptoms of major disruption of the liver necessitate prompt surgical therapy with aggressive blood product replacement and attempts to bring about hemostasis. Hepatic lobar resection, hepatic artery ligation, and large mattress sutures throughout the liver are often required to stop blood loss. Selective embolization of the liver with thrombotic agents may be helpful.[265–266] Expert surgical technique is essential for patient survival. There are several recent reports of favorable outcome when aggressive medical therapy was undertaken with apparent stabilization of the maternal condition so that surgery could be avoided.[251, 256, 258] However, if hemodynamic deterioration becomes evident despite aggressive blood replacement, prompt surgery to effect hemostasis is indicated.[245, 267]

Spontaneous hepatic rupture in 90% of reported cases has involved the right lobe of the liver.[248] This is associated with rapid, massive blood loss with hypovolemic shock. A sudden increase in abdominal distension is apparent. There is lack of unanimity about surgical therapy in patients with hepatic rupture. The obstetrician-gynecologist encountering such a patient should pack and place pressure on the site of rupture; he or she should proceed to evacuate the uterus and obtain consultation from a general or vascular surgeon experienced in hepatic surgery. No attempt should be made to repair the site of hepatic rupture by suturing the capsule or parenchyma. Pressure and application of topical thrombin may be of help.

Although the correct surgical approach to the liver is controversial, it is recommended that the hepatic artery supplying the ruptured and bleeding site be surgically ligated if possible.[232] If hemostasis is achieved with this ligation and is maintained following restoration of intravascular volume, nothing further is required. However, if there are multiple rapidly bleeding ruptures, a large, massively bleeding site, or if the ligation fails to arrest the bleeding, partial hepatic resection, usually by lobectomy, must be done.

Infrequently, gastric perforations related to peptic ulcer disease and gastric hemorrhage may cause an acute surgical abdomen during pregnancy.[268–275] In association with surgical repair of this area, cesarean section in the late stages of pregnancy is strongly advised.[271]

SUMMARY AND CONCLUSIONS

Optimal management of the gravid patient with a nonobstetric surgical disorder continues to challenge obstetricians and their consultants. The relative unfamiliarity of many general surgeons with the pregnant condition and of many obstetricians with disorders normally managed by general surgeons presents an experience and communications hurdle to be overcome by both parties for the benefit of the mother and the unborn child. Concern for the welfare of both parties in the pregnancy must not impede proper diagnostic evaluation and an appropriate surgical solution. The interpretation of individual patient findings in light of known physiologic changes of pregnancy is an important role for the obstetrician. Both groups of physicians must become comfortable with the concept that certainty of diagnosis preoperatively is an elusive, unrealistic, and potentially dangerous goal. Careful attention to the patient's history is as important as frequent reassessment of physical findings and diagnostic tests.

The incorporation of operative laparoscopy into the diagnostic and therapeutic approach to the pregnant patient with a probably surgical disorder of the abdomen should revolutionize current practice during the coming decade. Issues related to optimal nutritional support of the peripartal patient with enteral feeding, protocols for the suppression of preterm labor in postoperative patients, the expanded use of transcatheter embolotherapy, and better methods for maternal and fetal surveillance perioperatively await careful study.

ACKNOWLEDGMENT

The author wishes to express gratitude to Dr. Robert S. Rhodes, Professor and Chairman of the Department of Surgery at Mississippi, for his critical review of the manuscript.

References

1. Schnider SM, Webster GM: Maternal and fetal hazards of surgery during pregnancy. Am J Obstet Gynecol 92:891, 1965.
2. Hunt MG, Martin JN Jr Martin RW, et al.: Perinatal aspects of abdominal surgery for nonobstetric disease. Am J Perinatol 6:412, 1989.
3. Brodsky JB, Cohen EN, Brown BW, et al.: Surgery during pregnancy and fetal outcome. Am J Obstet Gynecol 138:1165, 1980.
4. Saunders P, Milton P: Laparotomy during pregnancy: An assessment of diagnostic accuracy and fetal wastage. Br Med J 3:165, 1973.
5. Kammerer WS: Nonobstetric surgery during pregnancy. Med Clin North Am 63:1157, 1979.
6. Pass HL, Hardy JD: The appendix. In Hardy JD (ed.): Hardy's Textbook of Surgery. Philadelphia: J.B. Lippincott Co. 1983, pp. 558–564.
7. Doherty GM, Lewis FB Jr. Appendicitis: Continuing diagnostic challenge. Emerg Med Clin North Am 7:537, 1989.
8. Weingold AB: Appendicitis in pregnancy. Clin Obstet Gynecol 26:801, 1983.

9. Rosemann GW: Acute appendicitis in pregnancy. S Afr Med J 49:1459, 1975.
10. Taylor JD: Acute appendicitis in pregnancy and the puerperium. Aust NZ J Obstet Gynaecol 12:202, 1972.
11. Frisenda R, Roty AR, Kilway JB, Brown AL, Phelan M: Acute appendicitis during pregnancy. Am Surg 16:503, 1979.
12. McComb P, Laimon H: Appendicitis complicating pregnancy. Can J Surg 23:92, 1980.
13. Kurtz GR, Davis RS, Spraul JD: Acute appendicitis in pregnancy and labor. Obstet Gynecol 23:428, 1964.
14. Punnonen R, Aho AJ, Gronroos M, Liukko P: Appendisectomy during pregnancy. Acta Chir Scand 145:555, 1979.
15. Allen JR, Helling TS, Langenfeld M: Intraabdominal surgery during pregnancy. Am J Surg 158:567, 1989.
16. Babaknia A, Parsa H, Woodruff JD: Appendicitis during pregnancy. Obstet Gynecol 50:40, 1977.
17. Finch DRA, Emanoel L: Acute appendicitis complicating pregnancy in the Oxford region. Br J Surg 61:129, 1974.
18. Hoffman ES, Suzuki M: Acute appendicitis in pregnancy: A ten year survey. Am J Obstet Gynecol 67:1338, 1954.
19. Sarason EL, Bauman S: Acute appendicitis in pregnancy: Difficulties in diagnosis. Obstet Gynecol 22:382, 1963.
20. O'Neil JP: Surgical conditions complicating pregnancy. Acute appendicitis: Real and simulated. Aust NZ J Obstet Gynaecol 9:94, 1969.
21. Mohammed JA, Oxorn H: Appendicitis in pregnancy. Can Med Assoc J 112:1187, 1975.
22. Brant HA: Acute appendicitis in pregnancy. Obstet Gynecol 29:130, 1967.
23. Gomez A, Wood M: Acute appendicitis during pregnancy. Am J Surg 137:180, 1979.
24. Horowitz MD, Gomez GA, Santiesteban R, Burkett C: Acute appendicitis during pregnancy. Arch Surg 120:1362, 1985.
25. McGee TM: Acute appendicitis in pregnancy. Aust NZ J Obstet Gynaecol 29:378, 1989.
26. Black WP: Acute appendicitis in pregnancy. Br Med J 1:1938, 1960.
27. Cunningham FG, McCubbin JH: Appendicitis complicating pregnancy. Obstet Gynecol 45:415, 1975.
28. Masters K, Levine BA, Gaskill HV, Sirinek KR: Diagnosing appendicitis during pregnancy. Am J Surg 148:768, 1984.
29. Moore GR, Smith CV: Schistosomiasis associated with rupture of the appendix in pregnancy. Obstet Gynecol 74:446, 1989.
30. Donnenfeld AE, Roberts NS, Losure TA, Mellen AW: Perforated adenocarcinoma of the appendix during pregnancy. Am J Obstet Gynecol 154:637, 1986.
31. Baer JL, Reis RA, Arens RA: Appendicitis in pregnancy with changes in position and axis of the normal appendix in pregnancy. JAMA 98:1359, 1932.
32. Bailey LE, Finley RK, Miller SF, Jones LM: Acute appendicitis during pregnancy. Am Surg 52:218, 1986.
33. DeVore GR: Acute abdominal pain in the pregnant patient due to pancreatitis, acute appendicitis, cholecystitis, and peptic ulcer disease. Clin Perinatol 7:349, 1980.
34. Alders N: A sign for differentiating uterine from extrauterine complications of pregnancy and puerperium. Br Med J 2:1194, 1951.
35. Humphrey MD, Ayton RA: Acute appendicitis complicating pregnancy and the puerperium: A study of 5 cases. Aust NZ J Obstet Gynaecol 23:35, 1983.
36. Markle GB: A simple test for intraperitoneal inflammation. Am J Surg 125:721, 1973.
37. Markle GB: Differentiating appendicitis from gyn conditions. Contemp Ob/Gyn 33(May):148, 1989.
38. Suidan JS, Young BK: The acute abdomen in pregnancy. In Rustgi VK, Cooper JN (eds.): Gastrointestinal and Hepatic Complications in Pregnancy. New York: Churchill Livingstone, pp. 30–45, 1986.
39. Hamlin E Jr, Bartlett M, Smith J: Acute surgical emergencies of the abdomen in pregnancy. N Engl J Med 244:128, 1951.
40. Puylaert JBCM: Acute appendicitis: US evaluation using graded compression. Radiology 158:355, 1986.
41. Puylaert JBCM, Rutgers PH, Lalisang RI, et al.: A prospective study of ultrasonography in the diagnosis of appendicitis. N Engl J Med 317:666, 1987.
42. Coady DJ, Snyder JR, Subramanyam B: Appendiceal abscess in pregnancy: Diagnosis by ultrasound. J Clin Ultrasound 14:70, 1986.
43. Babler EA: Perforative appendicitis complicating pregnancy. JAMA 51:1310, 1908.
44. Magarey CJ, Chant AD, Rickford CR, Magarey JR: Peritoneal drainage and systemic antibiotics after appendicectomy. Lancet 2:179, 1971.
45. Spirtos NM, Eisenkop SM, Spirtos TW, et al.: Laparoscopy: A diagnostic aid in cases of suspected appendicitis. Am J Obstet Gynecol 156:90, 1987.
46. Ragland J, de la Garza J, McKenney J: Peritoneoscopy for the diagnosis of acute appendicitis in females of reproductive age. Surg Endosc 2:36, 1988.
47. Reiertsen O, Rosseland AR, Hoivik B, Solheim K: Laparoscopy in patients admitted for acute abdominal pain. Acta Chir Scand 151:521, 1985.
48. Whitworth CM, Whitworth PW, Sanfillipo J, Polk HC Jr: Value of diagnostic laparoscopy in young women with possible appendicitis. Surg Gynecol Obstet 167:187, 1988.
49. Paterson-Brown S, Thompson JN, Teckersley JR, et al.: Which patients with suspected appendicitis should undergo laparoscopy? Br Med J 296:1363, 1988.
50. Fleming JS: Laparoscopically directed appendicectomy. Aust NZ J Obstet Gynaecol 25:238, 1985.
51. Semm K: Endoscopic appendectomy. Endoscopy 15:59, 1983.
52. Schreiber JH: Early experience with laparoscopic appendectomy in women. Surg Endosc 1:211, 1987.
53. Leahy PF: Technique of laparoscopic appendicectomy. Br J Surg 76:616, 1989.
54. Liu PL, Warren TM, Ostheimer GW, et al.: Foetal monitoring in parturients undergoing surgery unrelated to pregnancy. Can Anaesth Soc J 32:525, 1985.
55. Lowthian J: Appendicitis during pregnancy. Ann Emerg Med 9:431, 1980.
56. Kesarwani RC: Acute appendicitis complicating pregnancy. J Indian Med Assoc 82:316, 1984.
57. Doberneck RC: Appendectomy during pregnancy. Am Surg 51:265, 1985.
58. Ammerman KS, Toffle RC: Concurrent appendicitis and pregnancy at term. W V Med J 83:63, 1987.
59. Spitzer M, Kaiser IH: Perforative appendicitis in the third trimester of pregnancy. NY State J Med 84:132, 1984.
60. Law D, Law R, Eiseman B: The continuing challenge of acute and perforated appendicitis. Am J Surg 131:533, 1976.
61. Herczeg J, Kovács L, Keserü T: Premature labour and coincident acute appendicitis not resolved by betamimetic but surgical treatment. Acta Obstet Gynecol Scand 62:373, 1983.
62. Hill LM, Johnson CE, Lee RA: Cholecystectomy in pregnancy. Obstet Gynecol 46:291, 1975.
63. Simon JA: Biliary tract disease and related surgical disorders during pregnancy. Clin Obstet Gynecol 26:810, 1983.
64. O'Neill JP: Surgical conditions complicating pregnancy. Aust NZ J Obstet Gynecol 9:249, 1969.
65. Cooper AD: Cholelithiasis and biliary tract disease in pregnancy. In Rustgi VK, Cooper JN (eds.): Gastrointestinal and Hepatic Complications in Pregnancy. New York: Churchill Livingstone, 1986, pp. 124–137.
66. Bennion LJ, Grundy SM: Risk factors for the development of cholelithiasis in man. N Engl J Med 299:116, 1978.
67. Large AM, Lofstrom JE, Stevenson CS: Gallstones and pregnancy. AMA Arch Surg 78:966, 1959.

68. Stauffer RA, Adams A, Wygal J, Lavery PJ: Gallbladder disease in pregnancy. Am J Obstet Gynecol 144:661, 1982.
69. Chesson RR, Gallup DG, Gibbs RL: Ultrasonographic diagnosis of asymptomatic cholelithiasis in pregnancy. J Reprod Med 30:921, 1985.
70. Braverman DZ, Johnson ML, Kern F Jr: Effects of pregnancy and contraceptive steroids on gallbladder function. N Engl J Med 302:362, 1980.
71. Glenn F: Biliary tract disease. Surg Gynecol Obstet 153:401, 1981.
72. Friley MD, Douglas G: Acute cholecystitis in pregnancy and the puerperium. Am Surg 38:314, 1972.
73. Woodhouse DR, Haylen B: Gallbladder disease complicating pregnancy. Aust NZ J Obstet Gynaecol 25:233, 1985.
74. Landers D, Carmona R, Crombleholme W, Lim R: Acute cholecystitis in pregnancy. Obstet Gynecol 69:131, 1987.
75. Goodlin RC: Severe pre-eclampsia: Another great imitator. Am J Obstet Gynecol 125:747, 1976.
76. Weinstein L: Pre-eclampsia/eclampsia with haemolysis, elevated liver enzymes and thrombocytopenia. Obstet Gynecol 66:657, 1985.
77. Schwarz ML, Brenner W: Toxemia in a patient with none of the standard signs and symptoms of pre-eclampsia. Obstet Gynecol 66:19S, 1985.
78. Duffy BL, Watson RI: The HELLP syndrome mimics cholecystitis. Med J Aust 148:473, 1988.
79. Watson CJE, Thomson JH, Calne SR: HELLP: It's not cholecystitis. Br J Surg 77:539, 1990.
80. Hiatt JR, Hiatt JCG, Williams RA, Klein SR: Biliary disease in pregnancy: Strategy for surgical management. Am J Surg 151:263, 1986.
81. McKay AJ, O'Neill J, Imrie CW: Pancreatitis, pregnancy, and gallstones. Br J Obstet Gynecol 87:47, 1980.
82. Rabkin RN: Acute pancreatitis in pregnancy: Report of 2 cases with maternal survival. Obstet Gynecol 31:508, 1968.
83. Ferrucci JT Jr: Body ultrasonography. Part II. N Engl J Med 300:538, 1979.
84. Wengert PA, Metzger PP, Echer HA, Patterson LT: The use of ultrasonography in the diagnosis of calculus gallbladder disease. Am Surg 45:439, 1979.
85. Cintora I, Ben-Ora A, MacNeil R, Gilsdorf RR: Cholecystosonography for the decision to operate when acute cholecystitis is suspected. Am J Surg 138:818, 1979.
86. Dixon NP, Faddis DM, Silberman H: Aggressive management of cholecystitis during pregnancy. Am J Surg 154:292, 1987.
87. Printen KJ, Ott RA: Cholecystectomy during pregnancy. Am Surg 44:432, 1978.
88. Pritchard JA, MacDonald PC: Medical and surgical illnesses during pregnancy and the puerperium. In Williams' Obstetrics. New York: Appleton-Century-Crofts, 1980, pp. 701–786.
89. Johnson G Jr, Nuzum CT: The liver, gallbladder, and biliary tract. In Hardy JD (ed.): Hardy's Textbook of Surgery. Philadelphia: J.B. Lippincott Co., 1983, pp. 616–678.
90. Reddick EJ: Laparoscopic laser cholecystectomy. Laser Med Surg News Advances February:38, 1989.
91. Reddick EJ, Olsen DO: Laparoscopic laser cholecystectomy: A comparison with mini-lap cholecystectomy. Surg Endosc 3:131, 1989.
92. Cuschieri A, Berci G, McSherry CK: Laparoscopic cholecystectomy. Am J Surg 159:273, 1990.
93. Perissat J, Collet D, Belliard R: Gallstones: Laparoscopic treatment: Cholecystectomy, cholecystostomy, and lithotripsy. Our own technique. Surg Endosc 4:1, 1990.
94. Perissat J, Collet DR, Belliard R: Gallstones: Laparoscopic treatment, intracorporeal lithotripsy followed by cholecystostomy or cholecystectomy: A personal technique. Endoscopy 21:373, 1989.
95. Angel JL, Knuppel RA, Trabin J: Choledochal cyst complicating a twin gestation. South Med J 78:463, 1985.
96. Devoe LD, Moossa AR, Levin B: Pregnancy complicated by extrahepatic biliary tract carcinoma. J Reprod Med 28:153, 1983.
97. Vogelzang RL, Nemcek AA Jr: Percutaneous cholecystostomy: Diagnostic and therapeutic efficacy. Radiology 168:29, 1988.
98. Green J, Rogers A, Rubin L: Fetal loss after cholecystectomy during pregnancy. CMAJ 88:576, 1983.
99. Harary AM, Barkin JS: Acute pancreatitis. In Gleicher N (ed.): Principles of Medical Therapy in Pregnancy. New York: Plenum Publishers, 1985, pp. 853–857.
100. Wilkinson EJ: Acute pancreatitis in pregnancy: A review of 98 cases and a report of 8 new cases. Obstet Gynecol Surv 28:281, 1973.
101. Langmade CF, Edmonson HA: Acute pancreatitis during pregnancy and the postpartum period: A report on nine cases. Surg Gynecol Obstet 92:43, 1951.
102. Corlett RC, Mishell DR: Pancreatitis in pregnancy. Am J Obstet Gynecol 133:281, 1972.
103. Fischer EP, Dudley AG: Acute pancreatitis in pregnancy: A review and case report. Milit Med 136:578, 1971.
104. Young MKR: Acute pancreatitis in pregnancy: Two case reports. Obstet Gynecol 60:653, 1982.
105. Montgomery WH, Miller FC: Pancreatitis and pregnancy. Obstet Gynecol 35:658, 1970.
106. Klein KB: Pancreatitis in pregnancy. In Rustgi VK, Cooper JN (eds.): Gastrointestinal and Hepatic Complications in Pregnancy. New York: Churchill Livingstone, 1986, pp. 138–161.
107. Berk JE, Smith BH, Akrawi MM: Pregnancy pancreatitis. Am J Gastroenterol 56:216, 1971.
108. McKay AJ, O'Neill J, Imrie CW: Pancreatitis, pregnancy, and gallstones. Br J Obstet Gynaecol 87:47, 1980.
109. Block P, Kelly TR: Management of gallstone pancreatitis during pregnancy and the postpartum period. Surg Gynecol Obstet 168:426, 1989.
110. Jouppila P, Mokka R, Larmi TKI: Acute pancreatitis in pregnancy. Surg Gynecol Obstet 139:879, 1974.
111. Bartelink AKM, Gimbrere JSF, Schoots F, Dony JMJ: Maternal survival after acute haemorrhagic pancreatitis complicating late pregnancy. Eur J Obstet Gynecol Reprod Biol 29:41, 1988.
112. Geokas MC, Galtaxe HA, Banks PA, et al.: Acute pancreatitis. Ann Intern Med 103:86, 1985.
113. Toskes PP, Greenberger NJ: Acute and chronic pancreatitis. Disease-A-Month 29:1, 1983.
114. Spechler SJ, Dalton JW, Robbins AH, et al.: Prevalence of normal serum amylase levels in patients with acute alcoholic pancreatitis. Dig Dis Sci 28:865, 1983.
115. Kolars JC, Ellis CJ, Levitt MD: Comparison of serum amylase, pancreatic isoamylase, and lipase in patients with hyperamylasemia. Dig Dis Sci 29:289, 1984.
116. Nies BM, Dreiss RJ: Hyperlipidemic pancreatitis in pregnancy: A case report and review of the literature. Am J Perinatol 7:166, 1990.
117. Duncan JG, Imrie CW, Blumgart LH: Ultrasound in the management of acute pancreatitis. Br J Radiol 49:858, 1976.
118. Mattison DR, Angtuaco T, Miller FC, Quirk JG: Magnetic resonance imaging in maternal and fetal medicine. J Perinatol 9:411, 1989.
119. Lione A: Ionizing radiation and human reproduction. Reprod Toxicol 1:3, 1987.
120. Kazarian KK, Del Santo PB: Understanding the acute abdomen in pregnancy. Contemp Ob/Gyn 1985; Special Issue "Update on Surgery":26, 1985.
121. Weinberg RB, Sitrin MD, Adkins GM, Lin CC: Treatment of hyperlipidemic pancreatitis with total parenteral nutrition. Gastroenterology 83:1300, 1982.
122. Potter JM, Michael CA: Type I hyperlipoproteinaemia and pregnancy. Aust NZ J Obstet Gynaecol 22:155, 1982.
123. Gineston JL, Capron JP, Delamarre J, et al.: Prolonged total parenteral nutrition in a pregnant woman with acute pancreatitis. J Clin Gastroenterol 6:249, 1984.

124. Lee RV, Rodgers BD, Young C, et al.: Total parenteral nutrition during pregnancy. Obstet Gynecol 68:563, 1986.
125. Yamauchi H, Sunamura M, Takeda K, et al.: Hyperlipidemia and pregnancy associated pancreatitis with reference to plasma exchange as a therapeutic intervention. Tohoku J Exp Med 148:197, 1986.
126. Cameron JL, Capuzzi DM, Zuidema GD, Margolis S: Acute pancreatitis with hyperlipemia. Evidence for a persistent defect in lipid metabolism. Am J Med 56:482, 1974.
127. Corfield AP, Williamson RCN, McMahon MJ, et al.: Prediction of severity in acute pancreatitis: Prospective comparison of three prognostic indices. Lancet 2:403, 1985.
128. Hill LM, Symmonds RE: Small bowel obstruction in pregnancy: A review and report of four cases. Obstet Gynecol 49:170, 1977.
129. Beck WW: Intestinal obstruction in pregnancy. Obstet Gynecol 43:374, 1974.
130. Coughlan BM, O'Herlihy C: Acute intestinal obstruction during pregnancy. J R Coll Surg Edinb 23:175, 1978.
131. Svesko VS, Pisani BJ: Intestinal obstruction in pregnancy. Am J Obstet Gynecol 79:157, 1960.
132. Muguti GI: Intestinal obstruction during pregnancy and the puerperium at Mpilo Central Hospital. J R Coll Surg Edinb 33:156, 1988.
133. Donaldson DR, Parkinson DJ: Intestinal obstruction in pregnancy. J R Coll Surg Edinb 30:372, 1985.
134. Rachagan SP, Raman S, Sivanesaratnam V, Sinnathuray TA: Intestinal obstruction following previous myomectomy and the use of beta-sympathomimetics in pregnancy. Eur J Obstet Gynecol Reprod Biol 22:99, 1986.
135. Morris ED: Intestinal obstruction and pregnancy. J Obstet Gynaecol Br Commonwealth 72:36, 1965.
136. Pratt AT, Donaldson RC, Evertson LR, et al.: Cecal volvulus in pregnancy. Obstet Gynecol 57(suppl):37S, 1981.
137. Harer WB Jr, Harer WB Sr: Volvulus complicating pregnancy and puerperium. Obstet Gynecol 12:399, 1958.
138. Fanning J, Cross CB: Post-cesarean section cecal volvulus. Am J Obstet Gynecol 158:1200, 1988.
139. Graubard Z, Graham KM, Van Der Merwe FJ, Koller AB: Caecal volvulus in pregnancy. S Afr Med J 73:188, 1988.
140. Dunselman GAJ Jr: Intestinal obstruction in pregnancy. Trop Doct 13:174, 1983.
141. Davey WW: Companion to Surgery in Africa. Edinburgh and London: Churchill Livingstone, 1973, pp. 235–264, Appendix B.
142. Hofmeyr GJ, Sonnendecker EWW: Sigmoid volvulus in advanced pregnancy: Report of 2 cases. S Afr Med J 67:63, 1985.
143. Chang TH: Acute volvulus of the transverse colon: Report of an unusual case. W Va Med J 81:95, 1985.
144. Kohn SG, Henry AB, Douglass LH: Volvulus complicating pregnancy. Am J Obstet Gynecol 48:398, 1944.
145. Watson R, Quayle AR: Intussusception in pregnancy. Case report and review of the literature. Br J Obstet Gynaecol 93:1093, 1986.
146. Goldthorp WO: Intestinal obstruction during pregnancy and the puerperium. Br J Clin Pract 20:367, 1966.
147. Davis MR, Bohon CJ: Intestinal obstruction in pregnancy. Clin Obstet Gynecol 26:832, 1983.
148. Holbert TR: Intussusception in pregnancy. J Tenn Med Assoc 80:409, 1987.
149. Baker AH, Barnes J, Lister UG: Acute intestinal obstruction complicating pregnancy. J Obstet Gynaecol Br Emp 60:52, 1953.
150. Bourque MR, Gibbons JM: Intussusception causing intestinal obstruction in pregnancy. Conn Med 43:130, 1979.
151. Nkanza NK, King CS: Choriocarcinoma presenting as an intussusception: A case report. Cent Afr J Med 34:389, 1989.
152. Raf LE: Causes of abdominal adhesions in cases of intestinal obstruction. Acta Chir Scand 135:73, 1969.
153. Moore DT, Watts CD, Wilbanks GD: Intussusception complicating pregnancy: Report of a case. J Natl Med Assoc 59:20, 1967.
154. Matthews S, Mitchell PR: Intestinal obstruction in pregnancy. J Obstet Gynecol Br Comm 55:653, 1948.
155. Finn WF, Lord JW: Carcinoma of the colon producing acute intestinal obstruction during pregnancy. Surg Gynecol Obstet 80:545, 1945.
156. Putzki PS, Scully JH, Kotz J, et al.: Carcinoma of colon producing acute intestinal obstruction during pregnancy. Am J Surg 77:749, 1949.
157. Banner EA, Hunt AB, Dixon CF: Pregnancy associated with carcinoma of the large intestine. Surg Gynecol Obstet 80:211, 1945.
158. Sheld HH: Megacolon complicating pregnancy: A case report. J Reprod Med 32:239, 1987.
159. Ezem BU: Intestinal obstruction in pregnancy. East Afr Med J 63:483, 1986.
160. Graubard Z, Graham KM, Schein M: Small-bowel obstruction in pregnancy after Scopinaro weight reduction operation. S Afr Med J 73:127, 1988.
161. Kairuki HCM: Intestinal obstruction complicating the third trimester of pregnancy and labour: A report of 4 cases. East Afr Med J 55:125, 1978.
162. VanWingerden GI, Dons RF: Complete duodenal obstruction during pregnancy with intestinal nonrotation and painless midgut volvulus. J Reprod Med 26:265, 1981.
163. Kristoffersson A, Emdin S, Jarhult J: Acute intestinal obstruction and splenic hemorrhage due to metastatic choriocarcinoma. Acta Chir Scand 151:381, 1985.
164. Dan U, Rabinovici J, Koller M, et al.: Iatrogenic mechanical ileus due to over-distended uterus. Gynecol Obstet Invest 25:143, 1988.
165. Mansell RV, Beil AR: Postpartum intestinal obstruction following vaginal delivery. Am J Obstet Gynecol 82:872, 1961.
166. Coder DM, Schewitz LJ, Falls HC: Midgut volvulus following cesarean section. Obstet Gynecol 47:231, 1976.
167. Barber HRK, Graber EA: The intestinal tract in relation to obstetrics and gynecology. Clin Obstet Gynaecol 15:650, 1972.
168. McCorriston CC: Nonobstetric abdominal surgery during pregnancy. Am J Obstet Gynecol 86:593, 1963.
169. Uhland H, Parshley PF: Obscure intussusception diagnosed by ultrasound. JAMA 239:224, 1978.
170. Morin ME, Blumenthal DH, Tan A, Li YP: The ultrasonic appearance of ileocolic intussusception. J Clin Ultrasound 9:516, 1981.
171. Allen MJC: Sigmoid volvulus in pregnancy. J R Army Med Corps 136:55, 1990.
172. Malkasian GD, Welch JS, Hallenbeck GA: Volvulus associated with pregnancy. Am J Obstet Gynecol 78:112, 1959.
173. Keating JP: Sigmoid volvulus in late pregnancy. J R Army Med Corps 131:72, 1985.
174. Cowman RM, Davis L: An evaluation of cecal size in impending perforation of the cecum. Surg Gynecol Obstet 103:711, 1956.
175. Wanebo H, Mathewson C, Connolly B: Pseudo-obstruction of the colon. Surg Gynecol Obstet 133:44, 1971.
176. Wilmore DW, Smith RJ, O'Dwyer ST, et al.: The gut: A central organ after surgical stress. Surgery 104:917, 1988.
177. Page CP: The surgeon and gut maintenance. Am J Surg 158:485, 1989.
178. Vender RJ, Spiro HM: Inflammatory bowel disease and pregnancy. J Clin Gastroenterol 4:231, 1982.
179. Babson WW: Terminal ileitis with obstruction and abscess complicating pregnancy. N Engl J Med 235:544, 1946.
180. Abramson D, Jankelson IR, Milner LR: Pregnancy in idiopathic ulcerative colitis. Am J Obstet Gynecol 61:121, 1951.
181. Martinbeau PN, Welch JS, Weiland LH: Crohn's disease and pregnancy. Am J Obstet Gynecol 122:746, 1975.
182. Borcham PF, Soltau DH-K: Pregnancy and Crohn's disease. Br Med J 2:541, 1970.

183. Munro A, Jones PF: Abdominal surgical emergencies during the puerperium. Br Med J 4:691, 1975.

184. Georgy FM: Fulminating ulcerating colitis in pregnancy. Obstet Gynecol 44:603, 1974.

185. Watson WJ, Gaines TE: Third-trimester colectomy for severe ulcerative colitis. J Reprod Med 32:869, 1987.

186. Moeller DD: Crohn's disease beginning during pregnancy. South Med J 81:1067, 1988.

187. Imrie AH: Pregnancy and Crohn's disease. Br Med J 2:299, 1970.

188. Scudamore HH, Rogers AG, et al.: Pregnancy after ileostomy for chronic ulcerative colitis. Gastroenterology 32:295, 1957.

189. Hudson CN: Ileostomy in pregnancy. Proc R Soc Med 65:281, 1972.

190. Bohe MG, Erelund GR, Genell SV, et al.: Surgery for fulminating colitis during pregnancy. Dis Colon Rectum 26:119, 1983.

191. McEwan HP: Ulcerative colitis in pregnancy. Proc R Soc Med 65:279, 1972.

192. Heyworth B, Basu S, Clegg J: Crohn's disease and pregnancy. Br Med J 2:363, 1970.

193. Marshak RH, Korelitz BI, et al.: Toxic dilatation of the colon in the course of ulcerative colitis. Gastroenterology. 38:165, 1960.

194. Thomford NR, Rybak JJ, Pace WG: Toxic megacolon. Surg Gynecol Obstet 128:21, 1969.

195. Holzbach RT: Toxic megacolon in pregnancy. Am J Dig Dis 14:908, 1969.

196. Jalan KN, Sircus W, et al.: An experience of ulcerative colitis. Toxic dilatation in 55 cases. Gastroenterology 57:68, 1969.

197. Becker IM: Pregnancy and toxic dilatation of the colon. Dig Dis 17:79, 1972.

198. Peskin GW, Davis AV: Acute fulminating ulcerative colitis with colonic distention. Surg Gynecol Obstet 110:269, 1960.

199. Cooksey G, Gunn A, Wotherspoon WC: Surgery for acute ulcerative colitis and toxic megacolon during pregnancy. Br J Surg 72:547, 1985.

200. Anderson JB, Turner GM, Williamson RCN: Fulminant ulcerative colitis in late pregnancy and the puerperium. J R Soc Med 80:492, 1987.

201. Schofield PF: Toxic dilatation and perforation in inflammatory bowel disease. Ann R Coll Surg Engl 64:318, 1982.

202. Ojerskog B, Kock NG, Philipson BM, Philipson M: Pregnancy and delivery in patients with a continent ileostomy. Surg Gynecol Obstet 167:61, 1988.

203. Chang HB, Christal S, O'Sullivan T: Automobile passenger safety education in pregnant women and infants. J Reprod Med 30:849, 1984.

204. Crosby WM: Trauma during pregnancy: Maternal and fetal injury. Obstet Gynecol Surv 29:683, 1974.

205. Schoenfeld A, Ziv E, Stein L, et al.: Seat belts in pregnancy and the obstetrician. Obstet Gynecol Surv 42:275, 1987.

206. Sherer DM, Schenker JG: Accidental injury during pregnancy. Obstet Gynecol Surv 44:330, 1989.

207. Olusola OA, Oni EE, Okpere O, et al.: Severe road injuries in the third trimester of pregnancy. Injury 6:129, 1974.

208. Golan A, Sandbank O, Teare AJ: Trauma in late pregnancy. South Afr Med J 57:161, 1980.

209. London, PS: Injury and pregnancy. Injury 6:129, 1974.

210. Lavin JP, Polsky SS: Abdominal trauma during pregnancy. Clin Perinatol 10:423, 1983.

211. Patterson RM: Trauma in pregnancy. Clin Obstet Gynecol 27:32, 1984.

212. Fries MH, Hankins GDV: Motor vehicle accident associated with minimal maternal trauma but subsequent fetal demise. Ann Emerg Med 18:301, 1989.

213. Lavin JP, Mildovnik M: Delayed abruption after maternal trauma as a result of an automobile accident. J Reprod Med 26:621, 1981.

214. Bickers RG, Wennberg RP: Fetomaternal transfusion following trauma. Obstet Gynecol 61:258, 1983.

215. Rose PG, Strohm PL, Zuspan FP: Fetomaternal hemorrhage following trauma. Am J Obstet Gynecol 153:844, 1985.

216. Chibber G, Zacher M, Cohen AW, et al.: Rh isoimmunization following abdominal trauma: A case report. Am J Obstet Gynecol 149:692, 1984.

217. Higgins SD, Garite TJ: Late abruptio placenta in trauma patients: Implications for monitoring. Obstet Gynecol 63:10S, 1984.

218. Kettel LM, Branch DW, Scott JR: Occult placental abruption after maternal trauma. Obstet Gynecol 70:449, 1988.

219. Esposito TJ, Gens DR, Smith LG, Scorpio R: Evaluation of blunt abdominal trauma occurring during pregnancy. J Trauma 29:1628, 1989.

220. Higgins SD: Trauma in pregnancy. J Perinatol 8:288, 1988.

221. Franger AL, Buchsbaum HJ, Peaceman AM: Abdominal gunshot wounds in pregnancy. Am J Obstet Gynecol 160:1124, 1989.

222. Sakala EP, Kort DD: Management of stab wounds to the pregnant uterus: A case report and a review of the literature. Obstet Gynecol Surv 43:319, 1988.

223. Moss LK, Schmidt FE, Creech O: Analysis of 550 stab wounds of the abdomen. Am Surg 28:483, 1962.

224. Dudley DJ, Cruikshand DP: Trauma and acute surgical emergencies in pregnancy. Semin Perinatol 14:42, 1990.

225. Denehy T, McGrath EW, Breen JL: Splenic torsion and rupture in pregnancy. Obstet Gynecol Surv 43:123, 1988.

226. Barnett T: Rupture of spleen in pregnancy. J Obstet Gynaecol Br Emp 59:759, 1952.

227. Buchsbaum HJ: Splenic rupture in pregnancy. Obstet Gynecol Surv 22:381, 1967.

228. Ellis GF, Cantor B: Splenic rupture in pregnancy. Am J Obstet Gynecol 132:220, 1978.

229. Lamerton AJ: Spontaneous rupture of the spleen in early pregnancy. Postgrad Med J 59:596, 1983.

230. Sparkman RS: Rupture of the spleen in pregnancy: Report of two cases and review of the literature. Am J Obstet Gynecol 76:587, 1958.

231. Fletcher H, Frederick J, Barned H, Lizarraga V: Spontaneous rupture of the spleen in pregnancy with splenic conservation. West Indian Med J 38:114, 1989.

232. Nanda S, Gulati N, Sangwan K: Spontaneous splenic rupture in early pregnancy. Int J Gynecol Obstet 31:171, 1990.

233. Orloff MJ, Peskin GW: Spontaneous rupture of the normal spleen: A surgical enigma. Intr Abst Surg 106:1, 1958.

234. Barrett JM, Van Hooydonk JE, Boehm FH: Pregnancy-related rupture of arterial aneurysms. Obstet Gynecol Surv 37:557, 1982.

235. MacFarlane J, Thorbjarnarson B: Rupture of splenic artery aneurysm during pregnancy. Am J Obstet Gynecol 95:1025, 1966.

236. O'Grady J, Day E, Toole A, et al.: Splenic artery aneurysm rupture in pregnancy. A review and case report. Obstet Gynecol 50:627, 1977.

237. Mehrotra D, diBenedetto R. Theriot E, et al.: Spontaneous rupture of splenic artery aneurysm: Sixth instance of both maternal and fetal survival. Obstet Gynecol 62:665, 1983.

238. Lowry SM, O'Dea TP, Gallagher DI, Mozenter R: Splenic artery aneurysm rupture: The seventh instance of maternal and fetal survival. Obstet Gynecol 67:291, 1986.

239. Owens JC, Coffey RJ: Aneurysm of the splenic artery, including a report of 6 additional cases. Int Abstr Surg 97:313, 1953.

240. Barrett JM, Caldwell GN: Association of portal hypertension and ruptured splenic artery aneurysm in pregnancy. Obstet Gynecol 57:255, 1981.

241. Schoon I-M, Seeman T, Niemand D, et al.: Rupture of renal arterial aneurysm in pregnancy. Acta Chir Scand 154:593, 1988.

242. Cohen JR, Shamash FS: Ruptured renal artery aneurysms during pregnancy. J Vasc Surg 6:51, 1987.

243. Snir E, Levinsky L, Salomon J, et al.: Dissecting aortic aneurysm in pregnant women without Marfan disease. Surg Gynecol Obstet 167:463, 1988.

244. Neerhof MG, Zelman W, Sullivan T: Hepatic rupture in pregnancy. Obstet Gynecol Surv 44:407, 1989.

245. Bis KA, Waxman B: Rupture of the liver associated with pregnancy: A review of the literature and a report of two cases. Obstet Gynecol Surv 31:763, 1976.

246. Hakim-Elahi E: Spontaneous rupture of the liver in pregnancy. Obstet Gynecol 26:435, 1965.

247. Henny CP, Lim AE, Brummelkamp WH, et al.: A review of the importance of acute multi-disciplinary treatment following spontaneous rupture of the liver capsule during pregnancy. Surg Gynecol Obstet 156:593, 1983.

248. Bynum TE: Miscellaneous hepatic disorders. In Rustgi VK, Cooper JN (eds.): Gastrointestinal and Hepatic Complications in Pregnancy. New York: Churchill Livingstone, 1986, pp. 216–225.

249. Ekberg H, Leyon J, Jeppsson B, et al.: Hepatic rupture secondary to pre-eclampsia: Report of a case treated conservatively. Ann Chir Gynaecol 73:350, 1984.

250. Roopnarinesingh S, Jankey N, Gopeesingh T: Rupture of the liver as a complication of pre-eclampsia: Case report and review of the literature. Int Surg 66:169, 1981.

251. Goodlin RC, Anderson JC, Hodgson PE: Conservative treatment of liver hematoma in the post-partum period: A report of two cases. J Reprod Med 30:368, 1985.

252. Heller TD, Goldfarb JP: Spontaneous rupture of the liver during pregnancy: A case report and review of the literature. N Y State J Med 86:314, 1986.

253. Woodhouse DR: Conservative management of spontaneous rupture of the liver in pregnancy: Case report. Br J Obstet Gynaecol 93:1097, 1986.

254. Minuk GY, Lui RC, Kelly JK: Rupture of the liver associated with acute fatty liver of pregnancy. Am J Gastroenterol 82:457, 1987.

255. Roh LS: Subcapsular hematoma in fatty liver of pregnancy. J Forens Sci 31:1509, 1986.

256. Hibbard LT: Spontaneous rupture of the liver in pregnancy: A report of eight cases. Am J Obstet Gynecol 126:334, 1976.

257. Yen SS: Spontaneous rupture of the liver during pregnancy: A report of two cases. Obstet Gynecol 23:783, 1964.

258. Manas KJ, Welsh JD, Rankin RA, Miller DD: Hepatic hemorrhage without rupture in preeclampsia. N Engl J Med 312:424, 1985.

259. Katzeff TC, Moore PJ: Ruptured amoebic liver abscess in pregnancy: A case report. Cent Afr J Med 30:257, 1984.

260. Kent DR, Nissen ED, Nissen SE, et al.: Maternal death resulting from rupture of liver adenoma associated with oral contraceptives. Obstet Gynecol 50(suppl):5S, 1977.

261. Kent DR, Nissen ED, Nissen SE, et al.: Effect of pregnancy on liver tumour associated with oral contraceptives. Obstet Gynecol 51:148, 1978.

262. Monks PL, Fryar BG, Biggs WW: Spontaneous rupture of an hepatic adenoma in pregnancy with survival of mother and fetus. Aust NZ J Obstet Gynaecol 26:155, 1986.

263. Erb RE, Gibler WB: Massive hemoperitoneum following rupture of hepatic metastases from unsuspected choriocarcinoma. Am J Emerg Med 7:196, 1989.

264. Hayes D, Lamki H, Hunter IW: Hepatic cell adenoma presenting with intraperitoneal haemorrhage in the puerperium. Br Med J 2:1394, 1977.

265. Terasaki KK, Quinn MF, Lundell CJ, et al.: Spontaneous hepatic hemorrhage in preeclampsia: Treatment with hepatic arterial embolization. Radiology 174:1039, 1990.

266. Loevinger EH, Vujic I, Lee WM, Anderson MC: Hepatic rupture associated with pregnancy: Treatment with transcatheter embolotherapy. Obstet Gynecol 65:281, 1985.

267. Herbert WNP: Hepatic rupture and pregnancy. N Y State J Med 86:286, 1986.

268. Sandweiss DJ, Podolsky MB, Saltzstein HC, et al.: Deaths from perforation and hemorrhage of gastroduodenal ulcer during pregnancy and puerperium. Am J Obstet Gynecol 45:131, 1943.

269. Becker-Anderson H, Husfeldt V: Peptic ulcer in pregnancy. Acta Obstet Gynecol Scand 50:391, 1971.

270. Cunningham JT: The esophagus and stomach. In Gleicher N (ed.): Principles of Medical Therapy in Pregnancy. New York: Plenum Medical Books, 1985, pp. 813–819.

271. Fullman H, Ippoliti A: Acid peptic disease in pregnancy. In Rustgi VK, Cooper JN (eds.): Gastrointestinal and Hepatic Complications in Pregnancy. New York: Churchill Livingstone, 1986, pp. 87–103.

272. Paul M, Tes WL, Holliday RL: Perforated peptic ulcer in pregnancy with survival of mother and child: Case report and review of the literature. Can J Surg 19:427, 1976.

273. Honiotes G, Clark PJ, Cavanagh D: Gastric ulcer perforation during pregnancy. Am J Obstet Gynecol 106:691, 1970.

274. Dilts PV, Coopersmith B, Sweitzer C: Perforated peptic ulcer in pregnancy. Am J Obstet Gynecol 99:293, 1967.

275. Jones PF, McEwan AB, Bernard RM: Hemorrhage and perforation complicating peptic ulcer in pregnancy. Lancet 2:350, 1969.

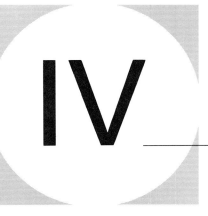

IV

Surgical Vaginal Delivery

UNIT ONE
Vertex Presentation

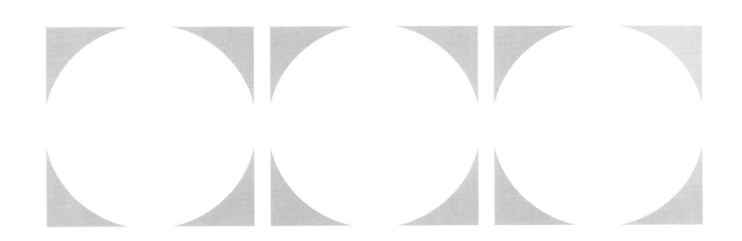

15

Forceps Delivery

Warren C. Plauché

Through all the generations of humankind, those entrusted with attending human births have agonized over the problem of obtaining some kind of purchase on the fetal head to help the mother in her birthing effort. Aberrations of position, rotation, and descent that interfere with fetal passage through the birth canal persist as management problems.

Two aberrations, deflexion and malrotation of the vertex, result in most of the position problems that cause difficult labors. Deflexions of the fetal head produce brow and face presentations that are difficult to surmount with any maneuver or device yet invented. Malrotations (persistent occiput posterior or occiput transverse) and problems of descent are more easily addressed by traction and rotation maneuvers.

HISTORICAL PERSPECTIVES

Centuries ago, when obstetric forceps were developed, the mechanisms of labor that caused malrotations and deflexion positions were not well understood. Severe abnormalities of pelvic architecture resulted from rickets and from the residua of neurologic and bone diseases. Fetal congenital anomalies were undetected during pregnancy. Reliable contraception was not available to women whose pelves were severely contracted or deformed. Labors were often long, exhausting events lasting many days. Mothers frequently lost their lives trying to deliver despite absolute fetopelvic disproportion or malpositioned or malformed babies. There were no drugs to enhance desultory labor. Intravenous fluids to combat dehydration and fatigue were not available. Blood loss could not be replaced. Prior to the late nineteenth century, cesarean section was almost uniformly fatal and not an option for the obstetrician.

The limitations of obstetric techniques led concerned birth attendants to seek mechanical ways to help mothers with difficult labors. Their deliberations led to the development of obstetric forceps. The earliest obstetric forceps were intended for use only on babies that had expired during labor. Many of these early forceps combined traction devices with destructive devices that were very bizarre by present-day standards.

One of the earliest recorded forceps that could have been used on live fetuses appeared in Persia in about 1500 B.C. This instrument consisted of leather straps that were moistened and slipped over the fetal head and fitted with handles for traction.

The most interesting story of obstetric forceps in Western medicine is that of the "secret method" of the Chamberlens of England. This family of accoucheurs gained fame and fortune and became obstetricians to royalty on the strength of their skill with difficult deliveries. Four generations of Chamberlens kept the secret sacrosanct.

William Chamberlen in about 1600 A.D. developed a crude metal forceps and passed the instrument and its technique on to his two sons, both of whom were named Peter. The younger son passed the skill and the instruments on to his three sons. It is perhaps unimaginable, within the ethics of current medical practice, that this family of obstetricians kept secret a useful, lifesaving technique for almost a century. No other physicians were allowed to see, use, or critique the mysterious secret of the Chamberlens until the entrepreneurial spirit of Hugh Chamberlen in the fourth generation broke the spell.

Hugh Chamberlen first tried to sell his family secret to Mauriceau of France. He eventually negotiated a sale to a consortium of Dutch physicians who had raised the considerable fee exacted. Extensive tests were planned by the Dutch, along with a grand scheme for franchising the device.

The Dutch were dismayed when preliminary trials failed to duplicate the amazing results of their English associate. One reason for this was that Hugh had not entirely revealed the Chamberlen secret. He had sold only one blade of his forceps.

Eventually, the "secret" of obstetric forceps became common knowledge and the famous obstetricians of nineteenth century France, England, Italy, and Germany produced many ingenious variations on the original instruments.

The basic idea was a crossed set of metal blades that fit inside the vagina and pelvis and around the baby's head. The blades allowed the obstetrician to add his pulling force to the mother's expulsive efforts. Once the knowledge of forceps became widespread, use of the device enjoyed the history common to many obstetric operations. Periods of praise and widespread use were followed by periods of disuse and criticism.

William Smellie (1697 to 1763) is credited with the introduction of the general use of forceps into the art of midwifery in his "Treatise on the Theory and Practice of Midwifery."[1] Although he recommended the instruments, his records indicate that he used them in only one delivery in a hundred.

Unfortunately, not everyone who read Smellie's book was trained or skilled in the use of forceps. The instruments were misused by unskilled obstetric attendants, to the detriment of many mothers and infants. Physicians quickly reacted to the forceps injury cases they were called on to attend. William Hunter, William Osborn, and Thomas Denman, all famous physicians of commanding opinion, spoke out against the use of forceps. By the early 1800s, forceps were little used in most of Europe.

This reticence to use forceps when no other effective, safe option was available was tragically illustrated by the labor and delivery of Princess Charlotte, only child of George IV, Prince Regent of England. The princess had an exhausting 50-hour labor. Her obstetrician, Richard Croft, son-in-law to the previously mentioned Thomas Denman, recorded a 24-hour unassisted second stage of labor. Prevailing opinion did not allow consideration of forceps to aid the delivery. Both the infant heir to the British throne and his mother died of the ordeal. The anguished obstetrician committed suicide. The history of Europe was changed because the absence of a male heir brought Queen Victoria to the throne. We can only speculate about the outcome if forceps had been used or if cesarean delivery had been available. This incident proved to be a turning point in the history of the use of obstetric forceps.

The incident related above was important, but it was the development of anesthesia for obstetrics in the early 1800s that again raised enthusiasm for instrumental delivery. Use of the instruments steadily increased until even a conservative obstetric unit like the Rotunda in Dublin reported that one delivery in ten was assisted by forceps in the decade ending in 1875.[2]

The popularity of forceps use peaked with DeLee's concept of "prophylactic forceps" in 1921.[3] DeLee held that the use of forceps in most deliveries would protect the baby's head from the rigors of perineal passage and result in a better outcome. Application of this principle at Chicago's Lying-In

Hospital resulted in an increase of forceps use from 28% in the 1930s to 68% in the late 1940s.[4]

Some obstetricians decried the increased use of forceps and continued to seek alternatives. Oxytocin use, as an effective alternative to forceps for the management of uterine atony, was another turning point in obstetrics in this century. Interest in this subject influenced Nicholson Eastman of Johns Hopkins to examine the role of obstetric forceps.[5] The concern of Eastman and others about the possible relationship between delivery events and cerebral palsy led to the famous Collaborative Study for Cerebral Palsy.[6]

Data from the extensive multicenter Collaborative Study of over 55,000 deliveries performed between 1959 and 1966 were minutely analyzed. The data collected supported books and papers 20 years after the study's completion. The conclusions derived from the data accumulated by this study were given great validity and had far-reaching influence. Flaws in this data pool recently have been pointed out by scholars.[7-8]

The study lacked intrapartal fetal assessment by electronic monitoring or scalp blood pH. There was no postpartal determination of fetal oxygenation and acid-base balance. The imaging technology of the time was inadequate for accurate diagnosis of cephalhematomas and intracranial bleeding. Absence of these parameters made it impossible to separate the effects of delivery methods from the effects of an adverse fetal environment prior to delivery. It is equally impossible to gauge the impact of modern neonatal intensive care techniques on the outcomes reported in the Collaborative Study.

The inadequacies of the Collaborative Study were not defects in its design. None of the described technologies were in use when the data were collected just 2 decades ago. One must be very careful when applying conclusions derived from the Collaborative Study to the present practice of obstetrics. The frequently quoted and influential study of Friedman and colleagues[9] reported diminished intelligence quotients in Collaborative Study babies delivered by midforceps. This report is an example of conclusions rendered suspect without knowledge of the intrapartal status of the babies. Another example is the conclusion of Bishop and colleagues[10] regarding the favorable influence of outlet forceps on the outcome of premature deliveries.

A downward turn in the popularity of forceps operations was presaged by E. Stewart Taylor's paper, "Can midforceps operations be eliminated," published in 1953.[11] Cesarean section began to replace vaginal delivery for breech presentation, multiple pregnancies, and disorders of labor. Forceps use for difficult midpelvic delivery came under particularly intense attack. Several symposia from the early 1980s relegate midforceps to the status of obstetric anachronism.[12, 13]

Once again, current psychosocial events exert strong influences on obstetric practice. Many families in the 1980s increasingly restricted themselves to one or two offspring, with the firm expectation that each would be a perfect specimen. Concern for the health and well-being of mothers shifted to concerns about infant outcomes. Immediate birth trauma and long-range birth deficits have become the obstetric topics of greatest interest to parents and their legal advisors. Obstetric instrumental delivery is held responsible for adverse birth outcomes that are not clearly attributable to delivery events.

There has never been convincing direct proof by controlled prospective studies of either the safety or the risk of forceps delivery. The available studies are voluminous and replete with biases and fervor for causes. One can easily find support for arguments for or against the use of forceps.

Richardson and colleagues[7] in their exhaustive literature survey of midforceps delivery, found conflicting studies at every turn and endless sets of confounding variables, with few controlled studies. He found it "impossible to conclude with finality whether the midforceps approach is a good obstetric option or an anachronism. However, it appears that the bulk of the evidence suggests that it can be a useful and safe tool in the armamentarium of the obstetrician, when properly indicated and skillfully applied."

Many recently trained obstetricians have little experience with the maneuvers possible with obstetric forceps. This fact adds new confounding variables of knowledge, experience, and skill to the evaluation equation.

Notwithstanding the cautious optimism of the most careful examiners of evidence relating to the use of forceps, litigation forces place intense pressures on the use of obstetric forceps.[14] The change in attitudes regarding the legitimate use of forceps for common delivery problems relates to the remarkable rise of cesarean delivery in the past 2 decades.

Parents have seldom sought redress for unfavorable obstetric outcomes if the obstetrician's choice was cesarean delivery. A consumer reaction to the high rate of cesarean delivery may lead to a reassessment of the use of obstetric forceps and of other delivery options. Devices that served generations of our obstetrician forebears may yet find a place in the new obstetrics.

FORCEPS INSTRUMENTS

A succession of special forceps have been designed for special circumstances. Obstetricians of the first half of the twentieth century were defined by their skill with a battery of these instruments. Several points of design and function must be understood in order to make an intelligent choice of forceps for simple traction, for rotation, for malpositions and asynclitism, and for the after-coming head of the breech presentation.

Forceps instruments are distinguished by their length, cephalic curve, pelvic curve, solid as opposed to fenestrated blades, parallel or crossed shanks, type of lock, and the presence or absence of an axis traction device (Fig. 15–1A to E). The more exotic designs feature hinged blades and knurled screws to separate the handles. We will not discuss these exotica because the vast majority of forceps maneuvers can be accomplished with three instruments: one for vertex traction, one for vertex rotation, and one for the breech. The instruments available under each category are largely a matter of individual choice, training, and preference. The obstetrician who intends to use forceps should make his or her choice and become skilled and comfortable with their use. Skill in deciding when to use the instrument is at least as important as technique.

The cephalic curve of obstetric forceps refers to the lateral curve in the blades that accommodates the diameters of the fetal vertex (see Fig. 15–1A).

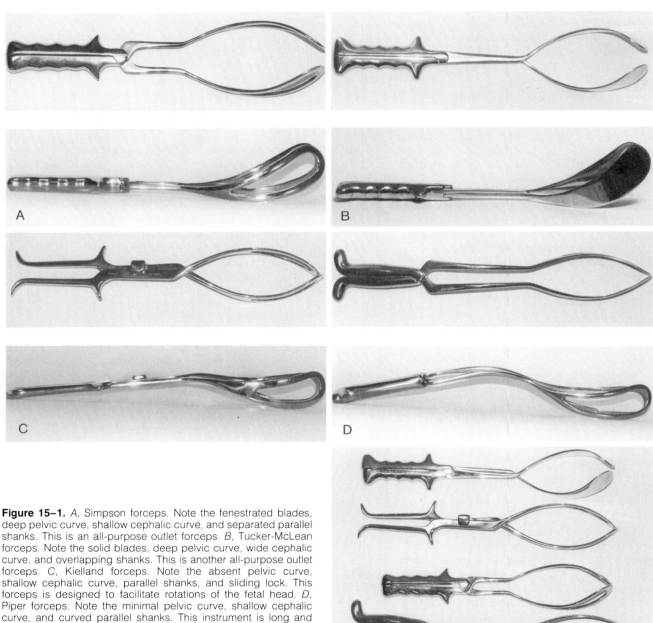

Figure 15–1. *A,* Simpson forceps. Note the fenestrated blades, deep pelvic curve, shallow cephalic curve, and separated parallel shanks. This is an all-purpose outlet forceps. *B,* Tucker-McLean forceps. Note the solid blades, deep pelvic curve, wide cephalic curve, and overlapping shanks. This is another all-purpose outlet forceps. *C,* Kielland forceps. Note the absent pelvic curve, shallow cephalic curve, parallel shanks, and sliding lock. This forceps is designed to facilitate rotations of the fetal head. *D,* Piper forceps. Note the minimal pelvic curve, shallow cephalic curve, and curved parallel shanks. This instrument is long and designed to facilitate delivery of the aftercoming head in breech presentations. *E,* Comparison of obstetric forceps in common use. From top to bottom: Tucker-McLean, Kielland, Simpson, and Piper forceps.

The exaggerated cephalic curve of Tucker-McLean (see Fig. 15–1B) forceps is most effective when the rounded vertex has little molding. Simpson-DeLee forceps (see Fig. 15–1A) have less cephalic curvature and are a good choice for application when the fetal head has elongated to fit a restricted maternal pelvis.

The pelvic curve of a forceps blade determines its fit within the birth canal according to the degree of curvature of the upper and lower edges of the blades. Forceps for simple traction have more pelvic curvature than those used for rotation. Blades with extensive pelvic curvature safely rotate within the pelvis only when the handles describe a very broad arc. Without this arc, the tips of the forceps follow a circular path that can damage maternal soft tissues. Forceps injuries to the maternal vaginal and paravaginal tissues and even to the bladder and rectum can be extensive and very difficult to repair.

Because of these difficulties, forceps with little pelvic curvature have been developed for rotation maneuvers. The classic rotation forceps are those of Kielland (see Fig. 14–1C).[15] Rotation with these forceps results in less risk of soft-tissue damage to the mother. Non-arcing maneuvers, such as "key-in-lock" rotations, can be safely accomplished.

Forceps with fenestrated blades offer a little better traction because of the additional purchase on fetal soft tissues offered by the fitting of these tissues into the openings in the blade. Additional traction security is obtained at the expense of increased incidence of minor fetal soft-tissue injury.

Luikart[16] developed forceps with solid blades, which he felt caused fewer superficial fetal soft-tissue injuries. Such injuries are actually more closely related to inaccurate placement of the forceps blades, the intensity and duration of traction, or the extent of rotation than to blade design. It is absolutely critical that the operator be certain of accurate placement of the forceps prior to any traction or rotation maneuver.

The design of the handles of the forceps may seem to be of little consequence; however, the wide separation of the parallel handles of the Simpson-type forceps necessitates much more stretching of the introital tissues than the overlapping handles of the Elliot, Luikart, or Tucker-McLean types of forceps. Overlapping shank blades are a little easier to use for arcing rotational maneuvers, for those who prefer not to use Kielland forceps.

The lock fitted to a forceps may also seem to have little special significance. In cases of mild asynclitism or deflection of the fetal vertex, the position may improve as traction forces are applied, provided that there is the opportunity for the forceps shanks to move a bit within the lock as the blade adjusts its position. This is possible only with the sliding lock fitted to overlapping shank forceps, as seen in Luikart and similar forceps.

Forceps assistance for delivery of the aftercoming head of the breech is a somewhat controversial subject, despite studies that show the efficacy of this procedure.[17]

Special forceps were designed by Piper that have little pelvic curve, modest cephalic curve, and long, backward-curving handles. These forceps serve to keep the fetal vertex in a flexed position during extraction (see Fig. 15–1D).[18] They are introduced in a straight-ahead fashion on each side of the aftercoming head to control the rate of descent and the amount of extension of the head. Sudden "popping out" of the fetal head, which has been associated with tentorial tears, can be prevented. Extension of the fetal neck, which has been associated with cervical cord injury, can be controlled.

The reluctance of modern obstetricians to use forceps is illustrated by a small study of the use of Piper forceps in vaginal breech deliveries on the Louisiana State University service at Charity Hospital of New Orleans between 1983 and 1984. This service encourages the placement of Piper forceps on the delivery table for use at all breech vaginal deliveries. The instrument was actually used in only one of 100 consecutive vaginal breech deliveries.

DEFINITION OF FORCEPS APPLICATIONS

Forceps applications are classified according to the station of the fetal head and the position of the sagittal suture at the time of forceps application.

Applications were redefined by the American College of Obstetrics and Gynecology's (ACOG) Committee on Obstetrics in February of 1988.[19] The definitions were modified slightly in August of 1989.

High Forceps

The definition of high forceps technique designates the application of forceps to a fetal vertex prior to its engagement in the maternal pelvis. Engagement implies that the biparietal diameter of the vertex is above the pelvic inlet. This condition is difficult to diagnose by examination, and a more practical description of engagement defines the bones of the advancing vertex to be at or below the level of the ischial spines.

There are currently no indications for obstetric high forceps.

Midforceps

The station of the fetal head defines the midforceps operation. Station is expressed as centimeters above (minus station) or below (plus station) the plane of the ischial spines. The definition of midforceps technique designates the application of forceps to the engaged fetal vertex, with the leading point of the skull presenting above station plus two but not above the ischial spines. The vertex must be engaged as defined previously. It may be lower in the pelvis, even at the introitus, but not in a position prescribed for low forceps.[19]

In the past, low forceps were very strictly defined as applying only to the vertex on the perineum, with the sagittal suture in exact anteroposterior position. A procedure was recorded as midforceps even when extraction occurred with the vertex on the perineum but in slightly oblique positions.

The extensive Collaborative Study data gathered in the 1960s was reanalyzed by Friedman and colleagues[9] 2 decades after its collection. These investigators condemned the use of midforceps. Vigorous responses in the literature raised doubts about the conclusions reached by Friedman's group. Little is known of the intrapartal status of infants in the Collaborative Study because it was done prior to the age of fetal monitoring. Outcomes related to the condition of the fetus in utero cannot be easily separated from those related to the use of forceps. This difficulty is critical, since forceps operations are often performed because of fetal distress.

All practicing obstetricians recognize that outlet delivery of a fetus in the oblique anterior position is a much easier operation than the rotation and extraction of a fetus in deep transverse arrest at the ischial spines. The former operation, by classic definition, was an "easy" midforceps delivery, the latter a "difficult" midforceps delivery. Infant morbidity was very different in the two instances.

Morbidity is not significantly different among outlet forceps, low forceps with minimal rotation, and classically defined "easy" midforceps cases. The redefinition of midforceps techniques by the ACOG verified this relationship.[19] The midforceps technique was essentially restricted to applications above plus two station.

Low Forceps

The revised definition of low forceps technique included applications of forceps when the leading point of the skull is at station plus two or more. Two subdivisions were identified: (1) rotations of 45 degrees or less (examples: left occiput anterior to occiput anterior, left occiput posterior to occiput posterior) and (2) rotations of more than 45 degrees.[19]

Extensive molding of the vertex accompanied by thick caput succedaneum is a trap set by nature for unwary or inexperienced obstetricians. The scalp may become visible at the introitus while the true biparietal diameter is still high in the

pelvis. If the obstetrician mistakes this condition for classic low forceps indications, he or she risks two errors. He or she may have a very difficult extraction or even a failure of the extraction procedure. There is also a risk of soft-tissue injuries to the mother and fetus.

Outlet Forceps

The ACOG committee added the category of outlet forceps technique, defined as the application of forceps when (1) the scalp is visible at the introitus without separating the labia; (2) the fetal skull has reached the pelvic floor; (3) the sagittal suture is in the anteroposterior diameter or in right or left occiput anterior or occiput posterior; and (4) the fetal head is at or on the perineum.[19] Rotation cannot exceed 45 degrees. This committee concluded that there was no difference in perinatal outcome and no increased morbidity when forceps rotation on the pelvic floor was 45 degrees or less.

Prerequisites for Forceps Application

Safety and success dictate that certain conditions be present when forceps operations are contemplated (Table 15–1). Amniotic membranes must be ruptured and the cervix fully effaced and dilated. The position and station of the fetus must be accurately known. The presenting part must be engaged in a vertex or face in mentum anterior position, with the exception of applications to the aftercoming head of the breech. The maternal pelvis must be adequate in size and architecture, and the fetus must be of appropriate size. Adequate anesthesia must be administered and an operator skilled in the use of forceps must be present.

Indications and Uses

Most babies enter the pelvis in occiput transverse position as labor begins. This position is dictated by the diameters of the pelvic inlet. The transverse diameter is almost always wider than

Table 15–1. PREREQUISITES FOR FORCEPS APPLICATION

1. Amniotic membranes ruptured
2. Cervix fully effaced and dilated
3. Position and station of the fetus accurately known
   a. Presenting part engaged
   b. Vertex or face in mentum anterior position (except for Piper forceps on breech aftercoming head)
4. Adequate maternal pelvis
   a. Size
   b. Architectural shape
5. Fetus of appropriate size
6. Adequate anesthesia
7. Operator skilled in the use of forceps

the anteroposterior diameter in the common types of pelves.

As descent continues and the vertex reaches midpelvis, it encounters a dramatic reduction in available transverse space. This narrowing of the birth canal is a result of the encroachment of the ischial spines. The vertex must rotate 30 to 90 degrees to the left or right so that its longest diameters may enter the larger oblique pelvic diameters.

Failure of the fetal vertex to rotate when its widest diameter encounters the ischial spines is a common cause of malrotation dystocia. This failure of internal rotation causes prolongation and eventual arrest of labor. Deep transverse arrest as the largest diameters of the vertex reach the level of the ischial spines is an important cause of true "failure to progress." It is the most common indication for classic midforceps rotation.

The obstetrician must choose a management method for deep transverse arrest from a short list of options. Options include observation for a judicious span of time, attempted manual rotation, midforceps delivery, and cesarean delivery. The most common current choice is cesarean delivery. As recently as 2 decades ago, cesarean delivery would have been the "last resort" decision after failure of the other three.

The risk of morbidity for mother and fetus in forceps deliveries increases under certain predictable conditions (Table 15–2). They include major rotations, vertex above plus two station, significant cephalopelvic disproportion, macrosomic infants, and advanced degrees of asynclitism or deflexion of the fetal vertex.[7, 19, 20]

Certain problems of pelvic architecture imply increased risk for malrotation and deflexion positions (Table 15–3). These architectural problems portend difficulty with forceps operations and are discoverable with careful clinical assessment of the pelvis.

Look for a shortened diagonal conjugate, prominent ischial spines, and a narrow interspinous diameter. A flat sacrum means reduced capacity of the posterior segment of the midpelvis. Other important unfavorable findings include a narrow subpubic arch, converging pelvic side walls, and narrow bituberous diameter. Chapter 6, "Clinical Pelvimetry," will prove helpful to the obstetrician

Table 15–2. FACTORS THAT INCREASE MORBIDITY RISK WITH FORCEPS DELIVERY

1. Major rotations
2. Vertex above +2 station
3. Significant cephalopelvic disproportion
4. Macrosomic or immature infant
5. Inadequate pelvic size or shape
6. Positional abnormalities of fetus
   Deflexion
   Asynclitism
   Malrotation

Table 15–3. CLINICAL PELVIMETRY: UNFAVORABLE PELVIC FINDINGS

1. Shortened diagonal conjugate
2. Prominent ischial spines
   Narrow interspinous diameter
3. Flat sacrum
   Reduced posterior segment of midpelvis
4. Narrow subpubic arch
5. Converging side walls
6. Narrow bituberous diameter of outlet

who wishes to sharpen his or her skills at clinical, manual evaluation of the pelvic capacity.

All of these risk factors must be evaluated by an experienced obstetrician before the decision to perform a midforceps delivery is made. Given any mix of risk factors, including the inexperience of the responsible operator, the wisest decision option is often cesarean delivery, providing personnel, facilities, anesthesia, and all other perioperative necessities are available.

Delivery decisions are seldom made on single issues. There is usually a constellation of problems vying for places in the decision matrix. Fetal distress, unavailable immediate cesarean delivery, severe maternal disease, the patient's wishes, or the physician's fear of lawsuit may influence the decision process.

The cold eyes of the legal system seldom see all the confounding variables that enter into an emergency obstetric decision. Some factors do not receive adequate attention. The weight of prevailing opinion is against heroic use of forceps. Given the possibility of intense stress and potential loss of reputation and practice in future court action, many obstetricians simply choose cesarean delivery.

Table 15–4 contains the indications for forceps delivery listed by the ACOG Committee in 1988.[19] It is a short list.

Many obstetricians feel that prolongation of the second stage of labor is not an indication for intervention as long as careful fetal monitoring indicates that the fetus is tolerating labor well. Others are concerned about the effect on the fetus of prolonged intermittent cranial pressure changes with long labors. Shortening of the second stage of labor by forceps delivery is most efficient when the criteria for outlet forceps are met, except in cases of fetal or maternal compromise.

Table 15–4. INDICATIONS FOR FORCEPS OPERATIONS

1. Shortening the normal second stage of labor in the best interests of the mother and fetus
2. Prolonged second stage of labor
3. Fetal distress
4. Maternal indications
   Cardiac disease
   Muscular dysfunctions (e.g., muscular dystrophy, myasthenia gravis)
   Physical exhaustion

(Adapted from the report of the Committee on Obstetrics, American College of Obstetricians and Gynecologists, 1988–1989.)

The second stage is prolonged in primigravidas after dilation is complete for 3 hours with regional anesthesia and for 2 hours without regional anesthesia. In multigravidas, the upper limits of normal second-stage labor are 2 hours with and 1 hour without regional anesthesia. Beyond these times, the risks and benefits of prolongation of labor versus prompt operative delivery should be evaluated.

Maternal indications for forceps delivery include cardiac disease, muscle dysfunctions such as myasthenia gravis or muscular dystrophy, and maternal exhaustion.

OCCIPUT POSTERIOR POSITION

Delivery methods for the vertex in occiput posterior position are controversial. In the past, these deliveries were commonly accomplished by 180-degree (Scanzoni) rotations. Scanzoni rotation operations usually fall into the "difficult" category of forceps deliveries. Risk of maternal and fetal injury is proportional to the degree of difficulty encountered. Most obstetricians currently believe that the majority of persistent occiput posterior positions are best delivered in that position with only minimal rotation.[26]

The operator should think of the forces required for direct occiput posterior extraction. The strong downward pull used to bring the occiput under the pubic symphysis in occiput anterior presentations is not efficient for the occiput posterior position. It places excessive force on the muscles of the posterior perineum. A generous episiotomy and a combination of direct outward and slightly upward traction deliver the vertex in flexion.

DEFLEXION POSITIONS

Large degrees of deflexion of the fetal vertex produce brow and face presentations. Brow presentation is recognized by palpation by the obstetrician of the anterior fontanelle, by the inability to reach the posterior fontanelle, and by feeling the root of the nose and supraorbital ridges.

The brow is almost never suited to the application of forceps and is usually best delivered abdominally. Most positions with this magnitude of abnormality signal themselves early in labor, either by the unusual feel of the presenting part or by an aberration in the labor pattern. Protraction and arrest patterns are common in such instances.

Face presentations present more normal diameters to the pelvis despite the abnormal extension of the fetal cervical spine. Face presentations are recognized by the inability of the obstetrician to feel either fontanelle and by palpation of the fetal nose, orbits, malar eminences, and mouth. The infant's edematous face is occasionally mistaken for a breech presentation.

Face presentations are delivered with a forceps technique not dissimilar to that described for occiput posterior positions. Many babies in face presentation can deliver vaginally if in mentum anterior position. Spontaneous rotation to anterior position usually takes place very late in the second stage of labor, and one must be very patient, in the absence of fetal distress, to await this late rotation before application of forceps. Both brow and face presentations are rare, and our discussion of forceps application is of the more usual flexed vertex, occiput anterior position.

FORCEPS APPLICATION

Low Forceps Application

Because most forceps applications are those that qualify for the designations low or outlet forceps, we will describe this basic application technique (Figs. 15–2A–H).

The first and most critical job of the forceps operator is to check the dimensions of the pelvis and the exact position of the fetal head. I refer the reader to Chapter 6 to review the methods of manually estimating the pelvic dimensions. The most important dimensions for low forceps extraction are the interspinous diameter, the curvature of the sacrum, the angle of the pubic arch, and the distance between the ischial tuberosities.

The operator must know that the fetal vertex is presenting with the sagittal suture in the anteroposterior position or an oblique position near the anteroposterior one. The degree of lateral asynclitism is important and can often be improved by manual manipulation prior to application of the forceps, when the infant's head is low in the pelvis. Any degree of deflexion of the head is important. Even the slight deflection represented by the position known as a "military attitude" offers a much larger object to the birth canal than when the vertex is tightly flexed.

Many obstetricians prefer to have both the rectum and the bladder of the patient empty prior to forceps operations. An empty bladder is particularly important if rotational maneuvers are to be attempted. Empty the bladder by catheterization under aseptic conditions. It may be difficult to introduce a soft catheter into the urethra and bladder when the head is large and low in the pelvis. Place two fingers in the anterior vagina, one on each side of the urethra, to relieve pressure on the urethra. This maneuver facilitates introduction of the catheter without trauma to the delicate and edematous urethral mucosa.

Forceps Application to Direct Occiput Anterior Position

Pick up the articulated forceps of choice and apply a bit of water or other lubricant. Recheck

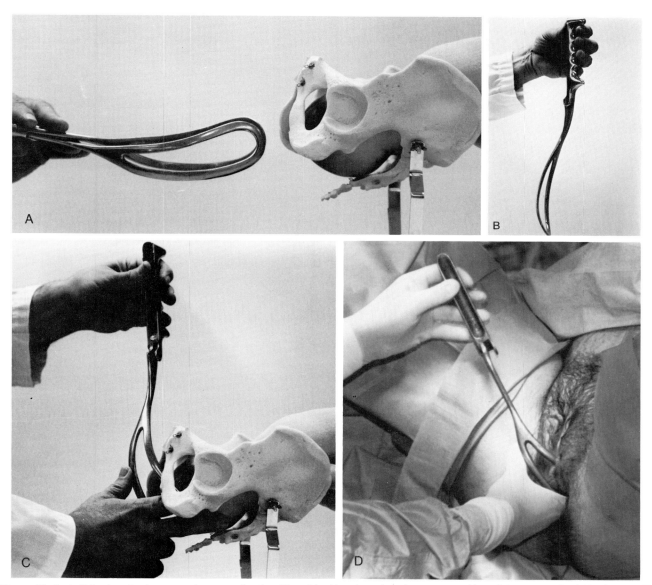

Figure 15–2. *A,* Orienting the forceps prior to application. To guide this orientation, the exact position of the vertex should be known. *B,* The forceps blades are held as delicately in the fingers as a pencil is held. *C, D,* Application of the right forcep blade. Introduce two fingers into the vagina. Slip the forcep blade into the vagina between the baby's head and your fingers. The thumb beneath the blade exerts guiding upward pressure. Note that the forceps handle is straight up.

Illustration continued on following page

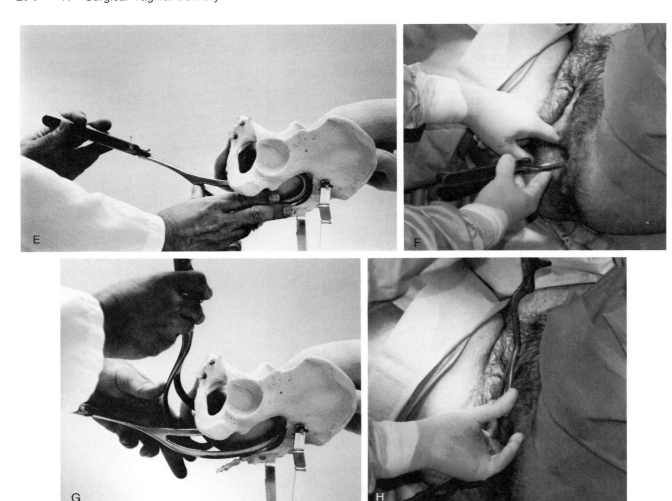

Figure 15–2 *Continued E, F,* Introduction of the right forcep blade. Rotate the forceps handle broadly to the left and downward as the forceps blade slips into the vagina. The operator checks the position of the forceps blade (courtesy Joseph Pastorek, M.D.). *G, H,* The right blade needs little support when the left blade is introduced in a fashion that is the mirror image of the right application. The two blades are articulated as shown in Figures 15–3 and 4. The position of the blades on the fetal head is carefully checked before traction begins.

the exact position of the fetal vertex. Hold the forceps for orientation in their expected final position and note the relative position of the handles (see Fig. 15–2A).

Disarticulate the forceps and take up the right blade, which is to be placed on the mother's left side. Hold the handle near its distal end by the thumb and the first two fingers of your left hand, as though holding up a pencil by its eraser end (see Fig. 15–2B). It is not held in the fist as though wielding a broadsword.

Introduce two or three fingers of the right hand between the left side of the vaginal wall and the baby's head (see Fig. 15–2C–E). The upper edge of the right thumb steadies the inferior curve of the forceps blade. The handle of the forceps is vertical and near the symphysis pubis. Introduce the blade slowly by pressing gently inward and downward with the left hand on the handle. The handle moves inferiorly toward a horizontal position and a bit to the mother's right as the blade of the forceps slips smoothly into the vaginal cavity, between the

operator's fingers and the baby's head. The right thumb presses inward and upward to guide the path of the forceps blade into place.

Check with the right hand to be sure that the blade placement is proper (see Fig. 15–2F). This forceps blade is supported in place while the other blade is introduced. If its position is unstable, it can be supported by an assistant or by pressing the handle lightly against the operator's thigh or abdomen.

The second forceps blade, which is to be placed on the mother's right, is now taken in hand and lubricated. Introduce this blade in a fashion that is the mirror image of the introduction described for the other side (see Fig. 15–2G, H). The right hand holds the handle straight upward, the fingers of the left hand enter the vagina, and the blade is guided between these fingers and the baby's head by the right hand bringing the handle down and in as the left thumb guides the blade into place. The left hand checks the position of the blade.

Before articulation of the two blades, check the

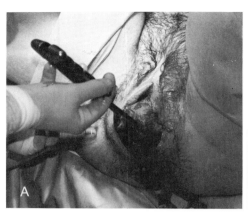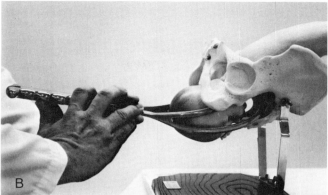

Figure 15–3. *A, B,* two methods of traction without compression. Both hands pull downward and outward on the shanks and handles of the forceps with no force squeezing the blades together.

position to be certain that the sagittal suture of the baby's skull is exactly midway between the two forceps shanks. If this is not the case, the forceps tip could endanger the fetal eye, nose, or other soft tissues. Forceps that are misapplied tend to slip with traction, imparting undesirable shearing forces.

Try to visualize where the tips of the forceps blades lie, although they can be neither seen nor felt. They should encompass the parietal bones, cradling the malar eminences of the baby's cheeks. Articulate the blades by their particular lock and make a final check of position. We seek an exact biparietal-bimalar application.

Dennen's[21] excellent treatise on forceps use recommended three checks of position. The posterior fontanelle should be midway between the sides of the blades and one finger's breadth above the plane of the shanks. The sagittal suture must be perpendicular to the plane of the shanks throughout its length. The fenestrations of the blades should barely be palpable. For forceps without fenestrations, no more than 1 to 1.5 cm of the forceps blade should be palpable below the fetal head. The tips of blades that extend further out than 1.5 cm may lie high on the baby's cheek, over the facial nerve, or over the ear. If all these criteria are met, biparietal-bimalar application is ensured.

There are two principal dangers of improper application of forceps: inappropriate pressure and slippage of the forceps. Pressure applied in the wrong location or excessive pressure may injure fetal soft tissues. The eyes, ears, facial nerves, and facial prominences are at special risk of injury. Both fetal and maternal soft tissues are at risk for lacerations if forceps slip during traction.

Forceps exert not only traction force but compression force. The obstetrician must guard against excessive compression by never squeezing the handles tightly together. Try putting your fist within a set of forceps and allow a trusted partner to squeeze the handles tightly together. It is possible to develop uncomfortably large amounts of compression.[22] Compressive forces are minimized

if traction is placed near the finger flanges of the forceps (Fig. 15–3A). These are near the fulcrum of the simple lever configuration of the forceps. Dennen[21] states that the maximum compressive force is under 5 pounds, with traction applied at the finger flanges.

Traction begins when the operator is certain of the accuracy of the forceps placement. Traction is most efficient when used to augment uterine contractions and the mother's own efforts, but this is not as critical as with vacuum extractions. One needs both a vector of force pulling outward and a vector pulling downward to bring the head under the symphysis pubis.

This author grasps the forceps with his thumbs beneath and his index and middle fingers above the shanks near their articulation and pulls both downward and outward simultaneously (see Fig. 15–3B). This maneuver gives the correct vectors of force and avoids compression of the forceps handles.

The Saxtorph-Pajot maneuver (Fig. 15–4) avoids undue compression in another way. The operator pulls outward with one hand and presses downward from above with the other hand. Some operators simply pull directly outward and allow the resistance of the perineal muscles to provide the downward force vectors.

Traction should be intermittent, slow, deliberate, and gentle. Rocking of the forceps from side to side occasionally seems to facilitate progress in difficult cases. However, rocking movements increase the risk of soft-tissue injury to the fetal structures near the tips of the forceps. Forceps delivery is not a test of strength. Resist the temptation to brace your feet and pull with maximum force.

The forceps handles are initially directed somewhat downward. As the occiput stems under the symphysis, the handles move to horizontal and gradually upward toward vertical as the baby's head is born in extension (Fig. 15–5).

Many obstetricians, including the author, remove the forceps blades after the occiput has come

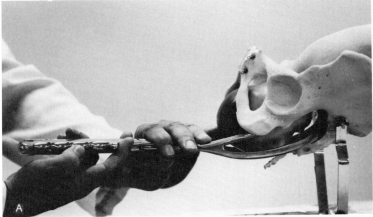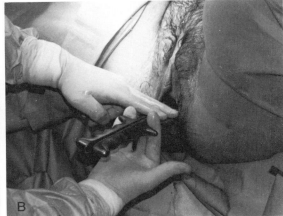

Figure 15–4. *A, B,* The Saxtorph-Pajot traction maneuver. The dominant hand exerts outward traction with two fingers on the flanges of the forceps handles. The other hand exerts downward pressure on the shanks of the forceps.

under the symphysis and complete the delivery manually with some modification of the Ritgen maneuver. This maneuver's upward pressure against the perineum aids the extension and expulsion of the vertex. The mother aids the expulsion effort by pushing while the obstetrician maintains control of the fetal head. Sudden expulsion risks maternal lacerations and sudden changes in fetal intracranial pressure.

The forceps blades are easily removed by disarticulating them and slipping out first one side and then the other. Bring each handle medial and upward toward the vertical while pulling gently outward in a maneuver the reverse of that of the insertion of the forceps.

Examine the baby immediately after delivery for any forceps marks or injuries and record your findings in the delivery record. If there was a reason why symmetric application was not possible, that reason should also be recorded. It is only by routinely inspecting the results of forceps application and traction that operators get direct feedback on the accuracy of their application technique.

Inspect the entire vaginal canal and cervix after delivery of the placenta for any lacerations or abrasions. If any rotation maneuvers have been performed, examine the cervix and vaginal fornices with meticulous care. The circumference of the cervix is not easily seen in its entirety. This can sometimes be accomplished by exerting upward pressure beneath the bladder with a ring forceps loaded with a rolled up 4 × 4 gauze square. This maneuver often brings the cervix pouting out into the field of vision.

If there is any doubt that the physician has seen the entire circumference of the cervix, particularly in the presence of postpartum hemorrhage, inspect the cervix more completely. Grasp the cervix between ring forceps in alternate quadrants until its entire circumference can be pronounced free of lacerations.

The posterior vaginal fornix is another area that notoriously hides from cursory efforts at inspection. Place the sponge-stick described above on or just behind the posterior lip of the cervix. Push the cervix upward and inward to reveal the posterior fornix. Failing this, ring forceps on each side of the posterior cervical lip elevate the cervix to reveal the fornix beneath it. Repair any lacerations that are revealed by these maneuvers, even though they may not appear to be bleeding at the moment they are visualized. It is not unusual for the operator to need retraction assistance for repairs in this area.

Midforceps Application

The most characteristic midforceps operation is rotation from an occiput transverse position. Cau-

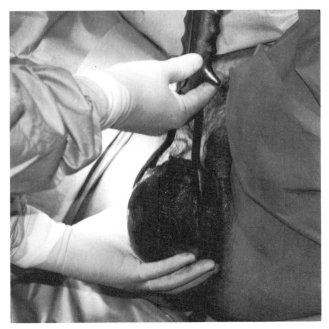

Figure 15–5. Forceps delivery is completed. Forceps handles are almost vertical as the vertex is born in extension.

tion and careful decision making should precede this operation. Most of the fetal injuries in midforceps deliveries are reported from rotational operations and extractions from high station.[20] Always carefully consider the alternative choice of cesarean delivery.

There are two methods of application of forceps to the fetal head in transverse position: a "wandering" technique and the so-called "classic" application. These methods apply whether the obstetrician chooses standard or Kielland forceps. Both techniques require that the operator be certain of the fetal position and the pelvic architecture. The operator must first orient himself or herself by holding the articulated forceps in the anticipated final position.

In the preferred wandering technique, the posterior blade is introduced directly posterior to the fetal head, over the examining fingers. The forceps handle begins in the vertical position and ends in the horizontal position. The blade then fits snugly over the posterior fetal parietal bone.

Introduce the anterior blade first laterally, much as described for low forceps application. At this phase of application, the blade is directly over the baby's face. Carefully and gently maneuver the handle of the forceps while guiding the blade with the internal hand so that the blade gently "wanders" across the face to come to rest anteriorly. The blade should be in position exactly opposite the posterior blade. Recheck the position of both blades. The sagittal suture must be exactly halfway between the shanks.

Articulate the forceps and begin to rotate to an occiput anterior or slightly oblique position. With standard forceps, the large pelvic curve of the blades requires the forceps handles to describe the widest possible arc in the process of rotation.

Sweep the initially horizontal handles in a wide lateral curve against the mother's thigh, then up and anterior, to almost vertical orientation. Slowly bring the handles back down to horizontal position. Try at all times to mentally visualize the location of the tips of the forceps and their movement.

The vertex is now occiput anterior and the forceps are in position exactly as they were after low forceps application, except for station. Traction proceeds.

Traction with midforceps is, by definition, from a higher station than that with low forceps. Supply a larger vector of downward force to bring the head down from high in the birth canal. This can be achieved manually or by the attachment of a special axis traction device to the flanges of the forceps handles. Examples are Cuikart's and Bill's traction devices.[30]

Often the required downward vector of force can be applied by a downward pull on a surgical towel draped over the forceps shanks at the level of the lock. Pressing downward at the same site accomplishes much the same result. The higher the

station, the more downward directed force is required and the more difficult the extraction becomes. Forceps are much better for outward traction than for downward traction.

Kielland forceps have very little pelvic curvature, and rotation can be safely completed without the wide sweep of the handles required with standard forceps (see Fig. 15–1C). With Kielland forceps, simply rotate the fetal head and forceps as when turning a key in a lock. Many operators first displace the head upward to make the rotation easier.

Traction begins once the occiput is in anterior orientation. The Kielland forceps are not very good traction instruments, but they usually suffice. They can be replaced, after rotation, with standard Tucker-McLean or Simpson-DeLee forceps if necessary.

The classic midforceps application technique differs from the wandering application in the introduction of the anterior blade. The anterior blade is turned so that the handle is vertical and the concave face of the blade is upward. Slip the blade into the vagina and cervix beneath the symphysis by bringing the handle down and pressing inward. The blade passes high into the uterus. Turn it over and withdraw somewhat to bring the blade to rest in normal position over the fetal parietal bone.

Classic applications are rarely performed because of the added risk of serious injury to the uterus and bladder from intrauterine manipulation of the forceps blade. The hinged blade of the Barton forceps was developed to avoid this problem. The Barton anterior blade can be introduced directly beneath the symphysis in position against the fetal head because of a hinge that allows the blade to angle sharply backward near its shank. Barton forceps are seldom used in modern operative obstetrics and have disappeared from the forceps cabinets at Charity Hospital of New Orleans.

PIPER FORCEPS

Piper and Bachman[18] developed special forceps with little pelvic curve, sufficient cephalic curve to accommodate the unmolded head of the breech, and long, curved handles to encourage flexion (see Fig. 15–1D). Milner[17] documented the utility of the use of forceps to maintain flexion and control of the aftercoming head in vaginal delivery of breech presentations.

Piper forceps are applied in a fashion very different from ordinary forceps. After delivery of the shoulders of the breech, clear the baby's nose and nasopharynx of blood and mucus. The baby can then breathe freely, and there is little urgency to the remainder of the delivery process. An assistant takes over control of the trunk and legs of the baby.

Orient the articulated Piper forceps, then disarticulate them. Drop to your knees and slip the right blade straight into the vagina between the protecting fingers of the right hand and the baby's head. Slip the left blade similarly straight in. Articulate the shanks and gently ease the head outward and upward over the perineum (Fig. 15–6). The handles remain slightly below horizontal during gentle traction and slowly rise toward the vertical to flex the head out.

Do not allow the head to be suddenly expelled or sharply deflexed. Sudden expulsion is associated with fetal tentorial tears and intracranial bleeding. Hyperextension of the fetal head is occasionally associated with injury to the cervical spinal cord.

Forceps Trauma

The ACOG Committee on Obstetrics stated in 1988 that "there is no difference in perinatal outcome when deliveries involving the use of outlet forceps are compared with similar spontaneous deliveries, and there are no data to support the concept that rotating the head on the pelvic floor 45 degrees or less increases morbidity".[19]

This statement should not be construed to mean that there are no soft-tissue and other injuries seen in low or outlet forceps deliveries. Dell and colleagues,[23] in 1985, recorded all soft-tissue changes and injuries to mothers and babies in prospectively matched groups of primigravidas delivered at term. These women were delivered while under epidural anesthesia by obstetric residents using either low forceps or one of two vacuum extraction instruments.

Superficial skin changes, most of which resolved quickly, were detected most often in the forceps

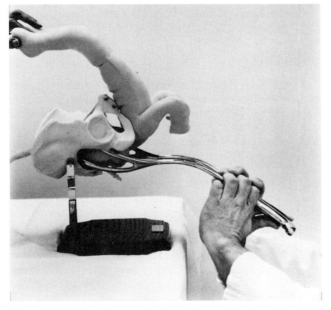

Figure 15–6. Piper forceps in place. Hyperextension of the fetal neck, shown here for clarity of illustration, should be avoided.

group (71%). One cephalhematoma was found by clinical inspection in 45 forceps cases. Maternal morbidity was minimal in this study, but some form of maternal soft-tissue trauma was identified in 48.9% of the forceps delivery group.

Be constantly alert to the possibility of extensive maternal soft-tissue damage when using midforceps. Keep a picture of the location and path of the distal tips of the forceps in your mind's eye. Constantly monitor the amount of soft-tissue resistance to rotation. The response to significant resistance must not be increased force but reassessment of the situation and delivery method.

Be cognizant of the possibility of forceps injury to the infant. Rotations are often performed in the presence of extensive molding of the fetal head and some degree of deflection and asynclitism. All of these factors make the identification of the exact fetal position difficult, even for the most experienced operator. The forceps may not be placed in the ideal anatomic position. The chance of fetal injury is correspondingly increased.

The flat surface of the blades should encompass the parietal bones, and the tips should lie just beyond the malar eminences of the fetal cheek. Displacement from the ideal bimalar, biparietal forceps position increases the chance of fetal injury. Misplaced forceps are poor traction devices, and a "difficult" delivery can be anticipated. When the most experienced operator available is uncomfortable with his or her ability to properly position the forceps, the choice of forceps for delivery should be reconsidered.

Forceps rotation maneuvers are among the risk factors for the unfavorable fetal outcomes identified by many authors. Chiswick and James[24] reported in 1979 a 15% rate of birth trauma and a 3.5% fetal mortality rate in Kielland forceps deliveries. Hughey and colleagues,[25] in 1978, found a 30% perinatal morbidity rate, including three deaths, among a group of 458 babies delivered by midforceps, in contrast to no perinatal mortality in a small group of 17 matched cases delivered by cesarean section. Bowes and Bowes,[13] in 1980, recorded 19.7% "morbid events" in 71 midforceps deliveries and only 5.4% in cesarean delivery of 37 similar cases.

Cardozo and colleagues,[26] in contrast, reported in 1983 that babies delivered by Kielland rotation had outcomes no different from those delivered by nonrotational forceps maneuvers or by emergency cesarean delivery. Dunlop,[27] reporting on midforceps deliveries at the University of Alberta Hospital in the late 1960s, found zero corrected mortality among 292 babies delivered by midforceps despite the fact that these cases embraced most of their difficult vaginal deliveries.

CONCLUSIONS

Most of the dangers from forceps delivery occur in the "difficult" cases. The difficulties are usually related to high station, rotational maneuvers, and emergency delivery of babies who are already compromised by some degree of intrapartal hypoxia.

The indications for midforceps delivery in modern obstetrics are relative ones in which the obstetrician chooses between instrumental vaginal delivery and cesarean delivery. The choice of forceps is influenced by a need for immediate delivery of infants in distress or by lack of prompt availability of the constellation of requirements for safe abdominal delivery.

The consultant obstetrician should be permitted the midforceps and other forceps operation options. Consultants should become comfortable with and expert in the performance of forceps operations. This implies continued training in forceps procedures in our residency programs.

A survey of forceps training in North America in 1981, reported by Healy and Laufe[28] in 1985, indicated that such training was indeed still available. The amount of midforceps training has decreased since the time of that report.

The next generation of obstetricians are becoming masters of abdominal delivery but are losing the skills of instrumental vaginal delivery by default. Dennen[21] stated that the decrease in forceps learning experiences, whether due to program director decree or to consumer pressure, results in inexperienced operators whose only safe option is abdominal delivery. A cesarean section rate edging toward 30% leaves few labor problems to be solved by other means.

Forceps instruction monographs and texts are being reissued. This marks a change in attitudes and training objectives by at least some leaders in the specialty.[21, 29, 30]

The next change must come through education of parents, their child care advisors, and their lawyers.[14] Considerable legal precedent must be overcome. Our neurology colleagues must be satisfied that our data really show that outlet forceps deliveries pose no greater fetal risk than do spontaneous deliveries. We need prospective studies of carefully matched and monitored cases to prove the statement that midforceps, in their new definition, impose no greater risk to mother and baby than does cesarean birth.

If the safety of forceps cannot be proved, the advocates of abdominal delivery for all dystocia events are right. If the proof exists but does not convince parents and their advocates, prudence remains on the side of those who choose cesarean delivery for cases of dystocia.

References

1. Smellie W: Treatise on the Theory and Practice of Midwifery. London: Wilson & Durham, 1752.
2. Kidd G: Discussion on the use of forceps and its alternatives in lingering labor. Trans Obstet Soc Lond 21:141, 1879.
3. DeLee J: The prophylactic forceps operation. Am J Obstet Gynecol 1:34, 1921.
4. Dieckmann WJ: Discussion in Tucker BE, Benaron HBW: The immediate effects of prolonged labor with forceps delivery, and natural labor with spontaneous delivery on the child. Am J Obstet Gynecol 66:540, 1953.
5. Eastman NJ: Pituitary extract in uterine inertia: Is it justifiable? Am J Obstet Gynec 53:432, 1947.
6. Niswander KR, Gordon M: The women and their pregnancies. DHEW Publ. No. (NIH) 73–379, 1972.
7. Richardson DA, Evans MI, Cibils LA: Midforceps delivery: A critical review. Am J Obstet Gynecol 145:621, 1983.
8. Gilstrap LC, Hauth JC, Schiano S, Connor KD: Neonatal acidosis and method of delivery. Obstet Gynecol 63:681, 1984.
9. Friedman EA, Sachtleben-Murray MS, Dahrouge D, Neff RK: Long-term effects of labor and delivery on offspring: A matched pair analysis. Am J Obstet Gynecol 150:941, 1984.
10. Bishop EH, Israel SL, Briscoe CL: Obstetrical influences on the premature infant's first year of development: A report from the Collaborative Study of Cerebral Palsy. Obstet Gynecol 26:628, 1965.
11. Taylor ES: Can mid-forceps operations be eliminated? Obstet Gynecol 2:302, 1953.
12. Chez RA, Ekbladh L, Friedman EA, Hughey MJ: Symposium on midforceps delivery, Contemp Ob/Gyn 15:82, 1980.
13. Bowes WA, Bowes C: Current role of mid forceps operation. Clin Obstet Gynecol 23:549, 1980.
14. Fineberg KS, Peters DJ, Willson RJ, Kroll DA: Obstetrics/gynecology and the law. Ann Arbor: University of Michigan Press, 1984.
15. Kielland C: On the application of forceps to the unrotated head, with description of a new model of forceps. Monstsschrift fur Geburtshilfs und Gynekologie 43:48, 1916.
16. Luikart R: A new forcep possessing a sliding lock, modified fenestra, with improved handle and axis-traction attachment. Am J Obstet Gynecol 40:1058, 1940.
17. Milner RD: Neonatal mortality of breech deliveries with and without forceps to the aftercoming head. Br J Obstet Gynecol 19:204, 1962.
18. Piper EB, Bachman C: The prevention of fetal injuries in breech delivery. JAMA 92:217, 1929.
19. Committee on Obstetrics, American College of Obstetricians and Gynecologists: Obstetric Forceps. Number 59, Feb. 1988.
20. Cosgrove RA, Weaver OS: An analysis of 1,000 consecutive mid forceps operations. Am J Obstet Gynecol 73:556, 1957.
21. Dennen PC: Technique of application. In: Dennen's Forceps Deliveries. Third Edition. Philadelphia: FA Davis Co. 1989, 43–55.
22. Kelly JV, Sines G: An assessment of the compression and traction forces of obstetrical forceps. Am J Obstet Gynecol 96:521, 1966.
23. Dell DL, Sightler SE, Plauché WC: Soft Cup Vacuum Extraction: A Comparison of Outlet Delivery. Obstet Gynecol 66:624, 1985.
24. Chiswick ML, James DK: Kielland's forceps: Association with neonatal morbidity and mortality. Br Med J 1:7, 1979.
25. Hughey MJ, McElgin TW, Lussky R: Forceps operation in perspective. I. Midforceps rotation operations. J Reprod Med 20:253, 1978.
26. Cardozo LD, Cooper DJ, Gibb DMF, Studd JW: Should we abandon Kielland forceps? Br Med J 287:315, 1983.
27. Dunlop DL: Midforceps operations at the University of Alberta Hospital (1965–67). Am J Obstet Gynecol 114:773, 1972.
28. Healy DL, Laufe LE: Survey of obstetric forceps training in North America in 1981. Am J Obstet Gynecol 151:54, 1985.
29. Laube DW: Forceps Delivery. Clin Obstet Gynecol 29:286, 1986.
30. Laufe LE: Obstetric Forceps. New York: Harper and Row, Hoeber Medical Division, 1968.

16

Vacuum Extraction

Warren C. Plauché

- ■ HISTORICAL INTRODUCTION
- ■ INSTRUMENTS
    - Mälmstrom cups
    - Bird cups
    - Other modifications
    - Plastic extractors
- ■ CONTRAINDICATIONS AND CAUTIONS
- ■ VACUUM EXTRACTION FORCES

- ■ VACUUM EXTRACTION TECHNIQUE
    - Mälmstrom cup technique
    - Soft cup extraction
- ■ INDICATIONS FOR VACUUM EXTRACTION
- ■ MORBIDITY AND MORTALITY
- ■ CONCLUSIONS
- ■ REFERENCES

Vacuum extraction is an obstetric operation "for the extraction of the fetal head from the mother by use of a vacuum extractor ("ventouse") applied to the fetal scalp."[1] The idea is ancient. Negative suction technology began with cupping, bleeding, and other rituals of medieval medicine. Ambrose Paré of France suggested negative suction to elevate depressed skull fractures in traumatic head injuries. Some modern pediatric surgery groups still use this technique.[2] James Yonge,[3] in 1706, combined the cupping glass with an air pump to obtain purchase on various objects, including the fetal head.

Obstetrics honors James Young Simpson from Edinburgh for his obstetric forceps and his advocacy of chloroform anesthesia for the pain of child-

birth. Simpson, in 1849, constructed an obstetric suction delivery device called the Air-Tractor, using the principles of the breast pump.[4] Simpson abandoned the device when he developed his obstetric forceps.

Credit for the modern vacuum extractor goes to Tage Mälmstrom of Sweden.[5] Mälmstrom's doctoral thesis contains the physical and mechanical principles that led to the extractor that bears his name (Fig. 16–1). The unique flanged mushroom shape of the Mälmstrom cup provided the first reliable suction-traction delivery instrument (Fig. 16–2). Mälmstrom published a series of monographs in the late 1950s detailing the use of his device. His descriptions of the limitations and complications of the device are classics.[5–7] All ex-

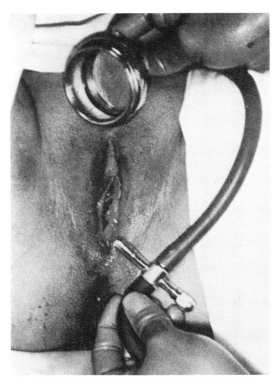

Figure 16–1. The Mälmstrom vacuum extractor with suction tubing and traction handle.

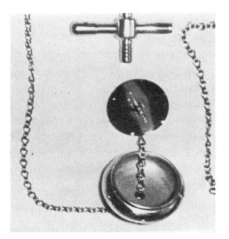

Figure 16–2. A 5-cm metal Mälmstrom cup with mushroom shape, traction chain, and traction handle.

tractors in current use, except for some of the plastic bells, are modifications of the Mälmstrom device.

The design history of the vacuum extractor is similar to the development of obstetric forceps. Obstetric inventors devised increasingly complex constructions to address the perceived weaknesses of the original design.

G. C. Bird[8] developed several of the most important design modifications. He moved the suction fitting from a central location to a peripheral one to facilitate occiput posterior and occiput transverse applications (Fig. 16–3). Inventors tried collars, cords, universal joints, and pulley devices to permit perpendicular force vectors during oblique traction (Figs. 16–4 to 16–9). In 1983, Bird joined this cadre with his "new generation" string traction cups (Fig. 16–8).

Perhaps Bird's most valuable contributions were improvements of extraction technique and codifi-

cation of a set of safety rules for extraction. Bird recognized the importance of fetal head position and extractor cup location in extraction problems.[9] He stressed the importance of maintaining flexion of the vertex and avoiding asynclitism and deflexion forces during vacuum delivery.[9–10]

Vacuum extraction (VE) became an important obstetric operation in Europe and Third World countries in the decades of the 1960s and 1970s. The instrument largely replaced forceps in some clinics and obstetric practices. The technique found broad use for indications that formerly required either difficult forceps manipulations or cesarean delivery.

The mechanics of placement of the vacuum cup and basic use of the instrument are simple. They are easy to teach to labor attendants with less sophisticated training than that of the certified obstetrician. Bird trained midwives and other non-physicians at Port Moresby in the South Pacific to use the technique. The reported experience of this group with 2452 extractions is among the most extensive available.[10] The mechanical simplicity of the instrument led to widespread use that eventually threatened the place of VE in obstetric history.[10, 11]

Selection of patients for VE is more complex than is the actual extraction. The management of labor forces, mechanisms, and positional aberrations necessitates detailed knowledge of obstetric

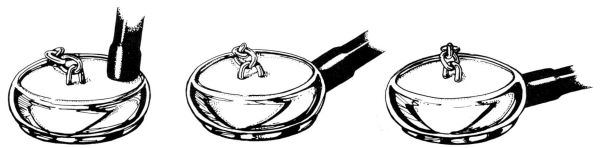

Figure 16–3. The Bird vacuum cups. *Left*, standard; *middle*, anterior; *right*, posterior.

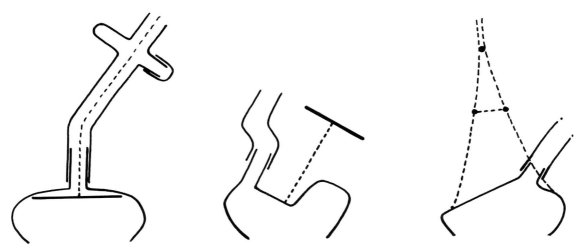

Figure 16–4. Cup configuration and traction elements of several vacuum delivery systems. *Left,* Mälmstrom; *middle,* Halkin; *right,* Lövset.

principles. The simplicity of application and traction with the VE led to its misuse. The instrument was used to manage problems that were beyond the capability of the technique.

Vacuum extraction enthusiasts tried to overcome significant cephalopelvic disproportion, dysfunctional labor, and difficult positional problems with the VE technique. Some applied vacuum cups to heads that bore the extensive molding and caput of obstructed labor. Even the breech presentation attracted the extractor enthusiast.[12] Some operators used the instrument at high station, a practice long discarded from forceps technique. Some attempted application through a partially dilated cervix, increasing the morbidity risk of the procedure. Reports of fetal injury began to accumulate as these questionable uses of the VE increased.

Bird decried misuses of the instrument that could be detrimental to the perinate.[10] Several changes in technique appeared during the past 30 years of experience with vacuum extraction. Mälmstrom abandoned application at high station, one of the original design intentions.[11] Other experts discouraged application when the cervix was dilated less than 7 cm. They recognized that deflexion of the fetal head, asynclitism, and relative cephalopelvic disproportion decreased the likelihood of successful outcome with the extractor. The recommended number of pulls and the duration of cup application progressively decreased over the years.

Vacuum extraction advocates recognize the importance of careful evaluation of problem labors by accepted obstetric principles. Individual case assessment and good obstetric judgment prevent misuse of the instrument.

Scalp damage and other injuries to the neonate limited the popularity of the vacuum extractor in the United States. The instrument arrived in the United States in the early 1960s, coincident with publication of several articles depicting severe scalp injuries.[13, 14]

Cosmetic scalp changes and even superficial scalp injuries are innate in VE use.[15] The mechanism of action transmits suction and traction forces directly to the fetal scalp. The characteristic chignon-like caput beneath the cup is intrinsic to the original technique. This artificial caput sometimes suffuses with blood and is mistaken for cephalhematoma by those who are not familiar with VE. Ultrasonography or computed tomography is necessary to differentiate hemorrhagic caput succadaneum from true cephalhematoma. Cephalhematoma describes a discrete collection of blood beneath the periosteum of a single skull bone.

Even minimal scalp injury is very obvious to new parents. The litigious society of the United States does not easily forgive perceived injury, even when it is clinically insignificant and incurred in the performance of a life-saving service.

The use of vacuum extraction became highly regionalized in the United States. A spectrum of response developed from enthusiastic support to

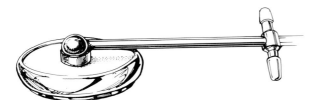

Figure 16–5. The Saling rigid handle vacuum cup with universal joint cup attachment.

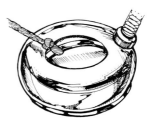

Figure 16–6. The O'Neil suction cup with rotating traction collar and nylon traction cord.

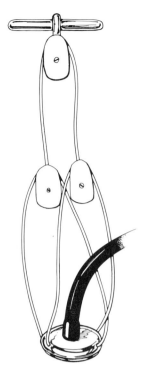

Figure 16–7. Vacuum cup with Lövset multiple pulley traction attachment.

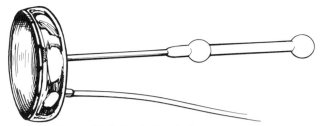

Figure 16–9. The Party plastic vacuum cup.

condemnation. Some obstetric training programs taught the procedure, some did not. In some regions of the country, the extractor became a common delivery instrument. Vacuum extraction was not acceptable to obstetric hospital staffs in other regions.

Extremely negative positions regarding VE use were often based on unfortunate individual outcomes in settings where few powerful staff members were familiar with the method. Neonatologists and child neurologists, struggling to explain intracranial bleeding and cerebral dysfunction to distraught parents, often express concern about instrumental delivery. Vacuum extraction and for-

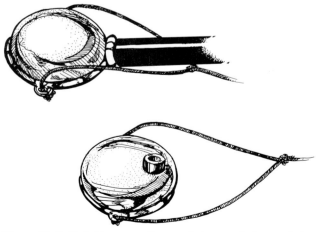

Figure 16–8. Bird string cups. *Top,* posterior cup; *bottom,* anterior cup.

ceps receive the brunt of this concern. We remain uncertain, even after decades of study, as to what portion of this criticism is justified.

It is difficult to differentiate between injuries related to obstetric prepartal emergencies and injuries from the delivery method used to address the emergency. Many parents, their advocates, and many obstetricians believe that cesarean delivery precludes untoward outcomes. They concede that the operator "did everything he or she could" when the choice was abdominal delivery. This same group quickly points to instrumental vaginal delivery as a causal agent for certain unfortunate outcomes.

Abdominal delivery solves many, but not all, obstetric difficulties. Cesarean delivery is not always atraumatic and does not always yield perfect obstetric results for mother or baby.

Some counselors for the legal defense of obstetricians advocate a delivery philosophy resembling "Once pregnant, always a cesarean." The profession should remain honest and open about the safety and efficiency of other emergency delivery methods.

Residents and junior staff are very enthusiastic about the VE when they are first introduced to the device. They immediately propose expanded indications and quick VE solutions to difficult labor problems. Failures and problems with the VE technique accumulate only with experience.

The capriciousness of fetal scalp injuries with VE has always been disturbing. Some very difficult extractions do not leave a mark, whereas some effortless extractions result in extensive scalp abrasions or cephalhematomas.

The place of vacuum delivery remains uncertain after 30 years of study and use because of the concerns described. The future of vacuum delivery may change with the introduction of new materials and instrument designs. Several new extractors utilize malleable plastic materials, which seem to cause fewer cosmetic scalp problems. New instrument designs attempt to distribute traction forces more evenly to increase extraction efficiency and decrease scalp damage.

Vacuum extraction exerts sufficient force to effect obstetric delivery by tugging on the fetal scalp. The vessels of the scalp of the fetus are fragile and connect directly with the dural sinuses via diploic veins (Fig. 16–10). Shearing VE forces can disrupt

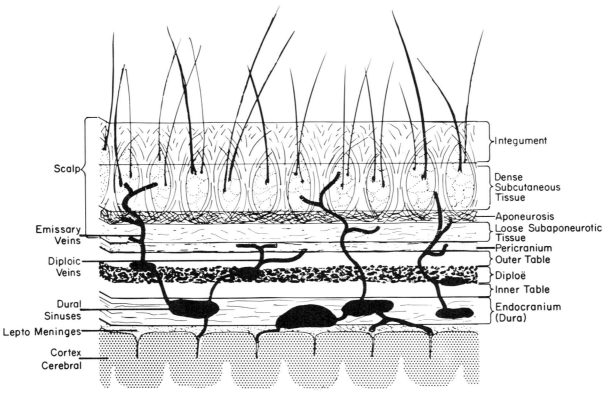

Figure 16–10. Anatomy of the fetal scalp. (Drawing by W.C. Plauché, M.D. Reprinted with permission from the American College of Obstetricians and Gynecologists. Plauché WC: Fetal cranial injuries related to delivery with the Mälmstrom vacuum extractor. Obstet Gynecol 53:750, 1979.)

these frail vessels. Rupture of a blood vessel beneath the periosteum results in a cephalhematoma. Rupture of a vessel beneath the galea aponeurotica results in a subgaleal hematoma.[16]

THE MÄLMSTROM CUP

Early attempts to develop a suction traction device for obstetric delivery failed. Even minimal traction forces pulled the cup off. Mälmstrom developed the first consistently successful cup for obstetric delivery. Mälmstrom's metal vacuum cup featured a mushroom shape. The diameter of the cup, where it attached to the scalp, was smaller than the widest inside diameter (Fig. 16–2).[5] The application of negative pressure enabled this device to draw the scalp into its interior mold. Edema developed in the scalp and created a chignon or doughnut-like deformation on which the cup exerted its pull. Operators could exert traction of sufficient magnitude to effect delivery without detaching the cup.

Manufacturers offered several sizes of Mälmstrom cups. The small 3-cm and 4-cm diameter cups were of little use except for the delivery of second twins or emergency extractions with incomplete cervical dilation. Mälmstrom's admonition to use the largest cup possible made the 5- and 6-cm

cups the most popular units. Metal cups are not flexible, and those of large diameter are difficult to introduce into the vagina.

The Mälmstrom extractor unit requires an awkward assembly process before placement of the cup on the fetal head. The cup is beautifully simple, but the accoutrements are complicated. A metal suction pipe exits the center of the dome of the cup. A pull chain attached to a metal disc threads through the suction pipe, a short length of flexible rubber hose, and a metal traction handle.

Early devices fixed the chain links in place with a gasketed nail. Later models fitted a small metal hook to fix the chain to the traction handle. More hose connected the traction handle to a rubber stoppered jar to collect fluids. Still another length of hose connected the vacuum jar to a suction pump. A pressure gauge occupied a third hole in the stopper of the vacuum jar.

Simple hand pumps developed the vacuum in early VE models. Later models featured electric pumps that controlled suction with foot switches to maintain constant negative pressures.

Users of these early complex systems had frequent problems with assembly and maintaining suction. Repeated sterilization stiffened the hoses. The inner bore of the rubberized hoses enlarged with frequent use. Instrument failure often occurred because a piece was either missing or worn.

BIRD'S ANTERIOR AND POSTERIOR CUPS

Bird found the placement and perpendicular traction on Mälmstrom cups particularly difficult in high applications and occiput posterior positions. He developed a cup with an eccentrically placed suction pipe for anterior presentations (see Fig. 16–3).[8] The lateral placement of the suction element enabled an oblique pull that remained perpendicular to the planes of the pelvis as descent progressed. Some correction of asynclitism was also possible. This modification was not ideal for the delivery of occiput posterior presentations. Bird developed a cup with the suction pipe on the lateral rim to solve this problem (see Fig. 16–3).

OTHER MODIFICATIONS

The same problems that Bird addressed puzzled other obstetrician inventors. Force vector studies indicated the need for more dispersion of traction forces. Efficient extraction necessitates constant perpendicular traction force despite changes in the direction of the pelvic axis as the head descends.

Halkin[18] developed a vacuum extractor cup with an unusual V-shaped profile and an eccentric position of the suction pipe. The traction chain attached at the center of a depression in the middle of the cup (Fig. 16–4). Lövset[19] also developed an offset suction pipe cup but used two chains to develop traction at the peripheral rim of the cup.

Saling and Rothe[20] attached a solid metal handle to their shallow cup by a universal ball joint (Fig. 16–5).

O'Neil's cup offered a movable traction collar that allowed two dimensions of movement of a nylon traction cord.[21] This ensured that force vectors always centered at the midpoint of the cup (see Fig. 16–6).

Lövset proposed a very complex traction setup consisting of two pulleys attached to loops of cord secured at four points along the rim of a standard cup (see Fig. 16–7). Strings from the first two pulleys passed to a third pulley fitted with a traction handle. This complicated construction proposed to distribute traction uniformly around the cup perimeter.

Bird's "new generation" extractor cups feature eccentric placement of suction pipes, as described previously. Nylon strings attach low on two sides of the cup (Fig. 16–8). This modification allows oblique pulls and distributes traction force. It eliminates the tedious threading of chains through tubes and handles.

PLASTIC EXTRACTORS

Plastic materials offer interesting opportunities to design new vacuum cups for obstetric delivery.

The Party extractor has a cup design similar to that of the Bird cup (see Fig. 16–9).[11] Cup and handle are made of rigid plastic, with an off-center suction pipe. The flexible traction handle attaches to the cup by a universal joint. This unit was developed in France and has not found its way to many sites in the United States. Obstetricians in the United States use two widely distributed plastic cups, the Silastic Soft Cup extractor and the firm plastic Mity-Vac or Columbia Medical Instruments (CMI) units.

THE SOFT CUP EXTRACTOR

Kobayashi of Japan originally developed the flexible plastic obstetric vacuum extractor (Fig. 16–11).[22] Dow-Corning Corporation currently produces and markets the bell-shaped 6.5-cm diameter Soft Cup. The Silastic material is firm but supple. The cup folds for introduction into the vagina. It is large enough and flexible enough to spread with negative pressure to encase much of the baby's head.

The Soft Cup offers several advantages; it develops symmetric, less cosmetically alarming caput succadaneum than is formed by other devices. Circular red scalp suction marks are more superficial. The Soft Cup causes fewer scalp abrasions and lacerations.

The Soft Cup has the disadvantage of pulling off with normal traction force more frequently than any other vacuum device we have tried. However, Soft Cup detachment does not carry the same threat of fetal injury as sudden detachment of metal cups.

The Soft Cup attaches to the traction handle by a firm plastic tube that contains concentric rings and longitudinal ribs to strengthen this extension of the cup. The metal traction handle contains a trumpet valve that allows control of pressures in the cup.

An electric pump is recommended to keep suction pressures constant at a preset value. The Silastic bell of the Soft Cup is reusable and must be sterilized before each use. The Silastic material resists deterioration quite well with repeated autoclaving.

The Mity-Vac/CMI Systems

The Mity-Vac and CMI units are small (4.5 cm), flared-lip cups of firm plastic. The cup is deep and relatively inflexible (Fig. 16–12). Its small size makes it easy to introduce into the vagina. The slight outward flare at the cup edge and straight interior walls of the cup result in a tall "top-hat" scalp caput.[17]

Our experience and research was with the Mity-Vac system. The Mity-Vac cup pulls off during

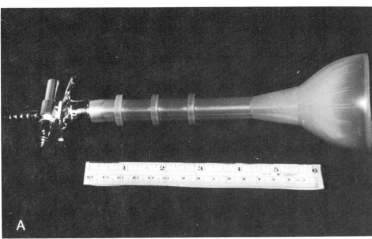
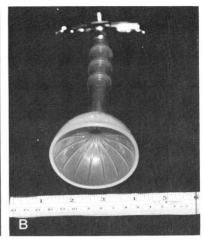

Figure 16–11. *A,* The soft-cup vacuum extractor. Lateral view showing from left to right: pressure-release valve, traction handle, flange connector, and 6.5 cm cup. *B,* The soft-cup vacuum extractor. Interior view showing the rounded edge, interior ribbing, and absence of a mushroom flange.

normal extraction less frequently than the Soft Cup but more frequently than the Mälmstrom metal cup.

The Mity-Vac cup is molded with a short, fixed, rigid traction handle. The handle attaches by clear plastic tubing to a fluid trap, then to an efficient hand pump with a pressure gauge. The Mity-Vac unit is small, effective, inexpensive, and the cup is disposable.[17]

Mälmstrom and Jansson,[7] Bird,[8] and Thiery[11] carefully described the standards for vacuum delivery. These obstetricians spoke with the authority of vast experience. They identified standard and special indications, prerequisites, and contraindications to the use of the VE (Tables 16–1 and 16–2). Table 16–3 outlines the important VE safety code developed by Bird.[10]

CONTRAINDICATIONS AND CAUTIONS

Absolute contraindications to the use of the vacuum extractor include severe cephalopelvic dis-

proportion, intact membranes, inadequately dilated cervix, face or breech presentation, and transverse lie.

Relative contraindications include brow presentation, extensive asynclitism, relative cephalopelvic disproportion, general anesthesia, absent uterine contractions, and uncooperative mothers (Table 16–1).

A few other considerations merit the attention of the attendant planning vacuum delivery. Hemorrhagic scalp problems with VE are much more likely in the presence of a coagulopathy in the baby. The obstetrician seldom knows the coagulation status of the infant, but disorders such as maternal autoimmune thrombocytopenia present the clear possibility of coagulopathy in the baby.

Scalp wounds from blood sampling or placement of electrodes potentially increase the chances of scalp bleeding. Thiery[23] described 4000 cases of fetal scalp blood sampling at full cervical dilation followed by completion of vacuum extraction. He found a very low incidence of scalp hemorrhage and no cases of extensive bleeding.

Bald babies and those with fine blond hair are

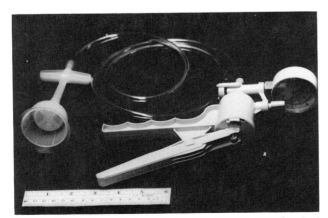

Figure 16–12. The Mity-Vac (Columbia Medical and Surgical, Inc.) vacuum extraction system. Disposable vacuum cup and handle, suction tubing, hand pump, and pressure gauge.

Table 16–1. CONTRAINDICATIONS TO VACUUM EXTRACTION

Absolute Contraindications
Face, breech, transverse lie
Moderate or severe cephalopelvic disproportion
Unknown fetopelvic relationships
Inadequate cervical dilation
Intact amniotic membranes
Missing or nonfunctioning devices

Relative Contraindications
Brow presentation
Severe asynclitism
Problems of fetal size
   Prematurity and immaturity
   Macrosomia
General anesthesia
Uncooperative mother

Table 16–2. PREREQUISITES FOR VACUUM EXTRACTION

Valid indication
Careful obstetric assessment
Ruptured amniotic membranes
Known occiput presentation without severe asynclitism or deflexion
Adequate cervical dilation—at least 7 cm, preferably complete
No significant cephalopelvic disproportion
  Absent fetal macrosomia
Adequate fetal maturity—34 wk or 2500 g
Informed permission for operation
Cooperative mother
Adequate labor mechanism
Complete and working equipment

more prone to cosmetic scalp lesions from VE than are babies with abundant hair. Bird[10] described very few scalp lesions in Melanesian babies examined in his Port Moresby studies. Abundance of hair protects the scalp without seriously interfering with adhesion of the cup.

American users of the extractor express concern over the placement of the vacuum cup over a fontanelle. They actively attempt to avoid such placement. Experiments show little deformation of the dura or brain resulting from placement of the vacuum cup over the posterior fontanelle.[6] The ideal placement of the cup encourages maximal flexion of the vertex. Mechanical considerations alone place the ideal cup site over the posterior fontanelle. Traction encourages deflexion in direct proportion to the distance of the cup forward of this ideal position.[10]

Asymmetric placement of the cup lateral to the midline creates asynclitism with traction. The ideal cup placement is directly in the midline, with the sagittal suture forming a diameter of the circular cup.

Oblique angles of pull, high suction pressures, cup rotation attempts, excessive duration of traction, and detachments of the cup foster scalp injury. The scalp is most fragile and prone to injury in areas of extensive caput succadaneum. Prolonged labor with extensive caput alone can cause desquamation of the skin of the scalp, even with spontaneous vaginal delivery.

Hypoxia increases susceptibility to traumatic injury to the infant's brain and intracranial ves-

Table 16–3. BIRD'S SAFETY RULES FOR VACUUM EXTRACTION

1. The head must be completely or almost completely delivered with no more than three pulls.
2. The head, not just the scalp, must at least begin to move with the first pull and must definitely advance with each subsequent pull.
3. In midcavity and high extractions, the head must be on the pelvic floor by the end of the second pull.
4. The cup must not be applied more than twice.
5. The head must be completely or almost completely delivered within 15 minutes of first applying the cup. Application time must never exceed 20 minutes.

After Bird GC: The use of the Vacuum extractor. Clin Obstet Gynecol 9:641, 1982.

sels.[10] Damage to the brain may already have occurred before the delivery process began. Gunn and colleagues[24] reported ultrasonographic evidence of fetal subdural hematoma in utero at 36 weeks' gestation, before the onset of labor.

Bejar and colleagues[25] reported echoencephalographic studies of neonates. They found cysts adjacent to the lateral ventricles, indicating white matter necrosis in 23 of 127 newborn premature infants. Eleven (9%) had cysts on the first day of life, indicating the antenatal onset of white matter necrosis. Neurodevelopmental examinations were abnormal in four of six of these patients who were re-examined at 26 months of age.

Neurologic deficits, such as those described in the last two paragraphs, are usually discovered long after labor and delivery. The possibility of antenatal onset is seldom considered. Labor and delivery are natural focuses for parents seeking redress for perceived damage to their child.

Technologic advances are just beginning to sort out which infants had pre-existing damage and which were damaged in transit. The technology is still inexact. Obstetric instrumental delivery may be mistakenly held responsible for the neurologic damage. For the present, one must take great care in affixing blame in any individual case.

The potential for injury to the fetus remains an obstruction to more widespread use of VE as a standard delivery instrument.

VACUUM EXTRACTION FORCES

The VE imposes both negative suction forces and positive traction forces on the fetal scalp. Working levels of suction force vary from 0.5 to 0.8 kg/cm^2 (400 to 600 mm Hg). Table 16–4 offers a conversion table for pressure measurement in vacuum systems.

The negative pressure component of VE force is distributed over a small area of scalp. Forces are particularly concentrated at the rim of rigid cups. The Silastic Soft Cup distributes the force over a wider area. Injury to the scalp has an inverse relationship to the size of the vacuum cup and a direct relationship to the duration of extraction.

Mälmstrom felt that positive traction forces distribute evenly around the circumferential attachment of the scalp at the base of the skull.[5] He estimated that normal extraction procedures exerted about 18 lb of traction force. Other authori-

Table 16–4. TABLE OF VACUUM CONVERSIONS

mm Hg	in Hg	lb/in²	kg/cm²
100	3.9	1.9	0.13
200	7.9	3.9	0.27
300	11.8	5.8	0.41
400	15.7	7.7	0.54
500	19.7	9.7	0.68
600	23.6	11.6	0.82

ties have measured the forces required to detach the cup and the head compression forces that occur with VE traction.[26–30]

Early studies hypothesized that the detachment of the vacuum cup at relatively low levels of traction force acted as a safety feature.[26] Saling and Hartung[27] found that the 6-cm Mälmstrom cup detached when traction exceeded 20 kg. Later investigators used electronic devices to measure directly the forces acting on the fetal head. Moolgaoker and colleagues[28] found that the 5-cm Mälmstrom cup evacuated to a negative pressure of 0.8 kg/cm^2 remained attached with traction of up to 51 lb (23.1 kg). The findings of these investigators were disturbing to those counting on detachment of the cup to signal when traction was excessive.

Duchon and colleagues[30] developed the most recent data on forces exerted by vacuum delivery. This group measured traction forces acting on a sphere covered with canine skin. Their findings confirmed those of the clinical groups. The maximal tractive forces were directly proportional to the degree of vacuum induced. The force necessary to cause cup detachment in the working range of 550 to 600 mm Hg of vacuum was approximately 22 kg (50 lb) for all cups 60 mm in diameter or larger.

Duchon and colleagues calculated the force concentrated on the scalp from data on relative deformation of the model. In the normal operating range of negative pressure, the greatest force was exerted on the scalp by the Mälmstrom cup (0.79 kg/cm^2). The Mity-Vac exerted an intermediate amount of force (0.68 kg/cm^2) and the Soft Cup the lowest amount of force (0.63 kg/cm^2).

The Soft Cup collapses onto the scalp at high negative pressures. The force per unit area theoretically increases dramatically with this phenomenon. Duchon's group concluded that all tested vacuum cups with a diameter of 60 mm or more provide "an appropriate, yet apparently safe (less than 22 kg) amount of force when operated at a vacuum of 550 to 600 mm Hg."[30]

Rosa[29] used complex mathematical formulas to calculate theoretical compression forces on the fetal head exerted by VE devices. Rosa estimated acceptable compression forces in the range of 1 to 2 lb/in^2.

Moolgaoker and colleagues' electronic system directly measured compression of the fetal head during traction with various delivery instruments.[28] The mean head compression recorded with the Mälmstrom cup was 11.2 lb/in^2 (0.77 kg/cm^2). This figure was ten times the level predicted by Rosa's calculations.

Comparative compression forces generated by obstetric forceps were even higher in the Moolgaoker series. His own obstetric forceps matched the force levels of VE. Other designs showed increased compression of up to 18.6 lb/in^2 (1.28 kg/

cm^2) for Kielland forceps. When he examined force/time relationships, vacuum devices developed significantly higher total compression forces because of longer traction times.[27] These figures indicate that all instruments that assist delivery exert considerable traction and compression forces on the fetal head.

A spectrum of unknown factors influence our thinking about the effects of delivery forces on the fetal head. Do we know the components of force that act on the fetal head during normal vaginal delivery? Is there agreement on the amount of force that is safe for the fetal head during delivery? Are Wylie's[31] estimates of 15.95-kg average forceps tractive forces for primigravidas and 11.33 kg for multiparous patients the acceptable, safe amount of force? Are McIntyre and Pearse[32] correct that 22.7 kg (50 lb) of force is the upper limit for fetal safety? Is Moolgaoker's[28] measured maximal traction force for certain forceps deliveries of 100 lb absolutely excessive? Do certain circumstances predispose babies to adverse outcomes from acceptable, normally safe, traction and compression forces during delivery?

We do not know what types, intensities, or directions of force may harm the individual fetus. We cannot quantify the effects of intrauterine events before and during delivery. Our goal should be to introduce as few negative variables into the equation of birth as possible. We must strive to help the baby in trouble by the safest means available under the prevailing circumstances. The safest, most effective delivery method for a given set of circumstances is the decision of the trained labor attendant on site.

VACUUM EXTRACTION TECHNIQUE

The application and traction techniques of vacuum extraction vary with the instrument and circumstances of its use. I will describe in this section the techniques for the classic Mälmstrom cup and for the Silastic Soft Cup. Nuances of technique vary from operator to operator. Basic principles and safety rules apply to all.

Mälmstrom Metal Cup Technique

For most applications, choose the largest metal cup that can be applied. Carefully assess the complete obstetric situation. Estimate the size of the pelvis and carefully evaluate pelvic architecture. Estimate fetal size and determine the exact position and attitude of the fetal vertex. Even minimal positional aberrations are important in difficult extractions. A decision to use the VE implies a valid indication and absence of any of the contraindications listed in Table 16–1.

Next, assemble the Mälmstrom instrument and test its function. Thread the chain attached to the metal disk through the suction pipe from inside the cup outward. Pass the chain through the short suction hose and through the metal traction handle. Pull the chain tight to bring the metal disk to the top of the cup. Push the hinged metal stop at the top of the traction handle through one link of the chain. Thread the long suction tubing onto the chain and onto the free end of the suction pipe in the traction handle. Attach the tubing to the intake fitting of a vacuum pump. The procedure is the same, to this point, for most modified metal cups.

A simple bicycle pump can induce negative pressure for VE. Many operators prefer one of the electric vacuum pumps, such as the one made by Egnel Corporation specifically for this purpose. These pumps develop more reliably controlled negative pressures than those achieved with most hand pumps. Top of the line models automatically maintain continuous negative pressure at a level predetermined by the operator.

Test the system by placing the cup on the gloved palm and developing a small amount of suction. If the system is not airtight, check each segment of the unit for a loose, worn, or cracked fitting.

Apply the cup to the fetal scalp once proper function is ensured. Apply a little lubricant to the cup. Water will do nicely. Spread the labia and carefully introduce one side of the rim of the cup into the vagina. Turn the cup as it enters the vagina so that the concave surface contacts the fetal vertex.

The location of the cup is a critical point of VE technique. Place the cup near the occipital fontanelle to ensure flexion of the vertex.[9]

Maintenance of flexion offers the smallest possible diameter to the birth canal. Traction on cup locations forward of the occipital fontanelle invites dystocia from deflexion.

Place the cup directly in the midline. The sagittal suture should form an exact diameter of the circle of the cup. Proper midline cup placement does not allow the head to become asynclitic during traction. Lateral cup placement encourages asynclitism.

Asynclitism, or lateral flexion of the fetal head, causes dystocia by presenting larger head diameters to the pelvis. A small amount of existing asynclitism can be corrected by placement of the cup in the midline, even though the sagittal suture is off center and less accessible. The head position then improves with traction.

Inexperienced VE users often place the cup on the most accessible presenting surface. Vacuum extraction works best if the head is well flexed and centered. It works poorly if any degree of deflexion or asynclitism develops. Careful preoperative assessment of fetal position allows the operator to properly place the cup for maximum traction efficiency.

Vacuum extraction has been suggested to treat the problem of deflexion of the fetal head. However, vacuum extraction does not perform at its best with even the mild deflexion of sincipital presentations (the so-called "military attitude"). Cesarean delivery is a better choice than VE for most brow presentations.[11, 15, 32] Bird[10] felt that brow presentation was not a contraindication to VE if a flexing application could be achieved. Do not use VE on face presentations.[11, 15]

Many deflexion problems occur in premature deliveries. Controversy surrounds the use of VE for premature babies. The propensity for scalp injury and intracranial bleeding increases in small infants. Prematurity plus a deflexion position creates a situation that calls for cesarean delivery.

Induce negative pressure in the system when the cup position is satisfactory.

Mälmstrom's early papers insisted on building up negative pressure slowly over a period of 10 minutes.[5, 6] Mälmstrom felt stepwise induction of vacuum was important to allow the slow development of sufficient caput to fill the inside rim of the cup. Well-formed caput distributes forces more evenly and guards against premature detachment of the cup.

Slow induction of caput lengthens extraction time. When extensive caput is subjected to prolonged negative pressure, it becomes suffused with blood. The purple, swollen caput can be mistaken for a cephalhematoma. The lesion is of minor clinical import but is cosmetically alarming.

Bird[10] and others[11, 34] encouraged rapid buildup of vacuum pressures and immediate extraction. This advice is particularly important under emergency conditions.

Induce the vacuum process initially with 200 mm Hg (0.2 kg/cm^2) negative pressure. Sweep a finger around the cup to be certain that no folds of vagina or cervix have become caught beneath the edge. Continue induction of vacuum to the average operating level of 600 mm Hg (range of 500 to 800 mm Hg or 0.5 to 0.9 kg/cm^2). Bird,[10] Thiery,[11] and Nyirjesy and co-workers[34] induced vacuum as rapidly as possible in one step to 700 to 800 mm Hg (0.8 to 0.9 kg/cm^2). They utilized lower negative pressures of 400 to 500 mm Hg (0.5 kg/cm^2) for premature infants.

With rapid induction of negative pressure, the operator relies only on the adhesion of cup suction for traction. The cup detaches at lower levels of traction. Traction forces need not be great, however, when there is no disproportion or positional abnormality to overcome. Traction begins with the next uterine contraction.

Traction concurrent with contractions is an important and enduring principle of vacuum extraction technique.[5] The VE assists the forces of uterine contraction. The pushing effort of the mother augments the VE forces.

To begin traction, pull gently on the traction handle with two fingers of one hand. The fingers of the other hand press the cup against the scalp and periodically sweep around the cup to be certain that no cervical or vaginal tissue slips beneath the rim of the cup. The thumb of the hand on the cup pushes downward to maintain flexion of the head. This posterior pressure encourages the utilization of all available room in the posterior segment of the pelvis.

Pull in a direction perpendicular to the pelvic plane through which the head is passing. Perpendicular traction usually requires a relatively sharp downward angle of pull early in the extraction. As the head descends, the direction of pull gradually becomes horizontal. Perpendicular traction at the outlet necessitates a gradually increasing upward angle. Avoid oblique traction angles that increase cup detachments and trauma to the scalp beneath the rim of the cup.[10, 11]

Some authors leave the cup on the fetal head throughout the delivery process. Others, including the author, recommend removal of the cup at the time the head crowns to minimize application time.[10]

Safe VE technique requires progress in descent of the fetal head at each pull. True downward movement of the head, not just elongation of the caput, must occur. Strive to complete the delivery with no more than three pulls. Two pulls often suffice. Failure of progressive descent results from application flaws, cephalopelvic disproportion, or positional abnormalities. Failure of descent in two pulls indicates the need for complete reassessment of the obstetric situation and the method of delivery.

Vacuum delivery with metal cups fails in 1.1 to 27% of trial extractions.[35] Table 16–5 outlines the principal causes of VE failure. Bird's series[10] provided good examples of mean failure rates. The Mälmstrom cup failed in 3.2% of extractions, and modified cups failed in 0.9% of extractions. If the cup pulls off, replace it only once in the same place or in a better one.

Spontaneous rotation of the fetal vertex from the occiput transverse to the occiput anterior position or from the occiput posterior to the occiput anterior position occurs in 96 to 98% of extractions.[10] Vacuum extraction devices do not occupy extra space in the pelvis. Rotations occur spontaneously as the head goes through the cardinal movements of labor. The operator's hand can cradle the fetal head and encourage rotation between contractions. Manual turning of the cup can develop "cookie cutter" scalp injuries. The little knob on vacuum cups acts as a pointer, not a rotator.

Soft Cup Extraction Technique

The standard Silastic flexible Soft Cup measures 6.5 cm in diameter (Fig. 16–13). Assemble the

Table 16–5. CAUSES OF VACUUM EXTRACTION FAILURE

Instrument failure—leaks, pump failure
Technique flaws
  Poor cup position
  Oblique traction
  Inappropriate intensity of pulls
  Failure to pull with contractions
  Maternal tissues caught beneath cup rim
Obstetric factors
  Cephalopelvic disproportion
  Position problems
    Deflexion—sinciput, brow, face
    Malrotations—occiput transverse, occiput posterior
    Asynclitism
Extensive caput and molding of vertex
Anencephaly or hydrocephaly
Macrosomic fetus
Cervical problems
  Incomplete dilation
  Cervical dystocia
Maternal factors
  Poor maternal effort or cooperation
  Inadequate contractions
  Anesthesia

instrument by simply attaching the traction handle to the vacuum pump hose. Fold the cup by pressing two sides of the rim together. Insert the folded cup into the vagina between the labia as they are separated by the operator's middle and index fingers. Allow the cup to unfold over the fetal occiput. Its 6.5-cm size encases much of the posterior fetal head.

The Soft Cup has a smooth bell shape with no internal mushroom-like flange.[38] A slow buildup of negative pressure offers no advantage with this instrument. Induce suction quickly to 600 to 800 mm Hg (0.6 to 0.85 kg/cm^2).

Early advocates of the use of the Soft Cup preferred to release the vacuum between pulls. Pressing downward on the trumpet valve in the traction handle rapidly releases pressure. Current authors maintain appropriate negative pressure throughout the delivery.[10]

The rules about the direction of pull and the number of pulls to accomplish delivery are the same with the Soft Cup as with the metal cup. Fewer scalp abrasions and lacerations occur with prolonged application of this instrument, compared with the metal cup.

The Soft Cup tends to pull off during extraction.[17] Pull-offs occur with less traction force than with the metal cups. Cup detachment happens most often with extensive caput and molding. The rolled edges of the Soft Cup do not accommodate well to the hills and valleys of the molded head. Oblique traction angles also readily detach the Soft Cup.

Dell, Sightler, and Plauché[17] reported a series of outlet deliveries in primigravidas under epidural anesthesia. The outcomes of deliveries with the Soft Cup, the Mity-Vac, and the outlet Simpson forceps were compared. The Soft Cup failed to complete delivery in 27.8% of cases, principally

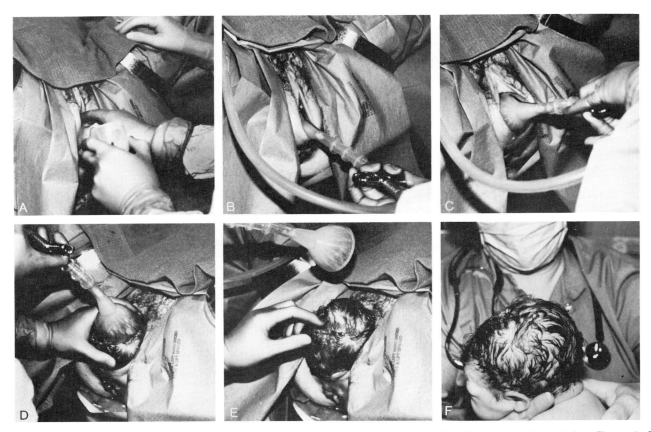

Figure 16–13. *A,* Soft-cup delivery. Folding the soft cup for introduction into the vagina. *B,* Initial traction at low station. First pull. *C,* Continued traction pull. Note change in direction from first pull. *D,* Continued traction. Third pull. Direction of pull much more vertical. *E,* Release of suction and removal of cup. *F,* The infant's head mmediately after soft-cup extraction. (Courtesy Sterling Sightler, M.D. and Diana Dell, M.D.)

because of detachment of the cup. Berkus and co-workers[38] found a 35% failure rate among 129 Soft Cup extractions.

Other Vacuum Cups

Cups with offset suction outlets facilitate occiput posterior applications. The new string traction arrangements help extractions that necessitate oblique traction angles, particularly those from higher stations. Traction that attaches to the periphery of the cup ensures continuous perpendicular traction forces.

The Mity-Vac/CMI semirigid plastic cup performs like a small metal cup without a mushroom flange. Its small size (4.5 cm) and slight flexibility facilitate insertion into the vagina. The short, rigid handle is fixed in perpendicular position on the relatively deep cup.

The straight sides of the Mity-Vac cup do not develop mushroom caput and thus limit the possible traction force. Dell and colleagues[17] reported pull-offs in 13 of 37 (35%) outlet Mity-Vac deliveries in primigravidas. The eventual instrument failure rate was 10.8%, compared with a 27.8% failure rate with the Soft Cup.

INDICATIONS FOR VACUUM EXTRACTION

The VE process developed as an aid to normal delivery. Its use quickly expanded to address diverse problems, from mild degrees of cephalopelvic disproportion to prolapse of the umbilical cord. Table 16–6 presents a summary of reported uses for the vacuum extractor.

The VE instrument became quite popular early in its history for emergency delivery for fetal distress. The delay required to develop caput in Mälmstrom cups limited VE use in emergency deliveries. Operators quickly learned to ignore the need for delay in emergencies. Several authors stated that VE helped avoid some emergency cesarean deliveries.[5, 11, 17, 33]

Many of the emergency cases that are candidates for vacuum delivery are associated with fetal hypoxia. Abruptio placentae and cord accidents late in labor are examples of such emergencies. Both vacuum delivery and forceps delivery are sometimes blamed for outcomes that may have been inevitable before the obstetrician picked up blade or cup. The fragile, hypoxic fetus deserves the gentlest possible delivery. However, prolonged hy-

TABLE 16–6. POSSIBLE INDICATIONS FOR VACUUM EXTRACTION

Second Stage of Labor, Vertex at or Below 0 Station
Secondary arrest of labor—no cephalopelvic disproportion
Fetal distress
  Prolapsed cord
  Other cord accidents
  Abruptio placentae
Need to reduce maternal effort
  Heart disease, hypertension, respiratory problems, exhaustion, distress
First Stage of Labor, Vertex Higher Than 0 Station
Prolonged first stage or arrest—no cephalopelvic disproportion
  Unresponsive uterine inertia
  Oxytocin contraindications
Fetal distress in first stage of labor
Maternal exhaustion or physical distress
  Severe pre-eclampsia, pulmonary edema, heart disease
Other Special Indications
Trial of VE in borderline cephalopelvic disproportion
Second twin delivery
Floating head at cesarean delivery
Delivery of pelvic tumor into incision

poxia is particularly devastating. If hypoxia cannot be corrected, speed of delivery becomes the overriding concern. When speed is essential, a quick vacuum extraction may have the advantage over a delayed cesarean delivery.

Emergency events causing fetal distress often happen early in labor with the infant at high station and the cervix incompletely dilated. This situation tempts inexperienced VE enthusiasts. Beware of this temptation. The highest incidence of injuries resulting from VE occur in the group of babies delivered from high station through an incompletely dilated cervix.[11] Few experienced operators continue to use the vacuum instrument under these conditions. They prefer cesarean delivery if it can be accomplished quickly and safely.

Vacuum delivery from low stations in the second stage of labor can be an easy and rapid method of managing the sudden appearance of fetal distress.

Injuries to the fetal scalp remain an occasional problem, even in elective outlet deliveries.[17] Vacuum extraction cannot overcome severe degrees of cephalopelvic disproportion. It cannot consistently correct advanced positional abnormalities. Use of the vacuum system in these circumstances invites not only failure of the process but damage to the fetus.

The vacuum cup can also deliver the fetal vertex during cesarean operations.[36, 37] It is particularly useful when the head is high above a transverse incision in the lower uterine segment. Manual delivery of such an infant is sometimes traumatic. Placing a vacuum cup on the floating head can bring it easily and quickly down into the incision. Similar application to the floating head has been recommended for the delivery of the second twin in vertex presentation.

MORBIDITY AND MORTALITY IN VACUUM EXTRACTION

Vacuum extraction is very safe for the mother. Our studies indicate that vaginal and cervical lacerations are significantly fewer with outlet VE than with outlet forceps delivery.[17] Berkus and colleagues[39] confirmed 50% less vaginal trauma during deliveries with VE than with forceps. The author's personal series of 228 consecutive Mälmstrom cup extractions contained only a 1.7% incidence of significant maternal vaginal trauma.[33] Sjostedt[35] reported a 0.7% incidence of maternal cervical laceration. No maternal death has been directly associated with vacuum extraction.

Fetal injuries are important considerations with vacuum extraction. Table 16–7 summarizes the experience in several Louisiana State University outcome studies for vacuum extraction and forceps deliveries. These various studies extend over a period of 18 years and are therefore not directly comparable. Persistent scalp injuries occurred in 18.7% of the author's Mälmstrom cup series.[33] Our literature survey of 14,276 Mälmstrom metal cup vacuum deliveries revealed a scalp abrasion or laceration rate of 12.6%.[15]

Multiple examinations recorded all scalp and facial trauma in the plastic cup outlet delivery series reported by Dell and colleagues.[17] Visible scalp lesions occurred in 46% of Mity-Vac deliveries and 44% of Soft Cup deliveries. Scalp or facial lesions were present in 71% of forceps deliveries. Many of the lesions recorded in this study were minor discolorations that disappeared in 24 to 48 hours. Some were much more serious, including one calcified cephalhematoma after VE.

Table 16–7. FETAL OUTCOME—VACUUM EXTRACTION AND FORCEPS: THE LOUISIANA STATE UNIVERSITY STUDIES

| | Mälmstrom Metal Cup VE | | Soft Cup VE | Mity-Vac VE | Outlet Forceps |
	Author's Cases *n = 228 (%)*	*Review Cases* *n = 14,276 (%)*	*n = 152 (%)*	*n = 37 (%)*	*n = 45 (%)*
Scalp or facial lesions*	18.7	12.6	44.0	46.0	71.0
Cephalhematoma†	10.7	6.0	13.9	16.2	2.2
Intracranial hemorrhage	0.35	0.8	1.3	0	2.2
Subgaleal hematoma	0.4	0.59	0.6	0.6	0
Perinatal mortality	1.3	2.6	0.6	0	0
Corrected‡	0	1.5	0.6	0	0

*Scalp abrasions or lacerations
†Clinical diagnosis only
‡Corrected for causes of death not related to delivery method

Clinically diagnosed cephalhematomas occurred in 10.7% of the author's personal series of 228 consecutive metal cup VEs.[33] Cephalhematomas occurred in 6% of the literature survey series of metal cup deliveries.[15] Dell and colleagues[17] recorded clinical cephalhematomas in 16.2% of outlet deliveries with the Mity-Vac cup, 13.9% with the Soft Cup, and 2.2% with outlet forceps.[17]

The diagnosis of cephalhematoma was not consistently investigated by ultrasonography or other imaging procedures in the above studies. Berkus and colleagues[39] found a comparable rate (14.3%) of cephalhematomas diagnosed by clinical means after Soft Cup delivery. Cranial ultrasonography confirmed only a third of these cases, for a true incidence of 5%.

Examiners rarely detect cephalhematomas at the time of delivery. Most cases are recognized on re-examination the day after delivery or later.[17] Evaluation by ultrasonography or radiologic imaging techniques distinguishes true cephalhematoma from hemorrhagic suffusion of the caput.

Intracranial hemorrhages affected 0.35% of the infants in a large survey of the VE literature.[15] Aguero and Alvarez[14] reported the highest incidence (8%) in 1962. Studies later in the 1960s and 1970s did not confirm this high figure. Bergman and Mälmstrom[40] found intracranial hemorrhages in 0.58% of metal cup VE deliveries. Bjerre and Dahlin[41] in 1974 reported a 1% incidence of intracranial hemorrhage associated with VE.

A 1980 study by Ludwig and colleagues[42] used computed tomography to scan infants after deliveries that included VEs. There was no correlation between the mode of delivery and intracranial hemorrhage. A similar ultrasonographic study in 1987 by Jeannin and co-workers[43] examined a small number of infants after difficult VE. They found no cases of intracranial hemorrhage. Berkus and co-workers[39] reported one subarachnoid hemorrhage in a child with a bleeding diathesis in their series of 78 Soft Cup deliveries.

Recent advances in cranial imaging methods show a very high general incidence of intracranial hemorrhage in babies born prematurely at 33 weeks' gestation or less.[43–45] Cartwright and colleagues[44] and Donat and colleagues[45] suggest that 40% of premature infants are subject to intracranial hemorrhage, compared with only 1% of term infants. Lebed and colleagues'[46] ultrasonographic studies in 1982 found evidence of some degree of intracranial hemorrhage in 90% of infants born before 33 weeks' gestation. Demir and colleagues,[47] in 1989, reported a fetal death in utero from an antepartal subdural hematoma. Occurrence of fatal intracranial hemorrhage before labor suggests caution when attributing causation to delivery methods or instruments.

Subgaleal hematomas develop from bleeding into the large subaponeurotic space between the scalp and the bones of the skull. Subgaleal hematomas are much more dangerous than cephalhematomas. A subgaleal accumulation of blood diffuses across the entire scalp from the forehead to the occiput. The capacity of the subgaleal space can exceed that of the infant's blood volume.[15]

Subgaleal hematomas are fortunately quite rare. They occur approximately once in 2500 instrumental deliveries.[15] We reviewed literature reports of 128 subgaleal hematomas in newborns in 1980.[16] Sixty cases followed vacuum extraction (48%), and 14 followed midforceps delivery (13.8%). Thirty-five cases happened after spontaneous vaginal delivery (28.4%) and 11 after cesarean delivery (8.9%). The mortality rate of 28% for subgaleal hematomas emphasized the severity of this rare complication.

Review articles by Bird[10] and Thierry[11] chronicle numerous studies of more subtle effects of VE delivery. Various investigators have examined newborns for retinal hemorrhages, electroencephalographic abnormalities, neurologic deficiencies, convulsions, and irritability.

Retinal hemorrhages are clearly more frequent with instrumental delivery than with spontaneous delivery. They are most common with VE. Schenker and Gombos[48] found retinal hemorrhages in 19% of babies from spontaneous vaginal deliveries, 31% from forceps deliveries, and 52% from VE deliveries. Ehlers and co-workers[49] reported a similar incidence of 38% after forceps delivery and 64% after VE. Retinal hemorrhages may be more closely related to the length and intensity of labor than to the method of delivery. No clear association exists between retinal hemorrhages after delivery and subsequent brain dysfunction.

Newborn electroencephalograms (EEG) are difficult to interpret. Majewski,[50] in 1963, reported abnormal EEG findings in 10% of infants after spontaneous delivery and 20 to 59% after VE. His evaluation of EEGs in these children at ages 3 to 5 years showed almost no abnormalities.

The findings of investigators using subjective tests of cerebral function in the newborn are also difficult to interpret. Conclusions must be questioned, given the nature of the data and the borderline analytic powers of the tests. Despite this disclaimer, most investigators examining these parameters find few differences between newborns of VE deliveries and other newborns.

Scanlon and colleagues[51] developed a behavioral examination of newborns to investigate the effects of maternal anesthesia on the newborn. Sarnat and Sarnat[52] described an encephalopathy staging method that Berkus and colleagues[39] felt could effectively assess ischemic-anoxic effects. Neither VE nor forceps had a negative effect on neurobehavioral function, as determined by these two modalities.[39, 51]

Thiery[11] evaluated babies during and after VE for evidence of anaerobic metabolism. He felt that oxygen supply was comparable during spontaneous and elective VE deliveries. Thiery stated that smooth, elective VE did not produce depressed infants, but prolonged extractions might have this effect.

The force-time integral measured by Saling and Hartung[53] was directly proportional to the risk of neonatal depression. These findings highlight the precaution to keep extraction times short and minimize the number of acceptable pulls.

Broekhuizen and colleagues[55] report more frequent occurrence of shoulder dystocia in their VE group as opposed to their forceps delivery group (3.1% versus 0.3%). Thiery[11] echoed this finding and felt that patient selection was the key to reducing this problem.

The perinatal mortality rate in our literature survey of over 14,000 VEs was 25.8 per 1000.[15] The perinatal mortality rate corrected to 15 per 1000 VE deliveries when deaths unrelated to the mode of delivery were excluded.

Long-term follow-up studies of children delivered by various methods are difficult and occupy the energy of many workers for extended periods. Reliable studies are therefore rare. A few have been carefully done by the same team of investigators over a time span that is sufficiently long to support the conclusions. Bjerre and Dahlin[41] studied infants delivered by VE and a control group for 4 years. They reported evidence of central nervous system damage in 5.3% of infants delivered by VE, compared with 5.9% of infants in the control group. Dongus and colleagues[54] followed infants for 7 to 9 years after instrumental delivery. This group's 1976 report showed a slight increase in psychopathologic sequelae after operative delivery. Forceps delivery preceded these sequelae more often than VE.

Groups studying cerebral dysfunction in children have not been able to separate the effects of maternal disease and predelivery events from those of delivery method. This fact limits the conclusions to be made from the examination of outcomes.

CONCLUSIONS

What is the place of vacuum extraction in the present and future of obstetrics? Responses to this difficult question are often tainted by personal and acquired biases about this controversial instrument.

Vacuum extraction techniques are easy to teach and easy to learn. Perhaps they are too easy. The obstetric principles governing proper patient selection for operative delivery are much more difficult to acquire and to apply. Some of the problems with VE stem from substitution of a facile new technique for sound obstetric judgment.

Obstetricians and their patients are becoming disenchanted with the rapid rise of cesarean delivery rates. If they turn to other modes of operative delivery, VE will be among the better alternatives. Its acceptance depends on the ability of consumers to accept cosmetic scalp changes in the infant and the risk of more serious fetal injuries in 6 to 15% of deliveries. The present medicolegal climate does not readily accept this level of risk when seeking redress for an unfortunate outcome.

Vacuum extraction was controversial on the Louisiana State University Charity Hospital obstetric service when we introduced the technique in 1976. A fetal death several years later from subgaleal hematoma after VE prompted extensive evaluation of fetal cranial injuries related to the technique.

This evaluation included a comprehensive literature review, examination of medicolegal precedent, and a randomized, prospective VE delivery study. The findings of these studies persuaded us to discontinue formal resident instruction in vacuum extraction in 1988.

References

1. Hughes EC: Obstetric-Gynecologic Terminology. Philadelphia: F.A. Davis Co. 1973, p. 409.
2. Tan KL: Elevation of congenital depressed fractures of the skull by the vacuum extractor. Acta Paediatr Scand 63:562, 1974.
3. Yonge J: An account of the balls of hair taken from the uterus and ovaria of several women. Philosophical Transactions 25:2387, 1706.
4. Simpson JY: On a suction tractor or new mechanical power as a substitute for forceps in tedious labours. Edinburgh Monthly J Med Sci 32:556, 1849.
5. Mälmstrom T: Vacuum extractor. An obstetrical instrument. Acta Obstet Gynecol Scand 33 (suppl 4):3, 1954.
6. Mälmstrom T: The vacuum-extractor. Acta Obstet Gynecol Scand 42 (suppl 1), 1964.
7. Mälmstrom T, Jansson I: Use of the vacuum extractor. Clin Obstet Gynecol 8:893, 1965.
8. Bird GC: Modification of Mälmstrom's vacuum extractor. Br Med J 2:526, 1969.
9. Bird GC: The importance of flexion in vacuum extraction delivery. Br J Obstet Gynaecol 83:194, 1976.
10. Bird GC: The use of the vacuum extractor. Clin Obstet Gynecol 9:641, 1982.
11. Thiery M: Obstetric vacuum extraction. Obst Gynec Ann 14:73, 1985.
12. Chalmers JA: Five years' experience with the vacuum extractor. Br Med J 1:1216, 1964.
13. Ahuja GL, Willoughby MLN, Ker MM, et al.: Massive subaponeurotic hemorrhage in infants born by vacuum extraction. Br Med J 3:743, 1969.
14. Aguero O, Alvarez H: Fetal injury due to vacuum extraction. Obstet Gynecol 129:212, 1962.
15. Plauché WC: Fetal cranial injuries related to delivery with the Mälmstrom vacuum extractor. Obstet Gynecol 53:750, 1979.
16. Plauché WC: Subgaleal Hematoma: A complication of instrumental delivery. JAMA 244:1597, 1980.
17. Dell DL, Sightler SE, Plauché WC: Soft cup vacuum extraction: A comparison of outlet delivery. Obstet Gynecol 66:624, 1985.
18. Halkin V: Une modification de la ventouse de Mälmstrom. Bull Soc Roy Belge Gynecol Obstet 34:145, 1964.
19. Lövset J: Modern techniques of vaginal operative delivery

in cephalic presentation. Acta Obstet Gynecol Scand 44:102, 1965.

20. Saling E, Rothe J: Modifikation der Vakuumetraktionsvorrichtung. Z Geburtshilfe Perinatol 182:93, 1978.

21. O'Neil AGB, Skull E, Michael C: A new method of traction for the vacuum cup. Aust NZ J Obstet Gynecol 21:24, 1981.

22. Maryniak GM, Frank JB: Clinical assessment of the Kobayashi vacuum extractor. Obstet Gynecol 64:431, 1984.

23. Thiery M: Fetal hemorrhage following blood samplings and use of vacuum extractor [Letter]. Am J Obstet Gynecol 134:231, 1979.

24. Gunn TR, Mok PM, Becroft DMO: Subdural hemorrhage in utero. Pediatrics 76:605, 1985.

25. Bejar R, Wozniak P, Allard M, et al.: Antenatal origin of neurologic damage in newborn infants. I. Preterm infants. Am J Obstet Gynecol 159:357, 1988.

26. Bergman P, Mälmstrom T: Natal and postnatal mortality in association with vacuum extraction and forceps deliveries. Gynecologia 154:65, 1962.

27. Saling E, Hartung M: Analyses of tractive forceps during the application of vacuum extraction. J Perinat Med 1:245, 1973.

28. Moolgaoker AS, Ahamed SOS, Payne PR: A comparison of different methods of instrumental delivery based on electronic measurements of compression and traction. Obstet Gynecol 54:299, 1979.

29. Rosa P: Defence de l'extraction par ventouse. Bull Soc R Belge Gynecol Obstet 7:10, 1955.

30. Duchon MA, DeMund MA, Brown RH: Laboratory comparison of modern vacuum extractors. Obstet Gynecol 71:155, 1988.

31. Wylie B: Traction in forceps deliveries. Am J Obstet Gynecol 29:425, 1935.

32. McIntire MS, Pearse WH: Follow-up evaluation of infants delivered by electronically recorded forceps delivery. Am J Obstet Gynecol 86:43, 1963.

33. Plauché WC: Vacuum extraction: Use in a community hospital setting. Obstet Gynecol 52:289, 1978.

34. Nyirjesy I, Hawks BL, Falls HC, et al.: A comparative study of the vacuum extractor and forceps. Am J Obstet Gynecol 85:1071, 1963.

35. Sjostedt JE: The vacuum extractor and forceps in obstetrics: A clinical study. Acta Obstet Gynecol Scand 46 (suppl 10), 1967.

36. Pelosi MA, Apuzzio J: Use of the soft silicone obstetric vacuum cup for delivery of the fetus at cesarean section. J Reprod Med 29:289, 1984.

37. Warenski JC: A technique to facilitate delivery of the high-floating head at cesarean section. Am J Obstet Gynecol 139:625, 1981.

38. Berkus MD, Ramamurthy RS, O'Connor PS, et al.: Cohort study of Silastic obstetric vacuum cup deliveries: II. Unsuccessful vacuum extraction. Obstet Gynecol 68:662, 1986.

39. Berkus MD, Ramamurthy RS, O'Connor PS, et al.: Cohort study of Silastic obstetric vacuum cup deliveries: I. Safety of the instrument. Obstet Gynecol 66:53, 1985.

40. Bergman P, Mälmstrom T: Natal and postnatal fetal mortality with vacuum extraction. Gynaecologia 154:65, 1962.

41. Bjerre I, Dahlin K: The long-term development of children delivered by vacuum extraction. Dev Med Child Neurol 15:378, 1974.

42. Ludwig B, Brand M, Brockerhoff P: Postpartum CT examination of the heads of full term infants. Neuroradiology 20:145, 1980.

43. Jeannin P, Afschrift M, Voet D, et al.: Cranial ultrasound after difficult vacuum extraction. Personal communication.

44. Cartwright GW, Culbertson K, Schreiner RL: Changes in clinical presentation of term infants with intracranial hemorrhage. Dev Med Child Neurol 21:730, 1979.

45. Donat JF, Akazaki H, Kleinberg F, et al.: Intraventricular hemorrhages in full term and premature infants. Mayo Clin Proc 53:437, 1978.

46. Lebed MR, Schifrin BS, Waffran F, et al.: Real-time B scanning in the diagnosis of neonatal intracranial hemorrhage. Am J Obstet Gynecol 142:851, 1982.

47. Demir RH, Gleicher N, Myers SA: Atraumatic antepartum subdural hematoma causing fetal death. Am J Obstet Gynecol 160:619, 1989.

48. Schenker JB, Gombos GM: Retinal lesions with vacuum extraction. Obstet Gynecol 27:521, 1966.

49. Ehlers N, Jensen JK, Hansen KB: Retinal haemorrhages in the newborn. Comparison of delivery by forceps and by vacuum extraction. Acta Opthalmol 52:73, 1974.

50. Majewski A: Elektroenzephalographische Kontrolluntersuchungen nach Vakuum-extraktion. Gynaecologia 156:187, 1963.

51. Scanlon JW, Brown WU, Weiss JB, et al.: Neurobehavioral responses of newborn infants after maternal epidural anesthesia. Anesthesiology 40:121, 1974.

52. Sarnat HB, Sarnat MS: Neonatal encephalopathy following fetal distress. Arch Neurol 33:696, 1976.

53. Saling E, Hartung M: Analyses of tractive forces during application of vacuum extraction. J Perinat Med 1:245, 1973.

54. Dongus W, Hartmann M, Lempp R, Pfleiderer A: Vergleichende Untersuchungen uber die Entwicklund der Kinder nach Vakuum- bzw. Zangenentbindung. Z Kinder-Jugend-Psychiatr 4:25, 1976.

55. Broekhuizen FF, Washington JM, Johnson F, et al.: Vacuum extraction versus forceps delivery: Indications and complications, 1979 to 1984. Obstet Gynecol 69:338, 1987.

17

Operative Vaginal Delivery of Abnormal Vertex Presentations

Warren C. Plauché

The fetal vertex enters the pelvis as the presenting part during labor in 95% or more of pregnancies. The inlet transverse diameter of the normal gynecoid pelvis is larger than the inlet anteroposterior diameter. This encourages the vertex to enter the pelvis in the occiput transverse position.

The head must execute the cardinal movements of labor as descent progresses. The fetal chin normally tucks tightly on the fetal chest in a fully flexed attitude. The forces of labor push the baby downward until it reaches the midpelvic level of the ischial spines. These spines offer an obstruction to the advancing head. The baby must rotate to bring its longest diameter into a more commodious diameter of the midpelvis.

The vertex must maintain its alignment in the pelvis during rotation and descent. A lateral bend to one side or the other risks dystocia from asynclitism. The head must stay well flexed as it descends into the cavity of the pelvis to avoid dystocia from deflexion attitudes. Internal rotation negotiates the obstruction at midpelvis presented by the ischial spines.

Failure of the fetal vertex to execute the cardinal movements of labor causes abnormal vertex presentations and difficult labors (Table 17–1). Malrotation results in deep transverse arrest and failure of descent. Canting of the head to one side or the other results in asynclitism. Deflexion of the vertex results in a sincipital (military attitude), brow, or face presentation.

Abnormal fetal lies or fetal anomalies can cause both deflexion and asynclitism. Occasionally, an extremity may enter the pelvis along with the vertex to form a compound presentation. The fetus with congenital abnormalities such as gastroschisis, omphalocele, hydronephrosis, or hydrocephalus presents fetopelvic relationships that require complex management decisions.

Vaginal delivery is an acceptable option in many of these cases. An important part of the training of every obstetrician is learning methods to accomplish vaginal delivery of difficult presentations. This chapter discusses the management of abnormal vertex presentations.

Discussion of these vaginal operative delivery methods does not imply endorsement of a particular method in any individual case. Cesarean delivery may be a better individual management choice for difficult labors caused by positional abnormalities. Heroic attempts at vaginal delivery risk injury to maternal soft tissue and the fetal cranium. Cesarean delivery has its own unique risks. Delivery decisions balance complex risk and benefit variables. The choice of delivery method depends on multiple individual circumstances present at the time of the decision. The choice is not easy, even for experienced obstetricians.

ISSUES OF INFORMED CONSENT

The delivery method chosen must have the informed consent of the mother and consensus among the family. The present trend of litigation risk increases pressure on physicians to delegate clinical decisions to their patients. Having them choose between operative vaginal delivery and cesarean birth is an example of this trend. Questions arise

Table 17–1. TYPES OF ABNORMALITIES OF VERTEX PRESENTATION

Rotation abnormalities
Transverse arrest
Occiput posterior position
Asynclitism
Deflexion attitudes
Military attitude
Brow presentation
Face presentation
Compound presentations

when patients are given the responsibility of making medical decisions.

What are the parameters of truly informed consent? Is the lay patient ever prepared to make difficult obstetrical decisions? Should the doctor place the lay patient in the role of front-line medical decision maker? What is the doctor's responsibility for outcome if the patient has chosen the delivery method? Is the physician really shielded from potential litigation if the outcome is unfavorable? Most of these questions remain unanswered.

The patient's wishes are important in any medical decision-making process. Each party involved in a critical nonemergency decision should understand the pertinent anticipated benefits and potential risks on all sides of the question. Truly informed choice by lay patients becomes increasingly difficult as the medical issues become more urgent and complex. Emergency medical decisions remain the responsibility of the physician.

The physician should try to present facts and not communicate biases during the informed consent process. If more than one solution is acceptable, the physician should explain the reasoning behind each choice. The full range of options open to the patient should be offered, and the risks assumed by each choice, even the unusual and grisly ones, should be explained. The risks and benefits of nonintervention should also be explained.

The physician must choose his or her words carefully and be certain the patient or responsible party understands them. Language appropriate to the ethnic background and education of the patient or responsible party should be used. If necessary, the services of a translator should be used. The physician must invite any questions and respond to them fully. Disclaimers are needed if the knowledge base is incomplete or controversial. The physician is the experienced, trained professional, and the patient is entitled to the physician's considered best judgment. The patient may then accept, discuss, or decline the doctor's choice or get another physician.

ROTATION ABNORMALITIES

Occiput Transverse and Occiput Posterior Positions

Internal rotation of the vertex is a cardinal movement of normal labor. Persistence of the occiput transverse or occiput posterior position represents a failure of internal rotation. Failure to rotate is often a matter of relative size. The fetus may be too large or the pelvis too small, or a combination of these two factors may exist. Tiny babies often present in unusual positions simply because of disparity between pelvic capacity and the size of the passenger. Failure of contractions to apply sufficient force to accomplish rotation also creates rotation abnormalities. Laxity of perineal resistance because of poor muscle tone or anesthesia may not provide the counterpressure that facilitates normal internal rotation and extension of the fetal head. For example, occiput posterior position persists more commonly in patients who have been administered epidural anesthesia.

Normal-sized babies usually adjust to the largest available pelvic diameter. Because the transverse diameter usually exceeds the anteroposterior diameter at the inlet, the most common positions at the time of engagement are right and left occiput transverse. The fetal head most commonly descends to the midpelvis during labor in one of these positions.

The ischial spines create an isthmus in the birth passage that makes it difficult for the fetal head to pass without rotation. The vertex must rotate 45 to 90 degrees to enter the largest oblique and anteroposterior diameters of the midpelvis. Proper rotation results in a right, left, or direct occiput anterior or posterior position. These are the positions commonly encountered in the second stage of labor.

Rotation to the anterior versus the posterior pelvic quadrant depends on the space available in these quadrants. The curvature of the sacrum and the shape and canting of the ischial bones determine the available posterior pelvic space. A flat sacral curvature and short sacrospinous ligament imply restricted posterior pelvic capacity.

The shape of the pubic arch and the distance between the symphysis pubis and the sacral promontory determine the available anterior pelvic space. Narrow subpubic angles and short diagonal conjugates imply restricted anterior pelvic capacity (see Chapter 6).

The delicate bone structure, deep sacral curve, and broad pubic arch of the gynecoid pelvis facilitate internal rotation. Android and anthropoid pelves, in contrast, have heavy bones, prominent ischial spines, narrow pubic arches, and flat sacral curves. These features limit the capacity of the fetal head to accomplish internal rotation.

The fetal head usually occupies the largest pelvic diameter at each pelvic plane. There is normally more room in the anterior quadrants of the pelvis than in the posterior quadrants at the levels of the middle and lower pelvis. Occiput anterior positions are therefore more frequent than occiput posterior positions.

The fetal head at midpelvis may fail to find adequate room into which to rotate into either the anterior or the posterior quadrant. The result is transverse arrest at the level of the ischial spines. When the spines are very prominent or the fetal head very large, there may be inadequate room for passage of the fetal head, despite rotation. This circumstance yields arrest of descent in a position other than transverse. Inadequate contraction forces can also result in failure of rotation and descent.

Transverse Arrest

The fetal head occupies a transverse position at some time during most labors. The head usually enters the pelvic inlet in the transverse position. Persistence of this transverse position implies failure of the fetal head to execute the cardinal labor movement of internal rotation. Transverse arrest occurs when progressive rotation and descent of the fetal head cease in the occiput transverse position. The cervical dilation curve usually reflects a protracted active-phase pattern or an arrest pattern.

ASSESSMENT OF TRANSVERSE ARREST

Arrest of the fetal head in the transverse position calls for complete reassessment of obstetrical conditions. The size of the baby must be rechecked, and its position in the pelvis and the size and architecture of the pelvis must be determined. Most of this assessment calls on manual skills. These skills are perfected by practice with feedback on outcome.

Transverse arrest of the fetal vertex most often occurs at the level of the ischial spines. The normal-sized, flexed occiput transverse vertex that fails to rotate offers an 11.5 to 12.5-cm object to an interspinous diameter of 9.5 to 10.5 cm. Passage of the normal head requires rotation of 45 to 90 degrees. Normal rotation fails if the pelvic capacity is too small, if the head is too large, or if the forces of labor are inadequate.

The adequacy of labor forces can be estimated by determining the intensity, frequency, and duration of uterine contractions. Contractions can be estimated by palpation, but intrauterine pressure transducers plot a more accurate record of pressure parameters over time.

The pelvic capacity should be reassessed by careful clinical pelvimetry (Chapter 6), with particular attention given to the diagonal conjugate, the size and closeness of the ischial spines, the depth of the sacral curve, the angle of the subpubic arch, and the convergence of the pelvic side walls.

Convergence of the pelvic side walls occurs in immature pelves and portends difficult vaginal delivery. A narrow subpubic angle indicates an unfavorable forepelvis. A short diagonal conjugate and wide subpubic angle identify the unfavorable platepelloid pelvis. Heavy, prominent ischial spines combined with a flat sacral curve and narrow subpubic angle identify the unfavorable android pelvis. On rare occasions, careful examination may reveal pelvic distortion from disease, tumor, or trauma.

The physician must obtain a new estimate of the size of the fetus. Estimates of fetal weight by either ultrasonography or manual methods are particularly difficult to make in late labor. Certain corollary signs help assess the presence of cephalopelvic disproportion.

The extent of molding of the fetal skull and the thickness of caput succadaneum should be assessed. Caput succadaneum results from the accumulation of edema in the tissues of the fetal scalp. Molding is the overlap of fetal cranial bones in response to attempts to fit into a restricted pelvic capacity. The extent of caput and the amount of molding closely correlate with the degree and duration of obstructed labor.

Caput may extend well beyond the true station of the fetal head. The physician must try to get an accurate impression of the true station of the head despite excessive caput. The fetal cranial bones may be impacted at zero station or above in a small pelvis even though the caput extends downward 2 cm or more.

Manual fundal pressure should cause some advancement of the vertex in the absence of obstruction (the Kristellar maneuver). The hand is pushed downward on the upper uterine fundus. With two fingers of the examining hand placed in the vagina, the physician tries to detect descent of the vertex. Failure to elicit any descent implies a degree of cephalopelvic disproportion. This finding is particularly ominous if extensive caput and molding are also present.

Finally, the physician must be certain that no anomaly of the fetus contributes to the failure to progress. Delivery decisions may be altered by the presence of hydrocephalus, megacystis, cystic hygroma, meningomyelocele, or other anomalies.

Management of Transverse Arrest

Management options for transverse arrest include both vaginal delivery maneuvers and cesarean delivery. Management decisions center around the likelihood of vaginal delivery. The assessment described above supplies the data with which to make these delivery decisions. The signs of obstruction are seldom absolute. Assessment of the pelvic capacity and fetal size is subjective and inexact.

Extensive molding or caput succadaneum indicates that strong contractions have been unable to accomplish rotation and advancement of the vertex. Confirmation of cephalopelvic disproportion comes from estimates of fetal size and pelvic capacity and from inability to manually produce descent of the presenting part with fundal pressure.

The obstetrician must be certain of the true station of the fetal head. Trouble accrues to the operator who attempts vaginal delivery thinking the vertex is at zero station, when in fact the cranium has not entered the true pelvis. Transverse arrest combined with signs of cephalopelvic disproportion should lead to cesarean delivery in most cases.

Transverse arrest without major degrees of cephalopelvic disproportion allows the obstetrician to consider vaginal delivery. The vertex must be rotated. Manual rotation of the vertex to an oblique (left or right) occiput anterior position may be tried first. The fingers of the appropriate hand are introduced into the vagina beside the fetal occiput. The right hand is used for left occiput transverse positions and the left hand for right occiput transverse positions.

The fingers cradle the occiput from beneath. Pronation of the hand encourages movement of the occiput into the anterior oblique or direct anterior diameters of the pelvis. Overlapping suture lines help obtain some purchase on the slippery scalp. The operator must be careful to exert only gentle pressure against these suture lines.

Oxytocin may be used as required to achieve uterine contractions of optimal quality after successful manual rotation. Rapid progress often occurs after manual rotation to a more favorable occiput anterior position. Manual rotation followed by spontaneous descent solves the problem of transverse arrest in the most ideal way, but manual rotation is not successful in many cases.

Two obstetric operations—vacuum extraction (VE) and midforceps rotation and delivery—are available to facilitate vaginal delivery of persistent transverse arrest. Anomalies and cephalopelvic disproportion must be ruled out before either modality can be considered. Complete cervical dilation is mandatory for forceps delivery and highly recommended for vacuum delivery.

Midforceps rotation and delivery from high station in the presence of transverse arrest is a prohibitively dangerous vaginal obstetric operation. Maternal soft-tissue damage occurs frequently. Most obstetric lacerations of the bladder, urethra, lower uterus, and upper vagina relate to difficult midforceps rotations (Chapter 23). Cranial and soft-tissue damage to the baby can result from forced rotation and extraction of the fetal head.

Forceps add 8% to the required pelvic capacity for delivery. Forceps can accomplish safe delivery of transverse arrest at lower stations if cephalopelvic disproportion and fetal macrosomia or anomalies are not present. It is difficult to be certain that all of these problems have been ruled out. Chapter 15 describes the details of midforceps procedure.

Vacuum extraction (VE) requires no extra pelvic space and allows spontaneous rotation of the fetal vertex. There is little risk of serious damage to maternal soft tissue with this modality. Vacuum cup application is not ideal when there is extensive caput or molding of the vertex. The cup will not fit snugly to the molded head and pulls off with minimal traction. Damage to the soft tissues of the fetal scalp is more likely with extensive caput succadaneum. The premature fetus is particularly prone to cranial soft-tissue injury with VE. Difficult VE occasionally results in cephalhematoma, subgaleal hematoma, or intracranial hemorrhage.

VE of occiput transverse positions can be effective with a mature fetus that is of average size and with no cephalopelvic disproportion. VE encourages descent when manual rotation has improved the position of the fetal head. Cup application is most secure and scalp injuries fewest when there is minimal caput or molding. The number of pulls should be limited to three, and the duration of the vacuum extraction effort should be no longer than 20 minutes. Traction must cease if no advancement occurs. Chapter 16 discusses vacuum instruments and extraction techniques in detail.

Persistent Occiput Posterior Position

Occiput posterior position is recognized at some time during the course of 49% of labors.[1, 2] Ninety percent or more of fetuses in the occiput posterior position rotate to a more favorable occiput anterior position as labor progresses. Occiput posterior position persists in 6 to 10%,[2, 3] making this position the most frequent malposition of the vertex.

Many cases of persistent occiput posterior position develop because of subtle abnormalities of pelvic architecture. Narrow transverse diameters or reduction in the space available for rotation predispose to occiput posterior position, and this position is particularly frequent in android and anthropoid pelvic configurations.[1, 2] Occiput posterior presentation commonly recurs with succeeding pregnancies because of its relationship to pelvic shape and size.

Conduction anesthesia relaxes the perineal muscles, whose resistance normally encourages rotation and extension of the vertex. Rotation abnormalities including occiput posterior position are more frequent with prolonged conduction anesthesia. Ineffective uterine contractions also contribute to the failure of the vertex to rotate from the occiput posterior position.

Persistent occiput posterior position is usually easy to recognize. Labor often lengthens by 1 to 2 hours.[1] Labor discomfort focuses in the low back. Examination reveals the triangular posterior fontanelle to be in one of the posterior quadrants of the pelvis. Moderate molding and caput succadaneum are common. The position of the posterior fontanelle and station of the vertex may be unclear to the examiner if caput and molding are extensive. The position of the ears adds information in cases of uncertain position.

MANAGEMENT OF PERSISTENT OCCIPUT POSTERIOR POSITION

The obstetrician confronted with a persistent occiput posterior position has several management options. Spontaneous delivery in this position may occur after a long labor. The vertex can be manually rotated to an anterior position. Vacuum cup traction can encourage spontaneous rotation and delivery. Application of forceps can directly assist delivery of babies in this position. A forceps rotation and extraction effects delivery in a variant of the occiput anterior position.

Phillips and Freeman[1] reported excellent results from Grady Memorial Hospital in Atlanta with a policy of nonintervention in cases of persistent occiput posterior position. Spontaneous or low-forceps delivery of the baby in an occiput posterior position over a generous episiotomy prevails for occiput posterior delivery on the Louisiana State University (LSU) Service at Charity Hospital in New Orleans.

Manual rotation can effectively assist occiput posterior delivery, particularly when the malposition results from poor perineal muscle tone because of conduction anesthesia. The obstetrician introduces the fingers of either hand beneath the fetal occiput. By turning his or her hand, the physician encourages the head to rotate in several stages. The occiput posterior position should be encouraged first into the transverse position and then into an anterior oblique position. Low forceps applied in the anterior position lend further assistance after manual rotation.

It is possible to manually rotate an infant in the occiput posterior position 180 degrees in a single step. This maneuver was taught by Dr. Leon Guillard at LSU for many years. The obstetrician turns his or her back to the perineum and reaches back to grasp the fetal head with the thumb on one side, fingers on the other. The palm cradles the occiput. The physician then turns toward the patient while suppinating the hand in one smooth motion. The resulting rotation, if successful, brings the occiput to an anterior position.

Modern obstetricians rarely use the classical Scanzoni midforceps rotation of occiput posterior to occiput anterior position. They seldom find sufficient reason to forcibly turn the vertex to a position that the fetus found unfavorable during labor.

Scanzoni applied standard forceps with the pelvic curve upward to the occiput posterior-positioned vertex. He rotated the forceps in a broad sweeping arc of 180 degrees. This resulted in the forceps' being upside down although the baby was in favorable occiput anterior position. He removed the blades and immediately replaced them in proper position for extraction. Extraction was performed with the baby in the occiput anterior posi-

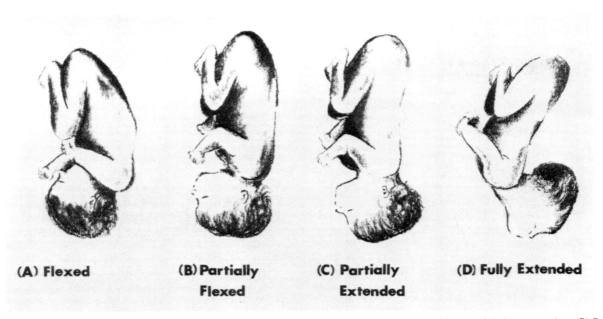

(A) Flexed   **(B) Partially Flexed**   **(C) Partially Extended**   **(D) Fully Extended**

Figure 17–1. Normal and abnormal flexion attitudes in vertex presentations. (A) Normal flexed position, occipital presentation. (B) Partially flexed position, sincipital presentation (military attitude). (C) Partially extended position, brow presentaton. (D) Fully extended position, face presentation. (From Iffy L, Kaminetsky HA: Principles and Practice of Obstetrics and Perinatology. New York: John Wiley & Sons, Inc., 1981.)

tion.

The sweeping arcs of Scanzoni rotations occasionally damage maternal and fetal structures. As a result, this procedural skill suffers the atrophy of disuse. Fewer Scanzoni rotations mean fewer trainees who are adept at its application. Cesarean delivery presents a better management choice than major midforceps rotation for many obstetricians facing delivery of a baby who is in a difficult occiput posterior position and cannot be delivered by manual rotation or direct extraction in the occiput posterior position.

MORBIDITY AND MORTALITY OF THE OCCIPUT POSTERIOR POSITION

Perinatal mortality rates for babies in the occiput posterior position are not greatly different from those for babies in the occiput anterior position. Phillips and Freeman[1] reported a perinatal mortality rate of 22 per 1000 in 552 consecutive cases of delivery of an infant in the occiput posterior

position. They found many episiotomy extensions requiring extensive repair. They recommended generous mediolateral episiotomies to facilitate delivery at the outlet. At LSU we find midline episiotomy to be adequate except for the patient who has a very short perineum. Slight diversion of the midline episiotomy lateral to the sphincter as described in Chapter 21 reduces tears into the rectum.

DEFLEXION ABNORMALITIES

Failure of the fetal vertex to maintain complete flexion of the chin on the anterior chest wall leads to complicated labors and deliveries (Figs. 17–1*B* through *D*). Minimal deflexion causes the sincipital position called "military attitude." Further deflexion results in brow presentation. Complete deflexion yields a face presentation.

Face Presentation

Face presentation is a condition of maximal deflexion of the fetal head in vertex position (Fig. 17–1*D*). Face presentation occurs once in 247 to 690 deliveries (mean 0.21%) (Table 17–2).[4–8] Rovinsky[9] stated that any factors that favor extension and reduce flexion of the fetal vertex encourage face presentation. Anencephaly is a natural cause of face presentation because of the absence of development of the cranium.[3] Conditions that enlarge the neck, such as goiters or cystic hygro-

Table 17–2. INCIDENCE OF FACE PRESENTATION

Author	Hospital and Year	% Face
Hellman	Hopkins 1950	0.21
Prevedourakis	Athens 1966	0.22
Cucco	Chicago 1966	0.14
Posner	Bronx 1957	0.20
Obstetric Collaborative Study	U.S. 1960	0.20
Cruikshank	Iowa 1973	0.17
Pritchard	Dallas 1985	0.30
Mean		0.21%

mas, are rare causes of face presentation.[5] Multiple loops of cord around the fetal neck may also cause deflexion of the head. Multiple loops of cord complicate 4.3% of face presentations.[4]

The contracted pelvis is a controversial etiologic factor. Seventeen to 39.4% of patients delivering a baby in the face presentation are reported to have some degree of pelvic contraction.[1, 6]

High parity was present in 10% of face presentations in the large studies of Prevedourakis[4] and Cucco.[5] Pritchard and co-workers[3] believed that the pendulous multiparous abdomen encouraged extension of the fetal head and increased the chances for face or brow presentation.

Face presentation increases with very large or very small baby size. Cucco[5] reported that 15% of face presentations occurred in premature babies and 37.5% in infants weighing more than 8 lbs. Prevedourakis[4] reported a 7.9% incidence of face presentation in babies weighing less than 2500 g and 13% of babies weighing more than 4000 g.

The usual development of face presentation begins when the forehead of the fetus strikes the tissues overlying either the promontory of the sacrum or the symphysis pubis. Descent gradually forces deflexion that progresses from brow presentation to face presentation. Face presentation is particularly associated with android maternal pelvic configurations.

The maximal deflexion of the fetal head seen in face presentations presents the submentobregmatic head diameter to the pelvis (Fig. 17–1*D*). This diameter averages 9.5 cm in length in mature infants. It is more favorable for vaginal delivery than is the occipitomental diameter of brow presentation, which averages 12.5 cm in length.

The face presentation can often negotiate a pelvic cavity of average size. The key to the passage of the face through the pelvis is the position of the chin. The fetus can be delivered vaginally if the occiput can rotate into the hollow of the sacrum so the chin can pass beneath the symphysis. The flat sacrum of the android pelvis does not easily accommodate this rotation.

Face presentations are identified by the position of the chin (mentum), not the occiput. Mentum anterior face presentation implies a favorable rotation. Mentum posterior presentations become wedged behind the symphysis and cannot be safely delivered per vaginum unless the baby is very small. One-third of face presentations begin as a mentum posterior presentation. Two-thirds of this number spontaneously rotate to mentum anterior presentation late in labor.[9]

Descent of the head is very slow because of the unusual position of the face in the pelvis. Uterine contraction forces normally act against the resistance of the perineal muscles to force rotation and extension of the presenting part. The face does not reach this muscular resistance until the head descends deep into the pelvis. Rotation does not usually occur until late in the second stage of labor.

Duration of labor is near normal with face presentations. Cucco found that 75% of patients delivered in less than 12 hours.[5] Prevedourakis[4] shortened the first stage of labor with oxytocin and made cesarean decisions early during labor. He reported labors of under 7 hours for primiparas and 4 hours for multiparas.

The examiner's fingers encounter the chin, mouth, bridge of the nose, and orbits in face presentations. The zygomatic arches and supraorbital ridges are particularly identifiable landmarks. Recognition is not easy when edema distorts facial structures after prolonged labor. The edematous face feels much like a frank breech presentation. The position must be confirmed with ultrasonography or x-ray imaging if necessary.

MANAGEMENT OF FACE PRESENTATION

The obstetrician must completely reevaluate the obstetric patient who is found to have a face presentation. The quality of contractions, pelvic capacity, size of the fetus, and exact position of the fetus in the pelvis must be determined. The physician should try to detect any anomalies that might cause difficult delivery or fetal compromise.

After this evaluation, the physician makes a preliminary choice of delivery method. Cesarean delivery may be chosen when the assessment reveals fetopelvic disproportion. Anomalies that are not incompatible with life often mandate abdominal delivery. Persistent mentum posterior position requires cesarean delivery in most instances.

Tiny premature babies in face presentation pose difficult decisions regarding vaginal versus abdominal delivery. Cesarean birth is often chosen to minimize trauma to these fragile infants. However, cesarean delivery is not always completely atraumatic and does not guarantee a perfect outcome.

Vaginal delivery is an appropriate option for face presentation in patients with normal labors, large pelves, and average-sized babies. The decision for vaginal delivery must be reevaluated periodically as labor progresses. Rotation to mentum anterior occurs very late in labor in many cases of face presentation. Conduction anesthesia relaxes perineal muscles and further delays rotation. The obstetrician must be patient, if no fetopelvic disproportion exists, and await late rotation to the mentum anterior presentation. He or she must watch for fetal distress and judge whether impaction of the fetal head impedes rotation or harms the fetus. The obstetrician must be prepared for prompt cesarean delivery in cases of fetal distress, failure to rotate to mentum anterior presentation, lack of descent, or another adverse turn of events.

Several maneuvers have been described to manually flex face or brow presentations to facilitate vaginal delivery. The Thorn maneuver is the most quoted of these conversion methods.[10] Prerequisite conditions include an adequate pelvis, normal fetal head size, ruptured membranes, and advanced cervical dilatation. The head should be relatively high in the pelvis. The lower uterine segment should not have become thinned out by excessively long labor. Flexion maneuvers require deep general anesthesia and disengagement of the vertex.

Thorn grasped the face or brow and pushed it upward above the inlet of the pelvis. He then pushed the face and brow forward with his internal hand while pressing backward on the baby's back with his abdominal hand. An assistant helped flex the fetal spine by pushing the buttocks forward. The fingers of the internal hand gradually worked their way posteriorly on the fetal head. Eventually two fingers reached the occiput. Thorn then pulled the occiput into the pelvic inlet while the assistant's fundal pressure forced the head into the pelvis.

Manual conversion of face presentations to occiput presentations is controversial and often fails. Such maneuvers pose considerable risk of cord prolapse and uterine rupture. Modern obstetrics has abandoned conversion of the mentum posterior face presentation in favor of cesarean delivery.[9]

Babies in the mentum posterior presentation can sometimes be rotated. The procedure for manual rotation is similar to that for occiput posterior presentation. The fingers of one hand are placed beside the face and the hand is swept broadly through an arc of 135 to 180 degrees. This maneuver usually is done in two stages, adjusting the hand position for each stage. Attempts at rotation must be very gentle to avoid soft-tissue injury to the fetus. The process stops immediately if there is resistance to rotation.

Forceps rotation of face presentation to mentum anterior presentation is not often attempted. Whitacre[11] researched this subject extensively and discouraged forceps rotation. Four and three-tenths percent (4.3%) of babies in Prevedourakis's[4] large series and 12.5% of Cucco's[5] series were delivered by forceps, but forceps were used as rotators in only one case.

There are several reasons to question forceps rotation and extraction of the face presentation. The obstetrician seldom knows all the conditions that have produced the face position. There is always a reason why the head has assumed this unusual posture. Recall the association with cephalopelvic disproportion, small pelves, and fetal anomalies. Even without hidden problems, the largest part of the head is relatively high in the pelvis at the time of forceps application to face presentations. The neck of the fetus is also in the pelvis and subject to injury. Forced rotations in the presence of cord entanglement or anomalies may precipitate acute fetal distress. Accurate application of the forceps is difficult. Inaccurate ap-

plication may injure fetal soft tissues. All of these factors mitigate against the use of forceps for rotation and extraction of the face presentation.

Use of outlet forceps without rotation does not increase the risk of injury to the baby or mother. Use of gentle outlet forceps when the face is low in the pelvis and is in mentum anterior presentation reduces the duration of labor pressures on the fetal face and neck.

Cesarean section provides the best management option for complicated face deliveries. There are geographic differences in the prevalence of cesarean delivery for face presentation. Cucco,[5] from Chicago, reported a prevalence of 70.6% cesarean deliveries, whereas Prevedourakis,[4] from Athens, Greece, had a cesarean rate of only 7.5%.

Transverse lower segment cesarean incisions usually provide adequate room for cesarean delivery of the face presentation. The position of the head in face presentation increases the likelihood of extensions of the transverse uterine incision. The head is often impacted in the pelvis when the decision is made to perform abdominal delivery. A gentle upward push from below by an assistant facilitates extraction of the baby. The obstetrician can avoid extensions of the incision by slowly elevating the head through the incision without applying leverage forces against the lower part of the incision.

A hand is introduced below the face in mentum posterior position and the occiput, the brow, and then the face are gently brought into the incision. The soft-cup vacuum extractor placed on the occiput can provide assistance with upward traction. The vacuum cup does not occupy additional space, as does the hand.

MORBIDITY AND MORTALITY OF THE FACE PRESENTATION

The infant loss reported with face presentation varies from 2.0 to 17.6%.[4, 5] In one large series 1 neonatal death per 163 cases was reported, for an overall perinatal mortality rate of 36.8 per 1000.[4]

The extensive edema of the face that develops during labor disappears without ill effect in a few days. It often takes many days for the infant to adopt a normal resting head position. The physician must watch for neurologic evidence of the rare injuries to spinal cord or brachial plexus. The extreme extension of the head in face position stresses these structures but only rarely causes permanent injury. The physician must be prepared to care for any associated congenital anomalies.

Brow Presentation

Brow presentation implies a moderate degree of cephalic deflexion (Fig. 17–1C). The small change of position in brow presentations results in a large increase in the size of the object presented to the birth canal. The persistent brow presents the large mento-occipital diameter of the fetal head to the pelvis. This diameter averages 12.5 cm at term. Few pelves can accommodate an object of that size.

Brow presentation occurs approximately once in 667 to 2000 deliveries (0.05 to 0.1%).[9, 12] The brow appears more often as a transient position during labor. Two-thirds of cases are unstable and spontaneously convert to either a face or an occiput presentation.[7] Additional deflexion produces a face presentation; further flexion produces an occiput presentation.

The causes of brow positions are the same as those listed for face presentations. Cephalopelvic disproportion and prematurity are prominent features of many cases.[13]

The obstetrician can recognize a brow at the time of pelvic examination by feeling the root of the nose and the supraorbital ridges. It is difficult to reach either fontanelle. If a fontanelle can be felt, it is the diamond-shaped anterior fontanelle. The forces of labor attempt to mold the head to shorten the large presenting diameter. Extensive molding and caput over the forehead make identification of the brow difficult late in labor.[14]

MANAGEMENT OF BROW PRESENTATION

Vaginal delivery is unlikely unless the baby is very small or the pelvis very large. Labor may be prolonged and exhausting.[9] The extreme amount of molding that develops even with small heads can damage the fetus.

The discovery of a brow presentation triggers reassessment of the entire case. The obstetrician must (a) reevaluate the size of the pelvis and the size of the baby, (b) rule out abnormalities of the fetal head and other organs, and (c) plan and prepare for cesarean delivery in most cases.

Vaginal delivery of the baby in brow presentation is occasionally possible. If discovered early in labor, the brow presentation may be manually encouraged toward further flexion. Manual flexion and rotation to occiput anterior presentation are occasionally possible if the pelvis is large and molding not severe. Cesarean delivery is necessary if descent does not progress after such a maneuver.[15] Ineffective or tumultuous labor or fetal distress also signals the need for abdominal delivery.[3]

Moore and Dennen[12] found 3 neonatal deaths in 36 persistent brow presentations for a perinatal mortality rate of 83 per 1000 births with attempts at vaginal delivery. They stated that forceps should be used with caution to deliver infants in the brow presentation unless manual conversion to an occiput presentation was successful. Cesarean birth is the delivery choice for most brow presentations.

Sincipital Presentation (Military Attitude)

Minimal deflexion of the fetal vertex results in a position of attention known as "military attitude." This position is more properly called *sincipital presentation* (Fig. 17–1B). This position offers the occipitofrontal diameter to the pelvis. This diameter averages 11 cm at term.[9] Sincipital presentation is usually a transient position found early in labor. The forces of labor acting against the pelvic side walls encourage increasing flexion as labor progresses. Most sincipital presentations flex into occiput positions. Only a few deflex further into either a brow or a face presentation.

As with any positional abnormality, upon discovery of a sincipital presentation the physician must reassess the fetus and pelvis. He or she must watch for progression into another presentation. Management options change as the position evolves to occiput, brow, or face.

COMPOUND PRESENTATIONS

Compound presentation implies that another anatomic part, usually an extremity, has entered the pelvis along with the principal vertex or breech presentation.

Transient compound presentations may occur frequently in early labor and are not recognized. Persistent compound presentations occur approximately once in 1000 deliveries. They occur when the pelvic inlet is not filled by the principal presenting part, as is the case with premature infants, abnormal positions and lies, fetal anomalies, and large pelvic capacities.

These same conditions predispose to prolapse of the umbilical cord. Prolapse of the umbilical cord fits the definition of compound presentation although it is rarely discussed in this context.

Almost every possible combination of presenting parts has been reported. The most common compound presentations are the vertex with a hand, vertex with a foot, and breech with a hand.

Collision of presenting parts in multiple gestations also constitutes a compound presentation. At times, the heads of both twins coincidentally enter the pelvic inlet. This most often happens when both babies are very small. On rare occasions, the head of one twin and the knee, foot, elbow, or hand of the other twin present as a compound presentation. Compound presentation complicates conjoined twins on rare occasions.

MANAGEMENT OF THE COMPOUND PRESENTATION

Compound presentation is usually discovered when a hand or foot is felt beside the fetal head.

The extremity can often be eased back up into the uterine cavity by gentle pressure. The condition can be simply observed. Labor often solves the problem by forcing the head past the extremity. Labor usually progresses normally.

The quality of labor and the condition of the fetus must be carefully monitored. The obstetrician should consider cesarean delivery in cases of fetal distress or arrest of labor progress.

On the rare occasions when the fetal hand or arm remains beside the head throughout labor, it becomes swollen and discolored (Fig. 17–2). This condition clears soon after birth, and permanent damage to the extremity is rare, although brachial plexus palsy has been described.

Compound presentations seldom cause serious delivery difficulties and add little to perinatal morbidity or mortality.

FETAL CONGENITAL MALFORMATIONS THAT AFFECT DELIVERY

Table 17–3 outlines malformations of the fetus that may affect the conduct of labor and delivery. Harrison and colleagues[16] classified those congenital malformations for which early vaginal or cesarean delivery is indicated.

Table 17–4 outlines anomalies usually managed by correction after elective early vaginal delivery. Many of these conditions are systemic disorders or less severe structural defects. These minor malformations do not often affect delivery methods. Corrective measures are begun promptly after birth.

Cases that require cesarean birth have extensive

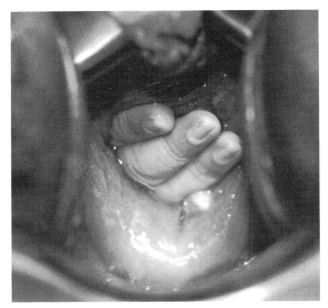

Figure 17–2. Compound presentation. The infant's hand precedes the vertex through a partly dilated cervix. (Courtesy Duane E. Neumann, M.D.; photographed by Rita L. Letellier.)

Table 17–3. FETAL ANOMALIES THAT MAY AFFECT DELIVERY DECISIONS

Head and neck
  Hydrocephalus
  Anencephaly
  Cystic hygroma
Ventral wall
  Gastroschisis
  Omphalocele
  Diaphragmatic hernia
Spine
  Meningomyelocele
  Sacrococcygeal teratoma
Limbs
  Atresias and conglutinations
  Amniotic band syndromes
Systemic disorders
  Osteogenesis imperfecta
  Thrombocytopenic purpura
  Hydrops fetalis
  Obstructive uropathies
  Urethral atresia
  Hydronephrosis
  Enteric cysts
  Bowel duplications and obstructions
  Ovarian cysts or tumors

structural anomalies that are potentially correctable and not incompatible with life (Table 17–5).

Clark and colleagues[17] described major congenital anomalies that require decompression procedures. All obstetricians dread procedures that are destructive to the fetus. Such instances are rare in modern obstetrics, but they still exist. A large hydrocephalic head presenting as a partly delivered breech requires decompression. Dystocia due to a large fluid-filled fetal abdomen may require transabdominal decompression.

Hydrocephalus

The ancient Greeks recognized hydrocephalus as a complication of pregnancy. Maternal morbidity and mortality from the delivery of such infants were extensive in the years before cesarean delivery. Mothers became exhausted by prolonged hopeless labors. Rupture of the lower uterine segment often caused death of the mother by exsanguination. Draining the cerebrospinal fluid from the spinal canal or ventricles of the infant saved some

Table 17–4. FETAL MALFORMATIONS FOR EARLY CORRECTION AFTER PRETERM DELIVERY

Obstructive uropathy
Isolated obstructive hydrocephalus
Amniotic band syndromes
Ventral wall defects
  Gastroschisis
  Omphalocele
Intestinal malformations
  Volvulus
  Ischemia
Hydrops fetalis

From Harrison MR, Golbus MS, Filly RA, et al.: Fetal surgical treatment. Pediatr Ann 11:896, 1982.

Table 17–5. FETAL MALFORMATIONS THAT MAY REQUIRE CESAREAN DELIVERY

Conjoined twins
Large omphalocele
Ruptured omphalocele or gastroschisis
Large hydrocephalus
Large sacrococcygeal teratoma
Large cystic hygroma
Large or ruptured meningomyelocele

From Harrison MR, Golbus MS, Filly RA, et al.: Fetal surgical treatment. Pediatr Ann 11:896, 1982.

of these mothers, but the baby died in most cases.[17, 18] Encephalocentesis was not the panacea.

The advent of ultrasonography brought reliable detection and tracking of antenatal hydrocephalus. By tracking ventricle size and cortical thickness, ultrasonography guides decisions about the timing of delivery, shunting of the fetal ventricles, or encephalocentesis.[17] Minor degrees of hydrocephalus may allow normal labor. As little as 280 mL of excess cerebrospinal fluid increases head size enough to create severe dystocia (Fig. 17–3).[17]

Chervenak and co-workers[18] reported 53 consecutive cases of fetal hydrocephalus from Yale University School of Medicine. They found that isolated hydrocephalus had the most favorable long-term prognosis. Hydrocephalus was an isolated finding in only 17% of their cases, however. Associated malformations in diverse organ systems occurred in 83% of cases. The most common associated abnormality was spina bifida.

Abnormal lies are common with large hydrocephalic heads. The physician must check for hydrocephalus and other anomalies in all breech or transverse presentations. Abdominal delivery may be necessary for the hydrocephalic baby in transverse lie, regardless of the prognosis for the baby.

Ultrasonography allows accurate detection of obstructive hydrocephalus early in pregnancy. Half of the fetuses with hydrocephalus in the study by Chervenak and co-workers[18] were confirmed before viability and were aborted. Just over half of the remaining cases had cesarean deliveries.

MANAGEMENT OF HYDROCEPHALUS

The physician faced with a hydrocephalic fetus has several management options. Some physicians offer pregnancy termination when the diagnosis is certain before viability or when other anomalies are present that are incompatible with life.[18] Selected cases benefit from placement of a shunt from the enlarged ventricle(s) to the amniotic sac.[19, 20] Unfortunately, shunt procedures have been less effective than anticipated. Encephalocentesis can be used to decompress the head to allow delivery.[17] Cesarean delivery can be performed with or without drainage of cerebrospinal fluid.[18]

Our neurosurgeons at LSU currently advocate elective cesarean delivery without encephalocentesis at the time of pulmonary surfactant maturity. Ventricular shunting is performed soon after birth for favorable cases. Cochrane and Myles[19] pointed out that optimal results followed shunting performed during the reversible stage of brain tissue damage. Delayed shunting cannot completely reverse advanced cortical loss. Infants with massive or asymmetrical ventriculomegaly have a poor prognosis and benefit little from atraumatic delivery.

Maximum benefit from planned atraumatic delivery accrues to fetuses with mild to moderate symmetrical ventriculomegaly and no other anomalies.[17] These favorable cases should be followed with serial ultrasonography. Cortical mantle thickness is a useful but not completely reliable indicator of later neurologic outcome.[21] Maximal brain damage occurs with acute, severe ventricular dilation.[18, 19]

The physician should begin serial amniocentesis for pulmonary surfactant maturity assessment at 34 to 36 weeks' gestation.[18] Elective cesarean delivery should be performed as soon as surfactant

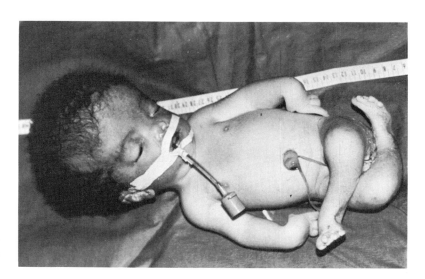

Figure 17–3. Hydrocephalic infant with multiple congenital abnormalities. (Courtesy Haywood Brown, M.D.; photographed by Rita L. Letellier.)

analysis indicates pulmonary maturity. A large vertical cesarean incision permits atraumatic delivery of the large head. Serial ultrasonography may reveal a sudden, rapid increase in hydrocephalus before surfactant maturity. Parenteral corticosteroids can be administered to attempt to induce surfactant production before cesarean delivery of these cases.[18]

Intrauterine ventriculoamniotic shunts showed promise in other primates but were not completely satisfactory in human pregnancies.[19, 20] These extracorporeal shunts frequently became dislodged or occluded. New ways of controlling the one-way shunt are under development.[20] Widespread implementation awaits improved technology.

Repeated transuterine ventricular taps are ineffective for advancing hydrocephalus.[19] Intrapartal encephalocentesis uniformly results in a poor outcome for the fetus.[18, 20] Part of the dismal outlook for intrapartal encephalocentesis stems from the fact that these are often the most severe and advanced cases.

A hydrocephalic fetus adds an element of risk for the mother during labor. Feeny and Barry[22] reported an increase in intrapartal rupture of the uterus before full dilation in these mothers. The lower uterine segment undergoes extensive thinning because of the size of the fetal head. Breech delivery of an infant with unrecognized hydrocephalus risks injury to maternal soft tissue because of frantic efforts to deliver the aftercoming head. Encephalocentesis reduces the chances of irreparable damage to the uterus but presages poor fetal outcome.

Encephalocentesis is most often performed in cases of hydrocephaly with fetal demise, hydroanencephaly, or severe associated anomalies. Draining the cerebrospinal fluid effectively collapses the head and allows delivery of the hydrocephalic head in breech presentation discovered after the body of the fetus has delivered.[17]

Tapping the ventricles in obstructed labor in vertex presentation allows vaginal delivery and prevents rupture of the thinned lower uterine segment. The ventricles can be drained by inserting a needle through the maternal abdominal wall under sterile conditions or by making a transcervical puncture.[17] The former technique probably reduces the chances of meningitis. This hypothesis has not been adequately tested because so few of these babies survive.

Neonatal ventriculoperitoneal shunting has so improved the prognosis for hydrocephalus that we must now be concerned with pregnancy in young women with shunts. Samuels and co-workers[23] reported 15 such cases from the literature and added 2 cases of their own. Malfunction of ventriculoperitoneal shunts commonly occurs in the third trimester of pregnancy as a result of increased intraperitoneal pressure and growth of the uterus. Shunts can be surgically revised during pregnancy.[23]

Ventriculoatrial shunts are seldom encountered, but they are not affected by the enlarging pregnant uterus. Normal vaginal delivery is usual for mothers with either type of ventricular shunt.[23]

Defects in the Ventral Wall

The major congenital defects in the fetal abdominal wall that cause obstetric delivery problems are gastroschisis and omphalocele. These are two distinct embryologic entities with very different outcomes.[24]

Gastroschisis is a paraumbilical, full-thickness defect of the abdominal wall (Fig. 17–4). Gastroschisis defects appear consistently to the right of the umbilicus and do not involve the umbilical cord. The bowel or other organs eviscerate through the relatively small defect without any covering

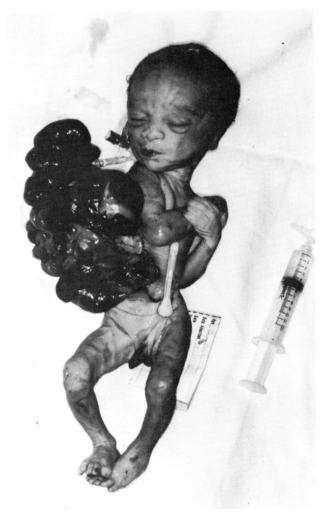

Figure 17–4. Infant with gastroschisis. Defect is lateral to the umbilicus. There is no covering membrane over extruded intestines. (Courtesy Haywood Brown, M.D.; photographed by Rita L. Letellier.)

sac.[24] The paraumbilical gastroschisis defect stems from abnormal involution of the right umbilical vein or omphalomesenteric artery.[25]

Omphalocele presents a dilated umbilical ring containing umbilical vessels and herniated viscera (Fig. 17–5A through C). The defect may be very large. The externalized viscera may or may not have a peritoneal sac but lack skin covering.[25] Omphalocele represents persistence of the body stalk and absence of the midabdomen somatopleure.[25]

There are three types of omphalocele. The common lateral-fold type is a midabdominal lesion that does not contain viscera of either the chest or the pelvis. Cephalic-fold omphalocele is located in the epigastrium and may involve the sternum, diaphragm, pericardium, or heart. The Pentology of Cantrell identifies the consortium of all these defects. Extrophy of the bladder and abnormalities of the hindgut complicate caudal-fold omphalocele.[24]

Defects in the ventral wall occur in 1 in 3400 (0.03%) live births.[24] This prevalence is approximately the same in the United States and the United Kingdom.[26] Gastroschisis occurs in approximately 1 in 9900 live births. Omphalocele occurs in 1 in 2280 to 1 in 10,000 live births.[26] Before 1963, gastroschisis and omphalocele were thought to be variants of the same defect. This may explain the wide range of reported prevalence.

Serum α-fetoprotein screening of mothers has increased the rate of antenatal diagnosis of defects in the ventral wall. Wald and co-workers[27] found that extensive screening in the second trimester in the United Kingdom identified 75% of fetuses with defects in the ventral wall. Ultrasonographic screening accurately identifies the type of defect in most cases.[28] An elevated α-fetoprotein level should trigger extensive sonographic scanning at any gestational age.[24]

Ultrasonographic scans differentiate defects in the ventral wall by their relationship to the umbilical cord, the presence of a covering sac, and the extruded organs. Intact omphalocele involves the umbilical cord insertion site. In the typical omphalocele, a membrane surrounds a compact mass of intestinal coils. The absence of viscera other than small bowel and stomach makes omphalocele the

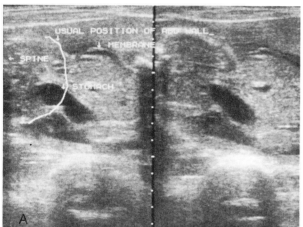

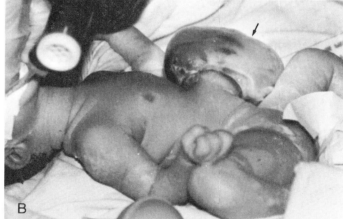

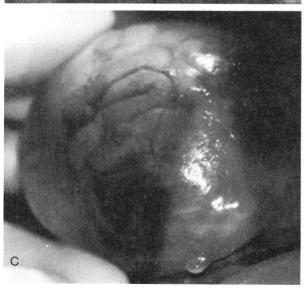

Figure 17–5. A, Ultrasound photo of omphalocele defect (courtesy Joseph Pastorek, M.D.). B, Infant with omphalocele (arrow). (Courtesy Mohammed Bey, M.D.; photographed by Rita L. Letellier.) C, Closeup of the omphalocele from Figure 17–5B. Note covering of peritoneal sac over extruded intestine. (Courtesy Mohammed Bey, M.D.; photographed by Rita L. Letellier.)

more likely diagnosis.[24] The obstetrician should look for filling of an intra-abdominal bladder. Its presence effectively rules out extrophy of the bladder.[24]

Gastroschisis is distinctly separate from the umbilical cord. Absence of any covering membrane over extruded organs suggests gastroschisis.

Sonographic examination of the entire fetus is indicated if the obstetrician suspects omphalocele. Infants with omphalocele have significant associated anomalies in 20 to 64% of cases. The obstetrician should check for defects involving the cranium and spine, heart, diaphragm, bowel, and bladder. Amniocentesis for karyotype reveals a 10% incidence of trisomy in babies with omphalocele.[24] Infants with gastroschisis have a smaller but still significant 5 to 30% incidence of associated anomalies.[25, 28]

MANAGEMENT OF DEFECTS IN THE VENTRAL WALL

Controversy continues over the ability of cesarean delivery to reduce mortality in infants with defects in the ventral wall. Several maternal–fetal medicine groups recommend abdominal delivery for such babies.[28–30] Outcomes with this plan of management are excellent.

Earlier studies failed to demonstrate improvement of outcome by cesarean delivery.[24, 25] Most of these cases were undiagnosed before delivery. Kirk and Wah[25] actually reported a 56% mortality rate in infants with gastroschisis delivered by cesarean section, versus an 8% rate mortality with vaginal delivery. The fact that few cases were discovered before delivery reduced the chance of selection bias in this study.

Current management encourages early screening by α-fetoprotein testing and ultrasonography. Diagnosed cases should be monitored with biophysical profile studies. The obstetrician can search for associated anomalies by karyotyping of amniocytes and obtaining high-resolution ultrasonographic scans of all systems. Growth curves and amniotic fluid quantity should be closely watched. As the time for delivery approaches, the physician may test for pulmonary surfactant maturity.

Fitzsimmons and co-workers[30] recommended a delivery protocol for all prenatally diagnosed defects in the ventral wall. The protocol suggests elective cesarean birth in a tertiary hospital at 36 weeks' gestation. This group believed that they presented babies in optimal condition to the pediatric surgeon for prompt repair of the defects. In 1988 this group reported 14 survivors among 14 candidates.[30]

The care of the baby immediately after delivery is critical to its survival. Hypothermia and injury to exposed organs should be avoided. A nasogastric tube should be inserted and adequate hydration should be provided.

Pediatric surgeons have described several management options, depending on the size and conformation of the defect and the prolapsed organs. They may choose expectant care when anomalies are incompatible with life. Smaller defects are suitable for primary closure. Larger defects require a two-stage repair with Silastic, Marlex, Goretex, or other sheeting material.[31, 32]

MORBIDITY AND MORTALITY OF DEFECTS IN THE VENTRAL WALL

Babies with omphalocele frequently have fetal distress during labor.[24] Omphalocele carries an overall perinatal mortality rate of 29 to 40%.[24, 25] Seventy-eight percent of infants with cephalic omphalocele die.[24] The presence of vital organs outside the body cavity is an ominous sign. The existence of associated anomalies or prematurity worsens the prognosis. The size of the defect and the possibility of surgical closure determine survival.

Early reports indicated that intrauterine growth retardation occurred frequently in babies with gastroschisis.[24, 25] Recent reports have not confirmed this finding.[29, 30]

Mortality rates from gastroschisis vary from 5 to 14%.[24, 29, 30] Fitzsimmons and co-workers[30] reported no deaths among a group without associated anomalies who delivered before term in tertiary hospitals by elective cesarean birth.

Massive Fluid-Filled Abdomen

Prenatal ultrasonography occasionally reveals a fetus whose abdomen is distended with fluid. This condition can be due to massive hydronephrosis, megalocystis, ascites, or large ovarian or other cystic tumors. Management depends on etiology.

Pediatricians apply the unusual eponym "prune belly syndrome" to the neonatal condition of babies with renal dysgenesis or massive hydronephrosis.[17] These babies often have hypoplastic lungs at birth. They also have other anomalies, such as hypoplasia of the muscles of the anterior abdominal wall, imperforate anus, and limb abnormalities. The prune belly syndrome associated with severe renal disease and other anomalies is rarely compatible with life.[17]

Megalocystis can be the cause of a massive fluid-filled abdomen (Fig. 17–6). Urethral atresia or stenosis results in massive distension of the bladder. This can be an isolated abnormality with a good prognosis. The kidneys can be normal in these cases or can be distended by hydronephrosis if vesicoureteral reflux exists. Ultrasonography helps differentiate between fluid-filled bladder and massive hydronephrosis. Hydronephrosis worsens

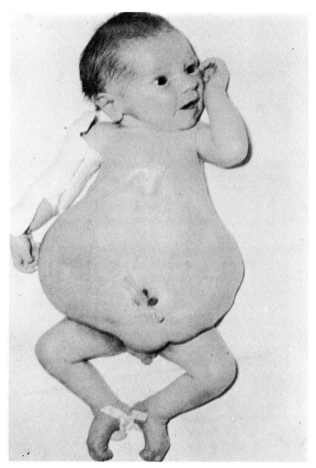

Figure 17–6. Infant with megalocystis as a result of urethral atresia.

the prognosis in proportion to the amount of reduction of renal function.[17]

Harrison and co-workers[16] reported 24 fetuses with renal dysgenesis or advanced hydronephrosis problems. The authors judged renal function by the quantity of amniotic fluid and by the filling of the bladder with urine. They inferred absence of renal function if the bladder failed to fill or if oligohydramnios was severe.

Harrison's group believed that term delivery was proper for fetuses with one multicystic or dysplastic kidney and good function of the other kidney. They considered termination of pregnancy if the disorder was bilateral and renal function poor.[33] Babies with these problems often have difficult deliveries because of massive enlargement of the abdomen and oligohydramnios.[16]

Hydronephrosis may be unilateral or bilateral. Prolonged, complete obstruction results in reduction of renal function, which may not be reversible. Harrison and colleagues[33] recommended early delivery to permit relief of the obstruction if renal function deteriorates.

Percutaneous aspiration of the renal pelves or bladder relieves the compression on the renal cortex for only a few hours. Vesicoamniotic or other urinary shunts help in a few selected cases.[16] These operations are discussed in greater detail in Chapter 29 on fetal surgery.

Aspiration of the bladder or renal pelves can decompress the abdomen sufficiently to allow safer delivery. Clark and colleagues[17] described needle aspiration before early cesarean delivery. Needle aspiration allowed vaginal delivery in another case of obstructed labor after delivery of the fetal head.

Preservation of long-term renal function is the critical point in cases of congenital hydronephrosis. Preterm delivery should be planned if renal function deteriorates. Surfactant maturity may be difficult to assess in cases with severe oligohydramnios. Corticosteroids administered to the mother help induce fetal pulmonary surfactant production. Corticosteroids are most effective between 30 and 34 weeks' gestation.

Other Masses

The obstetric surgeon occasionally encounters a fetus with a mass that obstructs normal labor progress. Sacral teratomas, cystic hygromas, meningomyeloceles, and ovarian cysts and tumors are examples of such masses. Obstetric ultrasonography permits discovery and accurate measurement of these masses. When masses are of sufficient size to obstruct labor, the obstetrician should perform atraumatic cesarean delivery. The obstetrician should try to get the baby to the pediatric surgeon in optimal condition for correction of the abnormality after delivery.

CONCLUSIONS

There are many ethical and legal implications to the procedures and decisions described in this chapter. These events affect fetuses and mothers in profound ways. Predelivery drainage of hydrocephalic heads and dysgenetic kidneys are examples of difficult management decisions. Pregnancy termination because of certain anomalies raises other moral, ethical, and legal problems.

Hospitals whose obstetrical services deal with these complex issues are wise to consider them before an emergency confronts them. Ethics committees should ponder the issues in detail. They should consider providing flexible guidelines to help physicians and families when these rare cases occur. Counseling patterns should be developed to aid parents and attendants faced with these medical crises.

Credentials and procedures committees have a particular responsibility to permit only those with special expertise to apply the more complex techniques described. They should define and revise the fine line between the latest accepted techniques and experimental therapy. The definitions must remain flexible to allow for inevitable progress. All recommendations must consider, respect, and protect the rights of all the participants in the problem: the fetus, the mother, the family, the obstetrical team, and the hospital.

References

1. Phillips RD, Freeman M: The management of the persistent occiput posterior: A review of 552 consecutive cases. Obstet Gynecol 43:171, 1974.
2. Quilligan EJ, Zuspan FP: Management of labor and delivery complications. In Douglas-Stromme—Operative Obstetrics, 4th Edition. New York: Appleton-Century-Crofts, 1982, pp. 392–396.
3. Pritchard JA, MacDonald PC, Gant NF: Dystocia caused by abnormalities of presentation, position or abnormalities of the fetus. In Williams Obstetrics, 17th Edition. New York: Appleton-Century-Crofts, pp. 659–660, 1985.
4. Prevedourakis CN: Face presentation: An analysis of 163 cases. Am J Obstet Gynecol 94:1092, 1966.
5. Cucco UP: Face presentation. Am J Obstet Gynecol 94:1085, 1966.
6. Posner AC, Lewis B, Rubin EJ, et al.: Face presentation. Obstet Gynecol 21:745, 1963.
7. Cruikshank DP, White CA: Obstetric malpresentations: 20 years' experience. Am J Obstet Gynecol 116:1097, 1973.
8. Hellman LM, Epperson JWW, Connally F: Face and brow presentations: The experience of Johns Hopkins Hospital 1896–1948. Am J Obstet Gynecol 59:831, 1950.
9. Rovinsky JJ: Abnormalities of position, lie, presentation and rotation. In Iffy L, Kaminetsky A (eds.): Principles and Practice of Obstetrics and Perinatology. New York: John Wiley & Sons, Vol. 2. pp. 912–913, 1983.
10. Thorn W: Zur Manuellen Umwandlang der Gesichtslagen in Hinter hauptslagen. Z Geburtshilfe Gynaekol 13:186, 1886.
11. Whitacre FE: Forceps management of face and brow presentations. Clin Obstet Gynecol 8:882, 1965.
12. Moore ETT, Dennen EH: Management of persistent brow presentation. Obstet Gynecol 6:186, 1955.
13. Meltzer RM, Sachtleben MR, Friedman EA: Brow presentation. Am J Obstet Gynecol 100:255, 1968.
14. Kovacs SG: Brow presentation at the Royal Hospital for Women 1950–1965, and a review of the literature. Med J Aust 2:820, 1970.
15. Stenchever MA: Normal vaginal delivery. In Iffy L, Charles D (eds.): Operative Perinatology: Invasive Obstetric Techniques. New York: Macmillan, 1984, pp. 524–526.
16. Harrison MR, Golbus MS, Filly RA, et al.: Fetal surgical treatment. Pediatr Ann 11:896, 1982.
17. Clark SL, DeVore GR, Platt LD: The role of ultrasound in the aggressive management of obstructed labor secondary to fetal malformations. Am J Obstet Gynecol 152:1042, 1985.
18. Chervenak FA, Berkowitz RL, Tortora M, et al.: The management of fetal hydrocephalus. Am J Obstet Gynecol 151:933, 1985.
19. Cochrane DD, Myles ST: Management of intrauterine hydrocephalus. J Neurosurg 57:590, 1982.
20. Platt LD, Devore GR: Modification of fetal intraventricular amniotic shunt. Am J Obstet Gynecol 152:1044, 1985.
21. McCullough DC, Balzer-Martin LA: Current prognosis in overt neonatal hydrocephalus. J Neurosurg 57:378, 1982.
22. Feeny JK, Barry AP: Hydrocephaly as a cause of maternal mortality and morbidity. Br J Obstet Gynaecol 61:652, 1954.
23. Samuels L, Driscoll DA, Landon MB, et al.: Cerebrospinal fluid shunts in pregnancy. Am J Perinatol 5:22, 1988.
24. Carpenter MW, Curci MR, Dibbins AW, et al.: Perinatal management of ventral wall defects. Obstet Gynecol 64:646, 1984.
25. Kirk EP, Wah RM: Obstetric management of the fetus with omphalocele or gastroschisis: A review and report of one hundred twelve cases. Am J Obstet Gynecol 146:512, 1983.
26. Baird PA, MacDonald EC: An epidemiologic study of congenital malformations of the anterior abdominal wall in more than half a million consecutive births. Am J Hum Genet 33:470, 1981.
27. Wald NJ, Cuckle HS, Barlow RD, et al.: Early antenatal diagnosis of exomphalos. Lancet 1:1368, 1980.
28. Hasan S, Hermansen MC: The prenatal diagnosis of ventral abdominal wall defects. Am J Obstet Gynecol 155:842, 1986.
29. Lenke RR, Hatch EI: Fetal gastroschisis: A preliminary report advocating the use of cesarean section. Obstet Gynecol 67:395, 1986.
30. Fitzsimmons J, Nyberg DA, Cyr DR, et al.: Perinatal management of gastroschisis. Obstet Gynecol 71:910, 1988.
31. Kim JH: Omphalocele. Surg Clin North Am 56:361, 1976.
32. Gilbert MG, Mencia LF, Brown WT, et al.: Staged surgical repair of large omphaloceles and gastroschisis. J Pediatr Surg 3:702, 1968.
33. Harrison MR, Golbus MS, Filly RA, et al.: Management of the fetus with congenital hydronephrosis. J Pediatr Surg, in press.

Identification and Delivery of the Macrosomic Infant

Joseph M. Miller, Jr.

Accuse not nature! She hath done her part;
Do thou but thine!

Paradise Lost, Book VI
Line 561

Infant weight is one of the first things parents want to know after delivery. Average birth weights vary greatly, from 2400 g among the Lumi of New Guinea to 3830 g among the Cheyenne.[1] Although low and high birth weights occur in 5 to 7% of newborns,[2, 3] the former has received far more attention. Over the last few decades, it appears that large babies have been delivered more often.[4, 5] The largest recorded American newborn, weighing 23 3/4 lbs, was reported more than a century ago. The birth was associated with polyhydramnios, and the mother had previously delivered an 18-lb stillborn.[6]

There is no single definition of excessive birth weight. A weight of either 4000 or 4500 g or more has been defined as macrosomia, although 4000 g or more appears to be more generally accepted.[7-9] An alternate definition, recently advanced, relates to the growth process: Fetal weight above the 90th percentile for gestational age (large for gestational age, LGA) has been identified as macrosomia.[10, 11] In this chapter, macrosomia is defined as birth weight of 4000 g or more.

Excessive fetal size carries risk for both the mother and the newborn. Difficulty in vaginal delivery may arise. Fetal/newborn complications include shoulder dystocia, low Apgar scores, and birth trauma. Shoulder dystocia occurs in 3 to 4% of vaginally delivered macrosomic infants, which is 3 to 20 times more often than in normally grown newborns.[12, 13] Low (less than 7) 1- and 5-minute Apgar scores are found 8 and 2% of the time, respectively.[12] Brachial plexus injury occurs in up to 2.4%, facial nerve injury in up to 7.2%, and clavicular fracture in up to 1.7% of deliveries.[3, 14]

Maternal complications of fetal macrosomia include a 50% increase in perinatal laceration, a threefold rise in postpartum hemorrhage, and a rise in operative delivery, especially cesarean section.[12, 15]

Aside from injury during birth, fetal complications include polycythemia and hyperbilirubinemia.[16] Hypoglycemia has been reported in 12% of heavy infants and is not confined only to the infants of diabetic women.[16] Birth asphyxia has been reported to occur more often,[7] but not all studies concur.[3] Meconium aspiration is more common among macrosomic infants.[3] This association stems from increased gestational age (post-datism) and probably not from post-maturity.

RISK FACTORS FOR MACROSOMIA

Multiple factors are associated with birth weight. Although many studies address more than one variable, in this section each variable is considered independently, relative to newborn size, with emphasis being placed on macrosomia.

Gestational Age

The relationship between birth weight and gestational age is well characterized.[17-20] Fetal growth curves, drawn from a variety of populations, have been developed. These curves are assumed to be representative of growth, although this assumption is misleading.[21] Nevertheless, median birth weights continue to rise at least through the 43rd week. Multiple-regression models indicate the strong influence of gestational age.[20, 22, 23] The incidence of macrosomia increased in a Canadian study from 8.2% if delivery occurred at 39 weeks to 12.3% if delivery was at 40 weeks, to 15.8% if delivery was at 41 weeks, and to 21.0% if delivery was at 42 weeks.[3] Among private middle-class patients in New York, 25.5% of babies delivered at more than 41 weeks were macrosomic.[24] In St. Louis, the occurrence of large infants increased dramatically as gestation lengthened. Among women who delivered at 38 to 40 weeks, 10.4% delivered infants weighing 4000 g or more. This increased to 23.8% of women who delivered at 41 to 42 weeks and 42.8% of women who delivered at 43 to 44 weeks.[25]

Sex

Male infants weigh more than female infants. Studies indicate that, for infants at term, males weigh approximately 70 to 150 g more.[17, 22, 23, 26, 27] Boys are twice as likely as girls to weigh more than 4000 g at birth.[2, 3, 16, 28]

Parity

Birth weight is associated with parity. Primigravidas have smaller infants, and grand multiparas deliver much larger ones.[17, 26] The range has been reported as 154 to 242 g at term. The effect of each successive pregnancy is less clear, with some authors showing a steady rise in birth weight[22, 23] and others showing a difference only between primigravid and multiparous patients.[17, 26] As a group, multiparas deliver macrosomic infants more often than do primiparas (10.9 vs. 8.5%).[3]

Maternal Habitus

Maternal height, weight, and height-adjusted weight have been correlated with infant weight. Larger, taller women have heavier babies.[3, 23, 27, 29] Maternal prepregnancy weight is an important determinant of birth weight.[30-32] Macrosomic newborns occur in only 1.0% of women with low prepregnant weight (less than 45 kg), as opposed to 20% of women with high prepregnant weights (more than 70 kg).[3] Even when adjusted for height, maternal prepregnancy weight remains significantly associated with birth weight.[33] When maternal delivery weight is considered, this too is correlated with newborn size. This correlation is nearly as strong as the association of birth weight with gestational age.[20] Because further evaluation has indicated that maternal weight gain is also important, this variable is discussed separately below.

Maternal height is a significant variable in identifying large babies.[34] In models of newborn size, maternal height has explained differences of up to 364 g.[23] Macrosomia increases from 6.1% if the mother is short (less than 153 cm) to 14.9% if the mother is tall (170 cm or taller).[3, 35]

Maternal weight for height has also been investigated because it is independent of height.[36] This variable is associated with newborn weight and explains an approximately 300 to 400-g difference in birth weight,[23, 26, 27] approximately the same as explained by height alone.[23, 26] Generally, this variable replaces maternal weight in regression equations.

Independent work on a white middle-class population, selected to deliver at term and to be without diabetes or toxemia, found that birth weight was the same among the weight-for-height groups.[34] There was, however, an interesting and varied relationship with more standard maternal variables. Among women who had low weight for their height, weight gain was important. Maternal height was the only significant variable studied that had a significant association among women who were heavy for their height.

Maternal Weight Gain

Maternal weight gain in pregnancy is strongly associated with size of the infant at birth.[3, 30, 37, 38] The relationship[39, 40] holds true under a variety of conditions, but the influence of weight gain does vary with prepregnancy body mass, age, parity, and level of education.[27, 29] In general, women who gain 20 kg or less have an 8.8% incidence of macrosomia, whereas women who gain more than 20 kg have a 2.1-fold increase (19.3%).[3] Weight gain appears to be more important for women of low weight at conception[34] and less important for very overweight women.[29]

Maternal Birth Weight

The birth weight of the mother is correlated with that of her child. Factors that influence intrauterine growth appear to be transgenerational.[2, 41, 42] In a study of white women, mothers who at their own birth had weighed more than 3500 g had infants who were 300 g heavier than those of women whose birth weight had been 2001 to 2500 g. This relationship was valid after correction for prepregnant weight and smoking.[41] A review of the Collaborative Perinatal Project data from Buffalo confirmed this association. Women who had weighed 8 lbs or more at birth were far more likely to deliver a macrosomic infant than those who had weighed 4 to 6 lbs (11.3% vs. 1.8%).[42] In a large study in Tennessee, researchers found a dramatic rise in newborn birth weight as mater-

nal birth weight increased; this association was valid for both white and black patients.[2] Mothers who themselves had weighed more than 4000 g at birth had infants who were 300 g heavier than infants of mothers who had weighed 3000 to 3499 g at birth.

Birth Weight of Prior Infant

Macrosomia is common in women who have had a large infant before.[28] Previous delivery of a large infant has a higher relative risk than maternal weight, height, parity, or smoking. Among mothers who delivered infants weighing more than 4500 g, previous delivery of an infant weighing more than 4000 g was found in 33%, far more often than in control populations (3%).[7] These findings were reinforced by the results of a study done in Australia, although the difference in the Australian study was less impressive (25% vs. 10%).[43]

Maternal Age

Older women are more likely to deliver a macrosomic infant.[37, 39, 44] In Jerusalem, women over the age of 30 had babies who were, on the average, 200 g heavier than the babies of women under age 20 without there being a significant difference in weight gain between the two groups of women. However, parity was greater in the older women.[27] In Australia, birth weight increased with the mother's age up to 40 and was important independent of parity.[23] Macrosomia is associated with advancing age in multiparas but not in primiparas.[3] Multiparous patients under the age of 20 delivered infants who weighed more than 4000 g far less frequently than did women over the age of 35 (7.5% vs. 14.5%).

Insulin-Dependent Diabetes

The incidence of fetal macrosomia in diabetic mothers ranges from 20 to 30%,[45–48] substantially higher than the general population. Within this subgroup, many of the other factors described in this section are independently associated with birth weight. The degree of overgrowth is greater in infants of diabetic mothers. Macrosomia tends to occur at an earlier gestational age in the fetuses of diabetic patients.[49]

The extent of diabetic control is related to the fetal growth process. Diabetic gravidas whose illness is tightly controlled have newborns whose birth weight distribution is no different from that of newborns of nondiabetic gravidas. The operative hypothesis is that maternal hyperglycemia produces fetal hyperinsulinemia, which in turn stimulates fetal growth. Evidence generated during the last decade reinforces this concept, and tight control of the diabetes should be sought. However, other factors, especially obesity and prior delivery of a macrosomic infant, also contribute to the likelihood of macrosomia.[48, 51]

Carbohydrate Intolerance during Pregnancy

Pregnant diabetic women also have a higher incidence of macrosomia than the general population, with up to 30% of their infants being overly large.[46, 52] Improved control of the diabetes appears important. Patients with a mean plasma glucose level higher than 105 mg/dl were 2.7 times more likely to deliver an LGA infant than were patients whose mean plasma glucose level was between 87 and 104 mg/dl.[53] LGA infants were found more frequently among women who had gained more weight and had previously delivered large babies.[53] However, maternal weight, as opposed to maternal age or fasting plasma glucose level on their glucose tolerance test, was of overriding importance.[54]

Even milder degrees of glucose intolerance have been found to influence infant size. Patients with one abnormal value of their glucose tolerance test (GTT) have come under careful scrutiny. Such patients have an increased risk of delivering an infant weighing 4000 g or more (10.7% vs. 6.7% for controls).[52]

Patients with a plasma glucose level of 135 mg/dl or higher drawn 1 hour after a 50-g glucose challenge who subsequently had normal GTTs were more likely to deliver infants weighing 4000 g or more than were women with a negative initial screen (11.9% vs. 6.4%).[8] This finding remained after correction for parity, obesity, race, and gestational age.

Macrosomia occurred more frequently as the 2-hour glucose level increased.[55] In a study of northern Italian women, infants weighing 4000 g or more were delivered to 9.9% of women whose 2-hour GTT value was less than 100 mg/dl, 15.5% of women whose value was between 100 and 119 mg/dl, and 27.5% of women whose value exceeded 120 mg/dl. In Philadelphia, among women with a normal GTT, macrosomia occurred in 8.6% of women whose 2-hour value was less than 140 mg/dl and in 24.4% of women whose 2-hour value was more than 140 mg/dl.[56]

Among nondiabetic pregnant women, change in glycosylated hemoglobin A_1 during the third trimester was positively correlated with relative birth weight,[57] although glycosylated hemoglobin itself has not been associated with relative birth weight or LGA newborns.[58]

Smoking

Reduction of fetal weight is observed in voluntary behavioral states. Smoking is such an example.[22, 27, 39, 40, 59] The strength of this association varies from 5 g per cigarette[27] to 108 g[22] if any smoking is done. Others have reported even higher reduction in birth weight: 160 to 250 g with smoking of more than a half pack per day.[38, 40, 60] This occurs despite the same or increased caloric intake.[40] Commonly, the effect of smoking is jointly shared with inadequate maternal weight gain.[59] In one study, smokers had a 6.6% incidence of macrosomia, as opposed to 11.2% if the mother was a nonsmoker. Others identified a doubling of the risk of macrosomia if the mother did not smoke.[28]

Social Status

Many investigators have reported differences in mean birth weight among socioeconomic classes.[26] This finding persists, even when corrected for maternal habitus[61] and gestational age.[26] A difference of 150 g exists between Classes I and II and Classes IV and V.[26] If addressed somewhat differently, patients in private hospitals have larger infants than do patients in public hospitals, the difference at term being 63 g.[23]

When years of formal education are considered instead of social class or income, a significant and independent association is found.[27]

Nutrition

The mother's nutritional state is an important consideration when looking at infant size.[20, 37, 60] Less well nourished mothers have smaller babies, a finding that is independent of other known variables.[60] Inadequate nutrition is associated with reduced weight gain and is important in explaining poor fetal growth.[40, 62]

Better nutrition is associated with improved pregnancy outcome.[63] Efforts to improve nutrition through diet supplementation had the expected benefit in Africa.[63] In the United States, entry of the at-risk pregnant patient in the Special Supplemental Food Program for Women, Infants, and Children is associated with fewer small-for-gestational-age newborns.[64, 65]

Ethnic Origin

Racial and ethnic background is an important influence on newborn weight. In a collaborative study done in the United States, median birth weights of black and white infants differed. Mean birth weights were 3286 ± 577 g for whites, as opposed to 3069 ± 565 g for blacks.[66] Significant differences remained after correction for socioeconomic factors; of the two factors, race is far more important in birth weight determination.[66]

IDENTIFICATION OF THE MACROSOMIC FETUS

Unless excessive size is considered, recognition of the large fetus is unlikely. Two methods exist to try to identify the newborn who weighs 4000 g or more before birth: clinical evaluation and sonography.

Clinical Evaluation

Both physical examination and risk assessment have been used. When palpation was employed, in one series only 43% of infants who weighed more than 4500 g were correctly identified. Moreover, for each infant diagnosed, 9 others were incorrectly so predicted.[43] In another series, the clinical diagnosis of excessive size was made in only 20%.[67] Although attention should be directed to macrosomia if the fundal height exceeds 40 cm, this criterion alone is clearly insufficient.[68]

Risk assessment has also been used.[3] When the factors of obesity (prepregnant weight of more than 70 kg), excessive weight gain (>20 kg), and gestational age (41 weeks or more) were considered, only 5.4% of patients with no risk factors delivered infants who weighed 4000 g or more. With one risk factor, macrosomia rose to 15.1%; if two or three risk factors were present, 31.5% delivered large infants. Unfortunately, 1/3 of mothers who delivered large infants had no risk factor, and only 1/5 of mothers with large infants had two or three risk factors. Clinical assessment, although helpful, does not allow accurate identification of the large fetus.

Ultrasonography

Ultrasonography has provided valuable insight in the area of fetal overgrowth. Depending on the analysis and endpoint, either the growth process (LGA) or the excessively sized fetus has been characterized. Because of the definition of macrosomia selected for this chapter, a birth weight of 4000 g or more shall be addressed first.

The ability to predict fetal size using ultrasonography has been established. In optimum circumstances, estimates are off by no more than 15% (2 standard deviations),[69] although many authors have reported greater ranges.[70, 71] The ability to predict weight before delivery requires that the established fetal weight formula apply to the population studied. Many formulas are available, although those from New Haven,[72] Chicago,[73] and Houston[69] are most commonly employed.

Large fetuses have not been well predicted by ultrasonography. Benacerraf and colleagues[71] found that only 65% of newborns who weighed more than 4000 g were so identified within 1 week of delivery; 90% of infants with lower weights were correctly identified. However, the predictive value of the positive test (fetal macrosomia) was only 68%, and that of the negative test was 89%.[71] The inherent limitation of ultrasonographic prediction of fetal weight estimates for macrosomia was reinforced by analysis of receiver-operative characteristic curves developed from patients in New Orleans.[74] Only 59% of macrosomic infants were so identified. Only 57% of those predicted to be large actually were. With 92% correctly assigned, infants with smaller weights were more accurately classified. When only diabetic patients were considered, the likelihood of macrosomia was 77% if the estimated fetal weight was more than 4000 g, but only 48% of macrosomic infants were correctly identified.[75]

Excessive size has been evaluated by other aspects of fetal biometry. The difference between the mean thoracic diameter and biparietal diameter was strongly correlated with macrosomia. Sensitivity was 87%, but the predictive value of the positive test was only 61%. The difference between the mean abdominal diameter and the biparietal diameter was similarly evaluated.[76] Sensitivity was only 46%, and specificity was 79%.

The ratio of the femur length to the abdominal circumference was found to be significantly correlated with birth weight of more than 3900 g.[10] With a cutoff of .205, specificity was 86% and the predictive value of a positive test was 68%. However, because both femur and abdominal circumferences are independently correlated with macrosomia, the use of this ratio is limited.[74]

Relative growth has also been evaluated. Among diabetic women, delivery of LGA infants was correlated with an abdominal circumference or estimated weight greater than the 90th percentile for the gestational age.[11] These factors were 78% sensitive, and the predictive values of the positive and negative tests were approximately 75% and 80%, respectively. This work, done at or near term, was repeated at the 30- to 33-week interval. In diabetic gravidas, an abdominal circumference above the 90th percentile was strongly associated with an LGA newborn.[77] Sensitivity and specificity were both about 85%, but the predictive value of the positive test was only 56%. This determination would seem to be of most benefit for identifying the non-LGA fetus, because the predictive value of the negative test was more than 96%.

Other attempts to identify the LGA newborn in late pregnancy have focused on shoulder width.[78] If the distance from the skin surface to the outer surface of the humerus was 12 mm or more, sensitivity was 83%, and specificity was 90%. If a shoulder width of 12 mm or more was combined with an abdominal circumference above the 90th percentile for gestational age, sensitivity rose to 96% and specificity was 89%.

The ratio of the femur length to abdominal circumference has been correlated with the occurrence of LGA newborns. Specificity was reported to be 90%, but sensitivity was only 65%.[78] Although statistical correlation has been substantiated, clinical utility has not.[76] Whereas specificity was high, sensitivity was only 24%, and the predictive values of the positive and negative tests were 70% and 63%, respectively. Even when a diabetic population was tested, use of this ratio was disappointing.[79]

Biparietal diameter alone was reported to be predictive of an LGA fetus.[80] Subsequent studies revealed this to be of very limited value.[74, 81]

The ratio of the biparietal diameter to the chest area was correlated with the delivery of an LGA newborn.[81] Only 57% of such infants were so identified, however.

Early studies indicated that umbilical cord velocimetry as measured by the Doppler effect provides insight into fetal growth.[82] Infants whose birth weight is above the 75th percentile for gestational age had a mean systolic to diastolic (S/D) ratio of 2.4, less than the group as a whole. In another study, the delivery of LGA infants was significantly more common if the S/D ratio was below 2.5, but sensitivity and specificity were limited.[83]

Serial ultrasonographic studies have been used to evaluate interval change. An abdominal circumference growth rate of 1.2 cm per week or more beyond the 32nd week of gestation was strongly correlated with LGA status of the newborn.[79] Both sensitivity and specificity were about 85%. These observations were better than excessive abdominal circumference corrected for gestational age.

To date, the abdominal circumference growth rate appears to be the most attractive assessment, but it does require at least two examinations in later pregnancy. From a single sonogram, relative weight assessment is probably best. Ultrasonic recognition of excessive fetal size is superior to clinical prediction.

DELIVERY OF THE MACROSOMIC INFANT

Vaginal delivery of the macrosomic infant is associated with an increased incidence of birth trauma. The question whether to perform cesarean section arises. Certainly, one could eliminate shoulder dystocia, with attendant neurologic injury, in this group by elective abdominal delivery of all mothers with a fetus weighing 4000 g or more. This is neither practical nor warranted. One would have to perform 27 cesarean sections to prevent each shoulder dystocia and 270 to avoid each severely affected infant.[3] Other strategies are appropriate.

The strong relationship among midpelvic delivery, prolonged second stage, and shoulder dystocia was pointed out a decade ago.[13] Avoidance of midpelvic delivery of macrosomic infants resulted in an incidence of shoulder dystocia of only 7% in a setting in which the cesarean section rate was only 31%.[84] Repetitive instruction in appropriate intraoperative management was instrumental in achieving a brachial palsy rate of only 0.7% of vaginally delivered macrosomic infants, with permanent palsy in only 0.1%.

It is difficult to be certain if the estimated fetal weight is more than 4000 g. Management decisions for infants of projected weights of 4000 to 4500 g should probably not be made on weight estimates alone. For infants who are indeed large (more than 4500 g), data suggest greater risks.[9, 67] Among infants of diabetic mothers, an estimated weight of more than 4000 g suggests increased risk. For such infants, abdominal delivery is already very likely and shoulder dystocia more common.[84] Cesarean section is probably indicated.[9, 67]

If a trial of labor is selected and shoulder dystocia occurs, prompt recognition and appropriate management, as outlined below, are indicated.

MANAGEMENT OF SHOULDER DYSTOCIA

Although infant size is important, it is primarily the delivery process itself in which difficulty is encountered. In vaginal delivery, once the head is out, there may not be sufficient room for the enlarged shoulders to emerge easily. Cord compression may follow, associated with reduced perfusion of the fetus. Shoulder dystocia may not be predicted with accuracy. Despite risk analysis, unexpected cases will arise. Careful and timely management is important in minimizing the sequelae of neurologic injury. Reduction of the interval from delivery of the head to delivery of the body is desirable. *Overly vigorous traction* on the head or neck or too much rotation of the body *may cause serious damage* to the newborn. However, injury to the brachial plexus may occur in the absence of shoulder dystocia and forceps delivery and does not automatically imply undue force by the obstetrician.[84a]

The deliverer should have a plan of action prepared. The usual steps presume a generous episiotomy. Adequate anesthetic coverage should be summoned. The infant's mouth or nose should be cleared. The inside of the birth canal is palpated to rule out thoracic or abdominal enlargement. Several techniques may then be used to reduce the impacted shoulder. Proscribed courses of action include desperate pulling on the fetal head and fundal expulsive efforts. The infamous fundal pressure serves only to worsen the impaction.[50] A good initial technique, while plans for additional efforts

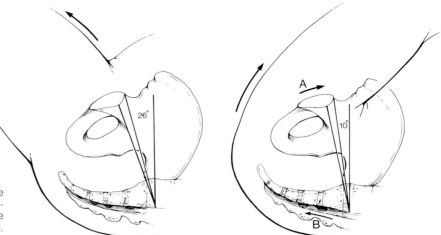

Figure 18–1. The pelvic configuration before *(left)* and after *(right)* the McRoberts maneuver. The symphysis rotates anteriorly (*A*), the angle of inclination is reduced to 10 degrees, and the sacral spine flattens (*B*).

are underway, is application of moderate suprapubic pressure.[85]

The McRoberts maneuver should be employed next.[86] The patient's legs are removed from the stirrups and sharply flexed on her abdomen. Additional mild traction will usually allow delivery of the impacted shoulder. The maneuver results in straightening of the sacrum relative to the lumbar spine. The symphysis pubis rotates toward the patient's head (Fig. 18–1). The angle of pelvic inclination decreases from 26 to 10 degrees.[86]

Although it does not increase the dimension of the maternal pelvis, this maternal repositioning reverses several factors promoting the dystocia. First, it elevates the impacted anterior shoulder of the fetus with respect to the mother. The fetus is carried anteriorly and the fetal spine flexes toward the anterior shoulder. This results in pushing the posterior shoulder over the sacrum and through the inlet. Second, with straightening of the maternal lordosis, the sacral promontory is removed as an obstruction. Third, weight-bearing forces are moved from the main pressure point of the pelvis in the lithotomy position, i.e., the sacrum. The inlet opens to its maximal diameter, allowing de-

livery forces to work more effectively. Traction forces needed for delivery are reduced. Success of the procedure is marked by relaxation of inward traction on the fetal head as the posterior shoulder traverses the inlet. Should delivery not easily ensue, the patient's repositioning should be maintained. This maneuver has been successful in more than 90% of cases.[88]

The critical problem encountered in shoulder dystocia is the excessive size of the shoulders relative to anteroposterior diameter of the pelvis. Because the maximal dimension of the pelvis is the oblique diameter, efforts to place the fetus in this alignment should be undertaken. The simplest is to push the anterior shoulder toward the anterior surface of the chest (i.e., partially rotate the fetus counterclockwise if left occiput anterior), as illustrated in Figure 18–2. If this is not successful, other efforts can be made.

Woods[89] described a method that uses the principle of a screw (Fig. 18–3). The posterior shoulder is rotated anteriorly toward the fetal chest wall. A half turn is accomplished. The anterior shoulder is released as it moves away from the symphysis. Descent of the shoulders occurs when the fetus is

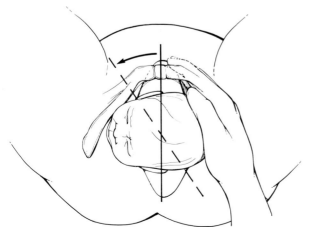

Figure 18–2. Rotating the shoulders to the oblique diameter.

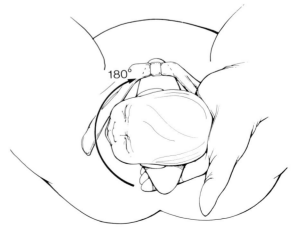

Figure 18–3. The Woods screw maneuver.

in the oblique diameter. The posterior shoulder passes beneath the symphysis and is delivered.

The Rubin maneuver is another procedure designed to relieve the impaction (Fig. 18–4). The shoulders are moved from the anteroposterior diameter by displacing the posterior shoulder toward the anterior surface of the fetal chest.[90] This often results in abduction of both shoulders. The smaller bishoulder diameter may allow the trapped anterior shoulder to escape from behind the symphysis, especially if suprapubic pressure is applied selectively. Adequate inhalation anesthesia with resultant uterine relaxation may assist in this effort.[91]

Many authors advocate delivery of the posterior shoulder either as an initial effort or as a backup when the previously mentioned efforts fail. The operator's hand passes into the vagina across the fetal chest and finds the elbow. The arm is flexed and swept across the chest and perineum. This frees room in the pelvis, and the anterior shoulder can often be readily delivered.[91] If not, the shoulder is placed in the oblique diameter or the fetus is rotated a full 180 degrees.[92, 93]

Deliberate fracture of the clavicle is possible and will promote collapse of the shoulders. Clavicular fracture may be accomplished by pressing this bone against the ramus of the pelvis. Force should be directed away from the lung, to avoid puncture. The fracture will heal rapidly with little significant sequelae.

Cleidotomy involves cutting the clavicle with scissors or another sharp instrument.[94] This is usually reserved for the dead fetus. Symphysiotomy has also been used successfully.[94]

A succession of methods will nearly always result in delivery with minimal trauma. Rarely, delivery cannot be accomplished because there is an obstructing tumor or the arms cannot be delivered. Cephalic replacement and immediate cesarean delivery have been used.[96, 97] The operator may replace the head by depressing the posterior perineum and applying the palm of his or her hand to the vertex. The head is returned to the occiput anterior or occiput posterior position. Uterine relaxation with subcutaneous terbutaline or anesthesia is beneficial.[98]

Rarely, shoulder dystocia will be encountered in a patient who unexpectedly delivers in bed. In this setting, the patient should be placed in the knee-chest position. This accomplishes two things: The patient stops pushing, and the pelvic girdle is rotated ventrally, just as with the McRoberts maneuver. Delivery can generally then be accomplished.

NEW THERAPIES

Several possibilities exist to reduce the likelihood of maternal or neonatal morbidity associated with delivery of the macrosomic infant.

Gestational Diabetes

The contribution of undiagnosed or poorly controlled gestational diabetes to excessive fetal size has been established. Accurate recognition is appropriate. Risk assessment is statistically well founded, but significant numbers of low-risk patients have glucose metabolic abnormalities.[99, 100] Universal screening is the only way to identify all potentially diabetic patients. The standard 50-g glucose challenge with measurement of plasma glucose 1 hour later is excellent, but the breakfast challenge test is also appropriate.[99, 101, 102] For clinical purposes, hemoglobin A_{1c} is probably not sufficiently accurate.[104]

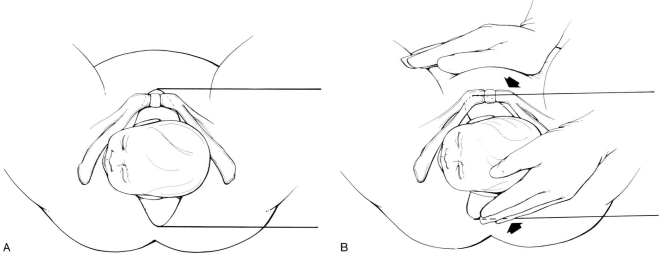

Figure 18–4. *A*, The shoulder-to-shoulder diameter is maximal, with the anterior shoulder trapped by the symphysis. *B*, Abduction of the shoulders by the Rubin maneuver. Both shoulders are pushed anteriorly.

Patients with one abnormal value on their GTT are at risk for macrosomia. Appropriate dietary management reduces the likelihood of this occurrence. Marginal glucose tolerance requires recognition and treatment. Liberal screening with attention to minor glucose metabolic abnormalities will reduce the occurrence of macrosomia.

Limited Length of Pregnancy

Macrosomia is strongly associated with postdatism.[25] Induction at term would limit excessive growth. With the use of agents to ripen the cervix, induction has higher success rates.[105] A large number of growing babies could have their size limited through limitation of pregnancy length. This process would be most appropriately applied to patients who were having an LGA fetus.

Universal Ultrasonography at Term

Ultrasonography provides useful information about the fetal growth process and fetal size. Ultrasonography can be conducted on women at term to identify (better than by risk factors alone) those with larger babies. Such information can forewarn the obstetrician of potential difficulties. If size is greatly excessive, vaginal delivery can be avoided.

SUMMARY

Careful attention to the patient, potential risk factors, clinical progress, and fetal size should allow obstetricians to reduce the occurrence of maternal and neonatal morbidity. No management plan is absolute, and, despite the best of plans, shoulder dystocia will occur. The attending health care providers should be skilled in effective and appropriate maneuvers to manage this condition.

References

1. Meredith HV: Body weight at birth of viable human infants: A worldwide comparative treatise. Hum Biol 42:217, 1970.
2. Klebanoff MA, Yip R: Influence of maternal birth weight on rate of fetal growth and duration of gestation. J Pediatr 111:287, 1987.
3. Boyd ME, Usher RH, McLean FH: Fetal macrosomia: Prediction, risks, proposed management. Obstet Gynecol 61:715, 1983.
4. Johar R, Rayburn W, Weir D, et al.: Birth weights in term infants: A 50 year perspective. J Reprod Med 33:813, 1988.
5. Brouillette LJ: Prediction and consequences of macrosomia. J La State Med Soc 33:139, 1987.
6. Barnes AC: An obstetric record for *The Medical Record.* Obstet Gynecol 9:237, 1957.
7. Modanlou HD, Dorchester WL, Thorosian A, et al.: Macrosomia—maternal, fetal, and neonatal implications. Obstet Gynecol 55:420, 1980.
8. Leikin EL, Jenkins JH, Pomerantz GA, et al.: Abnormal glucose screening tests in pregnancy: A risk for macrosomia. Obstet Gynecol 69:570, 1987.
9. Nelson JH, Rorner IW, Bartus RH: The large baby. South Med J 51:23, 1958.
10. Hadlock FP, Harrist RB, Feraneyhough TC, et al.: Use of femur length/abdominal circumference ratio in detecting the macrosomic fetus. Radiology 154:503, 1985.
11. Tamura RK, Sabbagha RE, Depp R, et al.: Diabetic macrosomia: Accuracy of third trimester ultrasound. Obstet Gynecol 67:828, 1986.
12. Golditch IM, Kirkman K: The large fetus: Management and outcome. Obstet Gynecol 52:26, 1978.
13. Benedetti TJ, Gabbe SG: Shoulder dystocia: A complication of fetal macrosomia and prolonged second stage of labor with midpelvic delivery. Obstet Gynecol 52:526, 1978.
14. Levine MG, Holroyde J, Woods JR Jr, et al.: Birth trauma: Incidence and predisposing factors. Obstet Gynecol 63:792, 1984.
15. Gould JB, Davey B, Stafford RS: Socioeconomic differences in rates of cesarean section. N Engl J Med 321:233, 1989.
16. Stevenson DK, Hopper AO, Cohen RS, et al.: Macrosomia: Causes and consequences. J Pediatr 100:515, 1982.
17. Brenner WE, Edelman DA, Hendricks CH: A standard of fetal growth for the United States of America. Am J Obstet Gynecol 126:555, 1976.
18. Lubchenco LO, Hansman C, Boyd E: Intrauterine growth in length and head circumference as estimated from live births at gestational ages from 26 to 42 weeks. Pediatrics 37:403, 1966.
19. Williams RL, Creasy RK, Cunningham GC, et al.: Fetal growth and perinatal viability in California. Obstet Gynecol 59:624, 1982.
20. Phillips C, Johnson NE: The impact of quality of diet and other factors on birthweight of infants. Am J Clin Nutr 30:215, 1977.
21. Wilcox AJ: Birth weight, gestation and the fetal growth curve. Am J Obstet Gynecol 139:863, 1981.
22. Petterson F, Melander S: Prediction of birth weight—Results of multiple regression analysis. Upsala J Med Sci 80:135, 1975.
23. Keeping JD, Chang A, Morrison J: Birthweight, analysis of variance and the linear additive model. Br J Obstet Gynaecol 86:437, 1979.
24. Chervenak JL, Dixon MY, Hirsch J, et al.: Macrosomia in the postdate pregnancy: Is routine ultrasonographic screening indicated? Am J Obstet Gynecol 161:753, 1989.
25. Arias F: Predictability of complications associated with prolongation of pregnancy. Obstet Gynecol 70:101, 1987.
26. Thomson AM, Billewicz WZ, Hytten FE: The assessment of fetal growth. J Obstet Gynaecol Br Commonw 75:903, 1968.
27. Seidman DS, Ever-Hadani P, Gale R: The effect of maternal weight gain in pregnancy on birth weight. Obstet Gynecol 74:240, 1989.
28. Scott A, Moar V, Oumsted M: The relative contribution of different maternal factors in large-for-gestational-age pregnancies. Eur J Obstet Gynecol Reprod Biol 13:269, 1982.
29. Abrams BF, Laros RK Jr: Prepregnancy weight, weight gain, and birth weight. Am J Obstet Gynecol 154:503, 1986.
30. Simpson JW, Lawless RW, Mitchell AC: Responsibility of the obstetrician to the fetus II. Influence of pre-pregnancy weight and pregnancy weight gain. Obstet Gynecol 45:481, 1975.
31. Eastman NJ, Jackson E: Weight relationships in pregnancy. I. The bearing of maternal weight and pre-pregnancy weight or birth weight in full term pregnancies. Obstet Gynecol Surv 23:1003, 1968.

32. Niswander KR, Singer J, Westphal M, et al.: Weight gain during pregnancy and pre-pregnancy weight. Obstet Gynecol 33:482, 1964.

33. Peckman CH, Christianson RE: The relationship between pre-pregnancy weight and certain obstetric factors. Am J Obstet Gynecol 111:1, 1971.

34. Winikoff B, Debrovner CH: Anthropometric determinants of birth weight. Obstet Gynecol 58:678, 1981.

35. Lazar S, Baile Y, Mazor M, et al.: Complications associated with the macrosomic fetus. J Reprod Med 31:501, 1986.

36. Billewicz WZ, Kemsley WFF, Thomson AM: Indices of adiposity. Br J Prev Soc Med 16:183, 1962.

37. Higgins AC: Montreal diet dispensary study. In Nutritional Supplementation and the Outcome of Pregnancy. Proceedings of a Workshop. Washington, DC: National Academy Press, 1972, p. 93.

38. Mitchell MC, Lerner E: Factors that influence the outcome of pregnancy in middle-class women. J Am Diet Assoc 87:731, 1987.

39. Weiss W, Jackson EC: Maternal factors affecting birth weight. In Perinatal Factors Affecting Human Development (PAHO Scientific Publication No. 185). Washington, DC: Pan American Health Organization, 1969, p. 54.

40. Beale VA: Nutritional studies during pregnancy II. Dietary intake, maternal weight gain, and size of infant. J Am Diet Assoc 58:321, 1971.

41. Hackman E, Emanuel I, van Belle G, et al.: Maternal birth weight and subsequent pregnancy outcome. JAMA 250:2016, 1983.

42. Klebanoff MA, Mills JL, Berendes HW: Mother's birthweight as a predictor of macrosomia. Am J Obstet Gynecol 153:253, 1985.

43. Svigos JM: The macrosomic infant. Med J Aust 1:245, 1981.

44. O'Sullivan JB, Gellis SS, Tenney BO, et al.: Aspects of birth weight and its influencing variables. Am J Obstet Gynecol 92:1023, 1965.

45. Johnson JM, Lange IR, Harman CR, et al.: Biophysical profile scoring in the management of the diabetic pregnancy. Obstet Gynecol 72:841, 1988.

46. Miller JM Jr: A reappraisal of "tight control" in diabetic pregnancies. Am J Obstet Gynecol 147:158, 1983.

47. Elliott JP, Garite TJ, Freeman RK, et al.: Ultrasonic prediction of fetal macrosomia in diabetic patients. Obstet Gynecol 60:159, 1982.

48. Small M, Cameron A, Luman CB, et al.: Macrosomia in pregnancy complicated by insulin-dependent diabetes mellitus. Diabetes Care 10:594, 1987.

49. Miller JM Jr, Brown HL, Pastorek JG II, et al.: Fetal overgrowth—Diabetic versus nondiabetic. J Ultrasound Med 7:577, 1988.

50. Gross SJ, Shime J, Fanine D: Shoulder dystocia: Predictors and outcome: A five-year review. Am J Obstet Gynecol 156:334, 1987.

51. William SP, Leveno KJ, Guzick DS, et al.: Glucose threshold for macrosomia in pregnancy complicated by diabetes. Am J Obstet Gynecol 154:470, 1986.

52. Al-Shawaf T, Moghraby S, Akiel A: Does impaired glucose tolerance imply a risk in pregnancy? Br J Obstet Gynaecol 95:1036, 1988.

53. Langer O, Levy J, Brustman L, et al.: Glycemic control in gestational diabetes mellitus—How tight is tight enough: Small for gestational age versus large for gestational age? Am J Obstet Gynecol 161:646, 1989.

54. Mares M, Beard RW, Bray CS, et al.: Factors predisposing to and outcome of gestational diabetes. Obstet Gynecol 74:342, 1989.

55. Tallarigo L, Giampietro O, Penno G, et al.: Relation of glucose tolerance to complications of pregnancy in nondiabetic women. N Engl J Med 315:989, 1986.

56. Herman G, Rainmondi B: Glucose tolerance, fetal growth, and pregnancy complications in normal women. Am J Perinatol 5:168, 1988.

57. Hanson V, Hagenfeldt L, Gagenfeldt K: Glycosylated hemoglobins in normal pregnancy: Sequential changes and relation to birth weight. Obstet Gynecol 62:741, 1983.

58. Yatscoff RW, Mehta A, Dean H: Cord blood glycosylated (glycated) hemoglobin: Correlation with maternal glycosylated (glycated) hemoglobin and birth weight. Am J Obstet Gynecol 152:861, 1985.

59. Rush D: Examination of the relationship between birthweight, cigarette smoking during pregnancy and maternal weight gain. J Obstet Gynaecol Br Commonw 81:746, 1974.

60. Metcoff J, Costiloe P, Crosby WM, et al.: Effect of food supplementation (WIC) during pregnancy on birth weight. Am J Clin Nutr 41:933, 1985.

61. Illsley R, Kincaid JC: In Butler NR, Bonham DG (eds.): Perinatal Mortality: The First Report of the 1958 British Perinatal Mortality Survey. Edinburgh: Livingston, 1963, p. 270.

62. Kennedy ET, Gershoff S, Reed R, et al.: Evaluation of the effect of WIC supplemental feeding on birthweight. J Am Diet Assoc 80:220, 1982.

63. Susser M: Prenatal nutrition, birthweight, and psychological development: An overview of experiments, quasi-experiments, and natural experiments in the past decade. Am J Clin Nutr 34:784, 1981.

64. Kennedy ET: A prenatal screening system for use in a community-based setting. J Am Diet Assoc 86:1372, 1986.

65. Schramm WF: WIC prenatal participation and its relationship to newborn medicaid costs in Missouri: A cost/benefit analysis. Am J Public Health 75:851, 1985.

66. Naylor AF, Myrianthopoulos NC: The relation of ethnic and selected socio-economic factors to human birthweight. Ann Hum Genet 31:71, 1967.

67. Parks DG, Ziel HK: Macrosomia—A proposed indication for primary cesarean section. Obstet Gynecol 52:409, 1978.

68. Posner AC, Friedman S, Posner LB: The large fetus: A study of 547 cases. Obstet Gynecol 5:268, 1955.

69. Hadlock FP, Harriet RB, Carpenter RJ, et al.: Computer assisted analysis of fetal weight based on sonographic measurement of fetal growth parameters. Radiology 150:535, 1984.

70. Ott WJ, Doyle S, Flamm S: Accurate ultrasonic estimation of fetal weight. Am J Perinatol 2:178, 1955.

71. Benacerraf BR, Gelman R, Frigoletto FD Jr: Sonographically estimated weights: Accuracy and limitation. Am J Obstet Gynecol 159:1118, 1988.

72. Shepard MJ, Richards VA, Berkowitz RG, et al.: An evaluation of two equations for predicting fetal weight by ultrasound. Am J Obstet Gynecol 142:47, 1982.

73. Birnholz JC: An algorithmic approach to accurate ultrasonic fetal weight estimation. Invest Radiol 21:571, 1986.

74. Miller JM Jr, Brown HL, Khawli OF, et al.: Ultrasonographic identification of the macrosomic fetus. Am J Obstet Gynecol 159:1110, 1988.

75. Benson CB, Doubilet PM, Saltzman DH: Sonographic determination of fetal weight in diabetic pregnancies. Am J Obstet Gynecol 156:441, 1987.

76. Miller JM Jr, Korndorffer FA III, Kissling GE, et al.: Recognition of the over grown fetus: In utero ponderal indices. Am J Perinatol 4:86, 1987.

77. Bochner CJ, Medearis AL, William J III, et al.: Early third-trimester ultrasound screening in gestational diabetes to determine the risk of macrosomia and labor dystocia at term. Am J Obstet Gynecol 157:703, 1987.

78. Mintz MC, Landon MB, Gabbe SG, et al.: Shoulder soft tissue width as a predictor of macrosomia in diabetic pregnancies. Am J Perinatol 6:240, 1989.

79. Landon MD, Mintz MC, Gabbe SG: Sonographic evaluation of fetal abdominal growth. Predictor of the large-for-gestational-age infant in pregnancies complicated by diabetes mellitus. Am J Obstet Gynecol 160:115, 1989.

80. Crane JP, Kopta MM, Welt SI, et al.: Abnormal fetal

growth patterns: Ultrasonic diagnosis and management. Obstet Gynecol 50:205, 1977.

81. Waldimiroff JW, Bloemsma CA, Wallenburg HCS: Ultrasonic diagnosis of the large-for-dates infant. Obstet Gynecol 52:285, 1978.

82. Fleischer A, Schulman H, Farmakides G, et al.: Umbilical artery velocity wave forms and intrauterine growth retardation. Am J Obstet Gynecol 151:502, 1985.

83. Miller JM Jr, Khawli O, Brown HL, et al.: Aberrant fetal growth: Doppler vs ultrasound (Abstract 312). Presented at the annual meeting of the Society of Perinatal Obstetricians, New Orleans, February 3, 1988.

84. Benedetti TJ, Wilson J, Pranger N, et al.: Avoidance of permanent brachial plexus injury without use of routine cesarean section for fetal macrosomia (Abstract 111). Presented at the annual meeting of the Society of Perinatol Obstetricians, New Orleans, February 4, 1989.

84a. Tan KL: Brachial palsy. J Obstet Gynaecol Br Commonw 80:60, 1973.

85. Resnik R: Management of shoulder girdle dystocia. Clin Obstet Gynecol 23:559, 1980.

86. Gonik B, Stringer CA, Hold B: An alternate maneuver for management of shoulder dystocia. Am J Obstet Gynecol 145:882, 1983.

87. Gonik B, Allen R, Sorab J: Objective evaluation of the shoulder dystocia phenomenon: Effect of maternal pelvic orientation on force reduction. Obstet Gynecol 74:44, 1989.

88. Pollack NB, O'Leary JA: McRoberts maneuver for shoulder dystocia: A survey (thesis). Jacksonville, FL: University Hospital of Jacksonville, 1985, p. 6.

89. Woods CE: A principle of physics as applied to shoulder dystocia. Am J Obstet Gynecol 45:796, 1943.

90. Rubin A: Management of shoulder dystocia. JAMA 189:835, 1964.

91. Dignam WJ: Difficulties in delivery, including shoulder dystocia and malpresentation of the fetus. Clin Obstet Gynecol 19:3, 1976.

92. Hopwood HG: Shoulder dystocia—Fifteen years' experience in a community hospital. Am J Obstet Gynecol 144:162, 1982.

93. Seigworth GR: Shoulder dystocia—Review of 5 years' experience. Obstet Gynecol 28:764, 1966.

94. Schramin M: Impacted shoulder—A personal experience. Aust NZ J Obstet Gynecol 23:28, 1983.

95. Hartfield VJ: Symphysiotomy for shoulder dystocia. Am J Obstet Gynecol 155:228, 1986.

96. O'Leary JA, Gunn DL: Cephalic replacement for shoulder dystocia. Am J Obstet Gynecol 153:592, 1985.

97. Sandburg EC: The Zavanetti maneuver extended: Progression of a revolutionary concept. Am J Obstet Gynecol 158:1347, 1988.

98. O'Leary JA, Gunn DL: Option for shoulder dystocia—cephalic replacement. Contemp Obstet Gynecol 27:157, 1986.

99. Coustan DR, Nelson NC, Carpenter MW, et al.: Maternal age and screening for gestational diabetes: A population based study. Obstet Gynecol 73:557, 1989.

100. Mestman JH: Outcome of diabetes screening in pregnancy and perinatol morbidity in infants of mothers with mild impairment of glucose tolerance. Diabetes Care 3:447, 1980.

101. Helton DG, Martin RW, Martin JN Jr, et al.: Detection of glucose intolerance in pregnancy. J Perinatol 9:259, 1989.

102. Coustan DR, Widness JA, Carpenter MA, et al.: Should the fifty-gram, one-hour plasma glucose screening test be administered in the fasting or fed state? Am J Obstet Gynecol 154:1031, 1986.

103. Coustan DR, Widness JA, Carpenter MA, et al.: The "breakfast tolerance test": Screening for gestational diabetes with a standardized mixed nutrient med. Am J Obstet Gyn 157:1113, 1987.

104. Miller JM Jr, Grenshaw MC Jr, Welt SI: Hemoglobin A_{1c} in normal and diabetic pregnancy. JAMA 242:278, 1979.

105. Hetni MA, Lewis GA: Induction of labour with vaginal prostaglandin E_2 pessaries. Br J Obstet Gynaecol 87:199, 1980.

UNIT TWO

Breech Presentation

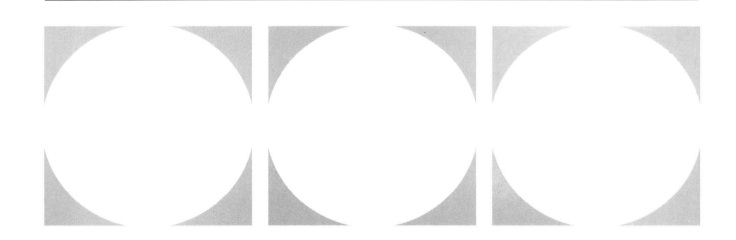

19

Assisted Breech Extraction

Salih Yasin
Mary J. O'Sullivan

During this century the management of breech presentation has undergone dramatic change, which is continuing. In this chapter, we review the risks and current management of breech presentation, reminding the reader that although times and management change, mechanisms do not.

INCIDENCE, TYPES, AND ASSOCIATED FACTORS

Breech presentation occurs in 3% of all singleton deliveries.[1] The earlier the gestational age, the higher the incidence, with 25 to 30% of all fetuses presenting as breeches before 28 weeks' gestation;[2, 3] yet the majority convert to cephalic presentation by 34 weeks.[1]

There are three major types of breech presentation (Fig. 19–1):

1. *Frank:* The hips of the fetus are flexed on the abdomen, and the knees are extended. This is the most common type in singleton breeches, occurring in 55% at term and in 38% of infants weighing less than 2500 g.[5]

2. *Complete:* The hips and knees of the fetus are flexed with the buttocks and knees at the same level. This is the least common type, occurring in 10% of preterm and term breeches.[6]

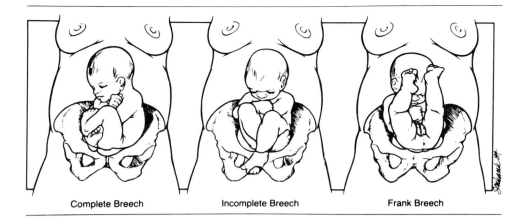

Complete Breech   Incomplete Breech   Frank Breech

Figure 19–1. Types of breech presentations. (From Seeds JW: Malpresentations: In Gabbe S, Niebyl JR, Simpson L [eds]: Obstetrics: Normal and Problem Pregnancies, 2nd ed. New York: Churchill Livingstone, 1991, in press.)

3. *Incomplete/footling:* One or both hips are extended so that one or both feet and/or knees are below the level of the fetal buttocks. This is most common in preterm singleton breeches (50%) and occurs in 20 to 24% of infants weighing more than 2500 g.

In the majority (80%) of breech presentations, no etiologic factors are found.[7] Reported associations include prematurity; uterine anomalies; abnormalities of amniotic fluid volume (hydramnios or oligohydramnios); multiple gestation; placenta previa; contracted pelvis; pelvic tumors; and skeletal, neuromuscular, or chromosomal fetal anomalies (Table 19–1). Other speculated contributors to this presentation include (a) a splinting effect of the lower extremities in the frank breech and (b) a short umbilical cord; possibly, the breech presentation is an adaptive measure to promote growth in multiple gestation.[8–11]

FETAL AND MATERNAL RISKS

Fetal and maternal risks in the breech presentation depend on many factors, including the type of breech, attitude of the fetal head, mode of delivery, intrinsic fetal abnormalities, gestational age, and maternal medical/obstetrical factors.

For breech-presenting infants, the perinatal mortality and morbidity are estimated to be three times that of comparable infants in the vertex presentation.[12] The uncorrected perinatal mortal-

ity for all breeches is 25 to 32%;[6, 13] corrected, the rate is 7 to 16%,[13, 14] and in preterm breeches it is 17 to 25%.[14]

Umbilical cord prolapse occurs at a ten times greater rate in the breech presentation (3.7%) than in the vertex presentation (0.3%).[15] The risk is further increased when the lower uterine cavity is not completely filled by the presenting part, when the infant is an incomplete breech (5 to 10%) or premature, or when the mother is multiparous.[12, 16, 17]

Extension of the fetal arm(s) above and/or behind the fetal head may cause nerve damage resulting in Erb's palsy and/or trauma to the muscles of the axilla, shoulder, and neck; fracture of the clavicle; torticollis; or a winged scapula with atrophy of the deltoid and biceps muscles.[18] Although such injuries might be avoided by cesarean section, improper management at surgery could result in a similar outcome.

The breech-presenting fetus may sustain other traumatic injuries, such as fractures of the clavicle, long bones, cervical spine, and skull during extraction, whether vaginal or abdominal. A lower extremity may be fractured during abdominal delivery, particularly if it is prolapsed through the cervix. Bony injuries may be associated with vascular injuries, resulting in hematomas surrounding the site. Trauma to intra-abdominal organs and/or soft tissues complicates vaginal breech delivery and, less frequently, cesarean births when the operator is not gentle handling the infant during extraction.

Hyperextension of the fetal head is one major contributor to neurologic injury, occurring in approximately 5% of breeches.[19] In breech deliveries conducted vaginally, hyperextension of the fetal head has been associated with intracerebral bleeding, tentorial tears, subdural hematomas, cervical cord lacerations, and hypoxia and the effects thereof.[20, 21] The same traumatic events may occur during the cesarean birth of an infant with a hyperextended head.[13]

Entrapment of the fetal head either at the pelvic

Table 19–1. FACTORS ASSOCIATED WITH BREECH PRESENTATION

Prematurity
Uterine anomalies
Abnormal amniotic fluid volume
Multiple gestation
Placenta previa
Contracted pelvis
Pelvic tumors
Fetal anomalies

inlet or by an incompletely dilated cervix is a potentially dangerous situation that may lead to traumatic and/or hypoxic injury and long-term neurologic sequelae or death. It is more common in the premature infant in whom the trunk is smaller than the head; however, it may also occur in an incomplete (footling) breech if the presenting part(s) and body pass through an incompletely dilated cervix. Obstruction at the pelvic inlet occurs in unrecognized fetopelvic disproportion including hyperextension of the head, hydrocephaly, macrocephaly, or a diencephalic fetus.

The incidence of fetal anomalies in breeches is generally estimated at 6 to 18%.[2, 6, 22, 23] Anomalies occur in the central nervous, genitourinary, skeletal, cardiovascular, gastrointestinal, and respiratory systems and in the chromosomes.[22] Many anomalies themselves are a cause of poor perinatal outcome that would have occurred regardless of the presentation and/or method of delivery.

A major contributing factor to the outcome of breech deliveries is the high incidence of prematurity and the complications thereof, such as hyaline membrane disease, necrotizing enterocolitis, intracranial hemorrhage, and other metabolic problems that may worsen the prognosis.[24] Between 16 and 33% of breeches are delivered before 37 weeks' gestation.[25]

Neurologic injury with or without hypoxia may occur during delivery. Mechanisms of these injuries in a breech include, but are not limited to, excessive longitudinal stretching of the spinal cord, torsional forces, and excessive flexion or extension of the fetal head at the level of the neck.[26] As a result, avulsion of the cervical nerve roots and/or partial or complete transection of the cervical cord, occasionally associated with tears in the dura and epidural hemorrhage, have occurred. These injuries may not be associated with bony trauma or vertebral fractures and most commonly affect the lower cervical region.[27] Even "average" traction or sudden hyperflexion of the head and cervical spine may result in damage to the vulnerable spinal cord.[20] Minor and major neurologic dysfunctions occur more often in the lower birth weight groups,[28] even after congenital anomalies are controlled.

With abnormal fetal heart rate (FHR) patterns at term, breech-presenting fetuses deteriorate more rapidly than vertex fetuses with similar FHR tracings.[29] Another possible mechanism of hypoxic brain injury is decreased blood supply secondary to obstruction of carotid and vertebral arteries.

Maternal risks stem from either vaginal or abdominal route of delivery. During vaginal breech birth, maneuvers used to deliver the infant may result in trauma to maternal soft tissue. These include vaginal tears, bladder or rectal injuries, and cervical lacerations or extensions. The latter may be a result of Dührssen incisions performed for an incompletely dilated cervix to allow the safe delivery of the aftercoming entrapped head. When the birth is cesarean, complications may arise from the procedure per se or from its post-operative course. There is increased blood loss during the surgery and an increased risk of major puerperal morbidity,[30, 31] as well as a longer hospital stay and higher cost.[32] Other sequelae include trauma to surrounding organs and a longer rehabilitation period before the patient can resume a normal lifestyle as compared with that after vaginal delivery. The rate of maternal death related to an abdominal delivery is ten times (0.07 in 1000 vs. 0.078 in 1000) that related to vaginal delivery.[33] In many cases it is the maternal medical/obstetrical complications requiring early delivery, often abdominally, that will increase maternal risks. Gestational age plus maternal/fetal compromise may further increase fetal risks.

MANAGEMENT

In this section, external cephalic version (ECV) is discussed first because of its potential role in decreasing the incidence of breech presentations in labor. Thereafter, the focus of the chapter is on safe vaginal breech delivery.

External Cephalic Version

After being advocated in the days of Hippocrates[34] and then falling into disrepute, the ECV has received renewed interest in the last decade. The purposes of the ECV are to

1. Correct the breech presentation to a vertex,
2. Lower the incidence of breech presentation in labor,
3. Decrease the cesarean section rate, and
4. Decrease the perinatal morbidity that may be associated with a breech vaginal birth.[35]

Because the majority of breech presentations spontaneously convert to vertex as pregnancy progresses and because there are potential complications, some do not favor the procedure.[36, 37] Others believe that in the properly selected patient the ECV is safe and has a role in modern obstetrics.[38–40] The reported success rate is 50 to 70%, with an ultimate (vaginal) delivery rate of 40%;[38, 40] abdominal deliveries are performed for cephalopelvic disproportion, fetal distress, failed progress, etc.

Complications of ECV include transient bradycardia,[41] fetal distress (1 to 2%) due to placental abruption or cord complications, fetomaternal hemorrhage with possible sensitization (1.5%),[42] premature rupture of the membranes and delivery,[43] failure of the procedure, antepartum hemorrhage, prolapsed cord, and, rarely, fetal trauma.

Factors associated with a decreased success rate

Table 19–2. CONTRAINDICATIONS TO EXTERNAL
CEPHALIC VERSION

Maternal
    Medical complications
    Bleeding or predisposing conditions
    Uterine anomalies
    Ruptured membranes
    Tocolytic contraindications
Fetal
    Compromise
    Anomalies
    Multiple gestation
    Growth abnormalities
    Nuchal cord

and increased complications include advanced gestation on initial attempt, repeated attempts, and labor.[44] Cornual implantation may decrease the chances of version.[45] Success appears best with parous patients, normal amniotic fluid volume, and nonfrank breech presentations.[46] Because uterine relaxation facilitates the procedure, some advocate prophylactic tocolysis,[44, 47] although others have not found that it affects the ability to rotate the fetus.[48] The best time to perform the procedure is when the chance of spontaneous rotation is decreasing and when, if a complication were to occur, a near-term neonate could be delivered. Therefore, 37 weeks or later seems ideal. At this time, the rate of success will depend on fetal size and amniotic fluid volume.

At the University of Miami/Jackson Memorial Medical Center, contraindications for ECV include the following (Table 19–2):

1. Maternal factors:
   a) Significant medical complications, e.g., insulin-dependent diabetes mellitus and severe hypertensive disorders.
   b) Vaginal bleeding or conditions predisposing to bleeding, e.g., placenta previa.
   c) Uterine anomalies.
   d) Ruptured membranes.
   e) Maternal contraindications to tocolytics.
2. Fetal factors:
   a) Fetal compromise or placental insufficiency, e.g., nonreactive nonstress test (NST), positive contraction stress test, and unexplained spontaneous decelerations in FHR.
   b) Fetal anomalies.
   c) Multiple gestation.
   d) Significant growth abnormalities: macrosomia and intrauterine growth retardation.
   e) Evident nuchal cord.

The protocol for ECV at the University of Miami/Jackson Memorial Medical Center is as follows:

1. ECV is done on labor and delivery.
2. An informed consent is obtained.
3. NST is reactive.
4. Ultrasonographic evaluation for adequate

fluid volume, confirmation of fetal position, placental location, and absence of a nuchal cord is performed.

5. Tocolysis is optimal but not required. It is started 15 to 20 minutes before the procedure, generally using terbutaline, 0.25 mg subcutaneously.

6. FHR is closely monitored between maneuvers.

7. A senior physician is in attendance, supervising the procedure.

8. Gentleness is essential, no force. Procedure: For the right sacrum position, the lower fetal pole is gently lifted cephalad and rotated laterally to the right, while the head is simultaneously guided to the left in a forward flip. As the breech moves transversely, the head is continuously guided to the left and down until it comes over the inlet (Fig. 19–2).

9. ECV is discontinued if contractions, bradycardia, pain, or resistance is encountered.

10. If patient is at term, and the cervix is favorable, induction is considered. The head is kept over the inlet through several contractions; membranes are ruptured early to facilitate descent.

11. Rh immunoglobulin is administered to candidates. (Some suggest a Kleihauer or similar test to detect whether one ampule is sufficient).

12. An NST is performed at the end of the

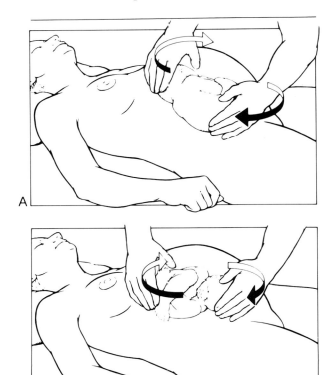

Figure 19–2. A, B, External cephalic version—forward flip. (From Seeds JW: Malpresentations: In Gabbe S, Niebyl JR, Simpson L [eds]: Obstetrics: Normal and Problem Pregnancies, 2nd ed. New York: Churchill Livingstone, 1991, in press.)

procedure. Findings are acted on if they are abnormal; e.g., a biophysical profile/contraction stress test may be done.

13. Instructions and labor precautions are explained to the patient if all tests are normal, and she has no evidence of contractions over the ensuing 20 to 30 minutes.

Cesarean Section or Vaginal Delivery?

Current statistics indicate that the breech presentation contributes to an increase in cesarean section rates. As many as 80 to 90% of all breeches are delivered abdominally.[49] Vaginal delivery was preferred until the late 1950s, when abdominal delivery gradually became more popular with the proclaimed purpose of minimizing perinatal morbidity and mortality.[50–52] This attitude became so widespread that some practitioners indiscriminately advocated cesarean sections for all breech presentations, regardless of the circumstances.[53] As a result, many young obstetricians have not been trained to do vaginal breech deliveries and do not feel competent to manage them, especially in an emergency situation.

Unfortunately, the confounding variables that affect the outcome of breeches were not taken into consideration. Nor was consideration given to the potential role of improvements in total perinatal care that have occurred in the last 25 years. Recent controlled studies[54, 57] have shown that for the appropriately selected patient with a breech presentation, whose delivery is performed by a skilled operator in the absence of contraindications, vaginal delivery of at least the frank breech is as safe as cesarean section.

Premature Breech

Entrapment of the fetal head may occur after passage of the proportionately smaller body through an incompletely dilated cervix. This will cause or aggravate hypoxia and increase intracerebral pressure, which in turn increases the risks of hyaline membrane disease and intracerebral bleeding. Cesarean birth may decrease trauma but will not eliminate it. Because the outcome is affected primarily by birth weight, controlled prospective studies have shown that the outcome of selected breech infants weighing more than 1500 g is not different whether they are delivered vaginally or by cesarean section.[24, 58–61] Infants weighing less than 1500 g appear to do better when delivered abdominally.[23, 54]

Diagnostic Imaging/Pelvimetry

Adequacy of the bony pelvis is a prerequisite for vaginal breech delivery. Accepted x-ray pelvimetry criteria include an inlet anteroposterior diameter of 11 cm, a transverse diameter of 12 cm, and a midpelvic interischial spinous distance of 10 cm.[62, 63] Conventional x-ray pelvimetry used to be the gold standard for assurance of pelvic adequacy. Because of the current trend in obstetric practice toward more liberal use of abdominal delivery, concerns regarding radiation exposure, and the inherent inaccuracies of the technique,[64] the role of conventional x-ray pelvimetry gradually faded, as did the ability of technicians to perform the procedure. Thus followed a rebirth of the technique of clinical pelvimetry to attempt to assess the structure and capacity of the pelvis.

More recently, digital radiography (computerized tomography [CT] scanner) has been used. With technologic improvements and skilled operators, radiography provides many advantages over conventional x-ray imaging. The International Commission on Radiologic Protection has recommended that the fetal radiation dose not exceed 1 rad (1 centiGray [cGy]). The conventional radiologic technique exposed the fetus to an average dose of 900 ± 100 mrads (0.9 ± 0.1 cGy),[65] whereas preliminary data show that the fetal dose for each radiograph by the CT scanner is in the vicinity of 20 mrads (0.02 cGy).[66] It provides accurate measurements at a competitive cost and is considered an improvement over the older techniques of x-ray pelvimetry.[64, 67]

Ultrasonographic evaluation is important in management of the breech birth to estimate fetal weight; to confirm the position of the breech, its type, the attitude of the fetal head, and the presence of nuchal arms; and to diagnose many major fetal anomalies.[68, 69] In our facility, we combine clinical pelvimetry with sonographic findings and follow the guidelines for vaginal delivery of the breech to determine candidates for vaginal delivery.

Guidelines for Vaginal Breech Delivery

The guidelines for vaginal breech delivery at the University of Miami/Jackson Memorial Medical Center are similar to those recommended by the American College of Obstetricians and Gynecologists.[70] They are listed in Table 19–3.

These guidelines take into consideration that we have full-time obstetric anesthesia coverage and an excellent neonatal intensive care unit, as well as the ability to perform a cesarean section within minutes. Because we do not do radiologic pelvimetry, evaluation of the pelvis is totally clinical. Occasionally a flat plate is obtained to confirm the location of the arms and attitude of the head, despite sonography.

It is important to stress that management needs to be individualized. Contraindications for vaginal delivery include those who do not meet the criteria

Table 19–3. GUIDELINES FOR VAGINAL DELIVERY OF THE BREECH INFANT

A. Sonographic* confirmation of
  1. Frank breech
  2. Flexed attitude
  3. No nuchal arms
  4. Estimated fetal weight ($\geq$1250 and $\leq$3750) g
  5. Estimated gestational age (36–42 weeks)
  6. Immature fetus (<24 weeks or <599 g)
  7. Intrauterine fetal death
B. Clinical evaluation for
  1. Adequate pelvis
  2. Progress of labor (Friedman curve)
  3. Absent fetal distress
C. Second twin

*Occasionally x-ray is necessary.

listed in Table 19–3, significant medical complications (moderate to severe hypertensive disorders, history of difficult delivery, and/or damaged infant), rupture of the membranes before labor, or an unengaged breech with meconium. A viable breech-presenting infant with hydrocephaly is delivered by cesarean section to prevent fetal trauma (decompression) and offer the best possible chances for the infant's survival.

Patients who have had a previous low segment transverse cesarean section may be considered for vaginal delivery when the malpresentation is the sole abnormality, the previous cesarean was performed for a nonrecurrent indication, and the patient satisfies all other criteria for a vaginal breech delivery. Using these guidelines, at our institution over the last 2 years (25,499 deliveries) we performed vaginal delivery in 313 (29.7%) of 1053 breech presentations. Fifty percent were at 33 weeks or earlier, 7.4% were at 34 to 36 weeks, and 41.9% were at 37 weeks or later. The majority were assisted (87.5%) or extracted (11.5%) without forceps. Almost invariably the latter were second twins. There was one death at term attributed to a difficult delivery.

Course of Labor

Maternal and fetal well-being is essential in managing the labor and delivery of a breech infant because of the known increased maternal and fetal risks. The course of labor must be normoprogressive, as measured by cervical dilatation and descent using the Friedman curve. The role of pitocin augmentation in a dysfunctional pattern is not a settled issue. Simple logic dictates that if labor is allowed, there is no real contraindication to pitocin in a dysfunctional pattern after dystocia is excluded. Continuous FHR electronic monitoring is interpreted with the same criteria as in a vertex to ensure fetal well-being. Because of the risk of cord prolapse and because they act as a good dilating wedge, membranes are not operatively

ruptured. However, when assessment indicates the necessity for intrauterine monitoring then amniotomy is performed. During the course of labor, variable (cord compression) decelerations may indicate cord prolapse; hence a pelvic examination is indicated if decelerations develop. As the breech-presenting infant descends through the birth canal, pressure on the fetal abdomen at the level of cord insertion may result in variable decelerations with contractions. Determination of fetal pH can be done by the usual technique, using the fetal buttocks. Meconium before the infant is in the pelvis should be considered a sign of fetal stress and is not "normal."

Anesthesia

Analgesia/anesthesia management is of paramount importance in breech presentations. Preoperative or early labor maternal assessment by anesthesia is necessary to plan management, because there is always the possibility of general anesthesia and/or a difficult intubation. Adequate oxygenation and optimal blood perfusion are needed for all obstetrical procedures, and more so with breech fetuses because they may deteriorate more rapidly than vertex fetuses.[29] Continuous communication between the obstetrician and anesthesiologist is essential during delivery to optimize outcome. Each must understand the other's problems and needs, especially during the actual delivery. Because of the possible hemodynamic side effects of β-adrenergic agents and the neuromuscular junction blockade of magnesium sulfate, it is important to inform the anesthesiologist of tocolytic therapies given to the patient, because these may affect the effects of anesthetic agents on the mother or fetus. Adequate analgesia and uterine relaxation when necessary for controlled delivery or intrauterine maneuvers will minimize the likelihood of birth trauma.

For vaginal delivery, the combination of narcotics for labor and local/pudendal anesthesia for delivery is often used. If there is neonatal depression secondary to the narcotics, this can be reversed with naloxone hydrochloride (Narcan). Ketamine, a potent intravenous analgesic with hallucinogenic and amnesic effects, may produce adequate perineal relaxation. However, it may result in neonatal depression when doses exceed 1 mg/kg,[71] and, of equal importance, it prevents effective maternal cooperation. Nitrous oxide or methoxyflurane can provide adequate analgesia for some patients. Uterine relaxation, when needed for intrauterine manipulation, can be achieved by halothane or small doses of intravenous nitroglycerine.[72] Spinal analgesia/anesthesia is rarely used in vaginal breech deliveries because it may interfere with the course of labor. Epidural anesthesia, given after the establishment of active labor with low (0.125 to 0.25%) concentrations of bupivacaine, does not interfere with labor and enables the mother to push effectively during the second stage of labor.[71] The recent use of anesthetic drugs resulting in less motor blockade may prove better for management in the second stage. However, these drugs will not eliminate the need for general anesthesia when intrauterine manipulation requires uterine muscle relaxation. In the absence of hypotension, epidural anesthesia is safe and has minimal complications. In the past, epidural anesthesia has been associated with an increase in the incidence of operative intervention,[73, 74] without fetal acidemia.[75] However, with the aforementioned advances in anesthetic techniques, operative intervention may be less. Indeed, epidural anesthesia (or at least placement of the catheter) is ideal, because if cesarean section is necessary the level of anesthesia can be easily adjusted.[76] Pumps allowing small-dose continuous analgesia (bupivacaine/fentanyl) make it possible to tailor the epidural analgesic technique to the specific patient's needs, labor course, and delivery.[77] Both techniques—repeated boluses and continuous infusions—are currently used on our service.

MECHANISMS OF DELIVERY

The methods of delivery for a breech include the following:

1. *Spontaneous:* The entire delivery occurs without assistance other than support of the body. This is a very rare event today.

2. *Assisted breech delivery or partial breech extraction:* The delivery occurs naturally without assistance to the umbilicus; thereafter delivery and/or extraction of the arms, shoulder, and head is assisted with or without forceps to the aftercoming head. This is the most common of vaginal breech deliveries.

3. *Total breech extraction:* The entire body is extracted with or without forceps, or delivery is assisted before birth of the umbilicus. Total breech extraction occurs most commonly in the second twin.

4. *Cesarean section:* Total breech extraction is carried out abdominally. In modern obstetrics, this is the most common method of delivery.

Spontaneous Breech Delivery

The spontaneous method of breech delivery is described first to help the reader understand the mechanisms of delivery. The most crucial time begins with descent in the second stage and ends with complete delivery of the infant.

When the sacrum reaches the pelvic floor, the umbilicus is entering the inlet (Fig. 19–3). This

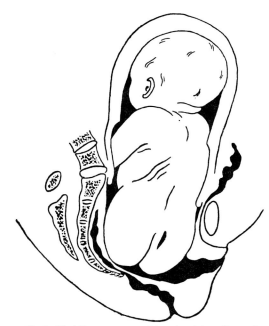

Figure 19–3. Umbilicus approaching the inlet. (From Beck AC, Rosenthal AH: Obstetrics Practice. London: Bailliere Tindall and Cassell, 6th ed, 1955, p. 477.)

may be accompanied by cord compression, which will be reflected by the FHR, and changes in oxygenation, manifested by decreasing fetal P_{O_2}, increasing P_{CO_2}, and progressive respiratory acidosis. Compression may progressively increase with delivery of the buttocks, shoulders, and head. At the same time, the space occupied by the placenta on the uterine wall decreases and early separation may occur, which will also affect gas exchange. If compression is prolonged, then significant metabolic acidosis will ensue. Therefore FHR monitoring is an essential component to management.

Equally important are a calm, comfortable, cooperative patient; a level-headed experienced physician conducting her delivery; an anesthesiologist prepared to manage her anesthesia; a pediatrician/ neonatologist for the newborn; an additional obstetrician to assist the delivery; and finally, but by no means least, an experienced obstetrical nurse. All equipment for neonatal resuscitation and general anesthesia should be in the room. On the delivery set, or easily available, should be the Piper forceps, two deep right-angle retractors, and at least four ring forceps.

At what point the patient should be moved to the delivery room varies, depending on her progress in labor, parity, and overall hospital practice. Generally, the nullipara should be moved as the baby is on the perineal floor, and the multipara by at least 8 to 9 cm cervical dilatation unless she is moving very quickly, in which case earlier will be better as long as the FHR is monitored. Once the patient is being moved, all previously mentioned personnel should be mobilized to the delivery room.

If the patient has had an epidural anesthesia, the perineal dose can be given if desired before moving her, or a pudendal block may be placed in the delivery room after the patient is prepared and draped. Certainly in a nullipara, and we believe also in a multipara, a generous episiotomy is desirable. This will give space for insertion of the operator's hand for manipulation of the arms should it become necessary, delivery of the shoulders through the outlet, and delivery of the aftercoming head. It will also allow for aspiration of the mouth and nasal passages if necessary before delivery of the head. The episiotomy is best performed in a frank breech presentation when the posterior buttock is presenting at the introitus. In a total breech extraction, the episiotomy is likely necessary before insertion of the operator's hand, and in the incomplete breech it is usually necessary when there is sufficient perineal distension or the buttocks are presenting. The choice of episiotomy is up to the individual preference of the physician and the size of the perineal body.

With the sacrum generally in a transverse position, and the intertrochanteric diameter occupying the anteroposterior diameter of the pelvis, the posterior buttock is born first, by lateral flexion of the infant's body. The anterior buttock is then born (Fig. 19–4). As the shoulders enter the inlet, the sacrum rotates 45 degrees anteriorly, reflecting the bisacromial diameter entering the inlet (engaging) in the oblique diameter (Fig. 19–5). The shoulders generally descend through the midpelvis in the oblique diameter, and as they reach the perineal floor rotation occurs so that the bisacromial diameter is anteroposterior and externally the sacrum is transverse (Fig. 19–6). The anterior shoulder impinges on the symphysis pubis, and the posterior shoulder and arm deliver first, again by lateral flexion of the infant's body followed by the anterior shoulder and arm. During the delivery, the fundus of the uterus is closely applied to the head, maintaining its flexion. The head engages in the oblique or transverse diameter of the

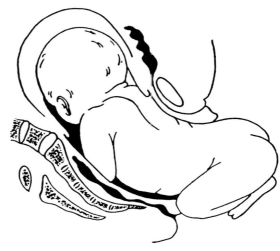

Figure 19–5. Shoulders entering the inlet in the oblique position. (From Beck AC, Rosenthal AH: Obstetrics Practice. London: Bailliere Tindall and Cassell, 6th ed, 1955, p. 479.)

inlet, usually with the occiput anterior or transverse (Fig. 19–7). The weight of the baby assists further descent through the midpelvis. The flexed head, face, and forehead fill the sacral curve as rotation occurs to the occiput anterior position (Fig. 19–8). Spontaneous delivery of the head occurs by flexion with the nape of the neck as the fulcrum under the symphysis (Fig. 19–9). The face is born first, followed by the forehead and the occiput.

In modern, in-hospital obstetrics, spontaneous delivery rarely occurs, but should be fully understood by anyone performing a breech delivery. By following the mechanism of the normal spontaneous breech delivery as previously described, the operator can minimize maneuvers and lessen risks during an assisted delivery or a total breech ex-

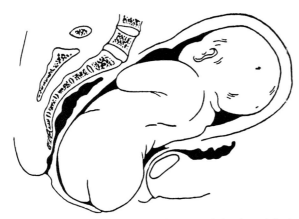

Figure 19–4. Delivery of the anterior buttock by lateral flexion. (From Beck AC, Rosenthal AH: Obstetrics Practice. London: Bailliere Tindall and Cassell, 6th ed, 1955, p. 478.)

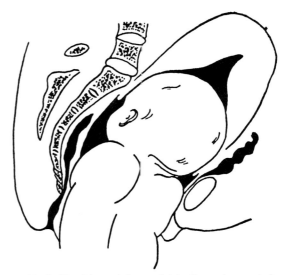

Figure 19–6. Shoulders at the outlet in the anteroposterior diameter. (From Beck AC, Rosenthal AH: Obstetrics Practice. London: Bailliere Tindall and Cassell, 6th ed, 1955, p. 480.)

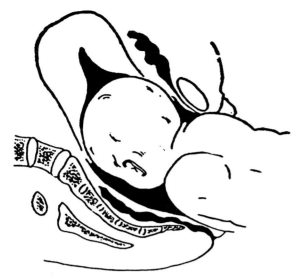

Figure 19–7. Head engages in the oblique position. (From Beck AC, Rosenthal AH: Obstetrics Practice. London: Bailliere Tindall and Cassell, 6th ed, 1955, p. 481.)

traction in most cases. The same principles also apply during cesarean extraction.

Assisted Breech Delivery

In the assisted breech delivery, the infant is allowed to deliver to the umbilicus spontaneously. Although it is most tempting to interfere earlier, it is wise to "keep your hands off." Some advocate gentle traction on the cord at delivery of the umbilicus to decrease stretching and pressure on the cord.[9, 78] Because compression of the cord is almost complete during delivery of the shoulders and head, decreasing this by loosening the cord is unlikely (Fig. 19–10). In fact, pulling down on the cord may tighten a loop around the arm, neck, etc. As mentioned earlier, not only may progressive

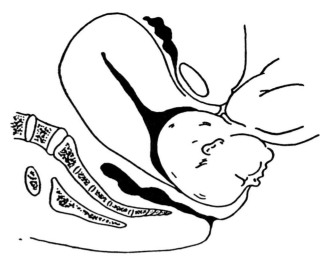

Figure 19–9. Delivery of the head by flexion. (From Beck AC, Rosenthal AH: Obstetrics Practice. London: Bailliere Tindall and Cassell, 6th ed, 1955, p. 483.)

fetal asphyxia develop because of cord compression by the shoulders and head, but placental separation may occur during delivery.[79] Delivery must be gentle—undue rushing or excitement invites fetal trauma. Therefore, clock watching from time of delivery of the umbilicus may be useful, because up to 4 minutes until complete delivery has been associated with 5-minute Apgar scores of 7 or higher.[80]

If the legs do not deliver spontaneously once the umbilicus is delivered, their delivery can be assisted using the Pinard maneuver. A finger is placed on the medial aspect of, and parallel to, the femur. The femur is rotated laterally on the infant's abdomen so the knee will bend, and the foot will fall against the back of the operator's hand, where the ankle can be grasped and the leg extended. If the sacrum is on the right, the operator's right hand would release the baby's right (or an-

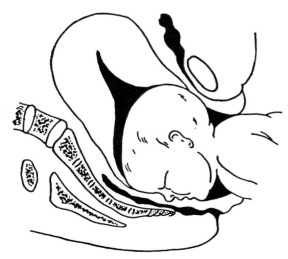

Figure 19–8. Rotation to the occiput anterior position. (From Beck AC, Rosenthal AH: Obstetrics Practice. London: Bailliere Tindall and Cassell, 6th ed, 1955, p. 482.)

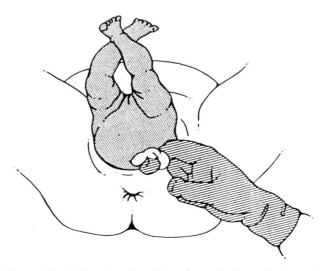

Figure 19–10. Cord traction. (From Oxorn H: Human Labor and Birth. Norwalk, CT: Appleton Century Crofts, 5th ed, 1986, p 251.)

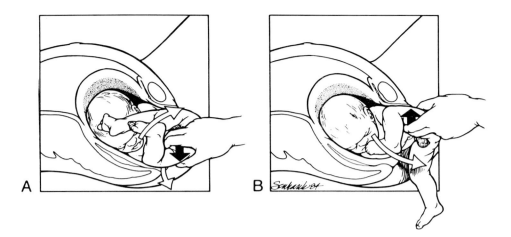

Figure 19–11. *A, B,* Pinard maneuver—lower extremities. (From Seeds JW: Malpresentations: In Gabbe S, Niebyl JR, Simpson L [eds]: Obstetrics: Normal and Problem Pregnancies, 2nd ed. New York: Churchill Livingstone, 1991, in press.)

terior) leg, which is on the left side of the mother, and vice versa (Fig. 19–11). The sacrum is usually to the right or left of the midline as the shoulders are descending through the inlet and midpelvis in the oblique diameter.

A towel may then be wrapped around the lower body. Both thumbs of the operator are placed on the sacroiliac synchondroses, and the fingers encircle the iliac crests and thighs of the infant (Fig. 19–12). Gentle steady downward traction, ideally with a contraction, is applied until the axilla is seen beneath the symphysis. Several maneuvers may be used to deliver the shoulders:

1. Either shoulder can be delivered by the operator's placing two fingers against the baby's back (e.g., for the right sacrum transverse, the left hand) across the shoulder parallel to the humerus, down to the elbow which is rotated laterally toward the infant's side, allowing the elbow to flex and the hand to drop out (Fig. 19–13). For delivery of the posterior arm, the infant's body is gently lifted up and toward the opposite maternal groin (flexed laterally). For the anterior shoulder, the infant is laterally flexed toward the floor. Care must be taken not to stretch the brachial plexus during lateral flexion (Fig. 19–14).

2. Once the axilla is seen, the lateroinferior border of the infant's scapula can be pushed up and posteriorly toward the infant's vertebrae, allowing the arms and shoulders to rotate across the chest and drop out (the Bickers maneuver; Fig. 19–15).

3. The procedures described in either 1 or 2 can be used to deliver the anterior shoulder, after which the infant is then rotated 180 degrees, bringing the posterior shoulder anteriorly and delivering it in a likewise manner.

4. If either arm is nuchal or raised above the head, rotation of the infant toward the direction of the fetal hand allows the resistance of the birth canal tissues to push the hand so it will move anteriorly, where it can be released. In a right sacrum anterior, if the right arm is nuchal, the

body should be rotated counterclockwise (Fig. 19–16).

5. The posterior shoulder can be rotated 180 to 210 degrees to become the anterior shoulder in a clockwise direction if the sacrum is on the left and counterclockwise if it is on the right. The shoulder is delivered spontaneously by this maneuver, which is repeated to allow delivery of the opposite shoulder. A modification of this Lövset maneuver

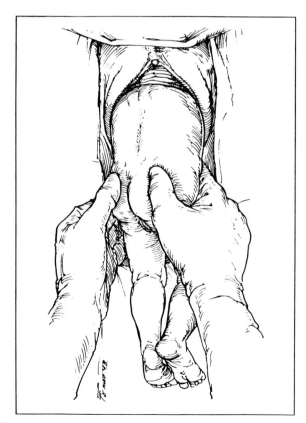

Figure 19–12. Placement of the fingers during extraction; a towel around the body prevents fingers from slipping. (From Cunningham FG, MacDonald PC, Grant NF (eds): Williams Obstetrics. Norwalk, CT: Appleton Lange, 18th ed, 1989, p 395.)

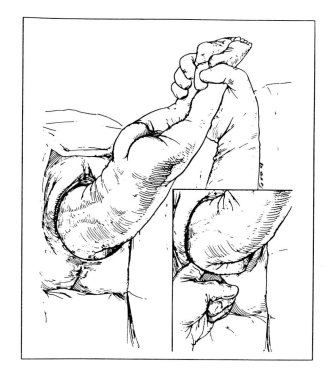

Figure 19–13. Upward traction to deliver the posterior shoulder and arm *(insert)*. (From Cunningham FG, MacDonald PC, Grant NF (eds): Williams Obstetrics. Norwalk, CT: Appleton Lange, 18th ed, 1989, p 396.)

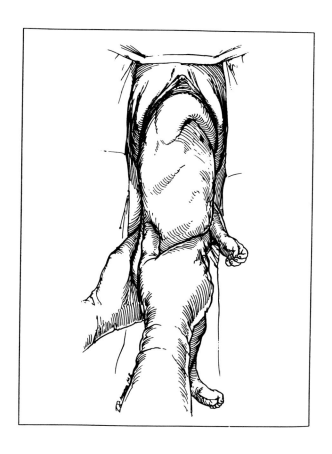

Figure 19–14. Downward traction to deliver the anterior arm and shoulder. (From Cunningham FG, MacDonald PC, Grant NF (eds): Williams Obstetrics. Norwalk, CT: Appleton Lange, 18th ed, 1989, p 396.)

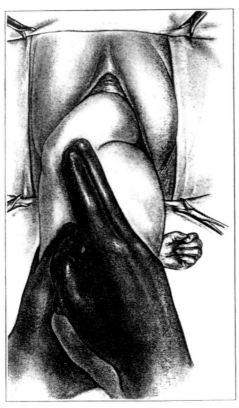

Figure 19—15. Delivery of the anterior shoulder by rotating the scapula posteriorly.

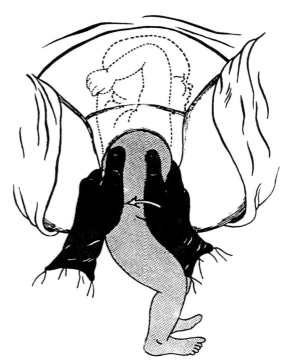

Figure 19—16. Rotation of the body toward the fetal hand to release a nuchal arm. (From Beck AC, Rosenthal AH: Obstetrics Practice. London: Bailliere Tincall and Cassell, 6th ed, 1955, p 499.)

is to deliver the anterior shoulder first and then rotate the posterior shoulder anteriorly, allowing the spontaneous or assisted delivery of the arms.

6. Occasionally, in order to release a nuchal arm, the infant has to be pushed upward into the uterus. The operator's hand is inserted into the uterine cavity to splint the humerus while rotating the arm across the head. As the arm descends, the operator exerts pressure in the antecubital space, which will help flex the elbow (Fig. 19–17). The hand should drop down and can be grasped and gently extracted.

Once the head has descended to the pelvic floor, delivery can be accomplished, generally easily, by flexion of the head assisted by the Mauriceau-Smellie-Viet maneuver. First described in the seventeenth century, this maneuver has stood the test of time. Before proceeding, if the mouth can be visualized by pressure on the perineum, it may be aspirated. Thereafter, the infant's body is supported by the assistant with a towel and held so that the body is only slightly elevated above the outlet. Overextension can result in cervical spinal cord injury and/or transection. Alternatively, the body may rest on the inferior arm of the operator, which will be used to reach the baby's face (Fig. 19–18). Two fingers, usually the index and third,

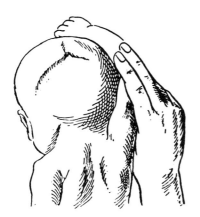
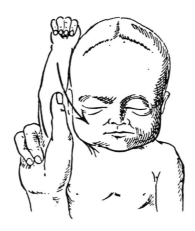

Figure 19—17. Graphic demonstration: displacing and flexing a raised fetal arm. (From Webster CJ: Textbook of Obstetrics. Philadelphia, WB Saunders, 1903, p 511.)

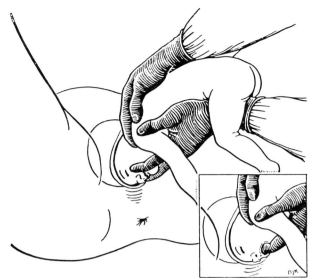

Figure 19–18. The Mauriceau-Smellie-Viet maneuver for delivering the head. (From Chassar Moir J, Myerscough PR: Munro Kerr's Operative Obstetrics. Baltimore: Williams & Wilkins, 8th ed, 1971, p 170.)

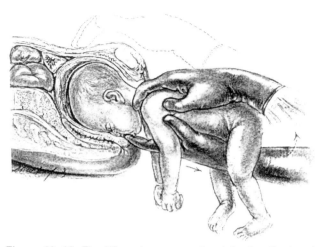

Figure 19–19. The Wigand maneuver for delivering the head. (From Titus P: The Management of Obstetrics Difficulties, 4th ed. St. Louis: CV Mosby, 1950, p 725.)

are placed on the malar eminences of the infant, or, as originally described, two fingers are inserted into the mouth. If the head is not in the midline, it can be rotated using the fingers in the mouth or along the malar region. The index and fourth fingers of the opposite hand are placed on either shoulder. The third finger may be pressed against the occiput to aid in flexion and act as a splint for the neck, preventing hyperextension and potential cervical spine injury. The head is then flexed and the body and head lifted out. Although it is ideal to use the malar eminences to aid flexion, it is easier to flex using the fetal mouth. Subluxation of the mandible and trauma to the floor of the mouth may occur. Counterpressure with the thumb against the chin may reduce these risks. When using the malar eminences, the operator should take care to avoid the orbital ridges. An alternative, the Wigand maneuver, involves suprapubic pressure applied by one hand of the operator or by an assistant to aid in descent of the head while the internal hand is in the infant's mouth to assist flexion of the head and direct the down, out, up maneuver for delivery of the head by flexion (Fig. 19–19).

The role of fundal suprapubic pressure is debated. As long as the delivery is slow and gentle, the fundus will stay applied to the head, keeping it flexed. Fundal pressure can cause head trauma and therefore should be gentle if used.

Although not commonly used in the United States, the Bracht maneuver is an alternative method of vaginal breech delivery.[9] The baby is allowed to deliver spontaneously to the umbilicus. With the back up, the baby is grasped in such a way that the operator's fingers encircle the buttocks and the thumbs are placed over the ischial

tuberosities. The thenar eminences of the operator exert gentle pressure against the femurs to extend the spine of the baby against the symphysis pubis. This maintains the hips in flexion and knees in extension. The shoulders deliver in the transverse position spontaneously. Maternal expulsive efforts during uterine contractions combined with suprapubic pressure by an assistant allow the head to deliver spontaneously along its axis, while at the same time there is no hyperextension of the neck but the spine itself is hyperextended (Figs. 19–20 and 19–21). The head can deliver without suprapubic pressure also (Burns-Marshall maneuver).

Forceps to the Aftercoming Head

In most cases, the Mauriceau-Smellie-Viet maneuver is used to assist delivery of the head in a controlled fashion to prevent intracerebral bleeding that may be precipitated by trauma from fundal pressure. Piper forceps are also used. Designed specifically for the aftercoming head, they have longer shanks than other forceps and lack a pelvic curve (Fig. 19–22). They should always be

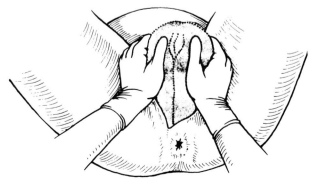

Figure 19–20. The Bracht maneuver—placement of the hands.

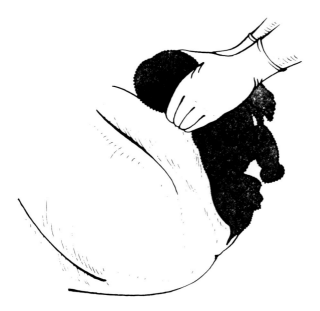

Figure 19–21. The Bracht maneuver—delivery of the body and head.

in the room, if not on the table. As in all forceps deliveries, the head should be in the pelvis and there should be adequate anesthesia—either a regional block or general anesthesia. If the operator is lifting only the head out, then a pudendal anesthesia is sufficient. To apply the forceps, not only should the operator be kneeling, but the body of the baby should be elevated slightly above the horizontal with the assistant taking care not to hyperextend the neck, which would cause either transection of the cervical cord or cord damage.

With the vertex anterior, the operator introduces the left blade laterally and slightly upward along the mento-occipital line of the fetal head, keeping the handle of the blade below the level of the perineum (Fig. 19–23A). The right blade is introduced similarly, taking care that there is no palpable cervix (Fig. 19–23B). Once applied satisfactorily, the blades are locked. In order to prevent hyperextension of the neck, the infant's body should rest on the shank of the forceps (Fig. 19–23C) or be held in a towel by an assistant so that the body and arms are slightly above the forceps

(Fig. 19–24). The head is extracted by flexion using continued downward traction on the forceps until the chin appears; traction is then outward and the handles of the forceps are elevated so that delivery is by flexion of the head.

Although the Piper forceps were traditionally used for the difficult delivery of the aftercoming head, Milner[81] demonstrated that prophylactic (elective) use decreased the mortality rate of vaginally delivered breech infants by 50%. This benefit was seen in all weight groups. The advantage of the forceps over the Mauriceau-Smellie-Viet maneuver is that traction is on the head, whereas the latter maneuver places traction on the axial skeleton, increasing the risks of trauma to structures in the neck and cervical spine, e.g., brachial plexus, muscles, jaw, and floor of the mouth.

Total Breech Extraction

Because we have already described the method of spontaneous and assisted breech delivery, this

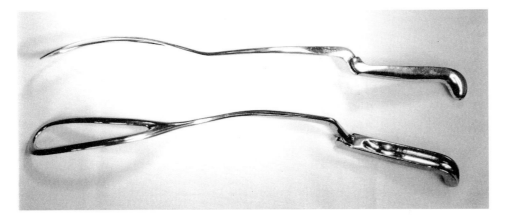

Figure 19–22. Piper forceps (cephalic curve above, absent pelvic curve below).

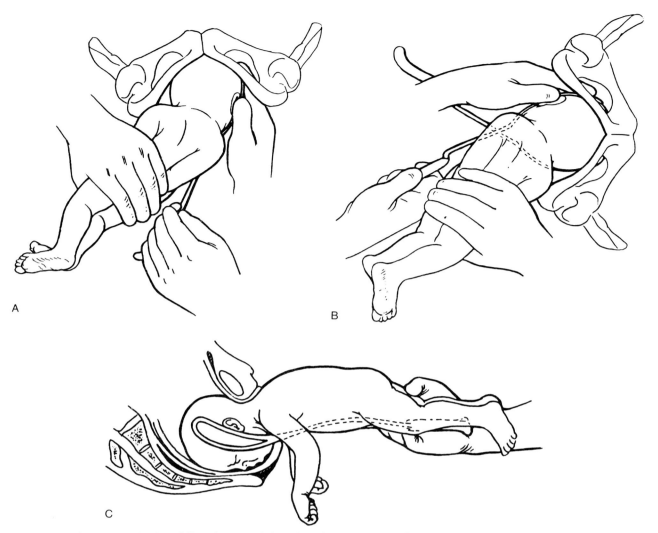

Figure 19–23. Graphic application of Piper forceps. *A,* Insertion of the right blade. *B,* Insertion of the left blade. *C,* Infant straddling the forceps. (From Dennen PC: Dennen's Forceps Deliveries. 3rd ed, Philadelphia, FA Davis, 1989.)

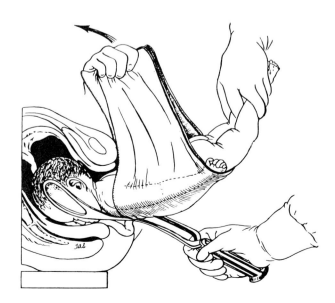

Figure 19–24. Piper forceps applied—infant's body supported by a towel for extraction of the head.

section describes the maneuvers used to "break up the breech" when it is in a frank presentation or there are other complications associated with extraction. Indications for total breech extraction in obstetric practice today include delivery of the second twin with fetal distress, where vaginal delivery may be accomplished more rapidly and as safely as a cesarean section; for the elective rapid delivery of the second twin; or as part of the procedure of version and extraction. It is rarely, if ever, indicated in a singleton breech delivery in American medicine. However, circumstances may be such that one is left with no real choice, e.g., prolapsed cord, fetal distress, or a fully dilated cervix where cesarean section might not be accomplished in enough time. In Third World countries facilities are limited, and singleton total breech extractions are performed where indicated because cesarean delivery may be more hazardous.

Procedures used for extraction of the lower extremities depend on whether the presentation is frank, complete, or incomplete. Adequate analgesia/anesthesia (epidural, spinal, or general) is essential unless one is dealing with a double-footling breech. If the feet are through the introitus, then a pudendal or local anesthesia may be sufficient,

but general may be necessary. Therefore, anesthesia personnel should be in the room ready to "crash" the patient. In the double footling, both feet should be grasped and brought down usually using the hand that is on the same side as the fetal back (for left sacrum transverse, the right hand is used). With a frank breech, the operator's hand facing the fetal abdomen is introduced to the anterior buttock and follows the thigh to the popliteal space. The fingers of the operator's hand are aligned parallel to the femur on its medial side, gently rotating the femur laterally against the fetal abdomen toward the fetal spine. This encourages flexion of the knee, by allowing the foot to fall against the posterior aspect of the operator's hand. The operator then keeps the index finger in the popliteal fossa and encircles the lower half of the leg, aiding flexion (the Pinard maneuver) and following the leg to the foot, which is grasped (Fig. 19–25) and gently extracted. In order to do this safely, the breech must be above the pelvic brim and there must be good uterine relaxations. The anterior leg is chosen because it will allow the back to remain anterior. If one cannot flex the anterior leg, then the posterior one can be flexed. As the posterior leg is brought down, the abdomen

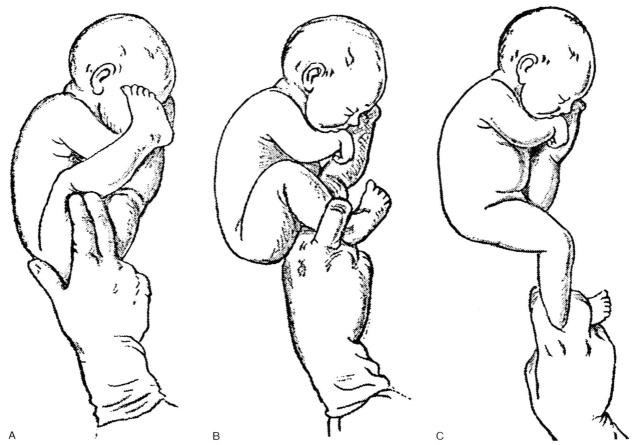

Figure 19–25. Pinard maneuver. *A,* Lateral rotation. *B,* Knee flexion. *C,* Extension of the hip and knee. (From Beck AC, Rosenthal AH: Obstetrics Practice. London: Bailliere Tindall and Cassell, 6th ed, 1955, p 500.)

may rotate anteriorly and/or the anterior buttock may get caught on the maternal symphysis pubis. Should this happen, a hand is inserted up to the anterior buttock, rotating it toward the fetal abdomen, i.e., to the right if the legs were on the right initially. An attempt should be made after rotation to extract the remaining leg. With continuous slow downward traction, the remainder of the delivery is conducted as an assisted breech extraction.

During any breech delivery, malposition of the arms may occur. The decision to attempt a vaginal versus an abdominal delivery should be based on clinical and/or x-ray pelvimetry, sonography to assess for anomalies, fetal weight, attitude of the head, and type of breech. In our opinion, it is wise to also assess the location of the upper extremities. Where one is raised to at least the level of the face, we do not electively attempt vaginal delivery because of the possible development of a nuchal arm with descent. Nonetheless, with the best planning, delivery may occur to the umbilicus or inferior scapula, after which the breech seems to resist further descent (Fig. 19–26). A nuchal arm is a definite possibility. Some factors that may contribute to a nuchal arm and/or further impede descent include an incompletely dilated cervix, extraction too early or too rapidly, a constriction ring, cephalopelvic disproportion (weight/hydrocephaly), or a deflexed head. Management demands accurate diagnosis as well as gentleness and care so as not

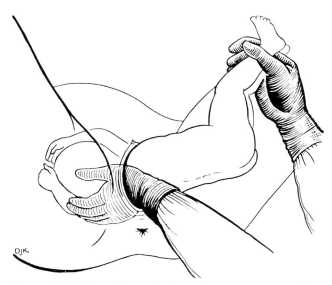

Figure 19–27. Internal examination to locate upper extremities. (From Chassar Moir J, Myerscough PR: Munro Kerr's Operative Obstetrics. Baltimore: Williams & Wilkins, 8th ed, 1971, p 162.)

to compound the problem by causing significant fetal trauma. Yet time is marching on. Delivery needs to be accomplished quickly because there is cord compression with its resultant hypoxic effects. While preparations are well underway for an emergency cesarean delivery, the operator may proceed to attempt vaginal delivery. He or she should examine the patient under general anesthesia if an epidural or spinal anesthesia is not already in place or there is insufficient uterine relaxation necessary for the intrauterine manipulation that will likely be required. If the cervix is fully dilated, the operator should introduce the hand facing the baby's back. The head and arms are usually above the brim (Fig. 19–27). The operator should gently push the body up a few inches and reach inside the uterus to the fetal arms to ascertain the problem. If one arm is not nuchal and can be easily delivered, this should be done to increase space. The arm should be followed upward with the examination fingers parallel to the humerus and the Pinard maneuver performed to deliver the arm. If the arms are high, using the hand facing the baby's abdomen may achieve easier access to the arm. When this does not or cannot work because of lack of space or because the arm is flexed behind the head, slow rotation of the body with the operator's hands on the thorax, in a direction opposite to the elbow toward the fetal hand, encourages the elbow as it meets the resistance of the maternal tissues during rotation to slip down, and the arm and hand follow (Fig. 19–16). Rotation may cause twisting of the neck and stretching of the brachial plexus, resulting in Erb's palsy.

A constriction ring as a cause of lack of descent is unlikely if labor was not protracted. Deep general anesthesia should relax this. Likewise, unless

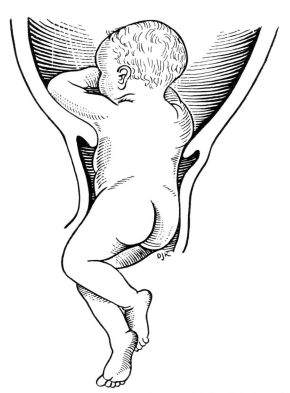

Figure 19–26. Raised arms and incompletely dilated cervix. (From Chassar Moir J, Myerscough PR: Munro Kerr's Operative Obstetrics. Baltimore: Williams & Wilkins, 8th ed, 1971, p 161.)

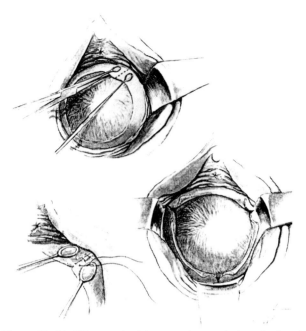

Figure 19–28. Dührssen incisions can be used when the head is trapped by an incompletely dilated cervix. *Top left,* cervix visualized at 2 o'clock for initial incision; *middle right,* first incision made; *bottom left,* repair.

the baby is small or presentation is an incomplete breech, an incompletely dilated cervix is unlikely.

If the cervix has trapped the head and the infant is alive, Duhrssen incisions may be performed to facilitate delivery. Adequate visualization using two deep right-angle retractors inserted into the vagina anteriorly is required to expose the cervix at 10 and 2 o'clock. Two ring forceps then grasp the cervix and pull it down slightly; incisions are made with a scissor to the depth of 1 to 2 cm. A third incision may be necessary at 6 o'clock (Fig. 19–28). Care must be taken not to hyperextend the fetal neck. Usually, two incisions are sufficient. Complications include extension of the incisions, uterine vessel lacerations, urethral or ureteral injury, and entry into the cul-de-sac/rectum. These are avoided by adequate visualization, at least two incisions, and gentle extraction of the head. After delivery, the incisions are repaired using usually interrupted chromic suture; the first stitch is placed above the apex.

Malposition of the head can occur when there have been multiple rotations of the body during delivery, when the head was initially malrotated in utero, or when descent occurred with the sacrum posterior. When the head is stuck and the back is anterior, a diagnosis is made by inserting a hand into the uterus alongside the fetal head to determine the location of the chin/face. If caught on the maternal symphysis, upward dislodgment will free it, and rotation of the chin posteriorly can be accomplished by gentle pressure of the operator's internal hand against the face or chin or by a

finger in the infant's mouth (Fig. 19–29). Flexion, descent, and delivery can be accomplished using the Mauriceau-Smellie-Viet maneuver or by Piper forceps once the head is in the pelvis. Forceps should not be applied in an unengaged head because this will only increase both maternal and fetal trauma. Should the shoulders be born with the back posterior, the occiput is posterior, with the chin facing the symphysis pubis. There are two options. First, the operator can rotate the body externally while *simultaneously* internally rotating the head. External rotation of the body alone will twist the neck and cause significant stretching of the brachial plexus and rotational injury to the cervical spine. If the head cannot be rotated with the body, then the operator can put one finger in the infant's mouth and place the fingers of the other hand on the infant's shoulders. The baby is pulled down posteriorly toward the floor, causing descent of the head to the perineum until the chin is under the inferior rim of the symphysis. The chin now acts as a fulcrum against the symphysis. With continued shoulder traction, and raising the infant's body anteriorly onto the maternal abdomen, the neck is flexed to allow the head to deliver by flexion (the Prague maneuver; Fig. 19–30).

With careful evaluation clinically, sonographically, and by x-ray where indicated; strict adherence to the guidelines for breech delivery; careful

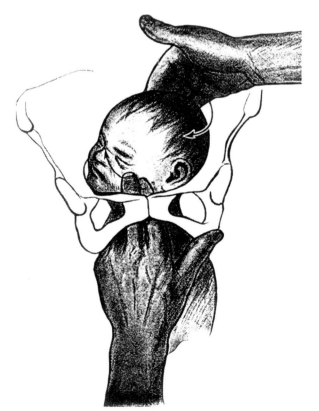

Figure 19–29. Rotation of the head off the symphysis pubis— here, a combined procedure is shown. (From Greenhill JP: Obstetrics. Philadelphia: WB Saunders, 12th ed, 1960, p 958.)

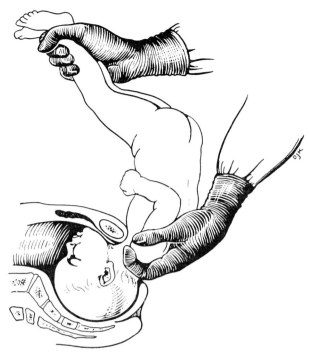

Figure 19–30. The Prague maneuver to deliver the head when the occiput is posterior.

assessment of the adequate progress of labor; and strict attention to management of the delivery itself, an operator rarely should encounter significant difficulty.

Cesarean section does not eliminate risks or trauma completely; although they are less for the fetus, there is a significant increase in maternal morbidity and mortality. The abdominal breech delivery is conducted as a total breech extraction, following the same maneuvers as for a vaginal delivery.

The Stat Breech

The patient who enters labor and delivery with a breech baby about to deliver (i.e., buttocks crowning or legs through the introitus) requires rapid mobilization of forces for delivery and a rapid survey of fetal status. To be notified and present urgently, in addition to anesthesia personnel, are an additional obstetrician, nursing assistance, and a pediatrician. If there is any chance whatsoever, a quick sonogram to determine the presence of a head, its attitude, and possible hydrocephaly is ideal because it would help in managing the delivery. How much can actually be accomplished and how rapidly everything will progress depend on the rate of descent of the fetus (i.e., how active the labor is), the FHR, the speed with which an abdominal delivery can be prepared, the experience of the obstetrician, and the ability to assess the attitude and normality of the fetus.

If delivery is already well on its way (i.e., the buttocks are born), the operator can proceed with a vaginal delivery unless there is definite evidence of a deflexed head or hydrocephaly and a chance of abdominal delivery. In many facilities in the United States, a cesarean section would not be a viable option at this point. In addition, the cord may be undergoing compression because the umbilicus is through the inlet. Ideally, the patient should be on a delivery table, where the anesthesiologist, if available, could be preparing her for general anesthesia if necessary, while the delivery was continuing. The lithotomy position is essential if at all possible. If the patient is on a bed or stretcher that will not allow this, she should lie across the bed or stretcher and have someone support her legs. Although it is often not the case, the obstetrician should at least try to remain as calm as possible while instructing the patient. Many maneuvers previously described may be necessary to accomplish delivery. If the fetus is dead, there is no risk of further fetal trauma, and concern is totally maternal. If the patient presented with a prolapsed cord and a FHR of 60 or lower, the fetus has probably already sustained significant hypoxia such that heroism may be unwarranted, and again concerns should be maternal. Finally, if the gestational age is less than 26 weeks or 600 g, even in a tertiary facility the survival rate is low. The patient's risks should be weighed against the minimal fetal benefit of aggressive management. Especially when the infant is premature, the cervix may not be completely dilated and the head may be entrapped. For this, general anesthesia and Duhrssen incisions may be warranted where the fetus has a reasonable chance of survival and facilities are available.

Although it should not happen in modern obstetrics because candidates for breech delivery are carefully screened, the management of the previously unrecognized trapped hydrocephalic head of the breech infant should be mentioned. If there is a concomitant meningocele, the membrane can be perforated and fluid drained. Additional methods for draining spinal fluid include insertion of a large-bore needle into the base of the fetal skull; separation, using sharp scissors, of the cervical vertebrae and exposure of the spinal canal; or introduction of a sharp large-bore needle suprapubically directly into the fetal head through the maternal abdominal wall, preferably under general anesthesia. In most cases, sufficient time may have passed that a live-born child is unlikely, because of severe metabolic acidosis that has developed because of prolonged cord compression and/or collapse of the skull. If abdominal delivery is required, it should be done under controlled circumstances, to do no more harm. Rushing will accomplish nothing but result in significant maternal trauma.

If the patient arrives in very active labor, and

on examination the cervix is fully dilated with a breech at 0 station or greater, but she is not delivering or the feet are presenting but the buttocks are still quite high, one can stop or slow contractions with a tocolytic while fetal and maternal assessment is carried out and forces are mobilized. Even in the presence of fetal distress, decreasing the frequency of contractions may be of fetal benefit. This will give everyone the opportunity to approach delivery more calmly and select the method that is in the best interests of the mother and infant. When the infant is already delivering, it is generally wiser to proceed with vaginal delivery, because the cord is already compressed. The anesthesiologist must be prepared to rapidly induce general anesthesia should intrauterine manipulations be necessary to facilitate delivery.

SYMPHYSIOTOMY

As a normal physiologic event in pregnancy, the sacroiliac joints widen by 0.6 to 0.9 mm and the symphysis pubis by 1 to 3 mm. Although rare, a pathologic separation of the symphysis pubis may occur.[82]

Although it is unlikely this procedure would be used to deliver the stuck aftercoming head in the United States today, it is described for its interest. The procedure is used in countries where obstructed (cephalopelvic disproportion) and prolonged (days) labor occurs. The indications are fairly rigid:

1. The fetus is live and weighs not less than 2500 g or more than 4000 g.
2. The labor is obstructed, and the head is not less than 1/5 or more than 2/5 above the pelvic brim on abdominal palpation.
3. The procedure is performed before signs of impending uterine rupture. In primigravidas this is usually after full dilatation unless there is significant fetal distress and the cervix is 8 to 9 cm dilated.

Besides an obstructed labor in a vertex presentation, the procedure is also used in arrest of the aftercoming head due to disproportion with a live fetus. One major benefit besides the immediate need for this delivery is permanent enlargement of the pelvis. Where access to medical care is a problem due to inadequate and distant services, it increases the chance for vaginal deliveries in future pregnancies.

With the patient in the dorsal lithotomy position, after adequate anesthesia (spinal, epidural, general, or local infiltration of the site of the incision and the joint), a catheter is inserted into the bladder. The urethra is retracted laterally with the vaginal finger to

1. Prevent urethral trauma,
2. Feel the point of the knife during incision of the symphyseal cartilage, and
3. Prevent the knife from cutting the vaginal wall.

Over the cartilage at its midportion, a 1-cm incision is made down to the cartilage with a scalpel. The instrument of choice is a solid bistoury-type knife because a disposable blade may break while one is cutting into the cartilage; however, a No. 23 scalpel blade on a Bard Parker handle is an alternate choice. It is important that the uppermost area of cartilage, as well as the lowermost, not be transected (Fig. 19–31). At the upper surface are fibers of the rectus sheath that support the incised joint if they are not cut, whereas at the lower edge there is a vascular plexus. The cartilage is completely transected to its full depth, which the operator can determine by feeling the point of the knife with the vaginal finger. After delivery is accomplished, either operatively or (usually) spontaneously, and perineal repair is completed, the thighs are kept together and the patient is maintained in the lateral position with a Foley catheter for continuous bladder drainage for 5 days. The patient may walk with help when she feels ready, and full mobility should be accomplished by Day 10.[83–86]

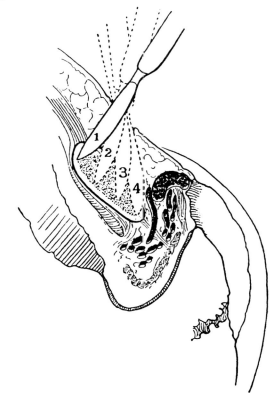

Figure 19–31. Symphysiotomy—demonstrating the fibers of the rectus superiorly and the venous plexus inferiorly. Numbers 1–4 demonstrate movement of the scalpel across the fibers in sequence. (From Greenhill JP: Obstetrics. Philadelphia: WB Saunders, 12th ed, 1960, p 920.)

SUMMARY

We have described the factors and complications associated with breech presentations. Because we believe there is a role for vaginal delivery, albeit in the selected case, we have attempted to cover this in detail by reviewing some maneuvers commonly used in the past when cesarean section was a rarity. The physician in training should develop the skills required for breech delivery and recognize that the more common abdominal delivery should be conducted with as much skill as is required for a vaginal breech delivery. To obtain a successful outcome in conducting a vaginal breech delivery, the operator must strictly adhere to the criteria described in this chapter, carefully assess and manage the progress of labor, undertake proper planning and use of institutional resources, and carefully conduct the delivery using the proper obstetrical skills. These skills are described in detail in several texts.[9, 78, 79, 81, 85–87]

References

1. Hughey MJ: Fetal position during pregnancy. Am J Obstet Gynecol 153:885, 1985.
2. Neligan GA, Prudham D, Steiner H: The Formative Years: Birth, Family and Development in New-Castle upon-Tyne. London: Oxford University Press, 1974.
3. Collea JV: Current management of breech presentation. Clin Obstet Gynecol 21:525, 1978.
4. Ralis ZA: Birth trauma to muscles in babies born by breech delivery and its possible consequences. Arch Dis Child 50:4, 1974.
5. Seeds JW: Malpresentation. In Gabbe S, Niebyl J, Simpson JL (eds.): Normal and Problem Pregnancies. New York: Churchill-Livingston, 1986, p. 465.
6. Brenner WE, Bruce RD, Hendricks CH: The characteristics and perils of breech presentation. Am J Obstet Gynecol 118:700, 1974.
7. Tompkins P: An inquiry into the causes of breech presentation. Am J Obstet Gynecol 51:595, 1946.
8. Cruikshank DP: Breech presentation. Clin Obstet Gynecol 29:225, 1986.
9. Weingold AB: The management of breech presentation. In Iffy L, Charles D (eds.): Operative Perinatology. New York: Macmillan, 1989, p. 537.
10. Seeds JW, Cefalo RC: Malpresentations. Clin Obstet Gynecol 25:145, 1982.
11. Blickstein I, Lancet M: Second breech presentation in twins—A possible adaptive measure to promote fetal growth. Obstet Gynecol 73:700, 1989.
12. Kuppila O: The perinatal mortality in breech delivery and observation on affecting factors. Acta Obstet Gynaecol Scand (Suppl) 39:1, 1975.
13. Rovinsky J, Miller JA, Kaplan S: Management of breech presentation at term. Am J Obstet Gynecol 115:497, 1973.
14. Fianu S: Fetal mortality and morbidity following breech delivery. Acta Obstet Gynaecol Scand (Suppl) 56:7, 1976.
15. Brant HA, Lewis BV: Prolapse of the umbilical cord. Lancet 1:1443, 1966.
16. De Crespigny LJC, Pepperell RJ: Perinatal mortality and morbidity in breech presentation. Obstet Gynecol 53:141, 1979.
17. Gimovsky ML, Wallace RL, Shifrin BS, et al.: Randomized management of the non-frank breech presentation at term: A preliminary report. Am J Obstet Gynecol 146:34, 1983.
18. Sherer DM, Menashe M, Palti Z, et al.: Radiologic evidence of a nuchal arm in the breech presenting fetus at the onset of labor. An indication for abdominal delivery. Am J Perinatol 6(3):353, 1989.
19. Wilcox HH: The attitude of the fetus in breech presentation. Am J Obstet Gynecol 58:478, 1949.
20. Bhagwanani SG, Price HV, Lawrence KM, et al.: Risk and presentation of cervical cord injury in the management of breech presentation with hyperextension of the fetal head. Am J Obstet Gynecol 115:1159, 1973.
21. Wigglesworth JS, Husenmeyer RP: Intracranial birth trauma in vaginal breech delivery. The continued importance of injury to the occipital bone. Br J Obstet Gynaecol 84:684, 1977.
22. Mazor M, Hagay ZJ, Lieberman JR, et al.: Fetal malformations associated with breech delivery—implications for obstetric management. J Reprod Med 30:884, 1985.
23. Karp LE, Doney JR, McCarthy T, et al.: The premature breech. Trial of labor or cesarean section. Obstet Gynecol 53:88, 1979.
24. Goldenberg RL, Nelson KG: The unanticipated breech presentation in labor. Clin Obstet Gynecol 27:95, 1984.
25. Morgan HS, Kane SH: An analysis of 16,327 breech births. JAMA 187:262, 1964.
26. Abroms IF, Bressnan MJ, Zuckerman JE, et al.: Cervical injury secondary to hyperextension of the head in breech presentation. Obstet Gynecol 41:369, 1973.
27. Daw E: Hyperextension of the head in breech presentation. Am J Obstet Gynecol 119:564, 1974.
28. Faber-Niholt R, Huisjes HJ, Touwen BCL, et al.: Neurological follow up of 281 children born in breech presentation—A controlled study. Br Med J 286:9, 1983.
29. Eilen B, Fleisher A, Schulman H, Jagani N: Fetal acidosis and the abnormal FHR tracing. The term breech fetus. Obstet Gynecol 63:233, 1984.
30. Hawrylyshyn PA, Bernstein P, Papsin FR: Risk factors associated with infection following cesarean section. Am J Obstet Gynecol 139:294, 1981.
31. Gibbs RS, Jones PM, Wilder CJ: Internal fetal monitoring and maternal infection following cesarean section. Obstet Gynecol 52:193, 1978.
32. Domowitz LG, Wenzel RP: Endometritis following cesarean section. A controlled study of the increased duration of hospital stay and direct cost of hospitalization. Am J Obstet Gynecol 137:467, 1980.
33. Bingham P, Lilford RJ: Management of the selected term breech presentation. Assessment of the risks of selected vaginal delivery versus cesarean section for all cases. Obstet Gynecol 69:965, 1987.
34. Hansen GF: Version of the fetus. In Iffy L, Charles D (eds.): Operative Perinatology. New York: Macmillan, 1984, p. 471.
35. Savona-Ventura C: The role of external cephalic version in modern obstetrics. Obstet Gynecol Surv 41:393, 1986.
36. Kasule J, Chimbira THK, Brown I: Controlled trial of external cephalic version. Br J Obstet Gynaecol 92:14, 1985.
37. Westgren M, Edvall H, Nordstrom L, et al.: Spontaneous cephalic version of breech presentation in last trimester. Br J Obstet Gynaecol 92:19, 1985.
38. Wallace RL, Van Dorsten JO, Eglinton GS, et al.: External cephalic version with tocolysis. J Reprod Med 29:746, 1984.
39. Marchick R: Antepartum external cephalic version with tocolysis. A study of term singleton breech presentation. Am J Obstet Gynecol 158:1889, 1988.
40. Robertson AW, Kopelman JN, Read JA, et al.: External cephalic version at term: Is a tocolytic necessary? Obstet Gynecol 70:896, 1987.
41. Hofmeyr GJ: Effect of external cephalic version in late pregnancy on breech presentation and cesarean section rate: A controlled trial. Br J Obstet Gynaecol 90:392, 1983.
42. Scaling ST: External cephalic version without tocolysis. Am J Obstet Gynecol 158:1424, 1988.
43. Bradley-Watson PJ: The decreasing value of external ce-

phalic version in modern obstetric practice. Am J Obstet Gynecol 123:237, 1975.

44. Morrison JC, Myatt RE, Martin JN Jr, et al.: External cephalic version of the breech presentation under tocolysis. Am J Obstet Gynecol 154:900, 1986.

45. Ferguson JE, Armstrong MA, Dyson DC: Maternal and fetal factors affecting success of antepartum external cephalic version. Obstet Gynecol 70:722, 1987.

46. Dyson DC, Ferguson JE, Hensleigh P: Antepartum external cephalic version under tocolysis. Obstet Gynecol 67:63, 1986.

47. Ferguson JE, Dyson DC: Antepartum external cephalic version. Am J Obstet Gynecol 152:297, 1985.

48. Van Veelen AJ, Van Cappellen AW, Flu PK, et al.: Effect of external cephalic version in late pregnancy on presentation at delivery: A randomized controlled trial. Br J Obstet Gynaecol 96:916, 1989.

49. Cesarean Childbirth. Report of a Consensus Development Conference Sponsored by the National Institute of Child Health and Human Development (DHHS Publication No. NIH 82-2067). Washington, DC: U.S. Government Printing Office, 1980.

50. Hall JE, Kohl SC: Breech presentation, a study of 1456 cases. Am J Obstet Gynecol 72:977, 1956.

51. Patterson SP, Mulliniks RC Jr, Schrier PC: Breech presentation in the primigravida. Am J Obstet Gynecol 98:404, 1967.

52. Victor-Lewis B, Seneviratne HR: Vaginal breech delivery or cesarean section. Am J Obstet Gynecol 134:615, 1979.

53. O'Leary J: Breech presentation: A defacto indication for cesarean section. Female Patient 10:95, 1985.

54. Tatum RK, Orr JW, Soong S, Huddleston JF: Vaginal breech delivery of selected infants weighing more than 2000 grams. Am J Obstet Gynecol 152:145, 1985.

55. Graves W: Breech delivery in 20 years of experience. Am J Obstet Gynecol 137:229, 1980.

56. Main DM, Main EK, Maurer MM: Cesarean section versus vaginal delivery for the breech fetus weighing less than 1,500 grams. Am J Obstet Gynecol 146:580, 1983.

57. Flanagan TA, Mulcahey KM, Korenbrot CC, et al.: Management of term breech presentation. Am J Obstet Gynecol 156:1492, 1987.

58. Nisell H, Bistoletti P, Palms C: Preterm breech delivery. Acta Obstet Gynaecol Scand 60:363, 1981.

59. Bowes W, Taylor E, O'Brian M: Breech delivery: Evaluation of the method of delivery on perinatal results and maternal morbidity. Am J Obstet Gynecol 135:965, 1979.

60. Gimovsky M, Paul R: Singleton breech presentation in labor. Experience in 1980. Am J Obstet Gynecol 143:733, 1982.

61. Mann L, Gallant J: Modern management of the breech delivery. Am J Obstet Gynecol 134:611, 1979.

62. Gimovsky ML, Petrie R, Todd D: Neonatal performance of the selected term vaginal breech delivery. Obstet Gynecol 56:687, 1980.

63. Todd WD, Steer GM: Term breech: Review of 1006 term breech deliveries. Obstet Gynecol 22:583, 1963.

64. Gimovsky ML, Willard K, Neglio M, et al.: X-ray pelvimetry in a breech protocol: A comparison of digital radiography and conventional methods. Am J Obstet Gynecol 153:887, 1985.

65. Osborn SR: The implication of the committee on radiologic hazards to patients: Variants in the radiation dose received by the patient in diagnostic radiology. Br J Radiol 36:260, 1963.

66. Federle MP, Cohen HA, Rosewein MF, et al.: Pelvimetry by digital radiography: A low dose examination. Radiology 143:733, 1982.

67. Kopelman JN, Duff P, Karl RT, et al.: Computed tomographic pelvimetry in the evaluation of breech presentation. Obstet Gynecol 68:455, 1986.

68. Bader B, Graham D, Stinson S: Significance of ultrasound measurements of the head of the breech fetus. J Ultrasound Med 6:437, 1987.

69. Feinstein SJ, Lodeiro JG, Vintzileos AM, et al.: Intrapartum ultrasound diagnosis of nuchal cord as a decisive factor in management. Am J Obstet Gynecol 153:308, 1985.

70. Management of the Breech Presentation (Technical Bulletin No. 95). Washington, DC: American College of Obstetricians and Gynecologists, 1986.

71. Dewan DM: Anesthesia for preterm delivery, breech presentation and multiple gestation. Clin Obstet Gynecol 30:566, 1987.

72. Willis D, Moffat E, Lai M, Helfgott A: Intravenous nitroglycerin for uterine relaxation (Abstract 49). Presented at the annual meeting of the Society of Perinatal Obstetricians, Houston, TX, 1990.

73. Crawford J: An appraisal of lumber epidural blockade in parturients with singleton fetus presenting by the breech. Br J Obstet Gynaecol 81:867, 1974.

74. Confino E, Ismajovich B, Rudick V, David M: Extradural analgesia in the management of singleton breech delivery. Br J Anaesth 57:892, 1985.

75. Breeson A, Kovacs G, Pickles B, Hill J: Extradural analgesia: The preferred method of analgesia for vaginal delivery. Br J Anaesth 50:1227, 1978.

76. James FM, Dewan DM, Floyd HM, et al.: Chloroprocaine vs bupivacaine for lumbar epidural analgesia or elective cesarean section. Anesthesiology 52:488, 1980.

77. D'Athis F, Macheboeuf M, Thomas H, et al.: Epidural analgesia with a bupivacaine-fentanyl mixture in obstetrics: Comparison of repeated injections and continuous infusion. Can J Anaesth 35:116, 1988.

78. Zuspan FP, Quilligan EJ (eds.): Douglas-Stromme Operative Obstetrics, 5th Edition. Norwalk, CT: Appleton & Lange, 1988, p. 463.

79. Reid D: Breech presentation. In A Textbook of Obstetrics. Philadelphia: W.B. Saunders, 1962, p. 539.

80. Collea JV, Chein C, Quilligan EJ: The randomized management of term frank breech presentation: A study of 208 cases. Am J Obstet Gynecol 137:235, 1980.

81. Milner RDG: Neonatal mortality of breech deliveries with and without forceps to the aftercoming head. Br J Obstet Gynaecol 82:783, 1975.

82. Moir JC, Myerscough PR (eds.): Symphysiotomy. In Munro-Kerr's Operative Obstetrics. London: Bailliere, Tindall and Cassel, 1971.

83. Seedat EK, Chrichton D: Symphysiotomy technique: Indications and limitations. Lancet 1:554, 1962.

84. Philpott RH: Obstructed labor. Clin Obstet Gynecol 7:601, 1980.

85. Webster JC: A Textbook of Obstetrics. Philadelphia: W.B. Saunders, 1903, p. 724.

86. Greenhill JP: Obstetrics. Philadelphia: W.B. Saunders, 1950, p. 920.

87. Reid D: Breech extraction and version. Eastman NH, Hellman LM (eds.): Williams Obstetrics, 12th Edition. New York: Appleton-Century-Crofts, 1961, p. 1162.

UNIT THREE

Multiple Gestations

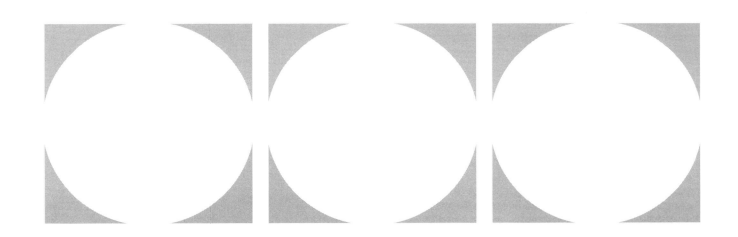

20

Vaginal Delivery of Twins

Robert Johnson
Mary J. O'Sullivan

Historically, multiple gestations evoked a sense of mythology, mystery, and controversy. Ancient and primitive societies regarded this occurrence with horror and wonder. Rarely were similar attitudes applied to a singleton birth. Corney[1] has reviewed the mythology of multiple gestation in detail. Although modern obstetrics has eliminated much of the mystery, controversy surrounding management of multiple gestation remains.

A review of the current understanding of occurrence of twin and higher order gestations will serve as a background to a discussion of the issues related to medical management.

TYPES OF TWIN GESTATION

Two types of twinning are generally recognized: *dizygotic* and *monozygotic*. In dizygotic twin gestations, two ova are released during the same menstrual cycle and are fertilized by two separate sperm. Laparoscopic evidence suggests that spontaneous multiple ovulations can occur in a cycle. Ovulation is under the control of gonadotropin release from the anterior pituitary. As follicle-stimulating hormone and luteinizing hormone begin to rise, peaking at midcycle, only one graafian follicle is usually selected for maturation and eventual ovulation. The mechanisms involved in a multiovulatory cycle have not been definitely described. Both systemic and local ovarian effects have been postulated.[2]

In any event, two or more viable fertilizable ova can be extruded during one ovulatory cycle from one or both ovaries and at different times in the cycle. Evidence for either phenomenon has been clearly demonstrated during laparoscopy for spontaneous twin ectopic gestation and ovum retrieval after gonadotropin-induced ovarian hyperstimulation. If both ova are released from one ovary, tubal transport and fertilization likely occur in the ipsilateral tube. However, if each ovary releases an ovum, transport and fertilization may occur in both tubes. Exceptions occur: Ovulation with transport and fertilization in the contralateral tube has been demonstrated in singleton ectopic gestations and in women whose ipsilateral tube was previously excised.

Even if multiple ovulation occurs at relatively close intervals, fertilization may not be by the same coital event. Fertilization of different ova within the same cycle by different coital events is referred to as *superfecundation*. This event is rare, but has been demonstrated by twins of different racial origins or who by blood group analysis were shown to have different fathers.[3] *Superfetation*

(ovulation and fertilization occurring in the subsequent month after fertilization of an initial ovum) is theoretical and has not been demonstrated in human reproduction. Suppression of normal corpus luteum response would have to be postulated.

The process leading to monozygotic twin gestation is entirely different from that described for dizygotic twin gestation. In monozygosity, one ovum is fertilized by one sperm, followed by zygotic division that creates two distinct individuals. It can be theorized that monozygotic twinning involves a teratogenic event, although its precipitants (genetic vs. environmental) are not clearly defined. Although one would hesitate to refer to a monozygotic twin gestation as a congenital malformation, the increased incidence of malformations among monozygotic twins compared with dizygotic twins suggests that a relationship exists, a continuum if you will.[4]

Timing is crucial in the development of monozygotic twinning. Post-zygotic division must occur within 15 days of fertilization. After this, twinning cannot occur. The exact timing determines placentation, chorioamnion formation, and whether the twins will be conjoined (Fig. 20–1). Division that occurs early in embryonic life (Days 1 to 3) results in dichorionic, diamniotic twins. Between Days 4 and 8, division will result in monochorionic, diam-

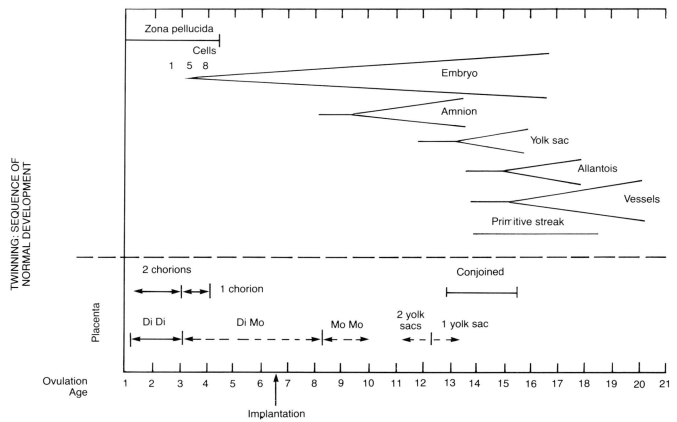

Figure 20–1. Embryogenesis and monozygotic twinning. Di Di—diamniotic, dichorionic; Di Mo—diamniotic, monochorionic; Mo Mo—monoamniotic, monochorionic. (From Benirschke K, Kim CK: Multiple pregnancy. N Engl J Med 288:1276, 1973.)

niotic twins. Splitting between Days 9 and 12 can result in monochorionic, monoamniotic twins. Finally, conjoined twins occupy one gestational sac, the result of incomplete division of the developing germ disk, occurring on Days 12 to 15. Although not absolute, monozygotic twins who divide earlier in this continuum generally fair better than their monochorionic, monoamniotic counterparts. Conjoined twins have the worst prognosis.

Conjoined twins are relatively rare (1 in 400 monozygotic or 1 in 1500 twin pregnancies), because of the overall low and stable incidence of monozygosity and the presumed high abortion rate among conjoined twins. They can be connected at any site, including, in decreasing frequency, (a) chest wall (thoracopagus, 70%), (b) abdominal wall from xiphoid to umbilicus (xiphopagus, 34%), (c) buttocks (pygopagus, 18%), (d) ischium (ischiopagus, 6%), and (e) the head (craniopagus, 2%).[5] The prognosis is poor. Most either spontaneously abort or are stillborn. However, some do survive delivery, with cesarean section being the preferred method. If anatomically feasible, surgical separation can be effected. Several conjoined twins have survived until old age unseparated (e.g., the "Siamese twins" for whom conjoined twinship is named lived for 63 years).

INCIDENCE

The true incidence of twinning may never be known, because of the increased rate of spontaneous abortion noted among twins. The rate of identified twin conceptions in 1000 first-trimester ultrasonograms varied from 3% to approximately 5% (two fetuses viewed vs. one fetus and an empty sac, respectively).[6] Of these, 21% went on to lose one fetus. Landy[6] referred to this as the "vanishing twin phenomenon." The loss rate may be as high as 63%.[7] For twin conceptions that progress to viability, there is a clear difference in incidence of zygosity. Monozygotic twinning is fairly constant across all studied populations, varying only between 3% and 5% of 1000 pregnancies. That this rate does not vary is consistent with the concept that monozygosity is a spontaneous teratogenic event affecting all populations equally.

Dizygotic twinning, on the other hand, displays a wide variation across populations, with several factors, such as race and ethnicity, influencing its incidence. Among Asians, the rate is approximately 3 to 5 per 1000; for Europeans and white Americans, approximately 10 per 1000; and for black Americans, about 15 per 1000. The highest rate is among black Africans: It has been demonstrated to be as high as 57.2 per 1000 in the Yoruba Nigerians.[8]

The reason for the differences in the rates of dizygotic twinning among different racial groups is not clear; however, differences in mean gona-dotropin levels among different racial groups have been demonstrated by researchers.[9, 10] Within all racial groups, age and parity exert a positive effect on dizygotic twinning rates, which steadily rise until approximately 37 years of age, and then fall as menopause approaches. Dizygotic twinning is highest among mothers of para 4 or greater. Monozygotic twinning rates are little influenced by these two variations. Multiple gestation rates overall (including monozygotic) are significantly increased by ovulation induction agents, which result in ovarian hyperstimulation and multiovulation.[11] The incidence of twins is 1.2% in the United States.[12] With ovulation induction using clomiphene, the rate increases to 6.8 to 17% and is even higher (18 to 35%) when gonadotropins are used.[13]

DIAGNOSIS

Theoretically, the earlier a clinical diagnosis is made in any medical condition, the more likely it is that interventional decisions can affect outcome. This concept certainly holds for multiple gestations. In the older literature, about 50% of twins were diagnosed at the onset of labor and even fewer were diagnosed before 32 weeks' gestation.[14, 15] With the liberal use of ultrasonography, antenatal diagnosis has increased to approximately 91 to 95%.[16] In Sweden, where all patients presenting for prenatal care were offered routine obstetrical ultrasonography from 1974 until 1982, 98% of 254 multiple gestations were detected by antenatal scan.[17] Compared with the previous 5 years at the same institution, a decrease in both perinatal mortality and major morbidity, as well as a decrease in the number of premature twin deliveries (less than 38 weeks) occurred in the group who underwent routine ultrasonography, suggesting that early diagnosis improves outcome.[17]

Although routine ultrasonography is more available, there are still settings in which it is not immediately available. The health care giver must keep the possibility of multiple gestation in mind when evaluating patients with both normal and abnormal findings. Some clinical factors that suggest the possibility of multiple gestation are listed in Table 20–1. If, however, there is any suspicion, ultrasonography should be performed to confirm the diagnosis and to determine fetal number, anatomy, placentation, and zygosity when possible.

In the first trimester, the diagnosis is confirmed by the presence of two actively beating fetal hearts. When one fetus and an empty sac are visualized, patients should be rescanned to either confirm or exclude the diagnosis (i.e., "vanishing twin" or yolk sac). Radiography has also been used to confirm multiple gestations in the second trimester or beyond after fetal calcification (14 to 16 weeks);

Table 20–1. FACTORS SUGGESTIVE OF MULTIPLE GESTATION

1. Age peak at 37
2. Parity of 4 or more
3. Race: black > white > Asians
4. Ethnicity African > Afro-American
5. Size greater than should be for dates
6. Increased fetal movement
7. Ovulation-induced pregnancy
8. Positive family history
9. More than one fetal heart
10. Abnormally elevated β-human chorionic gonadotropin levels for dates
11. Elevated maternal serum alpha-fetoprotein
12. Excessive weight gain
13. Anemia

however, sonography is preferred because of the risks of fetal radiation exposure.

Carlan and co-workers[18] reported on the use of computed tomography to exclude the diagnosis of conjoined twins in a monoamniotic twin pregnancy. Magnetic resonance imaging may hold some benefit in this regard as well.[19] Ultrasonography can quite clearly demonstrate the site of the union, most of the anatomy involved, and whether separation is feasible in many cases, predelivery. This is important for the obstetric and pediatric surgical team when planning delivery and possible surgical separation. Delivery should be in the same facility as the contemplated surgery.

MORBIDITY AND MORTALITY

Perinatal Mortality

The perinatal mortality rate in twins (and other multiple gestations) is increased compared with that of singletons. Even though 1.2% of all deliveries are twins, 11% of neonatal and 12.6% of perinatal mortalities occur in these babies.[16, 20, 21] In addition, the stillbirth rate is at least twice that of singletons.[22] The biggest reason for this high loss rate, at least in the liveborns and perhaps in some of the intrapartum stillborns, is the premature delivery of a physiologically unprepared fetus/ newborn. A comparison of data on singleton versus twin birth weights in the University of Illinois Perinatal Network from 1982 to 1986, showed that 10.4% of twin deliveries weighed less than 1500 g compared with 1.2% for singletons. The overall perinatal mortality rate was 54 in 1000 for twins versus 9.1 in 1000 for singletons, a sixfold increase.[20, 21]

In terms of gestational age, 42% of twins compared with 8% of singletons were at less than 37 weeks' gestation at delivery.[21] Zygosity, although not available in the Illinois data, also affects mortality. Monozygotic, monoamniotic twins (1.5% of all twins) have a perinatal mortality as high as 30 to 50%.[23, 24] Monozygotic, diamniotic-monochorionic twins have a higher loss rate than do dizygotic twins (186 vs. 151 in 1000).[25]

Despite these numbers, considerable improvement in the perinatal mortality rate of twins has occurred over the last 30 years, just as it has in that of singletons. This is largely due to a decrease in the mortality rate of neonates weighing between 1000 and 1500 g.[26] Using antepartal fetal evaluation, Rattan and co-workers[27] demonstrated a decrease in fetal deaths after 32 weeks from 23 per 1000 in 1975 to 1979 to zero in 1980 to 1983. Some of this decrease is due to improved antenatal care and early diagnosis.

For birth weights of 1500 to 2999 g, the twin perinatal mortality rate closely approximates that of singletons (Fig. 20–2). Below 1500 g, however, the neonatal death rate is significantly higher (p < 0.05) in twins, whereas the stillbirth rate is higher (but not statistically significant) in singletons (Fig. 20–3). Overall perinatal mortality in this weight group (i.e., below 1500 g) is only slightly higher in twins.[21] Chervenak and co-workers[16] showed that 81% of perinatal mortalities were at less than 29 weeks' gestation, or, by weight, 77% weighed 1000 g or less. In the Illinois Perinatal Network, 75% of deaths were in twins weighing less than 1500 g.[21] Therefore, a major problem is prevention of prematurity/immaturity, which eludes obstetricians even in singleton gestations. In contrast to some of the older reports, recent studies have shown no difference in perinatal mortality rates between the first and second twin infants.[16, 20, 21, 28, 29]

On the other side of the birth weight scale, in the Illinois study (Fig. 20–4) a significantly (p < 0.05) increased perinatal mortality rate was found in twin infants weighing more than 3000 g, contributed to by both stillbirths (p < 0.05) and neonatal deaths (p < 0.001).[21] The rate of respira-

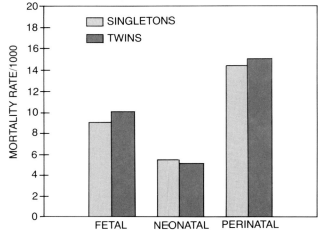

UNIVERSITY OF ILLINOIS PERINATAL NETWORK DATA FOR 1982–1986 MORTALITY RATES (PER 1000) BY BIRTHWEIGHT 1500–2999 g (SINGLETONS VERSUS TWINS)

Figure 20–2. Mortality rates of singletons versus twins at 1500 to 2999 g. birth weight. (Redrawn from Ghai V, Vidyasagar D: Morbidity and mortality factors in twins. Clin Perinatol 15:134, 1988.)

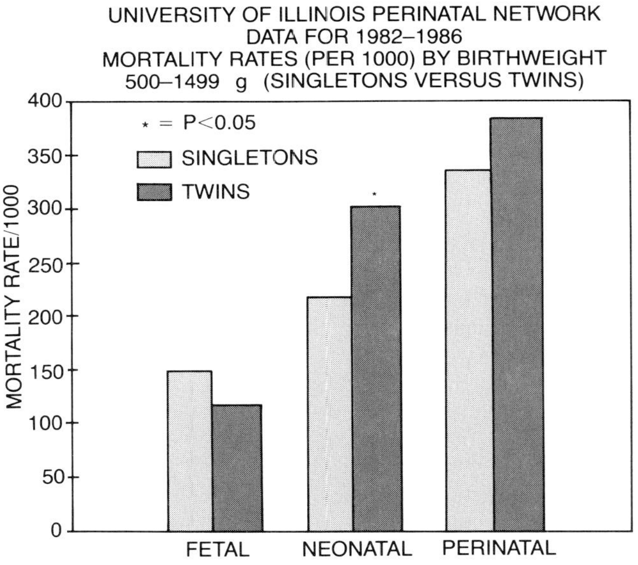

UNIVERSITY OF ILLINOIS PERINATAL NETWORK
DATA FOR 1982–1986
MORTALITY RATES (PER 1000) BY BIRTHWEIGHT
500–1499 g (SINGLETONS VERSUS TWINS)

Figure 20–3. Mortality rates of singletons versus twins at 500 to 1499 g. birth weight. (Redrawn from Ghai V, Vidyasagar D: Morbidity and mortality factors in twins. Clin Perinatol 15:134, 1988.)

tory morbidity in these infants was triple that for singletons. There was also a higher incidence (p < 0.001) of Apgar scores below 7 at 1 and 5 minutes compared with singletons.[21] Possible explanations include earlier placental maturation[30] and therefore earlier development of "post-maturity";[31, 32] an increased fetal mass relative to placental size that may result in acute uteroplacental insufficiency; and either fetal death or increased fetal distress in labor, hypoxemia, and/or meconium aspiration. Because optimum fetal survival is at 37 to 38 weeks' gestation,[32] and most twin gestations are delivered by 37 weeks (or 21 days earlier than the

UNIVERSITY OF ILLINOIS PERINATAL NETWORK
DATA FOR 1982–1986
MORTALITY RATES (PER 1000) BY BIRTHWEIGHT
3000+ GRAMS (SINGLETONS VERSUS TWINS)

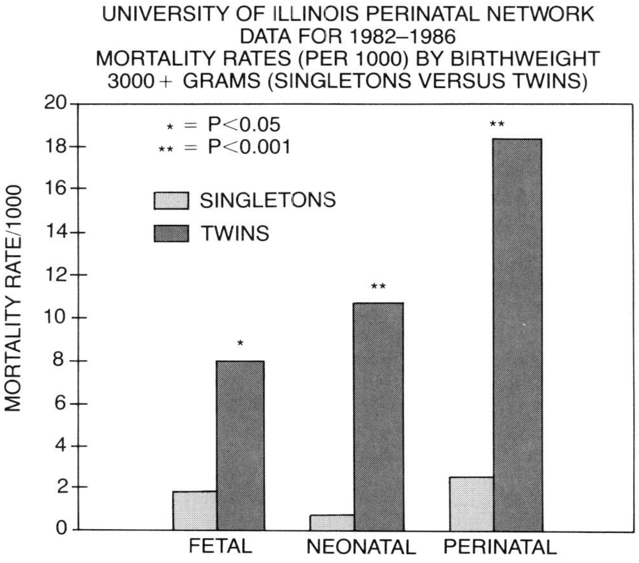

Figure 20–4. Mortality rates of singletons versus twins at 3000+ g. birth weight. (Redrawn from Ghai V, Vidyasagar D: Morbidity and mortality factors in twins. Clin Perinatol 15:135, 1988.)

calculated date of delivery),[33] perhaps twin gestation should be considered "term" at this time and management thereafter should be that of a postdate pregnancy.

Maternal Mortality

In a discussion of maternal mortality in twins in the twelfth edition of *Williams Obstetrics*, it is noted that in 2595 twin gestations compiled by five authors, there were 29 maternal deaths. This is a rate of 111.7 in 10,000. A compilation of three studies[34-36] in the 1950s mentions only one death in 2175 twin pregnancies (4.5 in 10,000). Since then, maternal deaths overall have declined considerably. There are no recent data; however, these women are at increased risk of morbidity and mortality due to complications such as premature labor and its treatment with tocolytics as well as an increased risk of preeclampsia, hemorrhage, and operative delivery. In 14 years at Jackson Memorial Hospital, only two maternal deaths have occurred in twin gestations—one was due to an amniotic fluid embolus, and the other was due to acute leukemia, with death occurring within 2 weeks of diagnosis.

Maternal/Fetal Morbidity

It is impossible to discuss all morbidities, their complications, and their treatments. Circulating fluid volume cardiac and renal workloads are increased with each additional fetus. So is the risk of fetal wastage and early delivery. With ovulation induction and resultant multiple gestations, hyperstimulation syndrome and its associated risks are increased, as are ectopic gestations. Any medical or obstetrical complication that is associated with pregnancy is aggravated by a multiple gestation, purely on the basis of physiology. For example, in the presence of underlying maternal cardiac disease, physiologic mechanisms are further stretched and risks increased.

There is an overall increased risk for operative abdominal delivery as a result of malpresentations, placenta previa, abruptio placentae, dysfunctional labor, and space-occupying congenital anomalies. All of those result in increased morbidity associated with surgery, e.g., infection, vascular, pulmonary, and wound complications.

The overstretched uterus that results from the multiple gestation and/or polyhydramnios (6% of twins[14]) increases maternal discomfort, causing pain, abdominal striae, pruritus, and compression of intra-abdominal contents leading to constipation, difficulty eating, and urinary frequency. Venous return decreases, sometimes resulting in vulvar and lower extremity edema and varicosities. Polyhydramnios is associated with preterm labor, increased risk of uterine dysfunction, and postpartum atony. If placenta previa concomitantly occurs, then the risk of hemorrhage is further increased secondary to atony of the lower uterine segment and marked varicosities in this area that may be encountered at cesarean section.

Premature rupture of membranes, as in singleton gestation, increases the risk of infection, preterm labor, and need for early delivery either by induction or cesarean section. The use of tocolytics to arrest preterm labor and/or hormones to stimulate fetal lung maturity increases the possibility of pulmonary edema.

Pre-eclampsia is increased regardless of previous parity,[37] occurring in 13% of twin gestations,[14] and is often earlier than in singleton gestations. Severe pre-eclampsia increases fivefold in primigravidas.[22] Because severe pre-eclampsia is treated the same as in a singleton gestation, preterm delivery is increased.

Maternal anemia relates both to increased fetal needs for iron and folate and to maternal needs to fulfill the physiologic increase in red cell mass. Furthermore, the risks of placenta previa or abruptio placentae and post-delivery uterine atony further aggravate the anemia postpartum.

Neonatal Morbidity

Just as mortality is related to premature/immature delivery, so is morbidity. Respiratory distress, intraventricular hemorrhage, necrotizing enterocolitis, and long-term neurologic sequelae are a function of preterm delivery and the increased risk of perinatal asphyxia associated with prematurity. There are, however, additional morbidities in twin gestations.

The incidence of congenital anomalies is increased in monozygous twins regardless of whether they are mono- or dichorial.[38, 39] The etiology of malformations appears to be related to whatever causes monozygotic twinning. The more severe manifestations are acardia and conjoined twins.[38, 40, 41] Other anomalies seen are neural tube defects; sirenomelia; gastrointestinal, renal, and cardiac anomalies; extrophy of the cloaca; and gonadal dysgenesis.[42] Twins are usually discordant for congenital defects, but more concordance exists for monozygotic than dizygotic conceptions.[39]

MANAGEMENT

Antepartum Management

Prenatal management focuses on reduction of prematurity and immaturity. Early diagnosis and aggressive management include frequent visits and clinical examinations to detect premature dilation. Education regarding the signs and symptoms of preterm labor; decreased work and increased rest; and aggressive treatment of threatened preterm labor with rest, fluids, and/or tocolytics/steroids may all decrease the risk of preterm delivery.

Routine hospitalization of patients with twin gestations grew out of the knowledge that middle-class women had a better perinatal outcome than lower-class working women. Hospitalization was an attempt to make up at least temporarily for the lack of social support.[43] However, in several studies in which patients admitted between 28 and 36 weeks' gestation were compared with a control group, no statistically significant improvement in length of gestation, incidence of preterm delivery, or perinatal outcome, was shown, although there was some increase in birth weight.[44–47]

Comparing a nonhospitalized group with a hospitalized group and an encerclage group, Weikes and colleagues[48] found no difference in outcome in the three groups. Others[49] have also shown that cerclage has not improved outcome.

In at least one study, hospitalization resulted in an increased incidence of preterm delivery, low birth weight, and very low birth weight in Finland.[50] Bed rest, however, did appear to decrease the incidence of hypertension.[44, 50]

β-mimetics have been used prophylactically in at least six studies with a placebo control group. Different drugs were used in almost all the studies. Yet, summarizing the studies, there is no evidence that β-mimetics were effective in preventing twin preterm labor, nor was there any improvement in the incidence of low birth weight.[51–56] However, there was a decreased incidence of neonatal respiratory distress syndrome in the drug group.[51, 53–55] The use of steroids to accelerate lung maturity may be less beneficial in twin than in singleton gestations, or larger doses may be necessary.[57]

Home uterine monitoring may be of benefit in the early detection of increased uterine activity. This allows earlier diagnosis of cervical change as a sign of preterm labor and earlier institution of tocolytic therapy, increasing the chances of success.[58, 59]

Although rare, maternal disseminated intravascular coagulation (DIC) associated with a second- or third-trimester intrauterine fetal death must be anticipated. Neither a first-trimester "vanishing twin" nor an early second-trimester loss that results in a fetus papyraceous is likely to be associated with DIC. The mother, however, will grieve the loss of this fetus, especially if she initially heard a fetal heart beat or felt fetal activity.

When an intrauterine fetal death occurs after 18 to 20 weeks, retention of the dead fetus is associated with a 25% risk of maternal DIC.[60] Therefore, early diagnosis of demise, serial assessment of maternal coagulation status, and surveillance of the remaining fetus or fetuses are essential to diagnose maternal DIC and/or the development of related fetal abnormalities. Treatment for mothers with laboratory diagnosed but not clinically evident DIC in the presence of a demise and at least one living preterm fetus begins with intravenous heparin, followed by either intravenous or subcutaneous heparin maintenance to correct maternal coagulation status. Delivery is accomplished when fetal lung maturity of the remaining fetus or other indications are established. The development of DIC in the other fetus can occur, especially in monozygous twins sharing vasculature, but under present clinical conditions it is essentially nonpreventable.[61, 62] Complications in the remaining fetus include death and the effects of vascular thromboses, e.g., hydranencephaly, porencephaly, digital anomalies, and bowel atresia.

Selective termination is discussed in the section on other multiple gestations. For fetal anomalies in twin gestations, selective termination can be considered.

Routine sonography in early pregnancy (16 to 20 weeks) decreases the incidence of undiagnosed twins. However, whether it is cost effective and whether early diagnosis ultimately affects outcome compared with diagnosis beyond 20 weeks have not been shown.[63]

Up to 21 weeks, the relationship of length to birth weight in twins is the same as that for singletons.[64] Figure 20–5 shows the growth of singletons compared with that of twins. Although the rates of growth are the same until 33 to 34 weeks, twins are in the lower range of the singleton curve. After 33 weeks, the rate of growth of twins declines compared with that of singletons.[21] Growth retardation in twins increases perinatal mortality 6.5-fold over that of normally grown twins. Serial growth studies during multiple gestations are part of fetal surveillance to evaluate fetal response to the environment[65] and detect discordant growth.

Discordant growth, defined as a 15 to 25% difference in birth weights, complicates 15 to 29% of twin gestations.[65–67] Discordance may be due to genetic variation, congenital anomalies, uteropla-

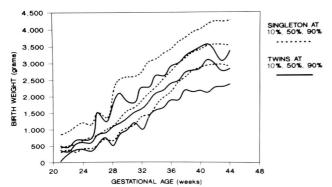

Figure 20–5. Intrauterine growth of twins and singletons. (Redrawn from Ghai V, Vidyasagar D: Morbidity and mortality factors in twins. Clin Perinatol 15:127, 1988.)

cental insufficiency, or twin transfusion. Sonograms should be done at least every 4 weeks, if the fetuses are thought to be dichorionic on the basis of a thick separating membrane, unlike sex, or separate placentas.[68] Otherwise, examinations should be performed at 2- to 3-week intervals.[68] The biparietal diameter of discordant twins, whereas parallel early in pregnancy, becomes divergent at 33 to 34 weeks. The abdominal circumference is often demonstrably different by 19 to 20 weeks. When head to abdominal circumference ratios are compared, there is a significant difference by 29 to 30 weeks.[69] If differences in estimated fetal weight of more than 25% are seen as early as 20 to 25 weeks, perinatal outcome is very poor.[70]

Because compromise can occur and growth deceleration is not uncommon, weekly nonstress testing is advisable. Contraction stress testing and/or biophysical profiles may be used as a backup for a nonreactive nonstress test. If these tests suggest fetal compromise, the decision to interfere will be based on gestational age, maturity status, and the risk of early delivery to the healthy fetus.

Clinically detectable twin to twin transfusion as a result of placental vascular anastomosis is relatively rare. It is suggested by a growth discrepancy on sonogram in like-sex twins with a single placenta and a thin separating membrane. Surprisingly few such syndromes occur in view of the high number of monochorionic twins with anastomotic circulations.[71] When the arterial circulation of one infant connects with the venous of the other in a common villous district, the potential for twin transfusion exists.[72] Management may be aided by continuous-wave Doppler studies to help distinguish genetic discordancy from placental insufficiency or twin to twin transfusion.[73, 74] The role of periumbilical blood sampling for diagnosis and/or intrauterine transfusion has yet to be determined.

The combination of oligohydramnios and polyhydramnios, especially at an early gestational age (less than 24 weeks), predicts a poor outcome[75] as is usually seen in twin to twin transfusion. We recently treated such a patient (diagnosed at 20 to 22 weeks with a fundal height of 34 cm) with indomethacin. It took 2 weeks to see a clinically significant difference. The fundal height decreased, and the infant with oligohydramnios started to collect amniotic fluid. Ultimately, both infants had normal fluid volumes, delivered at 34 to 35 weeks, and were monochorial with no obvious anastomosis seen. Indomethacin decreases fetal and neonatal urine production.[76–79]

Amniocentesis using an 18- or 20-gauge angiocath attached to intravenous tubing to allow drainage of amniotic fluid by gravity into a container at floor level can be used to decompress the uterus if there is maternal distress. Removal of 500 mL/hr to a total of 1500 to 2000 mL/hr is associated with maternal relief in a singleton gestation.[80] Because hydramnios with twin gestation frequently leads to preterm labor, amniocentesis, if used, should be combined with tocolytics.

Amniocentesis for genetic maturity, or diagnostic studies will often involve tapping both sacs, after identifying a separating membrane and leaving a dye, usually indigo carmine, in the first sac. When the second tap is attempted, the dye acts as a marker. If the fluid is clear, then the second sac has been tapped. For maturity studies, if both babies are the same size, only one sac need be tapped. When there is discordancy, it is best to try to obtain fluid from both babies or at the least the largest baby.[81–83]

Twin Labor

In modern obstetrics, 90 to 98% of multiple gestations receiving prenatal care are diagnosed before labor and delivery. The earlier in gestation the patient presents in labor, the less likely the diagnosis will have been made. Therefore, patients in preterm labor and those with discrepancies between size and date who have had no previous sonography should have a scan to help ascertain gestational age and rule out twins. Gestational age needs to be determined, as does the estimated fetal weights, possible discordancy, placentation, zygosity, cardiac activity, malformations, and presentation. Although this information will be available for twins previously diagnosed, confirmation of presentation in labor should be ascertained as well as attitude of the head if there is a breech presentation. When sonography is not available, an x-ray should be done. The risk of radiation exposure is not to be ignored; however, the benefit of accurate diagnosis of the position and attitude of the second twin for planning delivery management outweighs the risk. Even if a cesarean birth is planned, diagnosis of the position of the second infant is helpful in planning delivery. The risk of radiation exposure, however, may not be warranted if sonography is not available.

Preparations for delivery will depend to some degree on whether delivery is at term or before term. If the latter, the obstetrician must decide whether the nursery can handle two preterm or very preterm infants or whether maternal transport is required. In terms of perinatal survival, it is generally better to transport the mother before delivery than to transport the infants afterwards. Where maternal transport is planned, each receiving institution generally has its own protocols. These indicate whether a transport team is needed, what the method (land or air) of transport will be, the progress of labor, and who is responsible for the patient during transport if there is not a transport team.

In order to ensure adequate resources in the delivering hospital, two neonatal resuscitation teams and equipment must be available, especially for preterm infants. The delivery room personnel should have two types of cord clamps, one set for each infant so that after delivery of the placenta the proper cord for each infant is identifiable. If cord gases may be needed, four clamps of each kind should be available.

Where vaginal delivery is planned, the obstetrician should be skilled in intrauterine operative manipulation. An operative team should be available to perform a cesarean section at any time before delivery of the second twin. The anesthesiologist should see the patient to assist in planning the patient's analgesia/anesthesia management. Where possible, an epidural anesthetic is ideal. It provides analgesia in labor with minimal drug exposure to the infants and anesthesia for delivery, intrauterine manipulation, and/or cesarean section. With the new epidural techniques using continuous infusion of low-dose bupivacaine and narcotics, there is less hypotension, less interference with uterine activity, and less motor blockade. Patients can assist the delivery process by bearing down.[84, 85] As yet, there is very little in the literature regarding this technique in twin gestations. Our own experience over the last year has led us to be enthusiastic supporters of this type of epidural block.

The older literature reported increased hypotonic dysfunction in twin labors in patients who received epidural anesthesia (88%) compared with controls who did not (6.8%) and an increased perinatal death rate in the preterm epidural group (12% vs. 8%).[86] More recently, Crawford[87] reported that the acid/base status of the second twin was as good as or better than that of the first twin delivered vaginally under epidural block. In the nonepidural group, Twin A always had better acid/base status.[87]

The routine admission laboratory studies are sufficient. A recent blood type and screen should be available so that if hemorrhage occurs, blood is available on a quick crossmatch, or, if abnormal antibodies are present, blood can be obtained. Some patients prefer to donate their own blood before labor. Admittedly, patients with twins may have a lower hemoglobin/hematocrit level than patients with singleton gestations, because of the increased hemodilution. If they have taken their increased iron and folate supplements, it is unlikely they will be too anemic (unless there are other complications) for autologous donation. Instead of 500 mL, blood can be taken in units of 250 mL. In our facility, if the hemoglobin level is 11 g or greater, one unit is drawn, and this is repeated again in 10 days to 2 weeks. In patients whose hemoglobin level is 10 to 11 g, 250-mL draws are obtained. During blood drawing, we monitor the mother's blood pressure and the fetal heart rates and have had no problems to date, although the numbers are small. Autologous blood can be safely stored for approximately 28 to 35 days.

Monitoring of both fetuses during labor is required, either by auscultation every 15 minutes in the active phase and every 5 minutes in the second stage or by electronic monitoring. Twin machines are available to monitor both babies simultaneously. If a twin machine is not available, then two monitors can be used to accomplish the same purpose. If the times on both monitors are the same, contractions need only be recorded for one fetus and can be superimposed on the tracing of the second, especially where an intrauterine pressure catheter is not in place. Once membranes are ruptured, the latter can be hooked up with one catheter to two machines by linking the machines through a three-way stopcock.

Labor itself is managed as in a singleton gestation in terms of ancillary treatment for complications, e.g., pre-eclampsia, chorioamnionitis, dysfunctional pattern or abnormal progress, or abnormal fetal heart rate patterns.

Some controversy exists regarding whether vaginal delivery should occur in low-birth-weight infants, malpresentations of Twin B, previous cesarean section, and discordancy. The literature is developing in these areas and in the dynamics of obstetrical management. Vaginal delivery of twins is generally supported, especially if Twin A is a vertex, regardless of the position of Twin B.[14, 16, 20, 88–91] Although there appears to be no significant difference in outcome as measured by clinical parameters, in two studies a significant difference in pH level and cord gases was found between Twins A and B, although still within normal limits.[91, 92] With adequate monitoring of the heart rate of the second twin, Apgar scores do not correlate with the time interval between delivery of Twin A and Twin B.[16, 93, 94]

At least one author[91] has described vaginal deliveries when Twin A is a breech and Twin B is a vertex with no cases of interlocking. However, should interlocking occur, the outcome for both fetuses may be very poor.[95, 96] Therefore, cesarean delivery is the procedure of choice, as it is if Twin A is a transverse lie.

When Twin B is a nonvertex, after the birth of the first baby, delivery may involve external cephalic version (for breech or transverse lie), internal version and extraction as a breech, or cesarean section for any of these. When cesarean would be the choice for any malpresentation of Twin B, serious consideration should be given to a cesarean delivery for both. Either external cephalic version or intrauterine operative manipulation is safe in experienced hands.[90, 91, 97, 98] The liberal use of cesarean birth in twin gestations has not resulted in improved fetal outcome.[89, 99, 100]

In infants weighing less than 1500 g, the method of delivery may not affect outcome, and differences in outcome may be related to birth weight, not mode of delivery.[20, 101] Gilbert and colleagues[102] reviewed the literature and concluded that a previous cesarean section does not contradict vaginal delivery of twins. Facilities and physicians must decide their own capabilities and limitations. Tertiary care facilities generally have protocols that undergo frequent revision on the basis of their own or published studies.

The progress of labor is normal in twins, although it may seem slower. Many patients enter labor with some degree of cervical dilation, making the latent phase shorter while the active phase is longer than that of singletons.[103–106] Dysfunctional patterns are more frequent in the preterm twin labor. Dysfunction occurs in a third of nulliparas and in 16% of multiparas with twins, in contrast to 7% of nulliparas and 8% of multiparas with singletons. Therefore, the use of Pitocin to stimulate labor is increased. When Pitocin is properly used, there is no known increased risk of uterine rupture. In our institution, Pitocin is used to stimulate labor as needed in a twin gestation and is managed in the same manner as in singletons. A previous low-segment cesarean section is not a contraindication to stimulation of labor by Pitocin.[107]

Twin Delivery

In our patient population of 169 sets of twins (Table 20–2), 24.9% were delivered by 33 weeks, 30.8% were delivered between 34 and 36 weeks, and 44.3% were delivered at 37 weeks or later. Of the total, 51.4% delivered vaginally, and 10% required cesarean for delivery of Twin B. Before 33 weeks of gestation, 45% delivered vaginally, as did 53.8% of patients at 34 to 36 weeks, and 53% of patients at 37 weeks or later. It is general policy that if Twin A is vertex, vaginal delivery is attempted regardless of the presentation of Twin B. Management of Twin B is then individualized depending on individual preferences. Almost invariably, an infant in a breech presentation or transverse lie undergoes attempted external version under sonographic guidance. If unsuccessful, the breech infant is usually delivered vaginally either as a total breech extraction or as an assisted delivery. Extractions are done when the attending or chief resident has sufficient experience and

Table 20–2. DELIVERIES OF TWINS BY GESTATIONAL AGE AT JACKSON MEMORIAL HOSPITAL

	Gestational Age (Weeks)			
	<33	34–36	≥37	Total
Number of sets	42	52	75	169
% of total	24.9	30.8	44.3	
Vaginal delivery	19	28	40	87
% Delivered Cephalic vaginally	45	53.8	53	51.4

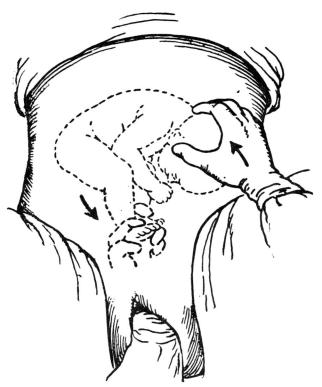

Figure 20–6. Left scapula (acromion) posterior. The anterior foot or both feet are grasped and gently extracted. Note the operator's right hand lifting the head toward the fundus. (From Beck AC, Rosenthal AH: Obstetrical Practice, 6th Edition, Baltimore: Williams & Wilkins, 1955, p. 915.)

comfort with the procedure. The transverse lie that persists is also managed on an individualized basis as described. A version and extraction are attempted under sonographic guidance. This is ideally attempted before membranes rupture, when adequate amniotic fluid facilitates fetal rotation.

Version is easiest when the back is up (scapular or acromion posterior) in a transverse lie; it is done in the following manner: The operator's hand that is on the same side as the fetal feet (Fig. 20–6) is introduced through the cervix, which must be fully dilated, to grasp both feet if possible. The extremities are grasped about the ankles and gently brought down, while at the same time either the operator or an assistant, using the sonographic transducer or a hand, lifts the head toward the fundus transabdominally.

Under sonography, the operator can easily see the feet or palpate along the upper side of the baby to identify the buttock, and then move down to grasp the feet. If both feet cannot be grasped, it is preferable to grasp the anterior foot so that during rotation and extraction the back will remain anterior (Figs. 20–6 and 20–7).

If the back is down (scapular or acromion anterior), the procedure is more difficult. The operator's hand is introduced this time behind the fetal back to the posterior foot (Fig. 20–8). Because both feet are toward the fundus, it may be difficult to grasp

them. It is best then to grasp the posterior or lower leg (Figs. 20–9 and 20–10) so the infant will rotate with its back anterior. If the abdomen rotates anteriorly, gentle pressure against the buttocks to rotate the breech is generally sufficient to rotate the back anteriorly. If membranes have not already ruptured, they can now be ruptured, and with a combination of steady gentle downward traction and maternal pushing, the infant is delivered as in a total breech extraction (see Chapter 19).

There is no reason to panic if the abdomen persists as anterior. The delivery is continued in the same manner until the shoulders are delivered. The head must now be born by flexion (Fig. 20–11). Using the Prague maneuver, the operator lifts the whole body onto the maternal abdomen, which flexes the head. The occiput will be born first, followed by the forehead and the rest of the face with the chin resting on the inferior symphysis pubis. If the head does not descend, the chin is likely caught by the superior border of the symphysis. The operator inserts one hand to make the diagnosis and rotates the chin into an oblique diameter, causing it to slip off the bone.

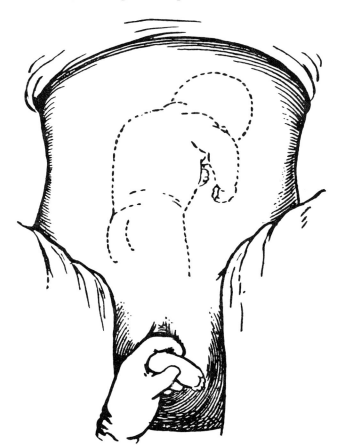

Figure 20–7. Left scapula (acromion) posterior. The version from a left scapular (acromion) posterior position is complete, with the back anterior having delivered what was the upper extremity (see Fig. 20–6). (From Beck AC, Rosenthal AH: Obstetrical Practice, 6th Edition, Baltimore: Williams & Wilkins, 1955, p. 915.)

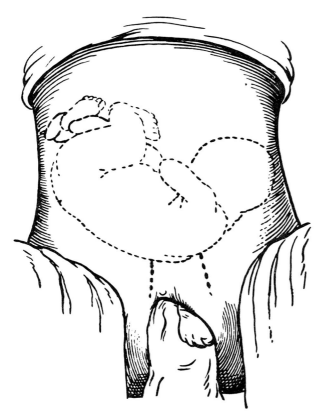

Figure 20–8. Left scapula (acromion) anterior. The operator's hand is inserted behind the fetal body to grasp the posterior foot. (From Beck AC, Rosenthal AH: Obstetrical Practice, 6th Edition, Baltimore: Williams & Wilkins, 1955, p. 918.)

It is wise to be prepared to make Dührssen incisions in case the cervix should clamp down, although this is unusual if the operator made certain before starting the extraction that the cervix was fully dilated and if membranes were intact at initiation of the procedure (see Chapter 19). Without an experienced obstetrician and/or sonographic guidance, attempting a version would be unwise.

If one waits after delivery of the first infant, the cervix may contract down, resulting in an entrapped head or raised arms or both. Attempting the version through intact membranes immediately after delivering the first infant eliminates the need for additional anesthesia because the uterus is still distended and contractions have not yet resumed. If the uterus is contracting or is not relaxed, general anesthesia with good uterine relaxation is required to do a version.

All vaginal twin deliveries are conducted in the atmosphere of a double setup. Piper forceps should always be in the room and on the table if one infant is vertex and the other is nonvertex before delivery.

If the operator has insufficient expertise with intrauterine manipulation or the status of Twin B is such that it may be more safely managed by cesarean section, then cesarean delivery is the procedure of choice. The operator must weigh the long- and short-term risks and benefits to mother and fetus in choosing the procedure for delivery. Some of these choices will, by necessity, be based on individual skills, hospital circumstances, and facilities.

Examination of the Placenta

It is every obstetrician's responsibility to carefully examine the twin placenta, document the findings at delivery, and obtain a pathologic examination. Chorionicity is important to help establish zygosity, which could be important in future tissue transplants. A monozygous pair will accept a transplant, whereas a dizygous pair will react as any two related individuals. If examination of the separating membranes reveals only the two amnions and one placenta, then the twins are monozygous. If there are two placentas and/or two chorions, the twins can be either monozygous or dizygous. Of course, if the babies are of different sex, they are dizygous. Twins who are of the same sex and have a dichorionic, diamnionic placenta should have further documentation of blood types to help determine zygosity for future use.

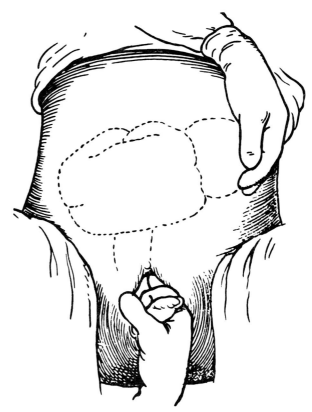

Figure 20–9. Left scapula (acromion) posterior. The posterior leg is brought down into the vagina, while the operator lifts the head toward the fundus to facilitate rotation. (From Beck AC, Rosenthal AH: Obstetrical Practice, 6th Edition, Baltimore: Williams & Wilkins, 1955, p. 918.)

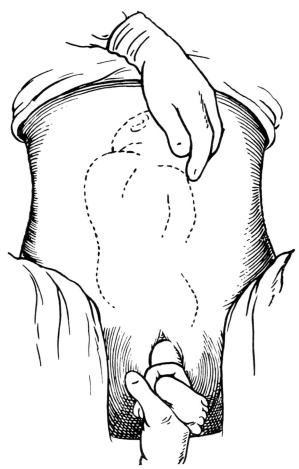

Figure 20–10. The version is complete, with the fetal back anterior; extraction now can be carried out. (From Beck AC, Rosenthal AH: Obstetrical Practice, 6th Edition, Baltimore: Williams & Wilkins, 1955, p. 918.)

OTHER MULTIPLE GESTATIONS

Ovulation-inducing agents have resulted in an increase of other multiple gestations such as triplets,[108–111] at least doubling the rate.[111] In a program of outpatient management of triplet pregnancy, the average gestational age and birth weight at delivery were 33 ± 3.5 weeks and 1869 ± 486 g, respectively (Fig. 20–12). Home uterine monitoring and frequent daily nursing contact seemed to contribute to a clustering of deliveries between 29 and 37 weeks. This management decreased the number of hospital days without significantly affecting delivery timing. Part of this decrease may be related to early diagnosis and decreased maternal activity.

The method of delivery of triplets increasingly has been by cesarean birth[108–113] in an attempt to decrease fetal trauma and acidemia associated with birth order. Biochemical studies suggest that, regardless of method of delivery, infants delivered within 10 minutes of each other show no significant acid/base differences in relation to birth or-

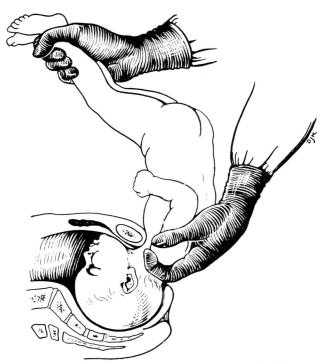

Figure 20–11. The Prague maneuver. The body is lifted into the maternal abdomen. (From Moir JC, Myercoualt PR: Munro Kerr's Operative Obstetrics, 8th Edition, Baltimore: Williams & Wilkins, 1971, p. 172).

der.[114, 115] Perinatal survival, as in all pregnancies, is related to gestational age. As expected, there is an increase in medical/obstetrical complications of pregnancy, some of which lead to early delivery[111] (Fig. 20–13).

The increasing number of cases of more than three fetuses in utero presents an even greater risk of complications and preterm delivery with the resultant complications. Such gestations were a medical oddity in the past, with minimal chance of survival. With modern treatment of infertility, the frequency of such gestations has increased,

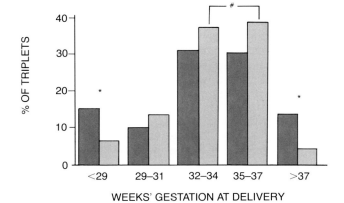

Figure 20–12. Gestational age in triplets. Grey bars—study population. black bars—literature survey. *—p = <0.01; #—p = <0.01. (Redrawn from Newman RB, et al.: Outpatient triplet management: A contemporary review. Am J Obstet Gynecol 161:551, 1989.)

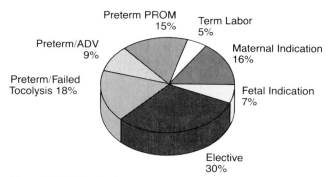

Figure 20–13. Indications for delivery in triplets. Fetal indications include intrauterine growth retardation, abruptio placentae, and fetal distress. Maternal indications include pregnancy-induced hypertension, pulmonary edema, abdominal pain, and chorioamnionitis. PROM—Premature rupture of membranes; ADV—advanced cervical dilatation. (Redrawn from Newman RB, et al.: Outpatient triplet management: A contemporary review. Am J Obstet Gynecol 161:547, 1989.)

just as that of twins and triplets has. In England and Wales, the perinatal and infant mortality rate for triplets was 31%, for quadruplets 45%, and almost 45% for quintuplets. Septuplets had a mortality rate of 91% from 1975 to 1983.[116]

A survey of the literature on multiple pregnancies by Petrikovsky and Vintzileos[117] revealed that for the reported cases of quadruplets, the average age at delivery was 31.08 ± 6.84 weeks. Of the 17 cases reported, 8 were delivered vaginally before 1980. More recently, the delivery of choice has been cesarean section because of second-stage complications such as cord prolapse, malpresentation, and fetal collision.

The reported incidence of quadruplets is 1 per 5370 to 600,000; quintuplets are more rare, at 1 per 15 to 20 million deliveries. Eight sets of quintuplets delivered at later than 27 weeks' gestation were collected from the literature. The majority (six sets) delivered vaginally, with an excellent outcome in infants at 32 weeks or greater. Vaginal deliveries included spontaneous, forceps, and breech extractions. All but one patient was managed on bed rest with no mention of tocolysis. One of two sets of septuplets resulted in five normal survivors. In the only set of octuplets, five infants survived, and none of the one set of nontuplets survived.[117]

Many multifetal gestations that occur as a result of ovulation induction and in vitro fertilization never reach viability. This is most unfortunate for the patients undergoing these procedures because they are then faced with a monumental new problem, i.e., pregnancy loss versus selective reduction of a multifetal gestation. It is essential that technology be perfected to reduce the number of multiconceptions. Technology is available to safely reduce the fetal number, a decision that is very difficult ethically and morally for the couples involved. Currently, transabdominal and transvaginal reductions have been successful, resulting in

few total losses. Most physicians will reduce to two fetuses, some to three, and some to one.[118–122] When faced with the alternative of total pregnancy loss, many couples choose to reduce the number of fetuses. Cerclages in a small group of triplets and quadruplets compared with a noncerclage group treated in the usual fashion (bed rest, β-mimetics, and dexamethasone) resulted in a significantly longer gestation (30.7 vs. 35 weeks) and a better perinatal outcome.[123]

Perhaps use of this technique combined with a very aggressive multidrug approach to decrease uterine irritability and prolonged bed rest is an alternate approach to selective reduction until multiconception can be avoided.

References

1. Corney G: Mythology and customs associated with twins. In MacGillivary I, Nylander PPS, Corney G (eds.): Human Multiple Reproduction. London: W. B. Saunders Co. 1975, p. 1.
2. Speroff L, Glass RH, Kase NG: Regulation of the menstrual cycle. In Speroff L, Glass RH, Kase NG (eds.): Clinical Gynecology, Endocrinology and Infertility, 3rd Edition. Baltimore: Williams & Wilkins, 1983, p. 75.
3. Harris DW: Letter to the editor. J Reprod Med 27:39, 1982.
4. Stockard CR: An experimental study of twins, double monsters and single deformities. Am J Anat 28:115, 1921.
5. Vaughn TC, Powell LC: The obstetrical management of conjoined twins. Obstet Gynecol 53:(Suppl)67, 1989.
6. Landy HJ, Weiner S, Corson SL, et al.: The "vanishing twin." Ultrasonographic assessment of fetal disappearance in the first trimester. Am J Obstet Gynecol 155:14, 1986.
7. Parisi P: Familial incidence of twinning. Nature 304:626, 1983.
8. Nylander PPS: Biosocial aspects of multiple births. J Biosoc Sci 3:(Suppl)29, 1971.
9. Nylander PPS: Serum levels of gonadotropins in relation to multiple pregnancy in Nigeria. J Obstet Gynaecol Br Commonw 80:651, 1973.
10. Creinan M, Keith L: The Yoruba contribution to our understanding of the twinning process. J Reprod Med 34:379, 1989.
11. Derom C, Derom R, Vlietinck R, et al.: Increased monozygotic twinning rate after ovulation induction. Lancet 1:1237, 1987.
12. Hrubec Z, Robinette D: The study of human twins in medical research. N Engl J Med 310:435, 1984.
13. Schenker JG, Yarkoni S, Granat M: Multiple pregnancies following induction of ovulation. Fertil Steril 35:105, 1981.
14. Farooqui MO, Grossman JR, Shannon RA: A review of twin pregnancy and perinatal mortality. Obstet Gynecol Surv 28:(Suppl)144, 1973.
15. Keith L, Ellis R, Berger GS, et al.: The Northwestern University multihospital twin study. A description of 588 twin pregnancies and associated pregnancy loss (1971–1975). Am J Obstet Gynecol 138:781, 1980.
16. Chervenak FA, Yoricha S, Johnson RE, et al.: Twin gestation: Antenatal diagnosis and perinatal outcome in 385 consecutive pregnancies. J Reprod Med 29:727, 1984.
17. Persson PH, Kullander S: Long term experience of general ultrasound screening in pregnancy. Am J Obstet Gynecol 146:942, 1983.
18. Carlan S, Angel JL, Sawai SK, et al.: Late diagnosis of nonconjoined monoamniotic twins using tomographic imaging: A case report. Obstet Gynecol 76:504, 1990.

19. Turner RJ, Hankins GD: Magnetic resonance imaging and ultrasonography in the antenatal evaluation of conjoined twins. Am J Obstet Gynecol 155:645, 1986.

20. McCarthy BJ, Sachs BP, Layde PM, et al.: The epidemiology of neonatal death in twins. Am J Obstet Gynecol 141:252, 1981.

21. Ghai V, Vadayasagar D: Morbidity and mortality factors in twins. An epidemiological approach. Clin Perinatol 15:123, 1988.

22. Mueller-Heubach E: Complications of multiple gestation. Clin Obstet Gynecol 27:1003, 1984.

23. Bernirschke EK: Twin placenta in perinatal mortality. NY State J Med 61:1499, 1961.

24. Myrianthopoulos NC: An epidemiologic survey of twins in a large prospectively studied population. Am J Hum Genet 22:611, 1970.

25. Nylander PPS: Perinatal mortality in twins. Acta Genet Med Gemellol (Roma) 28:363, 1979.

26. Kohl SG, Casey G: Twin gestation. Mt Sinai J Med 42:523, 1975.

27. Rattan PK, Knuppel RA, O'Brien WF: Intrauterine fetal death in twins after 32 weeks of gestation (Abstract 132). Presented at the annual meeting of the Society of Perinatol Obstetricians, San Antonio, Texas, 1984.

28. Desgranges MF, DeMuylder X, Moutquin JM, et al.: Perinatal profile of twin pregnancies: A retrospective review of eleven years (1969–1979) at Hopital Notre Dame, Montreal, Canada. Acta Genet Med Gemollol (Roma) 31:157, 1982.

29. Cetrulo CL: The controversy of mode of delivery in twins: The intrapartum management of twin gestation. Semin Perinatol 10:39, 1986.

30. Ohel G, Granat M, Zeevi D, et al.: Advanced ultrasonic maturation in twin pregnancies. Am J Obstet Gynecol 156:76, 1987.

31. Panel discussion: Outcome of twin birth. Acta Genet Med Gemellol (Roma) 28:369, 1979.

32. Petterson F, Smedby B, Lindmark G: Outcome of twin birth. Review of 1636 children born in twin birth. Acta Paediatr Scand 65:473, 1976.

33. McKeown T, Record RG: Observations on fetal growth in multiple pregnancy in man. J Endocrinol 5:387, 1952.

34. Eastman NJ, Hellman LM: In William's Obstetrics 12th Edition. New York: Appleton-Century-Crofts Inc. 1961, p 703.

34a. Aaron JB, Halpern J: Fetal survival in 376 twin deliveries. Am J Obstet Gynecol 69:795, 1955.

35. Bender S: Twin pregnancy. J Obstet Gynaecol Br Emp 59:511, 1952.

36. Guttmacher AF, Kohl SG: The fetus of multiple gestations. Obstet Gynecol 12:528, 1958.

37. MacGillivray I: Some observations on the incidence of preeclampsia. J Obstet Gynaecol Br Emp 65:536, 1958.

38. Melnick M, Myrianthopoulos NC: The effect of chorion type in normal and abnormal development variation in monozygotic twins. Am J Med Genet 4:147, 1979.

39. Myrianthopoulos NC: Congenital anomalies in twins. Acta Genet Med Gemellol (Roma) 25:331, 1976.

40. Hoyme HE, Higgenbotham MC, Jones KL: Vascular etiology of disruptive structural defects in monozygotic twins. Pediatrics 62:288, 1981.

41. Schinzel AA, Smith DW, Miller JR: Monozygotic twinning and structural defects. J Pediatr 95:921, 1979.

42. Jones KL, Bernirschke K: The developmental pathogenesis of structural defects: The contribution of monozygotic twins. Semin Perinatol 10:9, 1986.

43. Russel JK: Maternal and foetal hazards associated with twin pregnancy. J Obstet Gynaecol Br Emp 59:208, 1952.

44. Crowther CA, Verkuyl DAA, Neilson JP, et al.: The effects of hospitalization for rest in fetal growth, neonatal morbidity and length of gestation in twin pregnancy. Br J Obstet Gynaecol 97:872, 1990.

45. MacLennon AH, Green RC, O'Shea RT, et al.: Routine hospital admission between 26 and 30 weeks gestation. Lancet 335:267, 1990.

46. Saunders MC, Dick JS, Brown I, et al.: The effects of hospital admission for bedrest in duration of twin pregnancy: A randomized trial. Lancet 2:793, 1985.

47. O'Connor MC, Arias E, Raystan JP: The merits of antenatal care for twin pregnancies. Br J Obstet Gynaecol 88:222, 1981.

48. Weikes ARL, Menzies DN, DeBoer CH: The relative efficacy of bedrest, cervical suture and no treatment in the management of twin pregnancy. Br J Obstet Gynaecol 84:161, 1977.

49. Dor J, Shaler J, Mashiach G, et al.: Elective cervical suture of twin pregnancies diagnosed ultrasonographically in the first trimester following induced ovulation. Gynaecol Obstet Invest 13:55, 1982.

50. Hartikainen-Sorri AL, Jouppila P: Is routine hospitalization needed in the antenatal care of twin pregnancy? J Perinat Med 12:31, 1984.

51. Cetrulo CL, Freeman RK: Ritodrine HCL for the prevention of premature labor in twin pregnancies. Acta Genet Med Gemellol (Roma) 25:321, 1975.

52. Mathews DO, Friend JM, Michael CA: A double blind trial of oral isoxuprine in the prevention of premature labour. J Obstet Gynaecol Br Commonw 74:68, 1967.

53. O'Connor MC, Murphy F, Dalrymple IJ: Double blind trial of ritodrine and placebo in twin pregnancy. Br J Obstet Gynaecol 86:706, 1979.

54. Gummerus M, Halonen O: Prophylactic long term oral tocolysis of multiple pregnancies. Br J Obstet Gynaecol 94:249, 1987.

55. Skjaerris J, Abery A: Prevention of prematurity in twin pregnancy by orally administered terbutaline. Acta Obstet Gynecol Scand 108:39, 1982.

56. Marivate M, De Villiers KQ, Fairbrother P: Effect of prophylactic outpatient administration of fenoterol on the time and onset of spontaneous labor and fetal growth rate in twin pregnancy. Am J Obstet Gynecol 128:707, 1977.

57. Burkett G, Bauer CR, Morrison JC, et al.: Effect of prenatal dexamethasone administration in prevention of respiratory distress syndrome in twin pregnancies. J Perinatol 6:304, 1986.

58. Knuppel RA, Lake MF, Watson DL, et al.: Preventing preterm birth in twin gestation: Home uterine activity monitoring and perinatal nursing support. Obstet Gynecol 76:(Suppl)245, 1990.

59. Garite TJ, Bentley DL, Hamer CA: Uterine activity characteristics in multiple gestations. Obstet Gynecol 76:(Suppl)56, 1990.

60. Landy HJ, Weingold AB: Management of multiple gestation complicated by intrauterine fetal demise. Obstet Gynecol Surv 44:171, 1989.

61. DeLia JE, Cukierski MA, Lundergan DK: Neodymium yttrium-aluminum-garnet laser occlusion of rhesus placental vasculature via fetoscopy. Am J Obstet Gynecol 160:485, 1989.

62. DeLia JE, Cruikshank DP, Keye WR: Fetoscopic neodymium: YAG laser occlusion of placental vessels in severe twin transfusion syndrome (Abstract 28). Presented at the annual meeting of the Society of Perinatol Obstetricians, Houston, Texas, 1990.

63. Neilson J, Grant A: Ultrasound in pregnancy. In Chalmers I, Enkin M, Keirse M (eds.): Effective Care in Pregnancy and Childbirth Oxford, England: Oxford University Press, 1989, p. 425.

64. Iffy L, Lavenhar MA, Jakobovitz A, et al.: The rate of early intrauterine growth in twin gestation. Am J Obstet Gynecol 146:970, 1983.

65. Erkola R, Ala-Mello S, Piiroinen O, et al.: Growth discordancy in twin pregnancies: A risk factor not detected by measurements of biparietal diameter. Obstet Gynecol 66:203, 1985.

66. Leveno KJ, Santos-Ramos R, Duenholter JH, et al.: Sonar cephalometry in twin pregnancy: Discordancy of the bi-

parietal diameter after 28 weeks gestation. Am J Obstet Gynecol 138:615, 1980.

67. Baines ER, Romero R, Scott D, et al.: The value of biparietal diameter and abdominal perimeter in the diagnosis of growth retardation in twin gestation. Am J Perinatol 2:221, 1985.

68. Townsend RR, Simpson GF, Filly RA: Membrane thickness in ultrasound prediction of chorionicity of twin gestations. J Ultrasound Med 7:327, 1988.

69. Rodis JF, Vintzileos AM, Campbell WA, et al.: Intrauterine fetal growth in discordant twin gestations. J Ultrasound Med 9:443, 1990.

70. Abuhamad A, O'Sullivan MJ, Salman F, et al.: Sonographic evaluation of twin gestations at 20–25 weeks to predict discordance (Abstract 383). Presented at the meeting of the Society of Perinatol Obstetricians, Houston, Texas, 1990.

71. Robertson EG, Neer K: Placental injection studies in twin gestation. Obstet Gynecol 147:170, 1983.

72. Bernirschke K, Kim CK: Multiple pregnancy (first of two parts). N Engl J Med 288:1276, 1973.

73. Saldana LR, Eads MC, Shaefer JR: Umbilical wave forms in fetal surveillance of twins. Am J Obstet Gynecol 157:712, 1987.

74. Farmakaides G, Schulman H, Saldana JR, et al.: Surveillance of a twin pregnancy with umbilical arterial velocimetry. Am J Obstet Gynecol 153:789, 1985.

75. Chescheir N, Seeds JW: Polyhydramnios and oligohydramnios in twin gestations. Obstet Gynecol 71:882, 1988.

76. Cifuentes R, Oiley P, Balfe J, et al.: Indomethacin and renal function in premature infants with persistent ductus arteriosus. J Pediatr 95:583, 1979.

77. Gouyin JB, Guignard JP: Drugs and acute renal insufficiency in the neonate. Biol Neonate 50:177, 1986.

78. Cantor B, Tyler T, Nelson R, et al.: Oligohydramnios and transient neonatal anuria. A possible complication with the maternal use of prostaglandin synthetase inhibitors. J Reprod Med 24:220, 1984.

79. Hendriks SK, Smith JR, Moore DE, et al.: Oligohydramnios associated with prostaglandin synthetase inhibitors in preterm labor. Br J Obstet Gynaecol 97:312, 1990.

80. Pitkin RM: Acute polyhydramnios recurrent in successive pregnancies. Obstet Gynecol 48:(Suppl)42, 1976.

81. D'Alton ME, Dudly DRL: Ultrasound in the antenatal management of twin gestation. Semin Perinatol 10:30, 1986.

82. Hays PM, Smeltzer JS: Multiple gestation. Clin Obstet Gynecol 29:264, 1986.

83. Leveno KJ, Quirk JG, Whalley PJ, et al.: Fetal lung maturation in twin gestation. Am J Obstet Gynecol 148:405, 1984.

84. Cohen S, Tan S, Albright GA, et al.: Epidural fentanyl/bupivacaine mixture for obstetric analgesia. Anesthesiology 67:403, 1987.

85. Hunt CO, Naulty JS, Bader AM: Perioperative analgesia with subarachnoid fentanyl bupivacaine for cesarean delivery. Anesthesia 71:535, 1989.

86. Jaschevatzky OE, Shaht A, Levy Y, et al.: Epidural analgesia during labor in twin pregnancy. Br J Obstet Gynaecol 84:327, 1977.

87. Crawford JS: A prospective study of 200 consecutive twin deliveries. Anaesthesia 42:33, 1987.

88. Acker D, Lieberman M, Holbrook H, et al.: Delivery of the second twin. Obstet Gynecol 59:710, 1982.

89. Chervenak FA, Johnson RE, Berkowitz RL, et al.: Is routine cesarean section necessary for vertex-breech and vertex transverse twin gestations? Am J Obstet Gynecol 148:1, 1984.

90. Rabinovici J, Baikai G, Richman B, et al.: Randomized management of the second non vertex twin: Vaginal delivery or cesarean section? Am J Obstet Gynecol 156:52, 1987.

91. Laros RK, Dattel BJ: Management of twin pregnancy:

The vaginal route is still safe. Am J Obstet Gynecol 158:1330, 1988.

92. Young BK, Suidan J, Antoine C, et al.: Differences in twins: The importance of birth order. Am J Obstet Gynecol 151:915, 1984.

93. Cetrulo C: The controversy of mode of delivery in twins. The intrapartum management of twin gestation. Semin Perinatol 10:39, 1986.

94. Rayburn WF, Lavin JP, Miodovnik M, et al.: Multiple gestation: Time interval between delivery of the first and second twin. Obstet Gynecol 63:502, 1984.

95. Nissen ED: Twins: Collision, impaction, compaction and interlocking. Obstet Gynecol 11:514, 1958.

96. Cohen M, Kohl SG, Rosenthal AH: Fetal interlocking complicating twin gestation. Am J Obstet Gynecol 91:407, 1965.

97. Gocke SE, Nageotte MP, Garite T: Management of the non-vertex second twin: Primary cesarean section, external version, or primary breech extraction. Am J Obstet Gynecol 161:111, 1989.

98. Chervenak FA, Johnson RE, Berkowitz RL, et al.: Intrapartum external version of the second twin. Obstet Gynecol 62:160, 1983.

99. Medearis AL, Jonas HS, Stockbauer JW, et al.: Perinatal deaths in twin pregnancy: A five year analysis of statewide statistics in Missouri. Am J Obstet Gynecol 134:413, 1979.

100. Bell D, Johansson D, McLean FH, et al.: Birth asphyxia, trauma and mortality in twins. Has cesarean section improved the outcome? Am J Obstet Gynecol 154:235, 1986.

101. Morales WJ, O'Brien WF, Knuppel RA, et al.: The effect of mode of delivery in the risk of intraventricular hemorrhage in nondiscordant twin gestations under 1500 gms. Obstet Gynecol 73:107, 1989.

102. Gilbert L, Saunders N, Sharp F: The management of multiple pregnancy in women with a lower segment scar. Is a repeat cesarean section really the "safe" option? Br J Obstet Gynaecol 95:1312, 1988.

103. Friedman EA: Labor: Clinical Evaluation and Management, 2nd Edition. New York: Appleton-Century-Crofts, 1978.

104. Friedman EA, Sachtelben MR: The effect of uterine overdistention in labor: I. Multiple pregnancy. Obstet Gynecol 23:164, 1964.

105. Friedman EA, Sachtelben MR: The effect of uterine overdistention in labor: II. Hydramnios. Obstet Gynecol 23:401, 1964.

106. Friedman EA, Sachtelben MR: Preterm labor. Am J Obstet Gynecol 104:1152, 1969.

107. Leroy F: Oxytocin treatment in twin pregnancy labour. Acta Genet Med Gemallol (Roma) 28:303, 1979.

108. Loucopoulous A, Jewelewicz R: Management of multifetal pregnancies: Sixteen years of experience at the Sloane Hospital for Women. Am J Obstet Gynecol 145:902, 1989.

109. Holcberg G, Beale Y, Lewenthal H, et al.: Outcome of pregnancy in 31 triplet gestations. Obstet Gynecol 59:472, 1982.

110. Ron-El R, Caspi E, Schreyer P, et al.: Triplet and quadruplet pregnancies and management. Obstet Gynecol 57:458, 1981.

111. Newman RB, Hamer C, Miller MC: Outpatient triplet management: A contemporary review. Am J Obstet Gynecol 161:547, 1989.

112. Daw E: Triplet pregnancy. Br J Obstet Gynaecol 85:505, 1978.

113. Itzkowic D: A survey of 59 triplet pregnancies. Br J Obstet Gynaecol 86:23, 1979.

114. Antoine C, Kirshenbaum NW, Young BK: Biochemical differences related to birth order in triplets. J Reprod Med 31:330, 1986.

115. Creinin M, MacGregor S, Socol M, et al.: The Northwestern University triplet study IV. Biochemical parameters. Am J Obstet Gynecol 159:1140, 1988.

116. Botting BJ, Davies IM, MacFarlane AJ: Recent trends in the incidence of multiple births and associated mortality. Arch Dis Child 62:941, 1987.

117. Petrikovsky BM, Vintzileos AM: Management and outcome of multiple pregnancy of high fetal order: Literature review. Obstet Gynecol Surv 44:578, 1989.

118. Itzkowic J, Boedes R, Thaler I, et al.: Transvaginal ultrasonography-guided aspiration of gestational sacs for selective abortion in multiple pregnancy. Am J Obstet Gynecol 160:215, 1989.

119. Birnholz JC, Donowski WP, Binoi Z, et al.: Selective continuation in gonadotropin-induced multiple pregnancy. Fertil Steril 48:873, 1987.

120. Shalev J, Frankel Y, Goldenberg E, et al.: Selective reduction in multiple gestations: Pregnancy outcome after transvaginal and transabdominal needle guided procedures. Fertil Steril 52:416, 1989.

121. Evans MI, Fletcher JC, Zacor IE: Selective first trimester termination in octuplet and quadruplet pregnancies. Clinical and ethical issues. Obstet Gynecol 71:289, 1988.

122. Berkowitz RL, Lynch L, Chitkara U: Selective reduction of multifetal pregnancies in the first trimester. N Engl J Med 318:1043, 1988.

123. Goldman GA, Dicker D, Peleg D, et al.: Is elective cerclage justified in the management of triplet and quadruplet pregnancy? Aust NZ Obstet Gynaecol 29:9, 1989.

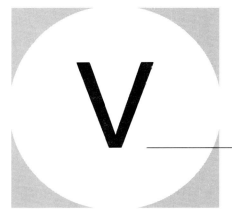

Complications of Vaginal Delivery

Episiotomy and Repair

Warren C. Plauché

- ■ HISTORICAL PERSPECTIVES
- ■ SURGICAL PRINCIPLES
- ■ MIDLINE EPISIOTOMY PROCEDURE
- ■ MEDIOLATERAL EPISIOTOMY PROCEDURE

- ■ MODIFIED MEDIAN EPISIOTOMY
- ■ POST-EPISIOTOMY CARE
- ■ SUMMARY

Episiotomy is an intrapartal incision of the perineum to increase the space available for delivery. It was developed to reduce (a) the risk of injury to maternal soft tissue during the birth process, (b) the resistance of soft tissue to delivery, and (c) the risk of birth injury to the child. In previous obstetric eras, large episiotomies increased the room available to accomplish vaginal delivery of babies who were large, in breech presentation, in a transverse lie, or rotated by forceps. These indications have become much less common in modern obstetrics.

The muscles and fascial planes of the pelvic diaphragm support the bladder, urethra, and rectum against the relentless pull of gravity. Obstetric injury to these structures causes cystocele, rectocele, and uterine prolapse. The symptoms of urinary incontinence, difficult defecation, and loss of introital constriction powers caused by these injuries have been a bane to womankind. Their treatment forms the basis for reparative gynecology. Efforts to prevent the problems related to

perineal soft-tissue injury led to prophylactic episiotomy and perineal reconstruction at the time of obstetric delivery.

The repetitive pressure of the fetal head against the heavy muscles of the pelvic floor may be responsible for some portion of infant birth trauma. Early proponents of episiotomy sought to reduce birth trauma to infants by incising the maternal perineum. Intrapartal hypoxia is a much more important cause of birth-related difficulties for the infant.

HISTORICAL PERSPECTIVES

The writings of Aristotle are evidence of early concern for the perineum at the time of obstetric delivery.[1] Salves, ointments, and immobilization of the mother's legs after delivery were the limits of early management of maternal perineal injury. Fielding Ould,[2] when second master at the Rotunda Hospital, wrote the first English-language description of episiotomy in 1742. Ould described the dangers of extraordinary soft-tissue dystocia. He recommended a "single Pinch with Probe-Sizars" to assist outlet delivery. He further recommended, "If the incision be made so near the rectum as to weaken its contraction, the wound must be united by a stitch."[2] These words launched the most common operation on women in Western medicine.

Episiotomy did not become a popular obstetric operation until obstetric delivery moved from the home to the hospital more than 150 years after Ould's book. Pomeroy[3] suggested routine median episiotomy and repair as early as 1918. Williams of Baltimore, who exerted a controlling influence on American obstetrics in his time, advocated noninterference. He recommended mediolateral episiotomies only for specific obstetric operative deliveries. DeLee of Chicago advocated routine mediolateral episiotomies and prophylactic outlet forceps for most deliveries. Because the widely flared shanks of DeLee's divergent forceps extended median episiotomy incisions, it is logical that he championed the mediolateral method.[4]

Eastman,[4] who succeeded Williams at Johns Hopkins Hospital, began in the 1940s to vigorously advocate median rather than mediolateral episiotomies. His influence resulted in marked reduction in the use of the mediolateral method. Barter and colleagues[5] recorded the rise in midline episiotomies at George Washington University Hospital from 62% of episiotomies in 1948 to 95% of episiotomies in 1958. Eighty percent of all deliveries in their series had episiotomies. Dallas[6] in 1953 further encouraged routine episiotomy as standard practice for obstetric delivery.

The controversy over median versus mediolateral episiotomy sprang from fear of potential complications with the midline procedure. Early investigators believed that median episiotomy resulted in a higher percentage of extensions through the rectal sphincter and mucosa than did mediolateral episiotomy. Harris[7] reported that such extensions occurred in 13% of 7477 median episiotomies studied in 1970.

Kaltreider and Dixon[8] reported a 4.5% incidence of third-degree extensions in more than 15,000 central (midline) episiotomies. The incidence of rectal lacerations among 799 mediolateral episiotomies was 5%, the same rate as for the central episiotomy group. The rate of spontaneous third-degree laceration for patients who recieved no episiotomy was 0.25%.

Laceration into the rectum was once a feared complication because it often resulted in permanent fecal incontinence. The risk of permanent sequelae, including fecal incontinence, is very small with modern repair techniques. Complete primary healing of median episiotomy extensions occurred in 96% of the cases in the Harris[7] study. Kaltreider and Dixon[8] found the incidence of rec-

tovaginal fistulae that required repair after central (midline) episiotomy to be 1 in 3055 episiotomies.

Some early investigators felt that median episiotomy did not sufficiently protect the supportive fascial planes of the perineum from delivery trauma.[8] The strongest proponents of this view advocated reconstruction of the perineum after a generous mediolateral episiotomy after each obstetric delivery.[9] I could find no definitive long-range follow-up study to fault or to verify this position.

Most pronouncements on the effectiveness of episiotomy in preventing maternal sequelae from obstetric trauma are anecdotal. A study of the anatomic changes and extended gynecologic follow-up of large, matched, randomized groups of patients over a period of at least 25 years is needed to reach firm conclusions.

The timing of episiotomy is another issue of sustained controversy. Episiotomy incision early in the second stage of labor results in increased blood loss and more rectal injuries but protects perirectal and perivesical fascial layers from tearing forces. Late episiotomy results in less blood loss, a thinner perineum to incise, and recession of the rectum from the line of incision. The fetal head and pelvic fascial planes are subject to more pressure trauma, however. If an episiotomy is performed, it should be done early enough to protect the structures of the pelvic floor from obstetric trauma.

Laufe and Leslie[1] in 1972 reported a dramatic (23 to 28%) reduction in the traction force necessary to extract a baby when episiotomy preceded outlet forceps delivery. These authors implied, but did not measure, a corresponding reduction in compression forces on the fetal head. This finding made a strong case for early performance of episiotomy before forceps delivery.

Blood loss related to the performance of episiotomy can be considerable. Odell and Seski,[10] in a careful examination of blood loss solely from the episiotomy site in 71 patients, found a mean loss of 253 mL, with a range of 50 to 300 mL. The length of time between incision and delivery and between delivery and completion of repair was the major factor related to blood loss. Blood loss was approximately 50 mL/min before delivery and 3 to 5 mL/min after delivery. Shortening the interval between incision and delivery most effectively reduced blood loss.

A renaissance of the obstetrics of minimal intervention arose in the 1970s. There was a resurgence of home deliveries, birthing rooms, and Lamaze coaching and little use of analgesia or anesthesia. Emollients to soften and "iron out" the perineum to prevent lacerations reappeared. Women who opted for delivery styles that relegated hospital facilities and obstetricians to standby roles often declined episiotomies.

In the 1980s cesarean delivery was the answer

to the management of fetal distress, soft-tissue dystocia, and "failure to progress." Forceps rusted on the shelf as cesarean rates soared. Few perinei were at risk for the trauma of prolonged labor or operative vaginal delivery.

Only time will tell what influences the last two decades have had on the incidence of genital herniation and prolapse. The preliminary indications are that advanced degrees of uterine prolapse, cystocele, and rectocele are becoming less frequent. Vaginal hysterectomy with anterior and posterior perineorrhaphy is performed for genital prolapse much less frequently than in the past.

SURGICAL PRINCIPLES

The surgical principles that apply to episiotomy and repair are straightforward. The surgeon seeks complete hemostasis and restoration of the perineum by anatomic approximation of muscles and fascial planes. Primary healing is aided by careful attention to aseptic technique. Primary healing of the perineum yields a near-perfect cosmetic result.

Pain from an episiotomy can be reduced by loose approximation of tissues to allow for edema formation. No suture knots should be left on the perineal skin or at the sensitive hymenal region. Some obstetricians combine repairs of pre-existing introital scarring, deformity, and rectocele with episiotomy repair. Extensive repairs, particularly those involving anterior herniation, should await resolution of the changes related to pregnancy and delivery.

MIDLINE EPISIOTOMY PROCEDURE

There are almost as many episiotomy and repair techniques as there are obstetricians. The method described below is a modification of the technique recommended by Barter and co-workers.[5]

For midline episiotomy, one blade of the scissors enters the vagina, and the other extends down the perineal midline raphe toward the anal verge (Fig. 21–1). Many operators place the scissors between the index and middle fingers of their nondominant hand, which presses outward, distending the introitus and thinning the perineum before incision. The scissor blades encompass vaginal epithelium, perineal skin, the transverse perinei muscles, and the medial fibers of the bulbocavernosus muscles. The tips of the scissors should not extend far enough to threaten the sphincter ani muscle or anal mucosa.

A firm snip of the scissor blades makes the incision. More snips are often necessary, but the operator should not produce a ragged wound. A modest cephalad extension of the apex of the inci-

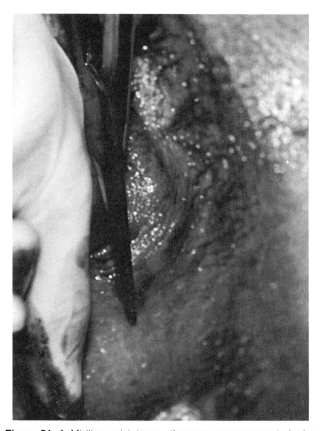

Figure 21–1. Midline episiotomy—the surgeon prepares to incise the perineum with the scissors. The surgeon's fingers tent the perineum and push the rectum downward.

sion in the vaginal epithelium prevents irregular tears in this direction.

Repair of midline episiotomy after delivery begins with a full inspection and palpation of the wound. A rectal examination is performed to check for damage to the anal sphincter or anorectal mucosa.

At midvagina, the vagina and rectum are separated by only a thin layer of areolar connective tissue. "Buttonhole" defects in the anterior anorectal wall high in the intravaginal portion of the episiotomy may develop rectovaginal fistulae if not recognized and repaired. This kind of injury is not necessarily due to a misplaced incision but may arise from delivery events.

Findley[11] first described injuries of the rectal wall without sphincter injury that were due to lacerations from passage of the chin, shoulder, or elbow of the fetus. Kaltreider and Dixon[8] also described this type of injury. Repair of the buttonhole rectal defect high in the incision requires a two-layer bowel closure, as described below. Kaltreider and Dixon[8] recommended treating rectal mucosal defects above an intact sphincter by incising the sphincter and mucosa to the level of the defect. They then repaired the entire defect as a complete perineal laceration. This technique creates a more extensive repair than is necessary in many cases.

The obstetrician should plan for any perineal scar revision or other repair that will accompany the episiotomy closure before the repair begins. Operating gloves should be changed, the wound irrigated with saline, and soiled drapes replaced. A small gauze pack is placed in the vagina above the upper extent of the episiotomy to control lochia flow. Absorbable suture of 00 or 000 chromic catgut or polyglycolic/polyglactin suture is satisfactory for episiotomy repair. Two lengths of suture suffice for all but the most complex repairs.

First, any extension of the episiotomy through the rectal sphincter or into the rectal mucosa is repaired. Exposure for rectal repair will be lost if the vagina and perineum are repaired first. Two layers of 000 absorbable suture swedged onto a gastrointestinal needle close lacerations of the rectal mucosa. There has been controversy about interrupted versus continuous suture and the placement of knots within or above the bowel lumen.

A very satisfactory two-layer closure was described by Barter and co-workers[5] in 1960. The first layer is a continuous Lembert suture of 00 or 000 chromic catgut suture in the submucosa of the rectal wall inverting the rectal mucosa into the bowel lumen (see Fig. 23–6A–C). Synthetic absorbable sutures are preferred by many modern obstetricians.

The operator exposes the apex of the tear and places the first stitch above this point. This suture continues onto the anal verge and is tied. This portion of the field will become obscured by the remainder of the repair. The bowel mucosa must be completely and securely closed at this step.

The operating field is irrigated with saline after restoration of bowel continuity. A second continuous suture imbricates the first layer. Elements of perirectal fascia should be deliberately included to add to the support of this closure (see Fig. 23–6B).

Next, the obstetrician retrieves the severed ends of the sphincter ani. The severed sphincter retracts laterally and inferiorly within its sheath. One end of the muscle is usually visible; the other is deeply retracted. Allis or similar clamps reach into the dimple left by the retracted muscle and grasp each end of the severed muscle. (see Fig. 23–6B).

Gently, the muscle ends are pulled together from each side. Two or three figure-eight sutures of the same material as the episiotomy repair loosely reapproximate the severed muscles (see Fig. 23–6C). Muscle tissue holds sutures poorly. Sphincter sutures should include fascial elements of the muscle sheath. The operating field is again irrigated with saline. Next, the repair of the vagina and perineum is addressed.

Exposure for episiotomy repair is usually adequate without the placement of retractors, which only distort the anatomic relationships and place tension on suture lines. The first suture is begun by passing the needle through the vaginal epithelium just above the apex of the incision. This anchors the suture and secures any apical arterial bleeders. The vaginal epithelium is closed with a continuous, locked suture that incorporates vaginal epithelium and the blood vessel–laden subepithelial layer. The obstetrician should guard against dragging sutures across contaminated areas on the drapes or perianal region. The dangling suture ends are flipped upward to rest on a fresh, sterile drape over the mons veneris.

A cavity forms beneath the vaginal suture line and the anterior rectal wall. The operator carefully secures all arterial bleeding points in this space by separate clamping and tying, not just covering over with sutured tissues. Some physicians prefer to obliterate this potential space by incorporating superficial bites of perirectal fascia in their suture line. Recalling the proximity of the rectum at this level, the operator avoids penetration of the rectal mucosa. The vaginal mucosal suture is carried to the level of the hymenal ring and then is laid aside on the abdominal drapes (Fig. 21–2).

A second suture reapproximates the muscles of the perineum. The purpose of this portion of the surgery is to restore the perineum to its predelivery state. The deepest muscle layer that may have been incised or separated is the pubococcygeus, the medial portion of the levator sling. One or two loosely tied simple sutures will bring these muscle bundles back to their midline location (Fig. 21–3). The physician should avoid building a midvaginal bridge of tissue that might later cause dyspareunia.

A single loosely tied suture brings the transversus perinei muscles back to their median insertion. An inverted mattress suture with the knot buried deep in the tissues causes less discomfort later.

In the literature on episiotomy repair, the crown stitch is frequently discussed. The crown stitch is

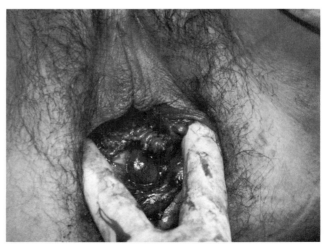

Figure 21–2. Steps in midline episiotomy repair. Step 1: Closure of the vaginal mucosa.

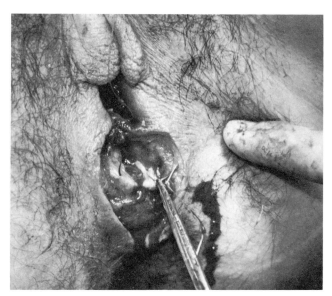

Figure 21-3. Steps in midline episiotomy repair. Step 2: Suture of the transverse perineal muscles.

a finishing suture at the introitus. This stitch is important to restore perineal anatomy. A misplaced, too generous, or too tight crown stitch is an important cause of post-episiotomy introital dyspareunia. Anatomic restoration requires loose reapproximation of the severed bulbocavernosus and superficial transverse perinei muscles (Fig. 21-4). It may take several sutures to accomplish this reapproximation. No single suture should incorporate excessive tissue or bear excessive tension.

One end of the bulbocavernosus muscle usually retracts more than the other, even when the episiotomy is in the midline. Its retraction pulls one or the other labium majorum upward. The operator brings the retracted muscle down to its insertion

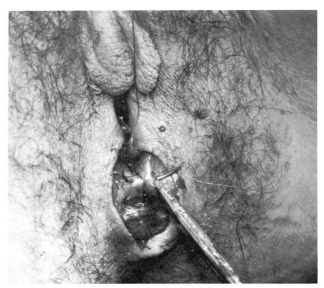

Figure 21-4. Steps in midline episiotomy repair. Step 3: Bulbocavernosus suture.

on the central perineal raphe and restores the symmetry of the vulva without creating tension in the tissues.

A single inverted mattress stitch sometimes suffices. The needle should pass deep into the retracted labium majorum to reach the retracted bulbocavernosus muscle bundles. When a single suture performs this task, it approximates the classical crown stitch. A layer of subcutaneous sutures helps relieve tension on the bulbocavernosus suture and builds perineal support (Fig. 21-5A). Dyspareunia may result if the bulbocavernosus or crown stitch constricts the introitus. Post-episiotomy pain increases if the sutures are under tension or tied too tight. The physician should allow for post-operative edema. Approximation, not strangulation, is key.

Dyspareunia from episiotomy scars frequently occurs at the hymenal ring. Suture material and knots should not be allowed to lie superficially at this sensitive location. The operator strives to achieve accurate approximation of skin and vaginal epithelium to allow primary healing with minimal scarring.

The last portion of the repair completes the perineal skin closure. The previous vaginal epithelium suture is passed deep under the hymenal ring. This suture proceeds as a continuous subcutaneous suture that brings together the superficial connective tissues of the perineum (see Fig. 21-5A). This suture is continued to the lower end of the perineal incision.

The same needle is passed through the dermis just under the skin at the inferior extremity of the perineal incision. This suture then continues up to the introitus as a subcuticular running mattress suture to close the perineal skin (see Fig. 21-5B).

The subcutaneous suture ends by passing through the perineal skin distant from the wound and being cut flush with the skin. It need not be tied. It will adequately approximate the skin and subcutaneous tissues. The complex course of the suture holds it in place. Because the suture is not fixed by a knot, it can retract if edema develops. This helps reduce pain and prevents excessive tension on individual suture lines. Loose tissue approximation and good hemostasis remain the secrets to minimal post-episiotomy discomfort.

MEDIOLATERAL EPISIOTOMY PROCEDURE

The scissors incise the perineum at a 45-degree angle inferiorly from the midline of the introital fourchette. The incision begins in the midline, not partway up one labium. A small error in incision placement when the crowning head distends the introitus is magnified when the tissues relax after delivery. Lateral placement of the episiotomy incision creates an unsightly and often painful scar.

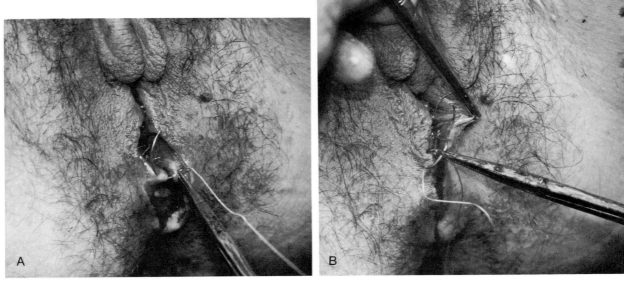

Figure 21–5. Steps in midline episiotomy repair. Step 4: Perineal suture. A, A subcutaneous suture run down to the inferior apex buries all other knots. B, A subcuticular suture running upward closes the perineal skin.

The properly placed mediolateral episiotomy incises the transversus perinei and bulbocavernosus muscles lateral to their midline attachments. This incision deeply incises the pubococcygeal portion of the levator muscle. Mediolateral episiotomy thus may develop more soft-tissue room for delivery than a median episiotomy.

A large mediolateral episiotomy incision sometimes enters the ischiorectal fossa at its most lateral and inferior extent. It should not involve the rectal sphincter.

Repair of mediolateral episiotomy requires more careful attention to anatomic reapproximation of perineal muscles. Otherwise, it is similar to the repair of midline episiotomy.

Mediolateral episiotomy repair begins with closure of the vaginal mucosa, as described previously. Two or more sutures close the defect in the levator sling by reapproximating the muscle fibers and sheath of the pubococcygeal muscle. Bulbocavernosus retraction is much more dramatic with mediolateral than with midline episiotomy. Several stitches are usually necessary to bring the bulbocavernosus muscle into anatomic position without tension.

The superficial portion of the perineal repair is no different from that of midline episiotomy, except in its direction. It is much more difficult to achieve cosmetic perfection and patient comfort with mediolateral incisions than with median incisions.

MODIFIED MEDIAN EPISIOTOMY

Problems with midline episiotomies occur when the perineum is short and when extra room is required for obstetric maneuvers. Under these cir-

cumstances, episiotomy extensions may damage the sphincter or rectum. Mediolateral episiotomies give more room and avoid the rectum, but they are more painful and are difficult to repair to cosmetic perfection. The obstetrician can achieve the cosmetic and post-operative comfort advantages of the midline episiotomy and the safety of a mediolateral episiotomy in one operation.

The incision in a modified median episiotomy begins in the midline fourchette of the introitus. The incision is directed in the midline toward the rectum for the length of the perineal body down to the rectal sphincter. If the operator needs more room than this midline incision affords, the incision is angled 20 to 30 degrees to the right or left. This incision takes a hockey-stick detour to avoid the rectal sphincter and rectum.

The modified median episiotomy affords almost as much soft-tissue room as the mediolateral episiotomy. If it extends from excessive introital distension, it does not tear the sphincter or rectum.

Repair of the modified median episiotomy resembles that of a midline perineal incision. The hockey-stick portion around the sphincter can be straightened during repair as the perineal muscles are brought together in the midline. This repair lengthens the perineal body and builds support for the lower vagina and rectum. The final cosmetic result closely resembles that of the midline episiotomy.

POST-EPISIOTOMY CARE

Many compulsive regimens have been proposed for the immediate post-delivery period. Few are more than meddlesome routines. An ice pack to the perineum immediately after delivery probably does reduce tissue edema. Anesthetic or antiseptic sprays are unnecessary. Heat lamps to the perineum do little to enhance healing. Antibiotics are unnecessary in all but the most contaminated of episiotomy wounds.

Soft seating painfully spreads the edges of the episiotomy incision and causes pain. For comfort, the patient sits on one buttock on the edge of a firm chair.

The initial phases of healing are usually complete in 6 to 7 days. Scar contraction and remodeling will continue for months. The patient should be warned to expect some degree of discomfort when first resuming intercourse and assured that this will improve with time. Adequate foreplay and lubrication are critical when vaginal intercourse resumes. Vaginismus can result if patients associate intercourse with introital pain.

The physician examines the episiotomy 4 to 6 weeks after delivery to confirm healing. At this visit, skin tag bridges are clipped and any granulation tissue tags are excised. Major revision of an unsatisfactory episiotomy should wait several months for completion of the healing process.

SUMMARY

Episiotomy was developed to allow room for obstetric maneuvers that are rarely performed in present-day obstetrics. Episiotomy also developed as a procedure to protect the perineum from stretching and tearing forces at delivery that result in a gaping introitus and genital herniation.

Many experienced obstetricians feel that patients who have careful episiotomy repairs with each delivery have little difficulty with laxity of the introitus, cystocele, urethrocele, or rectocele. This anecdotal experience is probably true, although large, matched, randomized studies with long-term follow-up do not exist. The principal justification for episiotomy in modern obstetrics is prevention of genital laxity and herniation.

Midline episiotomies suffice for almost all delivery requirements. Careful timing is required to gain the advantage of preventing fascial tearing while avoiding excessive blood loss that accompanies early perineal incision.

References

1. Laufe LE, Leslie DC: The timing of episiotomy. Am J Obstet Gynecol 114:773, 1972.
2. Ould F: A Treatise of Midwifery. Dublin: Milton and Head, 1742.
3. Pomeroy RH: Shall we cut and reconstruct the perineum for every primipara? Am J Obstet 78:211, 1918.
4. Eastman NJ: Median episiotomy. Obstet Gynecol Surv 3:828, 1948.
5. Barter RH, Parks J, Tyndal C: Median episiotomies and complete perineal lacerations. Am J Obstet Gynecol 80:654, 1960.
6. Dallas DA: The routine use of episiotomy with a description of the continuous knotless repair. West J Surg Obstet Gynecol 61:29, 1953.
7. Harris RE: An evaluation of median episiotomy. Am J Obstet Gynecol 106:660, 1970.
8. Kaltreider FD, Dixon DM: A study of 710 complete lacerations following central episiotomy. South Med J 41:814, 1948.
9. Inmon B: Mediolateral episiotomy. South Med J 53:257, 1960.
10. Odell LD, Seski A: Episiotomy blood loss. Am J Obstet Gynecol 54:51, 1947.
11. Findley D: An unusual birth injury. Am J Obstet Gynecol 42:1088, 1941.

22

Postpartum Hemorrhage

Randall C. Floyd
John C. Morrison

- ■ DEFINITION
- ■ INCIDENCE
- ■ PREDISPOSING FACTORS
- ■ PREPARATION OF AT-RISK PATIENTS
- ■ PREVENTIVE MANAGEMENT

- ■ TREATMENT
  Mechanical
  Pharmacologic
  Manipulative
  Surgical
  Topical Agents
- ■ SUMMARY

Obstetrics has one of the lowest transfusion rates in medicine. However, when hemorrhage does occur after abdominal or vaginal delivery, the loss of blood can be severe and may lead to maternal and/or fetal mortality or morbidity. Hospitalization for delivery, as well as the availability of blood, has dramatically reduced the risk of maternal mortality from postpartum hemorrhage in the United States.[1] Nevertheless, hemorrhage still remains the third leading cause of death in one series[2] and is said to account for 10.5% of non–abortion–related maternal deaths in the United States.[3]

Heavy bleeding after delivery is also associated with significant maternal morbidity, related to poor tissue perfusion of vital organs, and infectious complications.[4] Hypotension after severe postpartum hemorrhage may lead to panhypopituitarism, renal damage, or severe respiratory complications, such as adult respiratory distress syndrome.[1] Also, the morbidity associated with blood product infusion, such as hepatitis, transfusion reaction, and acquired immune deficiency syndrome, although infrequent, is still a significant risk.[2] Finally, postpartum hemorrhage can result in hysterectomy to control heavy bleeding, which may be life saving but results in lost fertility when performed in young women. Although most gravidas tolerate the relatively large volume of blood lost during

Supported in part by the Vicksburg Hospital Medical Foundation.

delivery very well, the obstetrician must detect patients at risk for postpartum hemorrhage because such cases may have severe morbidity and mortality.

DEFINITION

Postpartum hemorrhage is defined as loss of more than 500 mL of blood during the first 12 hours after delivery. The quantitative estimate is often as little as half the actual volume lost, however, because such hemorrhage is constantly underestimated.[4] The average amount of bleeding after delivery is more often approximately 1000 mL.

Most parturients increase their blood volume 30 to 40% (about 1000 to 1500 mL) during gestation. This physiologic alteration affords the woman a greater margin of safety in tolerating significant hemorrhage, but it also means that signs and symptoms of hypovolemia will not be apparent as soon in the parturient as in her nonpregnant counterpart. It is also wise to remember that equilibration after hemorrhage requires approximately 4 hours to be reflected in the hematocrit or hemoglobin level unless a large amount of intravenous crystalloid solution has been administered in the interim.[5]

An alternative definition, and one that is more physiologic, of postpartum hemorrhage is loss of more than 15% of the total estimated blood volume.[6] It characterizes the blood loss as a percentage of blood volume and can be related to patient symptomatology (Table 22–1).[6] In this way, a patient's symptoms are correlated with blood loss and volume depletion.

Table 22–1. CLASSIFICATION OF HEMORRHAGE

Class 1 hemorrhage—A loss of 15% of the blood volume, reflected by modest tachycardia. If the loss exceeds 15%, the tilt test becomes positive; i.e., in the sitting position for 60–90 seconds, the patient becomes weak, dizzy, or syncopal and experiences a fall in blood pressure.

Class 2 hemorrhage—A 20 to 25% loss of blood volume or more than 1200 mL in a 60-kg gravida. Tachypnea, tachycardia, decreased systolic blood pressure, reduced pulse pressure (less than 30 mm Hg), and delayed capillary filling become apparent.

Class 3 hemorrhage—A loss in excess of 30 to 35% of the blood volume or more than 1500 mL in a 60-kg patient at term. Hemorrhagic shock exists (best defined as inadequate perfusion of the microcirculation). The patient is cold and clammy, pale, restless and apprehensive, severely hypotensive, and oliguric. A combination of metabolic acidosis with superimposed respiratory alkalosis occurs.

Class 4 hemorrhage—A 40 to 45% blood loss or more than 2000 mL in a 60-kg gravida. There is profound hypotension. The only palpable pulse, the last to be felt before complete circulatory collapse, will be the carotid. Metabolic acidosis may rapidly induce "irreversible" shock unless appropriate resuscitation is undertaken immediately.

Table 22–2. CONDITIONS ASSOCIATED WITH POSTPARTUM HEMORRHAGE

A. Uterine atony	
Precipitous labor	Prolonged labor
Overdistended	Medications
uterus	Anemia
Amnionitis	Previous postpartum hemorrhage
Multiparity	Breech extraction
Midforceps	Fetal demise
Full bladder	
B. Lower genital tract lacerations	
Vulva	Vagina
Rectum	Cervix
C. Uterine abnormalities	
Rupture	Inversion
Placenta previa	Leiomyomata
D. Other	
Clotting disorders	Retained placenta

INCIDENCE

The incidence of postpartum hemorrhage is difficult to assess because of the multiple factors regarding its causes and quantitation. It is said to occur after vaginal delivery in approximately 5 to 8% of cases, although severe blood loss, such as Class 3 or 4 hemorrhage, occurs in less than 1%.[5, 7] On the other hand, postpartum hemorrhage is the most common cause of excessive blood loss during pregnancy. It is directly responsible for about one sixth of maternal deaths worldwide and in developing countries remains the leading cause of maternal demise.[7]

PREDISPOSING FACTORS

There are several conditions associated with postpartum hemorrhage (Table 22–2). Of these, uterine atony is most commonly associated with postpartum bleeding, accounting for 50%.[6] Uterine atony occurs when the myometrium does not contract persistently or firmly enough to constrict the tissue surrounding the blood vessels that supply the placental implantation site. Medications (e.g., magnesium sulfate) that interfere with contractions, overdistension of the uterus (twins, hydramnios, and macrosomia), or conditions in which the uterine musculature is fatigued (precipitous or prolonged labor, infection, etc.) are associated with a higher incidence of uterine atony. Excessive bleeding from the lower genital tract comprises approximately 20% of such cases and is discussed extensively in Chapter 22. Usually, lacerations of the lower genital tract follow instrumental delivery, although they can attend precipitate, spontaneous delivery.

A myriad of uterine conditions—notably, rupture of the lower uterine segment, persistent bleeding from placenta previa implantation after delivery, operative lacerations during cesarean delivery, and uterine inversion—cause approximately 20% of cases of postpartum hemorrhage.

Failure of complete placental separation as a result of accretic involvement of the myometrium is an uncommon but very severe problem and is discussed in Chapter 11. Even after placental separation from the lower uterine segment (partial or low-lying placenta previa), this area has sparse myometrium and frequently cannot contract sufficiently. This sequence of events is a common cause of hemorrhage due to placentation abnormalities.

Although uterine inversion may occur spontaneously, it has been related to inadequate separation of the placenta and inappropriate traction on the umbilical cord combined with fundal pressure. After delivery, a mass appearing at the introitus should raise the obstetrician's suspicion of uterine inversion. Uterine replacement as described in Chapter 12 should be undertaken as rapidly as possible. Rupture of the uterus should be suspected in patients with prior scarred uteri, although it can occur spontaneously without a previous surgical incision. The management of this condition is also discussed in Chapter 12.

The remaining 10% of cases of postpartum hemorrhage are related to late bleeding from retained placenta or coagulopathies that may occur at any time. Retention of placental fragments or delayed separation of the placenta can be a cause of early postpartum hemorrhage, but retained secundines are the most common cause of delayed hemorrhage.[8] Coagulation disorders can also be associated with postpartum hemorrhage. Idiopathic thrombocytopenic purpura and von Willebrand disease (Factor VIII deficiency) are usually known before delivery but can be diagnosed with hematologic consultation. Consumptive coagulopathy, which may follow abruptio placentae, severe infection, or the dead fetus syndrome, should also be considered in a patient who continues bleeding after delivery.

PREPARATION OF AT-RISK PATIENTS

It is important to remember that although life-threatening postpartum hemorrhage does not occur frequently, preventive management is of the utmost importance and accounts for much of the improved outcome in such patients during the past few years. Patients identified as being at risk for postpartum hemorrhage (see Table 22–2) should have blood available (type and screen) after admission to the delivery suite. If antibodies are present, blood should be crossmatched so that infusion may begin at a few minutes' notice. A large-bore intravenous catheter should be placed in the patient, and assessment of the subject's hemodynamic status during labor should be undertaken. The goal of intrapartum fluid management is that the patient be normovolemic during delivery and

when entering the postpartum period. A coagulation screen should be obtained in appropriate patients, and consistent monitoring of intake and output during and after delivery should be accomplished. If amniotic infection is noted, treatment with antibiotics may be helpful in preventing postpartum hemorrhage.[9] In addition, if oxytocin is being used for augmentation or induction, its infusion should be gradually reduced and finally discontinued during labor to allow the uterus to contract more effectively after delivery. Finally, it is wise to alert delivery room personnel (both nurses and physicians), as well as the anesthesiologist, recovery room personnel, and the pediatric staff, so that these personnel are aware of the patient's potential hemorrhagic problems.

PREVENTIVE MANAGEMENT IN THE THIRD STAGE OF LABOR

After delivery, the uterus should be gently massaged with the physician's hand on the maternal abdomen in a circular or back-and-forth motion, avoiding downward pressure on the fundus, until the uterus becomes well contracted. It has been shown that exceptionally vigorous massage of the uterus during the third stage of labor may impede its contraction.[7] Gentle traction on the cord may be applied during massage (Brandt-Andrews maneuver) until separation of the placenta occurs. The operator must avoid combining severe traction with fundal massage because this may result in uterine inversion.

If the placenta remains unseparated after 30 minutes or if profuse hemorrhage occurs at this point, the placenta should be manually removed. The operator accomplishes this (with appropriate anesthesia) by placing a hand inside the uterus and gently dissecting the edge of the placenta loose by sweeping the hand between the maternal surface of the placenta and the uterine wall (Fig. 22–1).

Once separation of the placenta has occurred (whether manually or spontaneously), the placenta is gradually led through the cervical canal with gentle cord traction and continued gentle uterine massage. Twisting the placenta several times as it appears in the vagina and at the vulva will cause the membranes to separate more completely, and ring forceps can be used to further assist definitive separation of the membranes. After removal of the placenta, the maternal surface should be inspected to detect areas that may not have separated completely or cotyledons that may have been retained. In addition, accessory vessels in lateral margins of the fetal membranes may indicate a succenturiate lobe that may remain in the uterus after delivery of the placenta.

If bleeding continues after the third stage of labor and retained placental fragments are sus-

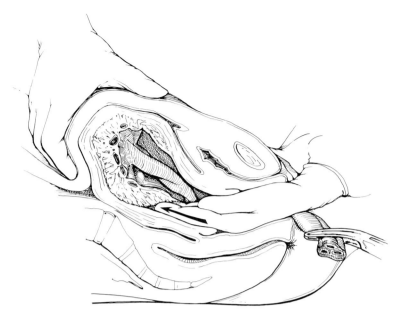

Figure 22–1. Manual removal of the placenta.

pected, manual exploration of the uterus is indicated. An unfolded 4-inch × 4-inch gauze wrapped over the gloved hand may expedite cleansing of the uterus. The fundus is stabilized by the physician's hand on the abdomen; once the physician's other hand enters the uterus, the first three fingers should be swept across the entire upper surface of the uterus, beginning at the fundus. Lacerations of the lower uterine segment as well as anterior-posterior and lateral aspects of the uterus may also be the cause of hemorrhage and should be assessed. The walls should be palpated by the palmar surface of one or two fingers to detect uterine defects as well as retained placental fragments. Such exploration should be gentle to avoid the possibility of uterine perforation. As for manual removal of the placenta, adequate anesthesia is necessary for examination of the uterine cavity. During the uterine exploration care should be taken to place waterproof gowns, extended gloves, or latex sleeves over the operator's arms so that contact with potentially infected blood will not occur.

LOWER GENITAL INSPECTION

Assuming that the third stage of labor has ended with the placenta removed intact, the lower vagina, cervical, vulvar, and perineal areas should be inspected for any lacerations. Small cervical lacerations that are not bleeding need not be repaired. After repair of the episiotomy (or lacerations), the patients are usually transported to the recovery room. It is during (a) delivery of the placenta and inspection of the lower vagina and (b) the recovery room period that most postpartum hemorrhage occurs.

TREATMENT FOR POSTPARTUM HEMORRHAGE

When postpartum hemorrhage occurs, there are several treatment methods that should be implemented in a sequential fashion (Table 22–3).

Mechanical Treatment

When placental fragments, uterine lesions, and lower genital lacerations have been ruled out,

Table 22–3. THERAPY FOR POSTPARTUM HEMORRHAGE

Mechanical
  Empty bladder
  Elevation of fundus
  Compression of uterus
  Uterine massage
Pharmacologic
  Oxytocin
  Ergot preparations
  Prostin/15-methylester, Hemabate
  Prostaglandin E_2 suppositories
Manipulation
  Foley balloon
  MAST* suit
  Aortal compression
  Uterine packing
Surgical
  Curettage
  Vascular ligation
    Uterine arteries
    Hypogastric arteries
    Ovarian arteries
  Hysterectomy
    Supracervical
    Total
Radiographic
  Hypogastric artery vasopressin (Pitressin) infusion
  Selective transarterial embolization
Topical hemostatic agents

*Military antishock trouser suit.

mechanical therapy should be employed. The bladder should be empty, because an atonic, overfilled bladder will prevent the uterus from effectively contracting. Elevation of the fundus and compression and massage of the uterus are all accomplished at the same time. The uterus is elevated gently by the operator's hand in the vagina and stabilized by the operator's hand on the maternal abdomen. Elevation of the uterus is important to allow adequate perfusion so that ecbolic agents can reach the myometrium. Care should be taken not to stretch the uterus too vigorously while attempting elevation because tears in the broad ligament may occur. Uterine massage is performed gently but firmly in a circular motion. A vaginal pack placed firmly against the cervix can aid in promoting uterine compression.

Pharmacologic Treatment

After delivery, most patients receive oxytocin. Routine administration of oxytocin during the third stage of labor has been shown to reduce blood loss after delivery.[9] It is usually administered by placing 10 to 20 units of oxytocin in a liter of isotonic saline or other crystalloid solution, delivered intravenously at the infusion rate of 200 mL per hour. The liter can be administered after delivery over a 30- to 40-minute period, if necessary, to correct hypovolemia and to ensure a contractile uterus. Oxytocin should not be rapidly injected intravenously as a bolus because it may cause hypotension or arrhythmias.[10]

Ergot preparations such as ergonovine maleate (Ergotrate) or methylergonovine (Methergine) are administered in dosages of 0.2 mg intramuscularly to patients who do not respond to oxytocin. These drugs may result in hypertension[11] and therefore should not be given to those who have a history or evince signs during labor and delivery of increased blood pressure. These agents cause a tetanic uterine contraction that usually occurs within a few minutes and may last for several hours. These myometrial contractions not only are stronger but last longer than those caused by oxytocin.

At this point, if hemorrhage continues and uterine defects as well as placental adherence and lower genital tract lacerations have been ruled out, several other pharmacologic approaches are available. Injection of the 15-methylester of prostaglandin (PG) $F_{2\alpha}$ (Hemabate) can be given intramuscularly or directly into the myometrium in doses of 250 µg every 30 to 60 minutes until a response is obtained or a maximum of 2000 µg is administered. This approach has been successful in treating hemorrhage unresponsive to oxytocic and ergot derivatives.[12, 13] $PGF_{2\alpha}$ has also been used by myometrial injection (transabdominally) at a dose of 1 mg.[14] This medication, more so than the 15-methylester, is associated with side effects

such as nausea, vomiting, and diarrhea. Finally, vaginal PGE_2 suppositories have been used with good success to control postpartum hemorrhage.[15] These agents have the disadvantage of vaginal placement where they may be diluted by continued bleeding. It may be efficacious to wrap the suppository in a 4-inch × 4-inch gauze and place it anterior to the cervix. In this fashion the drug is absorbed quite readily and is efficacious in contracting the uterus. Insertion of the suppository into the rectum is also an effective method of administration and may be used if heavy bleeding interferes with vaginal placement.

Manipulative Treatment

If the patient continues to bleed and uterine atony is the principal diagnosis, there are several manipulative therapies that can be advocated. A large Foley catheter balloon may control hemorrhage from the lower uterine segment, if this is thought to be the area of persistent bleeding. Such bleeding may result from a low-lying placenta or a cervical pregnancy (Fig. 22–2).[16, 17]

If the patient requires transportation to a Level III center after severe postpartum hemorrhage, the military antishock trouser (MAST) suit may be used.[18] The MAST is bulky, and proper fit and maintenance of normovolemia are essential. If the patient is not hemodynamically stable, pressure occlusion of the aorta through the abdomen frequently will provide temporary control of heavy postpartum hemorrhage so that organ perfusion and normovolemia may be achieved while preparing for surgery. In most patients, such occlusion

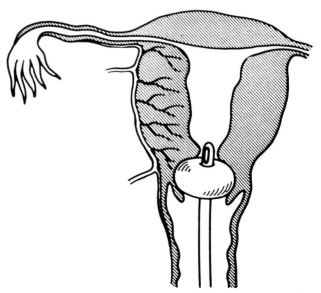

Figure 22–2. Use of a Foley balloon catheter to control bleeding from the cervix or lower uterine segment. (From Bowen LW, Beeson JH: Use of a large Foley catheter balloon to control postpartum hemorrhage resulting from a low placental implantation: A report of two cases. J Reprod Med 30:623, 1985.)

can be maintained for several minutes without any sequelae, although this method is recommended only for emergent treatment.

Uterine packing has recently enjoyed a resurgence in use, for several reasons. First, it is not associated with infection, as in the older studies when uterine packing was left in place for several days. Second, in our hands, it obviates the need for surgical intervention in at least 50% of the women with unresponsive postpartum hemorrhage. Most recently, Drucker and Wallach[19] have reported successfully avoiding laparotomy by using uterine packing in 11 of 13 patients. The other two subjects gained 30 to 60 minutes for stabilization before surgical exploration. Thus even in the most severe cases with continued bleeding, the operator is afforded 30 to 90 minutes to restore vascular volume and prepare for the surgical procedure. The deficiency of this method is that it requires considerable technical expertise.[19–21]

Uterine packing, as shown in Figure 22–3, is performed carefully and gently. Under general anesthesia the leading edge of a six-ply, 4-inch-wide gauze (a Kurlex or Kling 20-yard roll) is placed into one corner of the uterine fundus with a ring or uterine dressing forceps and is packed securely in the cornual area. The packing is then advanced across the dome of the uterus to the other cornu, and that area is packed securely. Care should be taken not to perforate the soft postpartum uterus. Some prefer to use dry gauze whereas others saturate the packs in Betadine solution.

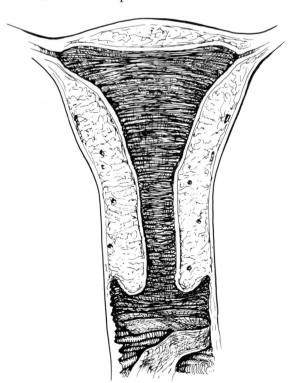

Figure 22–3. Uterine packing of a postpartum uterus.

The obstetrician continues packing, filling the corpus of the uterus in a "layered" fashion down to the isthmus, with each 20-yard roll tied sequentially to the next and a note made of the number of rolls used. Packing is continued into the lower uterine segment and down to the external cervical os until a tight configuration is obtained. Next, the vaginal fornices are tightly packed until the upper portion of the vagina is slightly distended. The lower vagina is then packed, and the procedure ends at the introitus.

It is important to continuously drain the bladder with a catheter because voiding will be difficult with the pack in place. A broad-spectrum antibiotic is administered, and the pack is removed in 6 to 12 hours. Intravenous oxytocin or other ecbolic agents are also continued.

Surgical Treatment

Patients who do not respond to the measures described above are usually candidates for laparotomy. One should consider curettage if it is possible that fragments of an adherent placenta are present. This etiology is rare after thorough exploration of the uterus. A dilation and curettage is more likely to be necessary in cases of late postpartum hemorrhage due to retained secundines.[8] Even several weeks after delivery, curettage should be performed gently to avoid uterine perforation. Care must also be taken during curettage to avoid denuding the entire endometrium because this can lead to the formation of adhesions and subsequent Asherman syndrome. The uterine adhesions do not respond to endogenous hormonal stimulation, and amenorrhea and sterility follow.

If laparotomy is indicated as an emergent procedure, direct pressure on the aorta while the obstetrician prepares for surgery can be a lifesaving measure when hypovolemia and hypoxia threaten perfusion of vital organs. A thorough exploration of the abdomen is performed to rule out rupture of the uterus, rents in the broad ligament, or retroperitoneal/broad ligament hematoma. If these problems are encountered, consideration of hysterectomy and/or drainage based on the patient's condition and desire for future fertility is carried out, as emphasized in Chapters 12 and 26.

For patients with normal pelvic anatomy, the next step is usually to occlude both uterine arteries and collateral veins. This technique appears to be effective in correcting hemorrhage by reducing the pulse pressure to the uterus because at least 90% of the blood flow emanates from the uterine arteries and collateral veins.[22] Occlusion of these vessels is technically less difficult than hypogastric artery ligation, and the risk of venous bleeding in the retroperitoneal space is avoided. This technique employs uterine artery ligation as popularized by O'Leary[22] (Figs. 22–4A and B). The site of the ligation is near the isthmus of the uterus and may be approximately 2 to 3 cm below the level of the uterine incision (if it is transverse).

The uterus is grasped and elevated with the left hand and is tilted to expose the vessels coursing through the broad ligament. A delayed-absorption type of suture (No. 1 chromic, 0-Vicryl, 0-Dexon, or 0-Maxon) on a large, atraumatic needle is passed through and into the myometrium from anterior to posterior about 2 to 3 cm into the uterine musculature medial to the vessels. In order to obliterate these vessels, 2 to 3 cm of myometrium must be included in the suture. The needle is brought forward through the avascular and visualized area of the broad ligament well lateral to the uterine artery and veins. Visualization of the ureter as shown in Figure 22–4C should be accomplished. The suture is then tied anteriorly, and the procedure is repeated on the contralateral side.

After this ligation, the uterus may appear to blanch and often will remain atonic; bleeding should be controlled, however. Collateral circulation and recanalization will occur in 6 to 8 weeks. Subsequent menstrual flow as well as future fertility have been unaffected.[22] Oozing from needle sites, suture line, or atony can be controlled with intramyometrial injections of oxytocin, 15-methylester of $PGF_{2\alpha}$, fibrin glue, or thromboplastin. Likewise, pressure over these sites with warm saline packs can control persistent oozing. O'Leary[22] has reported a success rate of approximately 95% in more than 200 cases.

Another surgical procedure for postpartum hemorrhage is ligation of the hypogastric arteries, which has a success rate of approximately 40%.[23] Ligation of the hypogastric arteries appears to reduce pulse pressure but may not absolutely control blood flow to the uterus. It has been shown that ipsilateral blood flow is reduced by approximately 50% whereas pulse pressure is decreased approximately 85%.[24] Although this operation is frequently advocated, it is potentially dangerous unless the surgeon has operative experience in the retroperitoneal space. This is particularly true

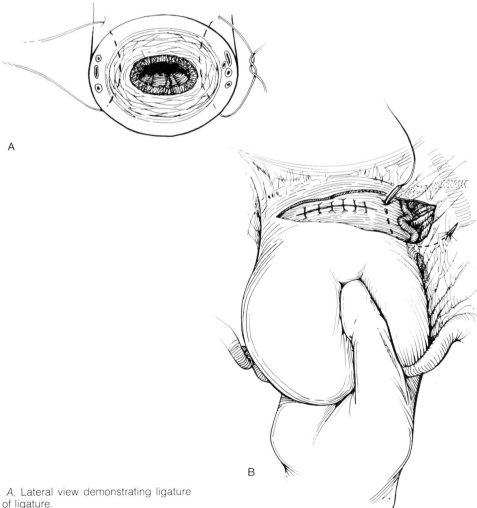

A

B

Figure 22–4. Uterine artery ligation. *A,* Lateral view demonstrating ligature placement. *B,* Anatomic relationship of ligature.

when the patient is hypovolemic and organ perfusion is poor. The principal risks of the procedure are damage to the iliac vein and ligation of the external or common iliac artery, which would compromise blood flow to the lower limb. In patients who are hemodynamically unstable or if the surgeon is inexperienced, hysterectomy may be considered. This is an acceptable treatment for those who do not respond to uterine artery ligation.

If ligation of the hypogastric artery is elected, the internal iliac artery is located at the bifurcation of the common iliac artery near the level of the sacroiliac joint (see Fig. 13–5). The safest approach to the artery is just below its origin from the common iliac. The peritoneum lateral to the infundibulopelvic vessels is opened, and the ureter is identified on the posterior medial leaf of the broad ligament and retracted medially. The bifurcation of the common iliac artery is identified. A right-angle clamp is passed around the hypogastric artery laterally to medially, with the nose of the clamp staying near the artery to avoid injury to the fragile hypogastric vein. Silk suture (No. 1) is used to tie the artery in two sites approximately 1 to 2 cm apart. The ureter is then reflected back to its normal position. Most surgeons do not favor closing the peritoneum over this area.

Although selective ligation of the anterior division of the hypogastric artery is performed by some, this may not be easily accomplished, and thus the anterior and posterior branches of the hypogastric artery are usually approached as one and ligated. Although there have been a few cases of gluteal hypoperfusion that resulted from ligation of the posterior branch of the hypogastric artery, collateral circulation in the pelvis is usually sufficient to allow perfusion of these areas within minutes of ligation.[4, 23] Another technique that has been useful in some cases is ligation of the ovarian artery. This procedure has been described in foreign literature and recently in the American literature as an adjunctive means for controlling hemorrhage not assuaged by hypogastric artery ligation or uterine artery ligation.[26]

When the uterus is thoroughly disrupted, hysterectomy is usually considered. In addition, when ligation of various vessels is ineffective in controlling hemorrhage, hysterectomy is a reasonable option.[27] During the performance of a hysterectomy for postpartum hemorrhage, attention must be directed toward meticulous hemostasis because of the large blood supply and vessel dilatation that exist during pregnancy. More complete descriptions of hysterectomy and uterine rupture are available in Chapters 13 and 27.

Other modalities for control of postpartum hemorrhage include radiographic invasive techniques. Femoral artery catheterization with vasopressin infusion or embolization of Gelfoam has been described in the treatment of severe postpartum hemorrhage.[28, 29] Gelfoam embolization usually allows for hemostasis within approximately 2 hours after beginning the procedure (Fig. 22–5). The material is gradually reabsorbed over a period of weeks but not until involution of the uterus has occurred. Pitressin is more immediate in its effect but both Pitressin and Gelfoam require the patient to be stable while this invasive procedure is performed. Pitressin has several side effects, such as hypertension, antidiuretic hormone secretion, and other problems. In some cases, the use of the MAST suit partially inflated on the contralateral side and across the abdomen may be helpful while the catheterization is performed. In general, these procedures are employed after continued bleeding has occurred in a patient on whom a laparotomy with ligation of vasculature has already been performed and the patient is relatively stable.

Topical Hemostatic Agents

A variety of topical hemostatic agents are available for control of bleeding at the time of surgery.[30, 31] Pressure and packs are time-honored means for controlling hemorrhage and usually are the first methods used to stop the bleeding. Oozing is usually treated first with digital pressure, which allows the clot to solidify within the vessel and adhere as a result of thrombus formation. Cold or warm packs have been used because cold promotes spasm and contractility of vessels while heat accelerates the formation of thrombin and clotting. Others prefer absorbable gelatinous sponge products (e.g., Gelfoam and Surgicel), which may be soaked in thrombin. These sponges are available in several sizes and may be cut to fit the desired area. Their use is contraindicated in contaminated wounds. After the sponges are placed on diffuse friable tissue, pressure is applied and a moist pack left in place for several minutes.

Microfibrillar collagen or Avitene is actually a sterile absorbable collagen. It promotes thrombin formation by stimulating platelet adhesion and aggregation. Avitene must be applied dry, and all instruments or materials, such as gloves, that come in contact with it likewise must be dry because its effectiveness is impaired by saline or thrombin. The Avitene is cut into the desired thickness and placed over the friable, bleeding areas. Such compounds have been incriminated in retroperitoneal fibrosis and ureteral obstruction. More recent literature suggests that such complications are more likely due to surgery than to problems with Avitene. Finally, the use of fibrin glue, a biodegradable tissue adhesive, can be helpful as a topical hemostatic agent.[30] Cryoprecipitate and bovine thrombin are placed at the bleeding sites; approximately 30 mL of each component is usually required. Equal volumes are drawn up into separate plastic syringes and sprayed along bleeding sites. The glue must be applied in a field as dry as possible. Therefore the glue is some-

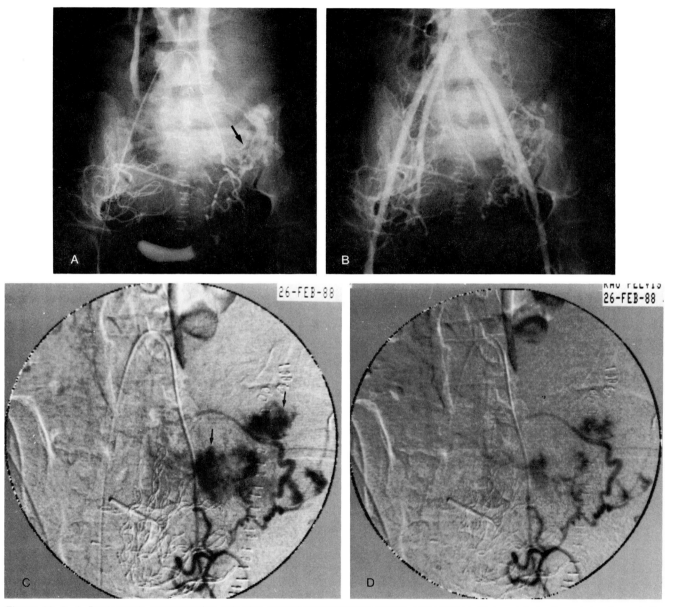

Figure 22–5. *A,* Radiograph demonstrating selective arterial catheterization before embolization. Note extravasation of dye *(arrow)*. *B,* Radiograph demonstrating selective arterial catheterization after Gelfoam embolization. *C,* Digital angiography demonstrating selective arterial catheterization before Gelfoam embolization. Note extravasation of dye *(arrows)*. *D,* Digital angiography demonstrating selective arterial catheterization after Gelfoam embolization.

times used in conjunction with Gelfoam or Avitene. The reaction begins immediately but is not complete for 2 minutes; suction or other debridement should not be employed during this time period.

SUMMARY

There are many ways to control postpartum hemorrhage. The best way is to (a) avoid such bleeding whenever possible by managing the first, second, and third stages of labor assiduously and (b) be prepared for torrential hemorrhage when it does occur. Identified risk factors should be noted on admission to the hospital and as they occur in labor. These patients should receive special attention at the time of delivery. Good obstetric judgment and surgical technique during the delivery process are vital. The use of sequential treatment for postpartum hemorrhage when it occurs and a "studied haste" with meticulous surgical technique at laparotomy are paramount. The obstetrician must remember that although obstetric hemorrhage is rare, it can be fatal if good technique and clinical judgment are not used.

References

1. Pritchard JA, MacDonald PC, Gant NF: Williams Obstetrics, 17th Edition. Norwalk, CT: Appleton-Century-Crofts, 1985.
2. Griffis KR, Wiener WB, Morrison JC: Maternal mortality in Mississippi: 1981–1986. J Miss State Med Assoc 28:305, 1987.
3. Kaunitz AM, Hughes JM, Grimes DA, et al.: Causes of maternal mortality in the United States. Obstet Gynecol 65:605, 1985.
4. Nelson GH: Consideration of blood loss at delivery as percentage of estimated blood volume. Am J Obstet Gynecol 138:1117, 1980.
5. Watson P: Postpartum hemorrhage and shock. Clin Obstet Gynecol 23:985, 1980.
6. Lucas WE: Postpartum hemorrhage. Clin Obstet Gynecol 23:637, 1980.
7. Kapernick PS: Postpartum hemorrhage and the abnormal puerperium. In Pernoll ML, Benson RC (eds.): Current Obstetric and Gynecologic Diagnosis and Treatment 1987. Norwalk, CT: Appleton & Lange, 1987, p. 524.
8. Thorsteinsson VT, Kempers RD: Delayed postpartum bleeding. Am J Obstet Gynecol 107:565, 1970.
9. Herbert WNP, Cefalo RC: Management of postpartum hemorrhage. Clin Obstet Gynecol 27:139, 1984.
10. Hendricks CH, Brenner WE: Cardiovascular effects of oxytocic drugs used postpartum. Am J Obstet Gynecol 73:1306, 1957.
11. Frederiksen MC: What place for ergot alkaloids in ob today? Contemp Ob/Gyn 31:37, 1988.
12. Hayashi RH, Castillo MS, Noah ML: Management of severe postpartum hemorrhage with a prostaglandin F2 alpha analogue. Obstet Gynecol 63:806, 1984.
13. Bruce SL, Paul RH, Van Dorsten JP: Control of postpartum uterine atony by intramyometrial prostaglandin. Obstet Gynecol 59:47S, 1982.
14. Jacobs MM, Arias F: Intramyometrial prostaglandin $F_{2\alpha}$ in the treatment of severe postpartum hemorrhage. Obstet Gynecol 55:665, 1980.
15. Hertz RH, Sokol RJ, Dierker LJ: Treatment of postpartum uterine atony with prostaglandin E_2 vaginal suppositories. Obstet Gynecol 56:129, 1980.
16. Bowen LW, Beeson JH: Use of a large Foley catheter balloon to control postpartum hemorrhage resulting from a low placental implantation. A report of two cases. J Reprod Med 30:623, 1985.
17. Nolan TE, Chandler PE, Hess LW, Morrison JC: Cervical pregnancy managed with hysterectomy: A case report. J Reprod Med 34:241, 1989.
18. Pearse CS, Magrina JF, Finley BE: Use of MAST suit in obstetrics and gynecology. Obstet Gynecol Surv 39:416, 1984.
19. Drucker M, Wallach RC: Uterine packing: A reappraisal. Mt Sinai J Med 46:191, 1979.
20. Douvas SG, Morrison JC: A guide to ob emergencies. Contemp Ob/Gyn 20:95, 1982.
21. Druzin ML: Packing of lower uterine segment for control of postcesarean bleeding in instances of placenta previa. Surg Gynecol Obstet 169:543, 1989.
22. O'Leary JA: Stop ob hemorrhage with uterine artery ligation. Contemp Ob/Gyn 27:13, 1986.
23. Clark SL, Phelan JP, Yeh S, et al.: Hypogastric artery ligation for obstetric hemorrhage. Obstet Gynecol 66:353, 1985.
24. Evans S, McShane P: The efficacy of internal iliac artery ligation in obstetric hemorrhage. Surg Gynecol Obstet 160:250, 1985.
25. Burchell RC: Physiology of internal iliac artery ligation. J Obstet Gynaecol Br Commonw 75:642, 1968.
26. Cruikshank SH, Stoelk EM: Surgical control of pelvic hemorrhage: Method of bilateral ovarian artery ligation. Am J Obstet Gynecol 147:724, 1983.
27. Clark SL, Yeh S, Phelan JP, et al.: Emergency hysterectomy for obstetric hemorrhage. Obstet Gynecol 64:376, 1984.
28. Sacks BA, Palestrant AM, Cohen WR: Internal iliac artery vasopressin infusion for postpartum hemorrhage. Am J Obstet Gynecol 143:601, 1982.
29. Pais SO, Glickman M, Schwartz P, et al.: Embolization of pelvic arteries for control of postpartum hemorrhage. Obstet Gynecol 55:754, 1980.
30. Malviya VK, Deppe G: Control of intraoperative hemorrhage in gynecology with the use of fibrin glue. Obstet Gynecol 73:284, 1989.
31. Helmkamp BF, Krebs HB, Loughner JE: Effectiveness of topical hemostatic agents. Contemp Ob/Gyn 25:171, 1985.

23

Obstetric Genital Trauma

Warren C. Plauché

Obstetric genital trauma encompasses a spectrum of maternal injury from minor contusions and abrasions to major lacerations and organ disruptions (Table 23–1). Some of the damage done to the birth canal at the time of obstetric delivery is subtle and unseen yet results in disability later in life.

Undetectable tears of fascial and ligamentous supports of the bladder, rectum, and uterus cause cystocele, rectocele, and uterine prolapse, as gravity exerts an inexorable pull on the pelvic organs. Damage to the cervix may be responsible for later cervical incompetence. Scarring can result in cervical dystocia. The ligamentous supports of the pelvis and lower back may be injured by the labor and delivery processes.

Obstetric genital trauma may also be overt and severe. There may be extensive cosmetic and functional damage, hematoma formation, and postpartum hemorrhage. Both the bladder and the rectum are subject to injury. The most tragic of obstetric genital injuries result in disabling fistulas between the genital and the urinary or intestinal tracts.

VULVAR AND PARAVAGINAL HEMATOMAS

Vulvar and paravaginal hematomas are uncommon complications of the puerperium. Eighty percent of cases appear immediately after delivery. Fifteen to 20% of cases do not appear until 1 to 3

Table 23–1. TYPES OF OBSTETRIC GENITAL TRAUMA

Hematoma Formation
Below pelvic diaphragm—vulvar and perineal
Above pelvic diaphragm—paravaginal, presacral, broad
ligament, lateral retroperitoneal spaces
Lacerations
Vulvar lacerations
First- to fourth-degree tears
Labial adhesion
Vaginal lacerations
Cervical or uterine lacerations
Vascular disruption—vulvar, pudendal, paravaginal,
paracervical, uterine vessels
Laceration of adjacent pelvic organs—rectum, bladder, ureter
Stress and Pressure Injuries
Tissue necrosis
Annular detachment of cervix
Fistula formation—vesicovaginal, ureterovaginal,
rectovaginal
Obstetric paralysis
Fracture of coccyx
Separation of symphysis pubis
Sacroiliac strain
Hip joint sprain

days after delivery. The few cases that seem to begin many days after delivery may represent delay in diagnosis or late bleeding from vascular pressure necrosis.

Incidence

Estimates of the incidence of postpartal hematomas of the vulva, vagina, and pelvis vary from 1 in 300 to 1 in 7000 deliveries, depending on the anatomic regions included. Romine[3] found the incidence of all postpartum hematomas at the University of Arkansas Medical Center to be 1 in 1018 deliveries for the decade ending in 1966 (0.1%). Few studies identify the prevalence of the various types of obstetric hematomas. Obstetric hematomas complicate approximately one delivery in 1000 in the current era.

Hamilton[1] reported the incidence of vulvar hematomas from the New York Lying-In Hospital in the 1930s to be 1 in 300 deliveries (0.3%). Paravaginal hematomas occurred much less commonly in 1 of 1671 deliveries (0.06%). These figures illuminate an era of frequent obstetric manipulations and forceps operations.

Fliegner,[2] in 1971, reported the incidence of postpartum broad ligament hematomas to be 1 in 3460 at Royal Women's Hospital in Melbourne (0.03%).

Classification and Causes

Vulvar and paravaginal hematomas are classified by their early or late appearance, etiology, extent, and anatomic location. Delivery events cause most of these hematomas. Instrumental delivery, precipitous spontaneous delivery, and in-

attentive hemostasis during episiotomy repair are the common culprits. Forty-eight percent of the postpartal vulvovaginal hematomas in Romine's series of 27 cases occurred in episiotomy sites.[3] Nineteen percent, however, occurred on the side opposite the episiotomy, indicating the importance of other events and forces. Two thirds of vulvovaginal hematomas, in a review by Quilligan and Zuspan,[4] occurred following forceps delivery and a prolonged second stage of labor. Primiparity and macrosomic babies are two other factors associated with peripartal hematomas.

Other proposed causal relationships are difficult to verify. Vulvar varices seem to be hematomas waiting to happen, but investigators, including DeLee,[5] found little relationship between vulvar varices and vulvar hematomas. Peridelivery coagulopathies were not confirmed etiologic factors in Romine's large series.[3] Pressure necrosis and blood vessel changes associated with hypertensive diseases of pregnancy are said to result in rare hematomas that appear spontaneously days or even weeks after delivery.[2]

Diagnosis—Signs and Symptoms

Vulvar hematomas cause intense, unremitting perineal pain. The surgeon should check episiotomy sites for hematoma formation during the first hours and days after delivery, particularly if the patient complains of unusual pain. Patients who have had forceps deliveries or traumatic or precipitous deliveries who complain of undue pain, swelling, or inability to void should be examined for hematoma formation.

Inspection reveals swelling of the vulva owing to an expanding hematoma mass with overlying edema. The vulvar skin is stretched to translucency and shows purplish discoloration that may extend to the inguinal and perianal area. Palpation reveals an exquisitely tender mass that displaces the vagina, rectum, or both, and fills the loose connective tissues of the labia.

Perineal and vulvar hematomas result from a bleeding site inferior to the pelvic diaphragm and levator muscles. These hematomas do not usually dissect into retroperitoneal spaces but may dissect into the ischiorectal fossa and thus gain access to commodious spaces between fascial planes. Venous bleeding into spaces restricted by fascial planes often stops spontaneously as a result of pressure on the open vessels by the expanding mass.

Paravaginal hematomas are initially less painful than vulvar hematomas but are more dangerous. They result from lacerated or torn paravaginal vessels bleeding above the restricting fascial planes of the pelvic diaphragm. These vessels communicate with the hypogastric, inferior hemorrhoidal, and inferior vesical arteries and veins. Arterial bleeding may occur when branches of the pudendal or uterine vessels are injured. Tamponade by a confined expanding mass does not occur, and blood loss may be massive (Fig. 23–1).

The presacral space, the spaces within the broad ligament, and the lateral retroperitoneal spaces can accommodate large collections of blood. Bleeding may not be suspected until the patient exhibits signs and symptoms of shock.

The patient with a small or moderate-sized paravaginal hematoma may have only unexplained fever or anemia. She often reports vague pelvic or rectal pressure sensations.

Patients with large retroperitoneal hematomas display shock, abdominal pain, and ileus. Those with advanced cases have unilateral leg edema, urinary retention, and occasionally hematuria. The diagnosis of paravaginal hematoma must be entertained whenever a postpartum patient has an unexpected fall in hematocrit level or an unexplained instability of vital signs.

Examination usually reveals a paravaginal mass with anterior and cephalad displacement of the bladder and uterus. In some instances, physical examination reveals no discrete mass. Blood dissects up the rectovaginal septum between the leaves of the broad ligament or into the large presacral and retroperitoneal flank spaces (see Fig. 23–1). Blood loss in these cases can be obscure, extensive, and life-endangering. Massive untreated hematomas eventually rupture into the peritoneal cavity as a preterminal event. These patients eventually develop irreversible shock and expire.

Computed tomography is a useful imaging technique to determine the location and size of large, dissecting pelvic hematomas. Computed tomographic scans are particularly useful for detecting collections of blood in inaccessible areas, such as the presacral space.[6] Pelvic ultrasonography and magnetic resonance imaging are becoming increasingly useful imaging tools in diagnosing and characterizing pelvic hematomas. Serial examinations can detect stability or expansion of hematomas.

Management

Small vulvar hematomas that are not enlarging may be observed and treated with ice packs and analgesic agents. There will be prolonged distortion and discoloration of the vulva. Many obstetricians first rule out coagulopathies and then manage all but the smallest hematoma cases by surgical drainage.

The patient returns to the delivery unit and is placed in the lithotomy position. Place her under light intravenous or general anesthesia and evaluate the hematoma for size, extent, and location. Take down any related episiotomy repair as an approach to the hematoma. If there has been no episiotomy, make an incision in the inferior portion of the mass, near the introitus. Evacuate the clots and irrigate the hematoma cavity with saline. Discrete bleeding vessels are seldom found in the wall of the hematoma. Secure any bleeding points that are identified by clamping and ligation or by electrocauterization.

Uncomplicated hematomas that appear immediately after delivery are clean wounds. Primary closure with absorbable suture is preferred. Attempt to obliterate any dead space without leaving a large amount of suture material in the depths of the wound. Repair the disrupted episiotomy or perineal incision.

Many surgeons close large hematoma cavities over dependent drains or suction drains. Remove drains in 24 to 48 hours or when drainage has ceased.

It is sometimes difficult to secure hemostasis in the base of a large hematoma cavity. Avitene,

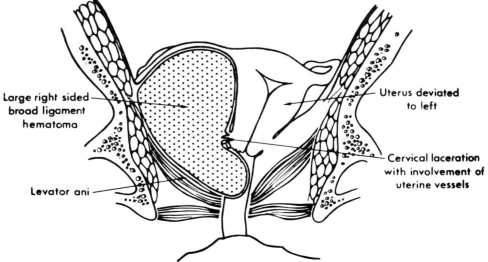

Figure 23–1. Paravaginal and broad ligament hematoma. (After Fliegner JRH: Postpartal broad ligament hematcmas. J Obstet Gynecol Br Commwlth 78:184, 1971.)

Large right sided broad ligament hematoma

Levator ani

Uterus deviated to left

Cervical laceration with involvement of uterine vessels

Gelfoam, oxycellulose sheets, or fibrin glue may be placed against the wound walls. These wounds may have to be packed open with gauze pressure packing. Pack the vagina with gauze for 12 to 24 hours to add opposing pressure. Perineal wounds that are packed open for an extended time quickly become colonized by ambient bacteria. The danger of infection in the wound site is greater than with primary closure. The wounds heal slowly by secondary intention. The eventual cosmetic effect is surprisingly good, although healing may take many weeks. Frequent hot sitz baths or whirlpool baths during secondary healing keep the area clean and comfortable.

Small, asymptomatic paravaginal hematomas that are not expanding may be observed without drainage as long as they are stable.

Incise moderate-sized, localized paravaginal hematomas over the most prominent portion of the bulge within the vagina. Retraction by assistants helps develop adequate exposure. Coagulate or tie small bleeding points in the incision and evacuate, irrigate, and inspect the hematoma cavity. Carefully search for bleeding points in the base of the cavity and ligate all bleeders. It is common to find no specific bleeding points. Drain the wound and close as described for vulvar hematomas. A vaginal pack for 24 hours applies pressure to the site. Pack infected hematomas open and allow them to heal by secondary intention with antibiotic therapy. They should be redressed daily until granulations are exuberant and clean.

Management of large paravaginal hematomas can involve much more complex decision processes. The problem cases have massive bleeding that dissects above the pelvic diaphragm into the retroperitoneal spaces (see Fig. 23–1). The patient with a large, expanding retroperitoneal hematoma, instability of vital signs, and a falling hematocrit level after transfusion may require a combined vaginal and abdominal surgical approach for control. The hematoma is evacuated by the vaginal approach, as described. The hypogastric arteries can be ligated to stop bleeding from pudendal or uterine artery branches. Alternatively, deep bleeding vessels may be embolized by radiologic catheterization techniques.

Pelvic hematomas can sometimes be drained by extraperitoneal approaches.[1, 4] However, extraperitoneal dissection denies the surgeon evaluation of the pelvic and abdominal organs. Exploratory laparotomy permits careful evaluation, better management decisions, and extended surgical procedures if required.

LAPAROTOMY TECHNIQUE FOR DRAINAGE OF PELVIC HEMATOMAS

Open the abdomen with a lower midline incision. Inspect the uterus to rule out uterine rupture or tearing of a major uterine blood vessel. Chapter 13 contains a complete discussion of the management of uterine rupture. Explore the other organs of the pelvis and the abdomen.

BROAD LIGAMENT HEMATOMAS

During evacuation of large broad ligament hematomas, always be conscious of the location and safety of the ureter. Open the broad ligament by incising the anterior leaf with scissors from the lateral third of the round ligament to the middle of the lower uterine segment (Fig. 23–2).

Carefully evacuate the blood clots with the fingers and suction tip. Inspect the uterine vessels for bleeding sites. Clamping and suturing in this area of distorted, obscured anatomy is most hazardous. Individually clamp and ligate any visible bleeding vessels. Do not rely on mass ligatures.

LATERAL RETROPERITONEAL HEMATOMAS

Obtain access to hematomas in the lateral retroperitoneal spaces by incision of the parietal peritoneum from the round ligament cephalad along the lateral end of the posterolateral pelvic wall. This incision is the same as that often used for dissection of the internal iliac (hypogastric) artery (Fig. 23–3). The ureter remains on the medial flap of this peritoneal dissection.

Evacuate blood clots and obtain hemostasis in the resulting spaces. It is often impossible to identify the vessel responsible for the hematoma. The uterine, pudendal, and cervicovaginal arteries are all subsidiaries of the internal iliac vessels. Ligation of the internal iliac arteries effects hemostasis in cases where branches of these arteries are responsible for the hematoma. Extensive collateral vessels make it necessary to ligate both internal iliac vessels to achieve hemostasis in most cases.

The need for adequate operating exposure and

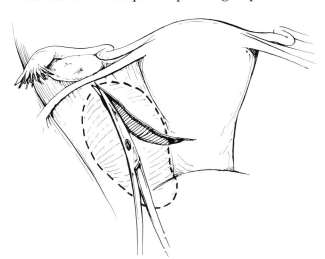

Figure 23–2. Broad ligament hematoma. Opening the anterior leaf of the broad ligament from the lower uterus to the round ligament for evacuation.

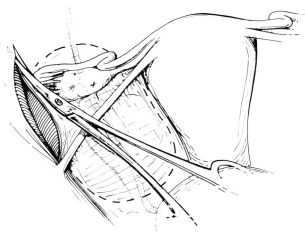

Figure 23–3. Retroperitoneal hematoma of the lateral pelvic wall. Opening the parietal peritoneum (for evacuation) from the insertion of the round ligament cephalad for evacuation.

hemostasis may necessitate removal of the uterus. The uterus is also removed if it is irreparably damaged. Hysterectomy serves no purpose, however, if the hematoma resulted from laceration of a distant branch of a pudendal or paravaginal vessel.

Once the internal iliac vessels are ligated and blood clots are removed, place perforated soft suction drains in the retroperitoneal space. The drains exit through stab wounds separate from the laparotomy wound. Close the posterolateral peritoneal incision with a continuous absorbable suture. Close the laparotomy wound with a Smead-Jones multilayer closure. Mass closure is more reliable when healing is likely to be poor. Replace blood loss and any deficient coagulation factors. Follow vital signs and serial hematocrit levels closely to be certain that the bleeding process is stable. Serial ultrasonographic studies are reassuring and help to identify recurrent hematomas.

PRESACRAL HEMATOMAS

Farkas and colleagues[6] described a method to manage isolated large hematomas in the presacral space. One of their patients developed a massive presacral hematoma following vaginal delivery, complicated only by a small laceration in the lateral vaginal wall. They approached the hematoma through a postanal extraperitoneal incision for evacuation, culture, and irrigation of the cavity, and closed suction drainage. Similar management can also be accomplished through a transperitoneal low abdominal laparotomy incision.

Management without evacuation has been recommended for nonexpanding retroperitoneal hematomas in stable patients. Farkas and colleagues[6] illustrated a complication of this conservative management with a second patient, who developed a chronic, symptomatic, calcified presacral mass. This lesion required excision many years after the original incident. Pedowitz and colleagues[7] described similar calcified retroperitoneal hematomas following management without evacuation. The author managed a patient with presacral calcified hematoma arising after presacral neurectomy for pelvic pain.

The preferred treatment for major pelvic hematomas is exploration, culture, evacuation, hemostasis, and closed drainage. Supportive fluids, blood products, and indicated antibiotics complete the regimen.

PERINEAL AND VULVAR LACERATIONS

The most common injuries incurred at delivery are lacerations of the perineum, vagina, and cervix. Factors that predispose patients to obstetric lacerations include first deliveries, births that are precipitous or unattended, forceps manipulations, and large babies.[8] The reason for the development of the episiotomy operation was prevention of the worst cases of genital laceration.

When the vaginal introitus stretches beyond its elastic capacity or expands too quickly, the tissues tear. These tears are often jagged and irregular in shape and may involve the urethra, bladder, rectal sphincter, or rectum. Obstetricians historically dreaded maternal birth injuries because of disabling late sequelae. These injuries resulted in urinary or fecal incontinence, sexual dysfunction, severe cystocele and rectocele, and vulvar deformity. Successful repair techniques for birth injuries and fistulas are among the triumphs of gynecology.

Classification

Perineal or vulvovaginal lacerations are classified by the extent of involvement of the tissue planes of the perineum (Table 23–2).[9] First-degree vulvovaginal lacerations involve only epithelial and subepithelial tissues of the vulva, perineum, or vagina (Fig. 23–4A).

Second-degree lacerations involve these same structures and the supportive muscles and fascia of the perineum. They may be extensive but do

Table 23–2. CLASSIFICATION OF SEVERITY OF OBSTETRIC VULVOVAGINAL AND PERINEAL LACERATIONS

First-Degree Lacerations
  Epithelial and subepithelial tears of the perineum and vagina
Second-Degree Lacerations
  Epithelial tears and superficial muscle and fascial tears
Third-Degree Lacerations
  Extensive epithelial, superficial muscle, and fascial tears and sphincter ani laceration
Fourth-Degree Lacerations
  All of the above plus tears into the anorectal cavity

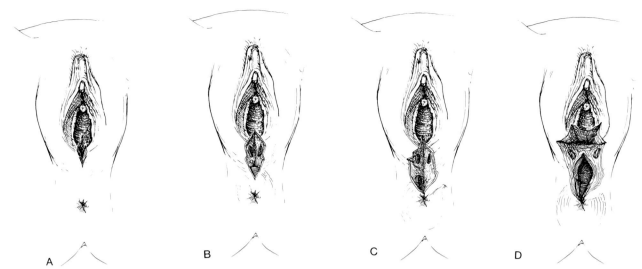

Figure 23–4. *A*, First-degree obstetric perineal laceration—tears of skin, subcutaneous tissue, and vaginal epithelium. *B*, Second-degree obstetric perineal laceration; the superficial perineal muscles are also torn. The rectal sphincter is intact. *C*, Third-degree obstetric perineal laceration; the rectal sphincter is also torn. The rectal mucosa is intact. *D*, Fourth-degree obstetr c perineal laceration; the rectal sphincter and mucosa are both torn by an extensive laceration.

not disrupt the sphincter ani or rectum (Fig. 23–4*B*).

Third-degree lacerations are more extensive and tear through the sphincter ani but not into the rectum (Fig. 23–4*C*). Large third-degree lacerations often extend in a Y or H shape up the posterolateral walls of the vagina and around the rectum. This creates a large defect.

Fourth-degree lacerations tear into the anorectal cavity and through the sphincter ani (Fig. 23–4*D*). Patients occasionally have tears through the rectal mucosa without disruption of the sphincter ani. Lacerations associated with episiotomy extensions are described in Chapter 21.

Principles of Perineal Laceration Repair

The surgical principles for successful primary healing of perineal obstetric lacerations are similar to those for successful episiotomy repair (Table 23–3).

Cleanliness and aseptic technique are important. Contamination of the operative field by feces during delivery is common. Irrigate the wound and drape with fresh drapes that exclude contaminated areas. Do not drag suture material over the anus or other contaminated sites as stitches are placed. Antibiotics are required only in obviously infected cases and repairs delayed 6 hours or more after delivery. By this time, extensive colonization of the wound by bacteria is certain.

Hemostasis is critical to primary healing. The consequences of missed bleeding vessels are vulvar and paravaginal hematomas. Clamp and tie all significant bleeding points. Covering over the bleeding areas with mass suturing techniques in-

vites vulvovaginal hematoma formation. Adequate visualization is critical. Redirect lighting and solicit assistance to reveal bleeding points and clear the operating field.

Anatomic reapproximation of muscular and fascial supports of the rectum and perineum is fundamental to functional success. Know the anatomy of the perineum and attempt to individually reconstruct each muscle group in the repair. Layer-by-layer reconstruction provides excellent cosmetic and functional results.

Understand the mechanisms of anal continence. The tiniest fistula causes embarrassing incontinence. Anal sphincter tone provides effective but only transient continence pressures. Long-term continence of feces and flatus depends on an adequate angle between the rectum and the anal canal. In the female, continence of the rectum operates much like continence of the bladder. Rebuilding the perineum establishes the proper anorectal spatial relationships.

The principle of approximation of tissues without tension or strangulation is important in perineal reconstruction. Perineal wounds fortunately are under reduced tension once the patient is out of lithotomy position. Allow for considerable edema in the vulva and perineum after delivery. Tighten sutures just enough to bring tissue layers into apposition. Several fine sutures in each layer yield better results with this plastic procedure than do tightly tied mass sutures.

Table 23–3. SURGICAL PRINCIPLES FOR SUCCESSFUL REPAIR OF OBSTETRIC LACERATIONS

Aseptic technique
Hemostasis
Anatomic reapproximation of tissues
Approximation without tension

Repair Procedure for Obstetric Lacerations

Repair first- and second-degree lacerations of the vulva, perineum, and vagina in a fashion similar to that described for midline episiotomy (see Chapter 21). Convert jagged skin edges into straight surgical incisions by trimming with Mayo scissors or a scalpel. Begin repair by approximating the vaginal mucosa with a running locked suture of 000 polyglycolic-polyglactin or chromic catgut suture (Fig. 23–5). The suture starts above the apex of the vaginal tear. Each bite incorporates vaginal epithelium and vascular subepithelial tissues. Continue to the hymeneal ring, then set this suture aside for later use.

Next, suture the transverse perineal muscles and bulbocavernosus muscles to their normal insertion on the median perineal raphe with several separate sutures of the same material.

Pass the previously set aside vaginal epithelial suture beneath the hymenal ring. Continue this stitch down to the inferiormost aspect of the perineal wound as a subcutaneous suture. Proceed with this same suture back up the perineal incision as a subcuticular skin closure. End the suture by pulling it just tight enough to approximate the skin edges and cutting it near the skin. No knots or suture ends are exposed on the perineum.

Extensive third- and fourth-degree lacerations challenge the ingenuity of the surgeon. The damage sustained in an H-shaped, deep, bilateral third-degree vaginal laceration combined with extensive perineal damage necessitates attentive repair (Fig. 23–6A).[8] For third-degree lacerations, first repair each arm of the vaginal epithelial tear to the level of the introitus with a running locked suture of 000 absorbable suture (see Fig. 23–6B).

Next, repair the damaged anal sphincter (see Fig. 23–6C). The torn sphincter ani muscle retracts within its sheath around the anus. Often one end of the muscle is visible as a torn edge of muscle, whereas the other end has disappeared within its circular sheath.

The muscle must be retrieved before attempts at repair. Use Allis or similar tissue clamps to dip into the dimple in the anal ring left by the retracted muscle, grasp the muscle edge, and pull it up into the field of operation (see Fig. 23–6B). Lieberman[9] used the needle of the repair suture to dip into the sphincter sheath and "fish out" the retracted muscle.

Approximate the muscle ends with two or more figure-of-eight stitches of fine-gauge absorbable suture. Sutures that reapproximate the sphincter should include portions of the muscle sheath to stabilize the suture line and not shred the muscle fibers. Approximation should be as free of tension as possible. In complicated cases, proctologists recommend a paradoxic relaxing incision of the sphincter at a site remote from the tear. We have not found this technique necessary in early repair of obstetric sphincter damage.

Extensive third-degree tears usually leave a gaping introitus and a torn perineum. Rebuild the perineum by careful reapproximation of the pubococcygeous muscle, which forms the medial portion of the levator sling. Two or three sutures of 000 absorbable material are sufficient. Bring the transversus perinei muscles back to the midline with two or three sutures of the same material. This step builds the length and thickness of the perineum and supports the lower rectum and re-establishes the normal anorectal angle.

The bulbocavernosus muscles usually retract far anteriorly within the labia majora. Bring them down on each side to their midline insertion with two or three sutures. These sutures pass boldly in a deep semicircular bite into the substance of the muscle. The entire labium majorum moves with traction on the suture if it is properly placed through the bulbocavernosus muscle. This suture then anchors the muscle down to the median raphe. Proper healing of these repaired muscle groups restores introital contractility.

Some trimming of the vaginal epithelium at the introitus may be necessary after this muscle repair to avoid the formation of a hummock of vaginal tissue at this site. The remainder of the repair of superficial tissues proceeds as described for the second-degree repair.

Fourth-degree laceration repairs begin with attention to the lacerations of the anorectal mucosa and anal sphincter (see Figs. 23–6B and C). Care-

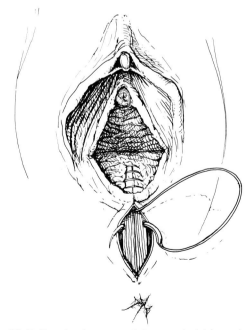

Figure 23–5. Repair of a second-degree obstetric perineal laceration. The vaginal epithelium has been closed. The suture now approximates the superficial perineal muscles.

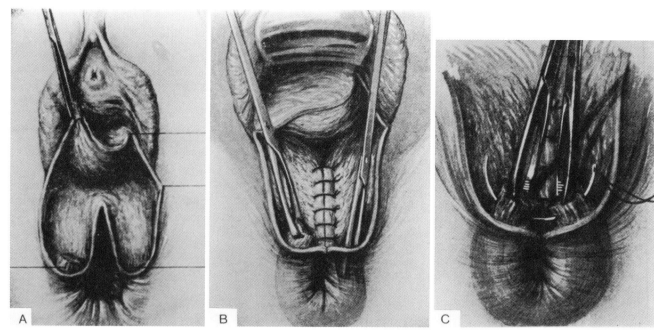

Figure 23–6. *A,* Fourth-degree perineal laceration demonstrating tearing of the rectal sphincter and the rectal mucosa. *B,* Fourth-degree perineal laceration repair: rectal mucosa has been closed in two layers. Allis clamps grasp the retracted ends of the sphincter ani muscle. *C,* Fourth-degree perineal laceration repair: suturing the sphincter ani. The remainder of the repair resembles episiotomy repair (see Figs. 21–1 to 21–5). (From Greenhill, JP: Obstetrics, 13th Edition, Philadelphia: W.B. Saunders Co., 1965.)

ful digital examination of the rectum ensures against unrecognized injuries to the upper rectum.

Closure of the anorectal mucosa begins above the apex of the defect. The first layer of 000 or 0000 polyglycolic-polyglactin or chromic catgut suture on a gastrointestinal needle turns the rectal mucosa into the bowel lumen with a running submucosal stitch. Irrigate the operating field with saline. Place a second continuous Lembert suture in the muscularis of the bowel to imbricate the first layer. This suture begins and ends a centimeter beyond the ends of the defect in the bowel. Irrigate the wound again. A third layer plicates perirectal fascial tissues over the repair. This layer continues as a subcutaneous suture at the anal verge to approximate the perianal skin before later repair work obscures this site.

The continuity of the bowel lumen is now restored. Irrigate the field copiously with saline. Repair the severed sphincter ani muscle as described under the section on third-degree laceration repair.

The postoperative period necessitates few special precautions. Constipating regimens offer no advantage. Stool softeners ease the early resumption of bowel function. Cold perineal packs in the first hours after repair reduce edema. Hot sitz baths during the healing phase make the patient more comfortable and simplify perineal hygiene. Encourage early ambulation. Advise return to intravaginal sexual function when re-examination shows complete healing. Edema and inflammation subside in 2 to 4 weeks. Wound remodeling continues for some weeks thereafter.

Special Problems

The obstetrician may occasionally encounter tears into the rectal lumen above an intact sphincter. Some authors recommend conversion of such a tear into a complete fourth-degree laceration if the tear is near the level of the sphincter. The laceration is then repaired as described for fourth-degree lacerations.[8, 10]

Small, high, buttonhole tears are related to the performance of large episiotomies or to overdistension of the vagina during delivery. Buttonhole injuries are repaired with two layers of absorbable suture, the first inverting the rectal mucosa, the second imbricating the first. The vaginal epithelium is closed transversely with a separate third layer of suture.

All wounds do not heal by primary intention. Despite the most careful technique and anatomic reconstruction, some obstetric laceration repairs break down. Infection, hematoma formation, hypoxia at the tissue level, and poor healing capacity contribute to these disruptions. Systemic diseases also inhibit the healing process. A patient on our service with Crohn disease had a perineal wound breakdown that proved very difficult to heal.

Long-neglected obstetric tears are allowed to heal by secondary intention. They require reconstruction by extensive perineorrhaphy after healing is complete.

Perineal wound dehiscences are infected wounds that should heal by secondary intention. Frequent, warm sitz baths add to the patient's comfort. Antibiotics are necessary if cellulitis is spreading.

An occasional case of necrotizing fasciitis begins in an episiotomy or obstetric laceration repair. Necrotizing fasciitis necessitates culture identification of the offending bacteria and courageous débridement beyond the extent of the process into healthy tissue. Such dissection seems cosmetically unacceptable at the time of surgery but is the only way to control the process. Apply skin grafts as required after clean granulation tissue covers the base of the wound. Obstetric traumatic wounds that heal by secondary intention often necessitate later perineorrhaphy to rebuild the perineum.

Neglected fourth-degree lacerations develop a cloacal deformity with no perineum. Both vaginal and rectal function are poor. Given and Browning[11] reported the repair of 32 cases of old, healed, complete perineal lacerations. Their article points out the reluctance of patients to mention incontinence of stool or flatus because of the social stigma of this dysfunction. They recommend an interval of 3 to 6 months between injury and repair. Earlier repair is often successful if infection is absent and granulation tissue is clean and mature. Preoperative bowel preparation, paradoxic sphincterotomy, colostomy, or cesarean birth for succeeding pregnancies are usually unnecessary adjuncts to these repairs. Vaginal delivery for the next pregnancy is successful in over 90% of cases.

Mattingly[12] offered an excellent discussion of anal incontinence in Telinde's Operative Gynecology textbook. He recommended the standard multilayer closure, as described previously. Mattingly recalled to service the century-old Warren flap technique of repair (Fig. 23–7). An apron-like flap of vaginal epithelium is mobilized from the posterior vaginal wall. This apron is pulled down and sutured over the rectovaginal defect.

The Warren flap technique fell into disuse but had an excellent record of success. Given and Browning,[11] Block and colleagues,[13] and Hibbard[14] offer 20 modern-era Warren flap cases that had complete success. Several major obstetric services in the United States use the Warren flap apron technique. It deserves the consideration of surgeons preparing to attack difficult or recurrent anal incontinence problems.

CERVICAL LACERATIONS

Laceration of the cervix at the time of delivery is second in frequency only to perineal laceration among obstetric traumatic events. Cervical lacerations vary from multiple small nicks in the epithelium to complete tears that extend into the lower uterine segment (Fig. 23–8). Deep lateral cervical lacerations cause massive bleeding and must be considered in the investigation of any postpartum hemorrhage. Unrepaired cervical lacerations result in a distorted, scarred cervix with eversion of the endocervical canal. Cervical incom-

petence or cervical dystocia may occur with later pregnancy.

The cervix may be torn during obstetric maneuvers or forceps applications attempted before complete dilation. Spontaneous cervical lacerations are more common and occur because of rapid dilation of a resistant cervix.

The cervix normally prepares for delivery by fragmentation of many of its fibrous circular collagen bundles. Prostaglandins, estrogens, progesterone, and possibly relaxin influence chemical changes in mature collagen and glyceroglycan ground substances. The cervix becomes hygroscopic, softens, and becomes more elastic and distensible as the time for delivery approaches. Cervical dystocia or cervical laceration may result if labor begins before these preparations are complete. Very rapid dilation may outstrip the elastic capacity of the cervix and result in laceration.

Diagnosis of cervical laceration depends on careful and complete inspection of the entire circumference of the cervix. The cervix after delivery appears as a floppy, edematous mass folded up at the apex of the vaginal vault. Large lacerations can hide among the folds. Torn blood vessels may be in spasm and not bleed immediately after delivery only to open up later with profuse hemorrhage.

Examine the entire circumference of the cervix after each delivery to be certain that the cervix is intact. Try placing a rolled gauze sponge held in a ring forceps in the anterior vaginal fornix and elevating the anterior wall of the vagina upward and cephalad. With luck, the cervix pouches out into full view. A more precise procedure is required to ensure that the entire cervix is seen.

Grasp the cervix with ring forceps at 12 and 2 o'clock (see Fig. 23–8). Inspect the cervix between the clamps to be certain there are no significant lacerations. Move the 12 o'clock forceps to 4 o'clock and examine the new segment of cervix between the clamps. Move the 2 o'clock forceps to 6 o'clock and "walk around the cervix" with alternate placements of the traction forceps until the entire cervix has been examined.

Small nicks in the cervix that are not bleeding require no repair. Suture larger lacerations with interrupted sutures of absorbable material that encompass most of the fibrous wall of the cervix. Attempt to avoid suturing through the endocervix (see Fig. 23–8).[9] The ring forceps inspection procedure described also provides ideal traction for repair of cervical lacerations.

Be certain to see and suture the upper extent of cervical lacerations. Lateral lacerations can extend into the lower uterine segment and involve descending branches of the uterine arteries. It is possible to safely suture some of these extensions from below. There is danger, however, that hemostasis will not be complete. Deep sutures placed blindly can distort or include the ureter or bladder base. Genitourinary fistulas can result from such

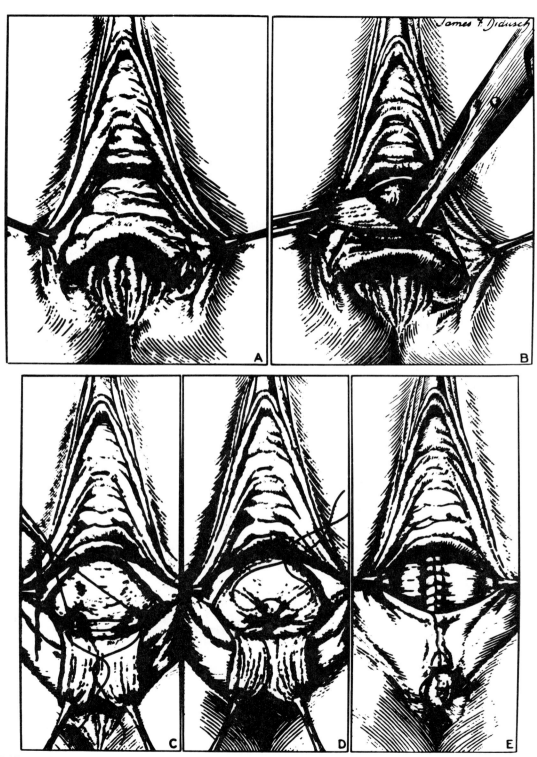

Figure 23–7. Warren flap technique for healed fourth-degree perineal laceration. *A,* The cloacal defect. *B,* Developing the vaginal epithelial flap. *C,* Anal sphincter repair. *D,* Plication of perirectal fascia. *E,* Completion of perineal closure. (From Mattingly RF: Anal incontinence and rectovaginal fistulas. In Mattingly RF [ed.]: Telinde's Operative Gynecology, 6th Edition, Philadelphia: J.B. Lippincott, p. 1679.)

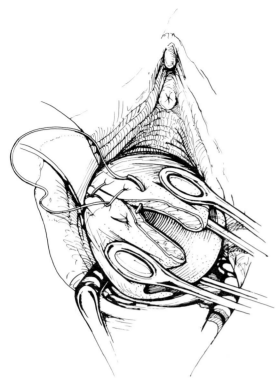

Figure 23–8. Repair of a cervical laceration. Ring forceps grasp the cervix on each side of the laceration and pull the cervix toward the operator. A running locked suture starting above the apex of the tear closes the defect.

inappropriately placed sutures or from undetected injuries.

Inadequate control of torn vessels in the upper cervix and lower uterus results in broad ligament hematoma formation. Instability of vital signs or hematocrit level or the appearance of a pelvic mass after repair of a cervical laceration calls for re-examination and diagnostic imaging. Laparotomy may be required.

ANNULAR DETACHMENT OF THE CERVIX

Avulsion of the cervix at the time of delivery may involve the anterior lip of the cervix or the entire cervix. Complete annular detachment of the cervix during delivery is quite rare. Ingraham and Taylor[15] found only 55 cases in a review of the world's English-language medical literature in 1947. Jeffcoate and Lister[16] added six personal cases in their review of the subject in 1952. We found no references to this topic in the literature of the past decade.

Annular detachment of the cervix implies sloughing of the cervix at the time of obstetric delivery. Pressure necrosis as a result of the fetal head's pressing the cervix against the bony pelvis is the most common cause of annular detachment of the cervix. Other causes include severe cervical dystocia, inappropriate suturing of an incompetent cervix, and application of vacuum extraction cups over an incompletely dilated cervix.[15–18]

Grant[17] identified labor patterns in which cervical detachment develops. The typical patient has a markedly prolonged labor with slow progress or arrest of cervical dilation. A purple edematous mass that is found to be the entire cervix is extruded after the baby and placenta are delivered. Modern management rarely allows such long labors, which explains the rarity of this syndrome in the recent literature.

Spritzer[18] described annular detachment of the cervix during a Mälmstrom cup vacuum extraction delivery. His report made it clear that the detachment was not caused by the vacuum instrument. We echo his admonition to be cautious about the use of the vacuum instrument when the cervix is not completely dilated and to not include cervical tissue in the vacuum cup.

The author has attended only one case of complete annular detachment of the cervix. Extrusion of the cervix occurred 6 weeks after a McDonald cervical cerclage was performed at 13 weeks' gestation. The attending obstetrician had placed the classic McDonald purse-string suture with bites through cervical tissue at 12, 9, 6, and 3 o'clock, using a single strand of polypropylene (Prolene) suture. A second suture was placed slightly above the first with bites at approximately 11, 7, 4, and 1 o'clock. The patient had few symptoms other than vaginal discharge. Six weeks later, she expelled the entire necrotic portio vaginalis of the cervix and the distal suture. We removed the remaining suture and ordered a course of broad-spectrum antibiotics. The pregnancy ended near term with a normal labor and vaginal delivery. The cervical os after delivery was flush with the vaginal vault.

Obstetric annular detachment of the cervix is alarming, but management is usually quite simple. Bleeding is minimal, since the process involves cervical devascularization. Postpartal sepsis after detachment has been involved in the several reported maternal deaths.[16, 18] Cultures at the time of delivery and intensive antibiotic therapy at the first sign of fever should control this problem. Healing takes place by secondary intention. Re-epithelization is usually complete in a few weeks.

The residual length of the cervical stump depends on the amount of cervix lost. The residual cervix after detachment can support later pregnancy.[17] Abdominal delivery after cervical detachment is not mandatory but several authors recommend cesarean birth.[18]

ACUTE OBSTETRIC URINARY TRACT INJURIES

Injuries to the supporting structures of the bladder and urethra occur frequently at the time of spontaneous vaginal delivery. The bladder, ureters, and urethra themselves are rarely injured directly except with extensive trauma that often includes rupture of the uterus. Lieberman[9] reported a 22% incidence of injury to the bladder with uterine rupture. Even extensive lacerations of the anterior vulva seldom injure the mobile urethral tube.

Urinary tract structures are at greatest risk at the time of operative delivery. Deep lacerations of the bladder and urethra may occur from midforceps rotations or other instrumental maneuvers. Laceration of the bladder and lower uterus at the time of classic internal application of Kielland forceps is a prominent historical example of such injury. This type of injury has thankfully disappeared from modern obstetrics.

Faricy and colleagues[19] reviewed reports suggesting that bladder injury occurs in 1 in 105 to 1 in 640 cesarean deliveries. Inadvertent incision of the bladder at the time of repeat cesarean delivery is the most common injury to the urinary tract on the obstetric services of Charity Hospital of New Orleans.

There are several reasons for this special risk. The bladder is often high on the lower uterine segment from previous cesarean operation. If there has been dehiscence of the uterine wound after a previous cesarean delivery, the bladder, the lower uterine segment, and the omentum adhere to the anterior abdominal wall. This places the bladder directly in the path of surgical entry into the abdomen.

Dense adhesions between the bladder wall and the lower uterine segment make for difficult dissection of the bladder flap at the next cesarean operation. Such dissection may inadvertently injure the posterior bladder wall or enter the bladder cavity.

Recognized entry into the bladder at the time of operation is seldom of clinical consequence. Proper repair yields uniformly good results. Unrecognized bladder injury may lead to fistula formation.

Introduce sterile milk or dye into the bladder whenever there is question about bladder injury to reveal any defects in the bladder wall. Sterile milk is available in most hospitals prepared as baby formula in the nursery. Draw up the formula directly from these sterile bottles into a bulb syringe and introduce it into the bladder through the indwelling catheter.

Use intravenous injection of indigo carmine to test the integrity of the ureters. When combined with intentional cystotomy, the dye reveals patency or obstruction of either or both ureters.

Intentional anterior cystotomy strikes fear in the hearts of some obstetric operators. Consider this procedure to explore the bladder for injuries or to ensure ureteral integrity. A repaired cystotomy wound heals readily. It adds no time to the patient's stay in the hospital and little extra effort to her postoperative care. The operator is always

wise to be certain that everything is all right along the urinary tract before closing the abdomen. This certainty is much preferred to worry and multiple imaging procedures in the postoperative period.

Repair of Cystotomy or Bladder Laceration

Visualize the entire extent of any laceration, incision, or other injury to the bladder before any attempts at repair. Be certain about the relationships of the injury to the ureteral orifices. Mobilize the bladder enough to place two rows of suture along the entire length of the bladder wound without tension and without compromising the ureters. Consultation with a urologist in the operating room is most helpful for obstetric surgeons who are not comfortable with surgical procedures involving the ureters and bladder.

Repair of a complete bladder laceration is similar to the repair of wounds to any hollow viscus. The closure is in two layers, the second imbricating the first (Fig. 23–9). Do not use permanent suture for bladder closure because it acts as a nidus for infection and calculus formation. Absorbable suture of small caliber, such as 000 polyglycolic-polyglactin or chromic suture on a small needle, is ideal.

Place the anchoring first stitch just beyond the

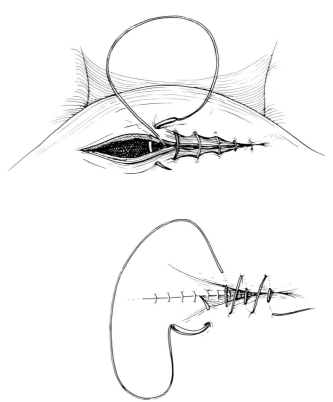

Figure 23–9. Cystotomy closure A first running suture of absorbable material closes all layers of the bladder wall. A second running suture imbricates the first layer.

apex of one end of the wound. A running suture plicates the muscularis layer of the bladder wall (see Fig. 23–9). This suture may encompass all layers, but many surgeons attempt to exclude and invert the innermost uroepithelial layer. This suture continues to the opposite end of the wound and is tied.

A second row of continuous sutures inverts the first layer, beginning and ending a centimeter beyond the wound (see Fig. 23–9). This imbricating second layer may be a Lembert stitch parallel to the wound or a Connell stitch at right angles to the wound. Watertight closure is not mandatory for accurate healing. Many surgeons check the suture line by filling the bladder with milk or dye before closure. This step also reveals other areas of unrecognized bladder injury in complicated cases.

Opinions vary about drainage of the wound site in cases of bladder injury. We place a soft suction drain near but not on the repair site. The suction drainage tubing exits through a separate stab wound in the anterior abdominal wall. We remove the drain in 48 to 72 hours or when drainage is minimal.

Keep the bladder empty for 7 to 10 days after repair with a suprapubic or transurethral catheter. Cystitis from prolonged transurethral catheterization must be anticipated and managed. Acidification of the urine is a common preventive measure. Culture the urine and employ appropriate antibiotics if infection is evident. Monitor urinary output carefully for the first few days after surgery. Hydrate the patient sufficiently to maintain a copious urine output. There may be some blood in the urine after bladder surgery. Keep bladder catheters free of clots by frequent, gentle irrigation with small volumes of a dilute solution of acetic acid.

Suprapubic transvesical catheters are becoming increasingly popular. They are effective and safe and offer the patient freedom from the discomfort of the Foley catheter.

Ureteral Injury

Injury to the ureters occurs rarely during obstetric operations. Ureteral injury is more common with severe traumatic events, such as uterine rupture or vehicular accident. Midforceps and high forceps operations involving rotations were formerly responsible for occasional ureteral injury. These operations are rare in modern obstetrics.

Injury to the ureter in obstetric cases usually occurs within the cardinal tunnel. The ureter may be transected, disrupted by trauma, or incorporated in a suture. It may be kinked or tented by suture placement. The delicate blood supply in the adventitial layer of the ureter may be stripped away by trauma or surgical dissection.

When ureteral injury is near the bladder, ureteroneocystotomy effects repair. The distal end of the ureter is ligated near the bladder. An intentional cystotomy is performed. A 2- to 3-cm angled tunnel is made in the muscularis of the bladder. The proximal end of the ureter is freshened. Guide sutures pass through the distal muscularis of the ureter. These sutures are then threaded through the new tunnel in the bladder wall. The ureter is pulled through the tunnel into the bladder. The distal ureter is sutured to the bladder mucosa with several fine absorbable sutures.

The site where the ureter exits the outside of the bladder wall is supported by sutures through the muscularis of the bladder and the ureter. There must be no tension on the implantation site. The bladder may be sutured to the psoas muscle on the posterior wall of the abdomen (the psoas hitch) to elongate and stabilize the implantation.

The site of ureteral injury may be too far from the bladder for direct reimplantation. A flap of bladder wall can be formed into a tube to gain an extra 2 or 3 cm of length. This maneuver is called the Boari flap, after its developer.

Ureteral injury higher in the pelvis requires ureteroureteral reanastomosis. The two ends of the ureter are spatulated and sutured end to end over a ureteral catheter. Both this procedure and the Boari flap are not operations for the occasional urinary tract surgeon. The obstetrician profits from consultation with his or her urology colleagues in these matters.

Urethral Trauma

Isolated acute urethral injury that requires repair is uncommon in spontaneous obstetric deliveries. Pressure necrosis from prolonged labor causes occasional late urethrovaginal fistulas. Instrumental deliveries, particularly rotation maneuvers, are the most frequent cause of urethral tears.

The first step in repairing the urethra is careful inspection of the extent of the injury. Lieberman[9] stressed identification of the ureters in cases of widespread periurethral damage and hematoma formation around the base of the bladder. Most urethral injuries can be repaired vaginally after careful delineation of the extent of damage.

Close the urethral epithelium first with 000 or 0000 interrupted absorbable sutures. Close the periurethral tissues over this repair with a second row of fine interrupted sutures. Suture the overlying vaginal epithelium with continuous or interrupted 00 absorbable sutures. Maintain bladder drainage by suprapubic catheter for 7 to 10 days.

OBSTETRIC GENITAL FISTULAS

Genital fistulas are chronic openings between the urinary or intestinal tracts and the genital tract. The passage of urine, flatus, or feces into the vagina signals their presence. Fistulas are particularly onerous to women and result in severe social, sexual, and functional disability.

The historical development of the specialty of gynecology in the United States began with efforts to address the disabilities caused by obstetric genitourinary fistulas. Sims'[20] report of successful fistula repair in 1852 was a milestone in the history of gynecology. Before cesarean delivery was a common and safe practice, prolonged and obstructed labor was common. Pressure necrosis resulted in large numbers of obstetric fistulas. Straining, difficult manipulations and forceps deliveries tore at the bladder, rectum, and their support structures.[21, 22] The resulting fistulas, genital prolapse, and herniations were responsible for much patient discomfort.

The dramatic reduction in the incidence of obstetric genital fistulas in the past 50 years resulted from changes in the management of obstructed labor and the liberalization of cesarean section. Many obstetricians now complete their training programs without seeing or repairing an obstetric genitourinary fistula. The most prevalent current obstetric fistulas are rectovaginal fistulas related to episiotomies.

Diagnosis of Genital Fistulas

Genital fistulas related to obstetric delivery include vesicovaginal, vesicouterine, vesicocervical, vesicocervicovaginal, urethrovaginal, ureterovaginal, rectovaginal, and anoperineal fistulas (Table 23–4). Complex diagnostic procedures, imaging techniques, and surgical management plans are often required to clarify complicated anatomic interrelationships. Simple procedures suffice for the initial assessment of the patient who complains of soiling of the perineum with urine or stool after delivery.

Rectovaginal fistula is signaled by the passage of flatus or stool through the vagina. Large fistulas are clinically obvious. Small fistulas can be detected by placing cotton balls in the vagina and then filling the rectum with tinted solution. Fine probes help localize small lesions. Radiologic procedures clarify the more obscure fistulas.

Table 23–4. OBSTETRIC GENITAL FISTULAS

Intestinal Tract
Rectovaginal fistula
Anoperineal fistula
Urinary Tract
Vesicovaginal fistula
Vesicouterine fistula
Vesicouterovaginal fistula
Vesicocervical fistula
Vesicocervicovaginal fistula
Ureterovaginal fistula
Ureterouterovaginal fistula

Vesicovaginal fistulas cause uncontrollable incontinence of urine. The patient is embarrassed by the odor and constant wetness. Large fistulas are clearly visible on the anterior vaginal wall. Small fistulas can be localized by placing cotton balls or tampons in the vagina and then filling the bladder with saline tinted with indigo carmine or other dyes. Cystoscopy and cystography clarify the position of fistulas in relation to the ureteral and urethral orifices.

The patient may complain of wetness and leakage of urine even when the above tests reveal no bladder defect. The obstetrician is then obligated to investigate the possibility of ureterovaginal fistula. Intravenous indigo carmine leaks through a ureterovaginal fistula and stains vaginal packing. Contrast pyelography can trace the course of complex ureterovaginal relationships. Obstetric ureterovaginal fistulas are rare. Investigation of urine leakage is not complete until this entity has been ruled out.

Vesicovaginal Fistula Repair

The literature of genital fistulas and their repair is extensive. Carter and colleagues[21] Counseller and Haigler,[22] Moir,[23] Bey,[24] Lescher and Pratt,[25] and others wrote important studies in the era when these lesions were more common. These reviews are still very useful to the modern physician faced with a fistula problem. Management of complex genital fistulas is not for the occasional operator. Fistulas often require the efforts of a team of bowel surgeons, urologists, and obstetrician-gynecologists for optimal management.

The timing of vesicovaginal fistula repair is important. Classic recommendations called for complete healing of the fistula over a period of months before attempted repair. The long interval resulted in great discomfort and embarrassment to patients. The current trend is toward early repair, provided that active infection is not present. Preoperative glucocorticoids were formerly recommended to improve the status of the tissues to be repaired. Steroids are seldom used in the current era.

The choice of operation for vesicovaginal fistula depends on the history of the lesion and the conditions found at the time of examination and dissection. Simple, mature, uncomplicated fistulas close easily using the layer technique described below. Very large defects or complex anatomic relationships are more difficult. Repair is doubly difficult when previous attempts at repair have failed or when the fistula is associated with radiation therapy or malignancy.

Dense, widespread scar tissue is an ominous prognostic finding. The broad dissection required to reach well-vascularized tissues inevitably enlarges the fistula opening. Extensive plastic procedures may be required to close the defect. Latzko[26] proposed a modified culpocleisis to close large fistulas using both anterior and posterior vaginal walls.

The interposition of vascular flaps of bulbocavernosus muscles or other tissues brings auxiliary blood supply to promote healing of tissues with reduced vascular supply. Such operations were first developed by Martius of Vienna and described in the American literature by McCall and Bolten.[27]

Layer Closure of Simple Vesicovaginal Fistulas

Table 23–5 outlines the principles of obstetric vesicovaginal fistula repair. Preoperative evaluation must clarify the condition of the upper urinary tract and the bladder. The relationship of the fistula to the ureteral orifices is particularly important. There must be room to dissect away scar tissue and place two rows of suture without compromising the ureters or ureteral orifices. An abdominal transvesical approach may be preferable if there is any question about adequate space for suturing.

Adequate exposure of the operating field necessitates proper patient position, directed lighting, and retraction by assistants. Urinary fistulas high in the vagina are difficult to approach in the lithotomy position. The Sims position or knee-chest position facilitates visualization of the anterior vaginal wall. The curved Heaney needle holder is useful for suturing when access is difficult.

Dissection begins by circumcision of the vaginal opening of the fistula. Dissection carries through the full depth of the fistula tract, including the bladder wall. The entire fistula tract is thus removed. The edges of the dissection should be free of dense scar tissue and should be well supplied with blood vessels. The bladder wall and the vaginal wall should separate easily.

Dissect the vaginal epithelium from the bladder around the circumference of the fistula for at least 2 cm (Fig. 23–10). In many cases this dissection is facilitated by incision of the vaginal epithelium at 12, 3, 6, and 9 o'clock. This creates four quadrant flaps, which are individually dissected.

Close the bladder opening in an anterior to

Table 23–5. PRINCIPLES OF VESICOVAGINAL FISTULA REPAIR

Complete healing prior to repair
Optimal preoperative condition of tissues
Aseptic surgical technique
Excision of entire fistula tract and scar tissue
Mobilization of tissue planes beyond scar tissue
Multilayer closure of bladder
Separate closure of vagina
Assurance of adequate or auxiliary blood supply to repair site
Bladder kept empty during healing process
Prompt treatment of local infections

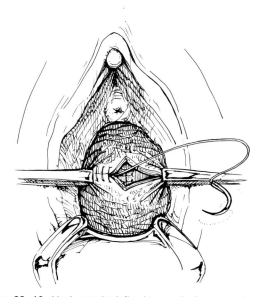

Figure 23–10. Vesicovaginal fistula—vaginal approach to closure. The fistula tract has been excised. The bladder has been closed in two vertical layers. The vaginal epithelium is now closed in a horizontal plane at right angles to the bladder closure.

posterior direction. The first layer of closure is a continuous 000 absorbable polyglycolic-polyglactin submucosal suture. Interrupted sutures are equally effective, as is chromic suture material. This layer turns the uroepithelium inward (see Fig. 23–9). A second continuous Lembert suture in the bladder muscularis layer imbricates the first layer. This suture begins and ends 1 cm beyond the fistula. These two layers must be closed without tension. Interpose a vascular flap if there is need for a supportive layer of tissue or additional blood supply (see Fig. 23–11). Complete the fistula repair by closing the vaginal epithelium. Trim the edges of the vaginal epithelial flaps and close the incision at right angles to the line of bladder closure (Fig. 23–10).

Place a loose vaginal pack to minimize early accumulation of tissue fluids between the layers of the repair. Suprapubic drainage is excellent for all urinary fistula repairs and preferred for those located in the lower trigone. Foley transurethral catheters provide adequate drainage if the bulb does not rest on the repair site.

Remove the pack in 24 hours. Maintain bladder drainage for 7 to 10 days.[23] At the end of this time, clamp the suprapubic catheter. Allow the patient to void spontaneously. Observe for any leakage of urine. Healing continues with prolonged bladder drainage despite the absence of a watertight seal at this time. Leakage of urine is an ominous prognostic sign, however, as is any inflammation or necrosis at the site of the repair.

Repair of Rectovaginal Fistulas

Rectovaginal fistulas are divided into those near the introitus and those higher up on the posterior wall. Very low fistulas may exit onto the perineum as anoperineal fistulas.

Low rectovaginal fistulas are those within a centimeter or so of the hymenal ring. These are often best managed by converting them into fourth-degree perineal lacerations and repairing the resulting defect as described in the section of this chapter on perineal lacerations.

High rectovaginal fistulas are those whose opening is in the mid-vagina or upper vagina (more than 1 cm above the hymenal ring). Close these fistulas in layers in a manner similar to that described for vesicovaginal fistulas. Order a standard bowel surgery preparation for the days preceding the operation.

In the operating room, completely outline the course of the fistula tract by passing a flexible probe along its length. Excise the entire fistula tract. Dissect the vaginal wall from the rectal wall for a distance of at least 2 cm around the circumference of the fistula defect.

Close the rectal defect in two layers. The first layer is a submucosal continuous suture of 000 absorbable material that proceeds from cephalad to caudad, beginning above the apex of the defect. A second layer imbricates the first.

Close the vaginal defect with a single layer of 00 absorbable suture at right angles to the rectal closure.

Stool softeners and a low-residue diet facilitate healing in the first week. Diversion of the fecal stream is not necessary except in recurrent or particularly difficult cases.

Complicated Fistulas

Coffey[28] described the process of transplantation of the ureters into the sigmoid colon with problem vesicovaginal fistulas. A functioning bladder could not be established in Coffey's cases, either because of the large size of the fistula or because the bladder was removed for tumor or other reasons. Serious urinary tract infections and chronic diarrhea are common after ureterosigmoid transplantation. Separate conduit pouches made of a loop of ileum or a combination of large and small bowel are more satisfactory long-term ureteral diversion methods.

The Martius bulbocavernosus interposition operation helps when there is decreased blood supply at the fistula repair site or when previous repairs have failed. Aartsen and Sindram[29] reported success in all of 14 radiation-induced rectovaginal fistulas.

To perform bulbocavernosus interposition, tunnel beneath the dissected vaginal epithelium mobilized for the fistula repair, deep to the labium majorum. Transect the distal bulbocavernosus muscle to create a vascular flap. The muscle, with its intact proximal blood supply, is rotated through the developed tunnel and sutured over the repair site as a pedicle graft (Fig. 23–11).

Fistulas that are very large or recurrent or that involve multiple organs are particularly difficult problems. Kelemen and Lehoczky[30] described an island flap technique to address vesicovaginorectal fistulas without having to divert the urinary or fecal stream. The fistula is widely dissected, as with other closures. A flap consisting of adipose tissue with an island of skin is raised from the labium majorum and genitofemoral sulcus. The development of this flap begins with a paravulvar gluteoinguinal incision on the side opposite the episiotomy incision used to expose the fistula. A 3- to 4-cm skin island with its underlying fat and blood supply is tunneled beneath the bulbocavernosus muscle. The fatty tissue covers the repaired bladder defect. The skin island covers the defect in the vaginal wall (Fig. 23–12*A, B*).

Difficult rectovaginal and vesicovaginal fistulas can be closed with myocutaneous flaps using the gracilis muscle. Fleischmann and Picha[31] describe an abdominal approach for gracilis muscle interposition for vesicovaginal fistula. Gorenstein and colleagues[32] utilized the gracilis muscle interposition procedure for difficult rectovaginal fistulas.

Endorectal flap advancement is advocated for difficult rectovaginal fistulas. Lowry and colleagues[33] report success in 83% of patients. This group used advancement flaps only for fistulas smaller than 2.5 cm in diameter below the mid-vagina. All fistulas were of infectious or traumatic origin, not the result of radiation or malignancy. Lowry's group recommended a muscle interposition operation for patients with failed previous repairs.[33]

Jones and colleagues[34] used transanal rectal ad-

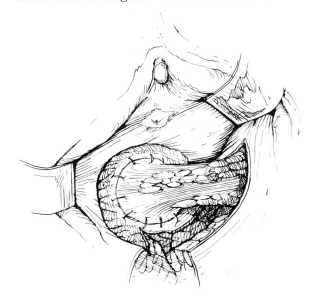

Figure 23–11. A Martius flap of bulbocavernosus muscle and fat covers the vesicovaginal fistula repair site to aid vascularization and healing. The vaginal epithelium will be closed over the flap graft.

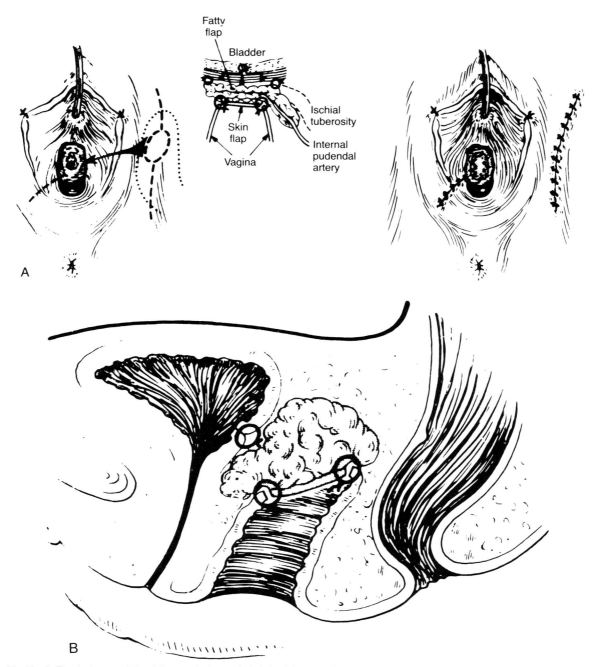

Figure 23–12. *A,* The Lehoczky island flap technique. *A, left:* Incision and flap development; *B, center:* positioning the flap of skin and adipose tissue; *C, right:* completed procedure. *B,* The Lehoczky island flap (lateral view). The flap of skin with underlying adipose tissue has been interposed between the vesicovaginal fistula bladder closure and the vagina. The skin portion of the flap closes the vaginal wall defect. (From Keleman Z, Lehoczky G: Closure of severe vesico-vaginal-rectal fistulas using Lehoczky's island flap. Br J Urol 59:154, 1987.)

vancement in a large group of patients with fistulas secondary to Crohn's disease. They eradicated the fistulas in 57.9% of these difficult cases.

SEPARATION OF THE SYMPHYSIS PUBIS

Symptomatic separation of the symphysis pubis at the time of obstetric delivery occurs in about 1 in 2200 deliveries.[35] We must make this diagnosis by clinical symptoms, since some separation of the symphysis is commonly demonstrated after obstetric delivery by imaging techniques. Symphyseal separation of over 1 cm is abnormal, but separations of 3 to 5 cm without symptoms have been reported (Fig. 23–13A, B).[35]

The pathologic defect is rupture of the tendinous anterior and posterior bands across the symphyseal joint. This allows separation of the joint cartilage and causes instability of the pelvic girdle. The causative factors are the intense forces of labor acting against the symphysis pubis. Associated factors include restraint of the laboring patient and excessive abduction of the thighs.[35, 36] Even patients with short, trouble-free labors can develop symphyseal separation.

Labor attendants in Third World countries and other remote areas perform intentional surgical division of the symphysis as an alternative to cesarean birth. The practice of symphyseotomy has hopefully all but disappeared from modern Western obstetrics.

Symphyseal separation is suspected when a postpartum patient complains of severe pain in the region of the symphysis pubis that intensifies with any movement of the pelvis. There is point tenderness and, occasionally, an indentation defect over the symphysis. Movement of the pelvic girdle evokes crepitation and duplicates the pain. The patient who is able to walk does so with extreme difficulty and pain. She has a wide, waddling gait. She may have sciatic pain and splinting of the extremities against any movement that causes pain.

Radiologic images of the symphysis reveal 1 cm or more widening of the joint space. The distance between the pubic bones may be as much as 3 to 5 cm. Advanced cases show ragged edges at the ends of the pubic bones.

Initial treatment consists of analgesics and bed rest with a pelvic sling or hammock type of support.[36] Maintenance of pelvic stability requires the support of an orthopedic girdle when ambulation resumes. This treatment seems simple but may be very difficult to accomplish. Orthopedic surgical fixation is indicated when joint stability cannot be maintained, when pain is severe, or when the symphyseal separation is vast.[37]

The symphysis occasionally sustains an open rupture accompanied by laceration of the bladder or urethra.[37] Immediate repair of injured structures and open fixation of the symphyseal joint are indicated. Acute septic arthritis with or without abscess complicates an occasional case. Other patients develop chronic osteoarthritis, osteomyelitis, and chronic pain, which are difficult orthopedic problems.

COCCYX FRACTURE

Fracture of the coccyx is an infrequent complication of vaginal obstetric delivery. Under ideal conditions, the sacrococcygeal joint is flexible enough to allow the coccyx to push backward out of the path of the advancing fetal head. Fixation of the sacrococcygeal joint may result in ligament tears or fracture. The J-shaped sacrococcygeal configuration, in which the coccyx protrudes sharply into the birth canal, is at particular risk for injury.

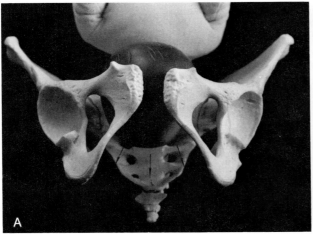 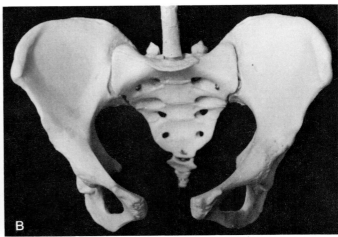

Figure 23–13. *A,* Separation of the symphysis pubis: The force of labor pressing the fetal head against the symphysis can result in tearing of support ligaments and separation of the pubic bones. *B,* The pubic symphysis may separate, creating a gap of 2 to 6 cm. This results in instability of the pelvic girdle and difficulty in walking.

The attendant at delivery may hear or feel a "snap" at the time the coccyx gives way. This does not always mean that a fracture has occurred. The paracoccygeal ligaments can be torn without fracture and yield the same sound and similar post-delivery symptoms.

The mother with coccygeal fracture or ligament tears experiences intense pain in the coccygeal region that may be mistaken for rectal or episiotomy pain. Any movement of the coccyx causes sharp discomfort. Walking, sitting, and defecation all cause pain. The pain of coccyx injury lasts many weeks and resists efforts to relieve the discomfort.

Treatment consists of analgesics, sitz baths, and avoidance of pressure on the buttocks and the sacrum. Some orthopedists recommend excision of the coccyx in severe cases. Injection of local anesthetics or corticosteroids into the area of the sacrococcygeal joint seldom offers long-term relief but may give temporary respite from intense discomfort.

MATERNAL OBSTETRIC PARALYSIS

Peroneal Nerve Palsy

The dorsal lithotomy position that American obstetricians most frequently choose for obstetric patients involves placing the legs up in stirrups. Pressure of rigid stirrups against the knee can injure the peroneal nerve, which occupies a fixed, superficial position in a shallow, bony depression lateral to the knee. Prolonged pressure on the lateral portion of the knee causes peroneal nerve palsy with loss of dorsiflexion of the foot (drop foot). This condition may be transient or permanent, depending on the duration and intensity of the nerve pressure. Neurologic consultation can rule out other causes of nerve palsy and drop foot.

The best management is prevention by careful padding of stirrups and adjustment of the legs to avoid pressure on the lateral aspect of the knees. Treatment is supportive and rehabilitative, with use of passive exercises and dorsiflexion foot splints.

Injuries to the Sacral Plexus

Whittaker's[38] dissertation in 1958 on neurologic injuries at the time of obstetric delivery estimated that some type of nerve injury occurred once in 2000 deliveries. Many of these injuries escape the attention of caretakers in the absence of paralysis or serious sensory disturbances, which occur only once in 5000 deliveries.

Obstetric paralysis sometimes results from pressure on the sacral plexus by the advancing fetal vertex. The majority of cases have been related to injuries by obstetric forceps in midpelvic operations.

The sacral plexus lies on the medial aspect of the piriformis muscle as it leaves the pelvis through the greater sciatic notch. Its two main branches are the pudendal and the sciatic nerves. The sciatic nerve has three principal components, a posterior trunk to the hamstrings, the medial popliteal nerve to the front of the lower leg, and the lateral popliteal nerve to the back of the lower leg. Motor fibers are least resistant to injury and are subject to loss of conductivity without break in the continuity of the nerve trunk. Even edema of the nerve trunk can produce transient impairment in nerve function.[38]

The clinical picture of nerve root injury appears immediately after delivery. The major complaint is weakness of the leg accompanied by numbness, tingling, or pain, most often located on the lateral aspect of the calf and the dorsum of the foot. There is impairment of sensation to pin prick and light touch in 70% of cases. Weakness or paralysis of the tibialis anterior muscle is a common feature that results in inability to dorsiflex the foot (drop foot).

Treatment is expectant, with a foot board, drop-foot splints, and passive exercises. Sensory function usually returns within 4 weeks and motor function within 12 weeks.[38] Muscle atrophy occurs if recovery is delayed. Muscle paralysis can be permanent but may continue to improve for up to 2 years.

HIP AND BACK STRAIN

The major complaint of discomfort related to childbirth for some patients is postpartal hip or back pain. Such patients complain of sacroiliac pain and tenderness or pain near the greater trochanter of the femur when walking.

Sacroiliac strain can occur from joint instability because of physiologic pregnancy changes combined with the pressures of normal delivery. The sacroiliac joint and the hip capsule can be injured from bearing-down efforts in the lithotomy position during expulsion of the baby. These joints are also at risk when the patient moves on and off the delivery table and when the legs are taken in and out of delivery stirrups. The patient with an epidural or spinal anesthetic offers little help or resistance when moved into or out of delivery position. The leverage offered by the legs can result in strains to the hip and back.

Care must be taken not to abduct or externally rotate the thighs excessively or twist the back when taking patients down from stirrups. The thighs should be flexed and the knees brought together in the midline. The legs are then extended

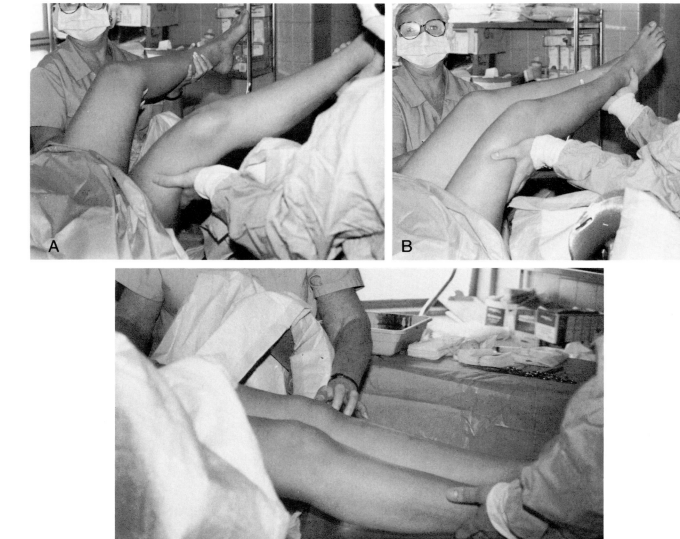

Figure 23–14. *A,* Taking the legs from the delivery table stirrups. Method to avoid hip and back strain. Step 1: Lift the legs simultaneously, flexing a little at the hips and knees. *B,* Step 2: Bring the knees together in the midline. *C,* Step 3: Simultaneously bring the legs to the level of the table top. (Courtesy Glenn Aucoin, M.D.)

and brought down to the table (Fig. 23–14). No stress is placed on either the hip joint or sacroiliac joints by this procedure.

ALLEN-MASTERS SYNDROME

Allen and Masters,[39] in 1955, described 28 patients with a clinical syndrome they believed resulted from previous traumatic laceration of uterine supports at the time of spontaneous obstetric delivery. The symptoms reported included deep dyspareunia, dysmenorrhea, pelvic pressure, and tiredness. Physical findings included a hypermobile cervix that appeared to have no attachments and pain on upward motion of the cervix.

They described retroversion of the uterus, fluid in the pelvis, and healed laceration of one or both broad ligaments and one or both uterosacral ligaments. They recommended repair of the broad ligament defects with a double layer of sutures combined with repair of torn uterosacral ligaments and uterine suspension. Perineorrhaphy and cystocoele repair were included in some cases. Relief of pelvic pain was reported to be prompt and consistent and was followed by gradual resolution of other symptoms.

Gynecologic surgeons occasionally see broad ligament defects such as those described by Allen and Masters. They are rare and do not seem consistently related to traumatic obstetric events.

Some seem to be congenital variants of normal pelvic anatomy.

One must remain skeptical of an operative procedure designed to relieve tiredness and other vague symptoms.

POSTPARTAL LABIAL ADHESION

Adhesion of the labia minora after delivery results from abrasion or laceration of both labia. Post-delivery immobilization of these structures permits healing in rare instances by agglutination of the apposed injured surfaces. Shaver and colleagues[40] reported the failure of topical applications of estrogen to improve postpartal labial adhesion in the manner expected with pediatric labial adhesions. This finding was anticipated because the causes of the two entities are different.

Postpartal labial adhesions are composed of relatively dense scar tissue that must be separated by sharp dissection. The labia are then kept apart with soft, nonadhesive dressings until surface healing is advanced.

Regular vulvar hygienic measures and rapid return to ambulation after delivery prevent most instances of labial adhesion.

SUMMARY

We have reviewed a portion of the spectrum of disorders related to trauma at the time of obstetric delivery. Many injuries result from the forces required for normal delivery of large, firm infant heads through restricted pelvic passages lined with friable tissues. Some of these disorders result from obstetric manipulations or emergency delivery procedures.

Some injuries are unavoidable. Many maternal obstetric injuries are avoidable by judicious labor management, wise delivery decisions, and meticulous obstetric habits and technique. The obstetrician's job is to minimize the incidence of maternal injuries and disabilities resulting from these injuries.

References

1. Hamilton HG: Post-partum labial or paravaginal hematomas. Am J Obstet Gynecol 39:642, 1940.
2. Fliegner JRH: Postpartal broad ligament hematomas. J Obstet Gynecol Br Commwlth 78:184, 1971.
3. Romine JC: Postpartum Hematoma. J Ark Med Soc 64:155, 1967.
4. Quilligan EJ, Zuspan FP: Management of delivery trauma. In Douglas-Stromme Operative Obstetrics, 4th Edition. New York: Appleton-Century-Crofts 1982, pp. 692–742.
5. DeLee JB: Vulvar hematomas. In Principles and Practice of Obstetrics. Philadelphia: WB Saunders Co., 1927, p. 783.
6. Farkas AM, Quevedo-Bonilla G, Gingold B, et al.: Presacral

7. Hematomas: Diagnosis and Treatment. Dis Col Rect 30:130, 1987.
8. Pedowitz P, Poser S, Adler NH: Puerperal Hematoma. Am J Obstet Gynecol 81:351, 1961.
9. Frisoli G: Maternal Birth Injuries. In Iffy L, Kaminetsky HA (eds.): Principles and Practice of Obstetrics and Perinatology, Vol. 2. New York: John Wiley & Sons, 1981, pp. 975–989.
10. Lieberman BA: Repair to injuries of the genital tract. Clin Obstet Gynecol 7:621, 1980.
11. Royston GD: Repair of complete perineal laceration. Am J Obstet Gynecol 19:185, 1930.
12. Given FT, Browning G: Repair of old complete perineal lacerations. Am J Obstet Gynecol 159:779, 1988.
13. Mattingly, RF: Anal incontinence and rectovaginal fistulas. In: Mattingly RF (ed.): Telinde's Operative Gynecology, 5th Edition. Philadelphia: JB Lippincott Co., 1977, pp. 611–626.
14. Block IR, Rodriguez M, Olivares AL: The Warren operation for anal incontinence caused by disruption of the anterior segment of the anal sphincter, perineal body, and rectovaginal septum. Dis Col Rect 18:28, 1975.
15. Hibbard LT: Surgical management of rectovaginal fistulas and complete perineal tears. Am J Obstet Gynecol 130:139, 1978.
16. Ingraham CB, Taylor ES: Detachment of the cervix: A review. Am J Obstet Gynecol 53:873, 1947.
17. Jeffcoate TNA, Lister UM: Annular detachment of the cervix. J Obstet Gynaecol Br Emp 59:309, 1952.
18. Grant FG: Annular detachment of cervix. Br Med J 2:1539, 1955.
19. Spritzer TD: Annular detachment of the cervix during delivery by vacuum extraction. Am J Obstet Gynecol 83:247, 1962.
20. Faricy PO, Augspurger RR, Kaufman JM: Bladder injuries associated with cesarean section. J Urol 120:762, 1978.
21. Sims JM: On the treatment of vesico-vaginal fistulae. Am J Med Sci 23:59, 1852.
22. Carter B, Palumbo L, Creadick RN, et al.: Vesicovaginal fistula. Am J Obstet Gynecol 63:479, 1952.
23. Counseller VS, Haigler H: Management of urinary-vaginal fistula in 253 cases. Am J Obstet Gynecol 72:367, 1956.
24. Moir JC: Personal experience in the treatment of vesicovaginal fistulas. Am J Obstet Gynecol 71:476, 1956.
25. Bey NM: A new technique in dealing with superior rectovaginal fistulae. J Obst Gynecol Br Emp 41:579, 1934.
26. Lescher TC, Pratt JH: Vaginal repair of the simple rectovaginal fistula. Surg Gynecol Obstet 124:1317, 1967.
27. Latzko W: Behandlung hoch sitzender blasen und mastdarmscheiden fisteln nach unteruextirpation mit hohem scheiden verschluss. Zntrbl Gynak 25:905, 1914.
28. McCall ML, Bolten KA: Martius Gynecological Operations. Boston: Little, Brown, 1956.
29. Coffey RC: Transplantation of the ureters into the large intestine in the absence of a functioning urinary bladder. Surg Obstet Gynecol 47:367, 1956.
30. Aartsen EJ, Sindram IS: Repair of the radiation induced rectovaginal fistulas without or with interposition of the bulbocavernosus muscle (Martius procedure). Eur J Surg Oncol 14:171, 1988.
31. Kelemen Z, Lehoczky G: Closure of severe vesico-vaginorectal fistulas using Lehoczky's island flap. Br J Urol 59:153, 1987.
32. Fleischmann J, Picha G: Abdominal approach for gracilis muscle interposition and repair of recurrent vesicovaginal fistulas. J Urol 140:552, 1988.
33. Gorenstein L, Boyd JB, Ross TM: Gracilis muscle repair of rectovaginal fistula after restorative proctocolectomy. Dis Col Rect 31:730, 1988.
34. Lowry AC, Thorson AG, Rothenberger DA, et al.: Repair of simple rectovaginal fistulas. Influence of previous repairs. Dis Col Rect 31:676, 1988.
35. Jones IT, Fazio VW, Jagelman DG: The use of transanal

rectal advancement flaps in the management of fistulas involving the anorectum. Dis Col Rect 30:919, 1987.

35. Callahan JT: Separation of the symphysis pubis. Am J Obstet Gynecol 66:281, 1953.

36. Cibils LA: Rupture of the symphysis pubis. Obstet Gynecol 38:407, 1971.

37. Blum M, Orovono N: Open rupture of the symphysis during spontaneous delivery. Acta Obstet Gynecol Scand 55:77, 1976.

38. Whittaker WG: Injuries to the sacral plexus in obstetrics. Can Med Assoc J 79:622, 1958.

39. Allen WM, Masters WH: Traumatic laceration of uterine support: Clinical syndrome and operative treatment. Am J Obstet Gynecol 70:500, 1955.

40. Shaver D, Ling F, Muram D: Labial adhesions in a postpartum patient. Obstet Gynecol 68:24s, 1986.

VI

Cesarean Delivery

Cesarean Section: History, Incidence, and Indications

Karen A. Raimer
Mary J. O'Sullivan

DEFINITION AND HISTORY

Cesarean section or cesarean birth is defined as an operative procedure to deliver the fetus through an incision in the abdominal and uterine walls. Therefore, delivery of an extrauterine abdominal pregnancy or a fetus after uterine rupture does not fulfill the definition of cesarean delivery.

Many theories explain the origin of the term *cesarean section,* none of which can be substantiated by review. One of the three most popular theories is that Julius Caesar was delivered via cesarean section.[1] If this were true, it is surprising that his mother was still alive when he invaded Britain. For her to have survived a cesarean section would have been unlikely, because the knowledge of human anatomy at the time was minimal. The second theory implicates a Roman law created by Numa Pompeleus in the eighth century B.C. called "lex cesarea," which dictated that the procedure be performed after fetal maturity to save an infant whose mother was dead or dying. The last theory of this trilogy posits that the term originated in the Middle Ages when the Latin words *caedere* and *seco,* both meaning "to cut," were used.[2] Although this origin is speculative, the operative procedure has been documented and has progressed through three different periods as operative skills and knowledge have improved.

Before the latter part of the sixteenth century, the procedure was performed only on dead and dying mothers to save the fetus. More often than not, however, the infant was stillborn. In 1581, Francois Rousset[3] first recommended the procedure for the living mother after several of his friends reported their experience, although there is no documentation of his friends' cases. The first documented reports of cesarean section being performed on living patients were published by Francois Mauriceau in 1668, at which time it was used only as a last resort to accomplish delivery but always resulted in maternal death.[4]

The first physician whose patient survived the procedure was an Englishman named James Barlow.[5] In 1779 he performed the operation on Jane Foster, a gravida eight, para seven, with a pelvic deformity. After laboring for 4 days, Jane was delivered of a dead fetus. She completely recovered and reportedly returned to work 17 days after surgery.

Around the beginning of the nineteenth century, cesarean sections were a controversial issue. There were two schools of thought and much debate over the management of difficult labors. The choices were cesarean section versus forceps delivery, craniotomy, or embryotomy. As the maternal survival rate of the cesarean operation improved, more physicians began to favor cesarean delivery over craniotomy of the fetus. During this era, it was noted that the cesarean operation had a better outcome if the procedure was performed on a healthy patient early in labor, before rupture of the membranes, with limited vaginal examinations, and all of these conditions are still true today.

Cavalline,[1] in 1768, first suggested that infection was the principal cause of maternal death and that if the source of infection was removed the mortality rate would be greatly reduced. Although Porro did not perform the first procedure that bears his name, he performed the first successful cesarean section, subtotal hysterectomy, and bilateral adnexectomy in 1876 on a dwarf with pelvic contracture secondary to rickets.

The emergence of the modern era and, therefore, the turning point in the evolution of the cesarean section occurred with a monograph published by Sanger in 1882.[6] He was the first to recommend closure of the uterine incision. His technique included stripping the peritoneum from the uterine wall and resecting a 2-cm, wedge-shaped portion of the uterine wall, resulting in a thick edge adjacent to the peritoneum and a thin edge adjacent to the uterine cavity. The mobilized peritoneum was then folded over these edges of the uterine incision and sutured in two layers. The deep layer was closed using silver wire with interrupted sutures of silk on the superficial layer. This modification revolutionized the procedure by reducing maternal mortality and morbidity while maintaining reproductive capability. Leopold[1] suggested that, after delivery of the infant, the uterus should be exteriorized to place a ligature around the cervix to decrease blood loss during uterine

closure. Sanger approved of this modification and used it successfully, further increasing his maternal survival rate.

Toward the end of the nineteenth century, cesarean section was gaining acceptance as an option in the management of difficult labors. The principle of timely operation[7, 8] (i.e., early in labor), reemphasized by Williams[9] in 1930, further improved the mortality/morbidity rate.

Whereas earlier the indications had been only maternal, just before World War II, with the introduction of blood transfusions, antibiotics, and safer anesthesia increasing the safety of the operation, indications shifted toward the fetus, as is the case today.

CESAREAN SECTION RATE IN THE UNITED STATES

The rising cesarean section rate in the United States is one of the major concerns facing obstetricians today. For many years, the rate remained relatively stable at 3 to 5%. This began to change in the 1960s. In 1965, the cesarean section rate was reported to be 4.5%, it increased to 16.5% in 1980,[10] and data from 1988[11] indicate a 24.7% rate. Table 24–1 lists the total and estimated cesarean live births and suggests a leveling off of the cesarean deliveries in the last 3 years, with rates of 24.1%, 24.4%, and 24.7%, respectively, in 1986, 1987, and 1988.[11] In 1987, 65% (601,000) were primary cesareans and 33% (328,000) were repeat procedures. Attempts to lower or stabilize the cesarean section rate are aimed at the two most common indications, namely, repeat procedures and the diagnosis and management of dystocia (Table 24–2). In 1985, the American College of Obstetricians and Gynecologists issued relaxed guidelines to promote vaginal births after cesarean sections (VBAC).[12] The VBAC rate for 1988 was 12.6%, increased over a rate of 9.8% for 1987 (Table 24–3). This is the largest annual increase ever observed, implying a stabilization in the cesarean rate and an increase in VBACs.

There have been similar increases worldwide in

Table 24–1. TOTAL NUMBER OF LIVE BIRTHS AND ESTIMATED NUMBER OF LIVE BIRTHS BY CESAREAN DELIVERY[11]

Year	Total No. of Live Births	No. of Live Cesarean Births	%
1970	3,731,000	205,000	5.5
1975	3,144,000	327,000	10.4
1980	3,612,000	596,000	16.5
1985	3,761,000	854,000	22.7
1986	3,757,000	905,000	24.1
1987	3,809,000	929,000	24.4
1988	3,913,000*	967,000*	24.7

*Provisional data.
From National Center for Health Statistics: National Hospital Discharge Survey[11]

Table 24–2. INDICATIONS FOR CESAREAN BIRTHS IN 1987[11]

35%—Elective repeat
28%—Dystocia (difficult and prolonged labor)
10%—Breech presentation
10%—Fetal distress
17%—Other obstetrical and medical complications, including premature rupture of membranes, multiple births, prolonged pregnancy, premature labor, other malpresentations, hypertension, and diabetes

the cesarean section rates. Figure 24–1 shows that Brazil reports the highest rate (32%), with Japan and Czechoslovakia reporting the lowest at 7%.[13] Several nations have mounted efforts to decrease their rising rates, and apparent stabilization has occurred in England, Bavaria, Canada, the Netherlands, and Sweden[13] (Fig. 24–2).

It is often difficult to study a population as diverse as that of the United States. A homogenous population such as that in Dublin, Ireland, offers some interesting observations. Unlike other countries, Ireland has not experienced a sharp rise in cesarean births. The cesarean section rate in 1979 was 5.5%, compared with 6.1% in 1988[14] (Table 24–4). Why is there such a discrepancy between the rates of the United States and Ireland?

It has been proposed that the rise in cesarean sections in the United States over the past 15 years occurred concomitantly with an improved perinatal mortality rate.[15, 16] Recent data have not supported this hypothesis.[17, 18] In a Consensus Development Statement, the National Institutes of Health indicated that the sharp rise in cesarean rates could be arrested and even reversed without affecting the improving perinatal mortality rate.[19]

Table 24–3. CESAREAN SECTION RATES[11]

Year	Cesarean Section Rate (%)	Primary Cesarean Section Rate (%)	Vaginal Birth after Cesarean Delivery Rate (%)
1970	5.5	4.2	2.2*
1975	10.4	7.8	2.0*
1980	16.5	12.1	3.4*
1981	17.9	12.5	3.6*
1982	18.5	13.3	4.8
1983	20.3	14.3	4.6
1984	21.1	15.0	5.7
1985	22.7	16.3	6.6
1986	24.1†	17.4	8.5
1987	24.4†	17.4	9.8
1988‡	24.7†	17.5	12.6

*Figure does not meet standards of reliability of precision because the weighted numerator is less than 10,000 deliveries.
†The rises in rates between 1986 and 1987 and 1987 and 1988 were the smallest increases in 5 years (0.3% each year).
‡Provisional data.
—The average length of hospital stay for cesarean delivery is 5.0 days for a primary cesarean and 4.5 days for a repeat cesarean. The average length of stay for a normal vaginal delivery is 2.5 days.
—Previous studies have shown that 50 to 80% of patients with low transverse uterine scars who attempt vaginal delivery have a successful vaginal birth.
—The average cost for cesarean delivery in the United States in 1989 was $7,186.00 versus $4,334.00 for normal vaginal delivery, according to the Health Insurance Association of America.

This is supported by the Dublin data[14] (Table 24–4).

To what does the National Maternity Hospital in Dublin owe their low cesarean section rate? First, they practice aggressive management of labor directed at "early detection and prompt treatment of dystocia by non-surgical means."[20] Second, they have allowed patients with a previous low transverse cesarean scar a trial of labor that proved to be successful 60% of the time. Third, they permit a liberal trial of labor in breech presentations.[18, 20–22] The population served is 99% white and Irish.

The Dublin data seem impressive; however, perinatal morbidity is not addressed. Leveno and co-workers[23] demonstrated a sevenfold decrease in intrapartum fetal death and a twofold decrease in neonatal seizures with liberal use of cesarean sections (rate 10.1%), especially in cases of dystocia or fetal compromise.

It seems unlikely that the low cesarean section rate seen in Dublin will ever again be achieved in the United States. Still, attempts should be directed toward active management of labor and encouragement of VBACs.

INDICATIONS

The broadening of indications certainly has had a dramatic impact on the rise in the cesarean birth rate. Indications are easily categorized into maternal or fetal. Efforts to reduce the cesarean section rate may be aimed at certain of these indications, provided neither maternal nor fetal health is compromised.

Maternal Indications

Maternal criteria for cesarean sections are listed in Table 24–5.

In abruptio placentae, expeditious vaginal delivery with a live fetus is the preferred route for the mother, especially if a coagulopathy has developed. If the bleeding is moderate, maternal vital signs remain stable, and the fetus is showing no compromise, vaginal delivery in a reasonable period of time is a viable option. When the fetus is dead, despite a coagulopathy one can often keep up with blood and coagulation replacement while attempting a vaginal delivery.

Where a complete placenta previa is present, delivery almost invariably will be via cesarean section. Much controversy has surrounded the route of delivery with a partial or marginal placenta previa. If vaginal delivery is considered, a double setup examination should be performed with the operating team and anesthesia and pediatrics personnel present in the event that an emergency procedure becomes necessary.

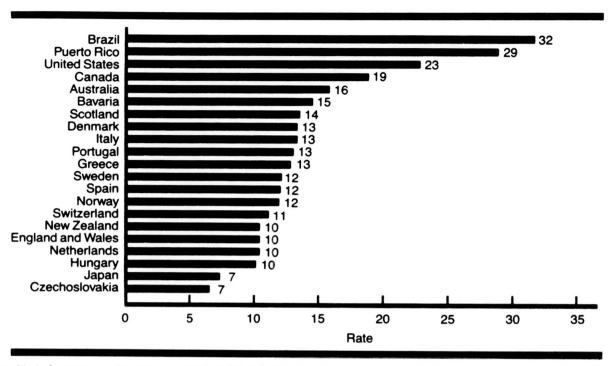

Figure 24–1. Cesarean section rates per 100 hospital deliveries in selected countries for 1985 or the most recent year for which data were available (1981 through 1986 for Brazil, 1984 and 1985 for Puerto Rico and Canada, 1982 for Italy, 1987 for Portugal, 1983 for Greece, 1983 through 1986 for Switzerland, and 1986 for Czechoslovakia). There was incomplete coverage of cesarean section rates for Australia, Bavaria, Portugal, Spain, and Switzerland. (From Notzon FC: International differences in the use of obstetric intervention. JAMA 263:3287, 1990.)

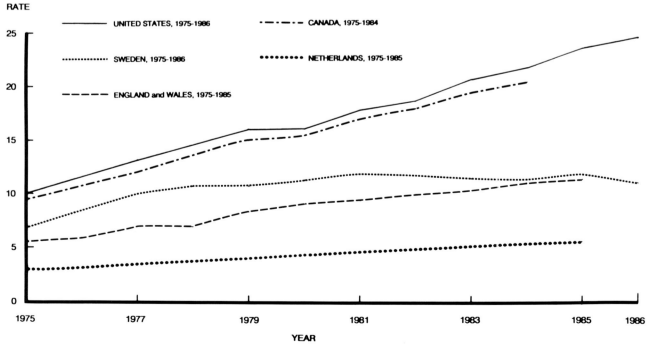

Figure 24–2. Trends in cesarean section rates per 100 hospital deliveries in five countries. (Adapted from Notzon FC: International differences in the use of obstetric intervention. JAMA 263:3290, 1990.)

Table 24–4. NATIONAL MATERNITY HOSPITAL, DUBLIN, IRELAND: COMPARATIVE TABLE FOR 10 YEARS

	1979	1980	1981	1982	1983	1984	1985	1986	1987	1988
Cesarean section (%)	5.5	4.9	5.5	5.2	6.0	4.2	5.1	5.3	5.9	6.1
Perinatal mortality rate (%)	15.6	14.2	12.2	11.3	13.1	15.2	16.1	15.4	14.7	13.3
Perinatal mortality rate, excluding congenital anomalies (%)	11.0	10.3	8.8	7.4	9.8	9.9	11.2	10.4	10.6	9.5

Adapted from National Maternity Hospital, Dublin: Clinical Report for the Year 1988. Dublin: National Maternity Hospital, 1988.

Previous vaginal reconstructive surgery is considered an indication for a cesarean section on the basis of the hypothesis that stretching of the vagina and pressure exerted by the descending fetus may interfere with a reconstructive procedure, especially after repair of vesicovaginal fistulae. Cesarean section is only rarely indicated after successful repair of rectovaginal fistulae (i.e., only if the repair is unusual or difficult or more than one repair is needed).

Pelvic tumors may obstruct the progress of labor. Cervical myomas are an indication for elective cesarean section. However, pedunculated myomas or myomas that involve the lower body of the uterus may be drawn up and out of the pelvis as the uterus enlarges. Deciding the route of delivery in a case of pedunculated myoma may be delayed until the onset of labor. If the pelvic tumor is ovarian, and the diagnosis is made early in pregnancy, surgical extirpation is recommended in the second trimester. Tumors diagnosed in the third trimester are best managed with a cesarean delivery, followed by removal of the tumor. Other pelvic masses believed to obstruct the progress of labor include large cystorectoceles, enteroceles, bladder tumors, and congenital pelvic kidneys. In these unusual cases, decisions should be based on the progress of labor.

Cervical carcinoma in situ is not an indication for a cesarean delivery. However, Stage I invasive carcinoma of the cervix, after fetal viability, is best managed by classic cesarean section with radical hysterectomy, including pelvic lymphadenectomy.[24]

The patient who has a cerebral aneurysm or an arteriovenous (A-V) malformation causes much concern among obstetricians. Vaginal delivery can be attempted in corrected A-V malformation, provided the second stage is modified by regional (epidural) anesthesia and a forceps delivery to obviate cerebrovascular stress.[25, 26] Elective cesarean sections, however, are indicated in patients with untreated A-V anomalies.

An aortic root evaluation should be done in patients who have Marfan's syndrome. If there is no dilatation or the defect has been surgically repaired with a graft, vaginal delivery is an option and should be managed in a similar fashion as in patients with cerebral aneurysms or A-V malformations.

Few maternal medical conditions are themselves an indication for cesarean section, although severe hypertensive disorders may be if delivery is remote. At the University of Miami, Jackson Memorial Hospital, a retrospective review of 38 primigravidas at 34 weeks' or earlier gestation with severe pre-eclampsia necessitating delivery revealed that a Bishop score of 4 or higher was associated with vaginal delivery.[27]

The most difficult indication to define is "dystocia." It is for this reason that diagnoses such as "failure to progress" are so widely used. This indication is listed for nearly ⅓ of cases and is a major contributor to the rapid rise of primary cesarean rates. More satisfactory terms should be employed that define the actual reason for failure to progress, such as "arrest of dilatation" or "arrest of descent." When a patient's labor fails to progress, it is often difficult for obstetricians to distinguish between cephalopelvic disproportion (CPD) and uterine dysfunction.

In 1982 Friedman[28] published his labor progress curve (Fig. 24–3) from observations of normal patients in labor. The latent phase can last to 20 hours in nulliparous women and 14 hours in parous women. When do patients reach the active phase of labor? In a retrospective study, Peisner and Rosen[29] determined that 25% of patients reached the active stage at 4-cm dilatation and 90% by 5-cm dilatation. Many cesarean sections are performed in the latent phase with the diagnosis of failure to progress made before the patient ever reaches the active phase of labor.[28, 30] Oxytocin augmentation, observation, and/or ambulation may be more appropriate[31] at this stage of labor.

CPD may be a function of one of the "3 *p*s": passage, passenger, and power. The "power" of uterine contractions can be assessed directly with intrauterine pressure catheters. Before these catheters, overestimation of the strength of uterine contractions may have been a contributing factor in the premature diagnosis of CPD. Caldeyro-Barcia and Poseiro[32] described the "Montevideo

Table 24–5. MATERNAL INDICATIONS FOR CESAREAN SECTION

Antepartum hemorrhage
Previous vaginal surgery
Pelvic tumors
Cervical carcinoma
Aneurysms or cerebral arteriovenous malformations
Marfan syndrome
Pelvic malformations
Severe hypertension—selected cases
Perimortem

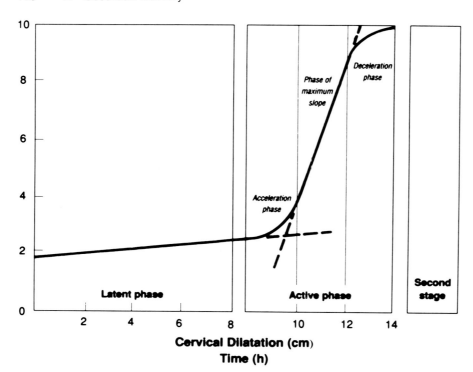

Figure 24–3. Composite graph of cervical dilatation for nulliparous women. (From the American College of Obstetricians and Gynecologists. Dystocia. Washington, D.C.: ACOG Technical Bulletin #137. 1989.)

unit" as a method of quantitating the strength of uterine contractions. The number of contractions in 10 minutes is counted and multiplied by the average intensity of the contractions in millimeters of mercury above the baseline tone. At least 200 Montevideo units are considered adequate to effect cervical dilatation.[33] If contractions are not adequate, oxytocin augmentation should be considered if pelvic measurements are clinically adequate.[34] Clinical assessment of the pelvis has been shown to be as reliable as x-ray pelvimetry.[35] A diagram suggesting management of dysfunctional labor is shown in Figure 24–4.

Historically, post-mortem cesarean sections were performed only after maternal death with the aim to deliver a live infant. However, the neonatal survival was at best poor. Today there are few maternal conditions due to either chronic or acute illness or trauma in which the maternal prognosis is so grave that a post-mortem cesarean may be necessary. After examining cases of the past century plus using current knowledge of fetal physiology, Katz and co-workers[36] concluded that optimal neonatal survival could be achieved if delivery were initiated within 4 minutes of maternal cardiac arrest. Occasionally, such as in massive trauma, maternal survival may be enhanced by performing a perimortem cesarean delivery before maternal cardiac arrest, allowing for more effective cardiopulmonary resuscitation without the hindrance of a gravid uterus, especially where chances of maternal survival are very low and there is a viable fetus that has a reasonable chance of survival.

Although optimal survival is achieved within 4 minutes of cardiac arrest, if there is evidence of fetal life, physicians are justified in doing a post-mortem section regardless of the time interval after cardiac arrest.

Fetal Indications

Some fetal criteria for a cesarean section are listed in Table 24–6. An abnormal fetal lie occurs in 1 in 300 (.33%) deliveries.[36–40] Persistence of a transverse, oblique, or unstable lie beyond 35 to 36 weeks is of major clinical significance and demands a cautious clinical plan. If spontaneous rupture of the membranes occurs without a fetal part filling the pelvic inlet, there is an increased risk of cord prolapse and fetal distress, which in turn increases maternal morbidity and mortality

Table 24–6. FETAL INDICATIONS FOR CESAREAN SECTION

Abnormal presentation
The VLBW* infant
Macrosomia
Fetal anomalies
Fetal distress
Active materna genital HSV†
Maternal thrombocytopenia

*Very low birth weight (<1500 g).
†Herpes simplex virus.

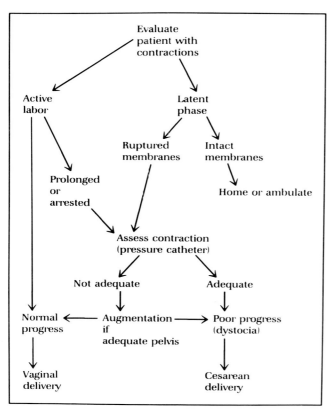

Figure 24–4. Management of abnormal progress of labor. (Iams JD, Reiss R: When should labor be interrupted by cesarean delivery? Clin Obstet Gynecol 28:745, 1985.)

resulting from emergency procedures. The most commonly reported clinical settings associated with abnormal lie include grand multiparity, prematurity, pelvic contracture, and abnormal placentation.[37–42]

External cephalic version of the abnormal lie is still controversial. Some believe that it carries a higher fetal loss rate than cesarean delivery.[40, 42, 43] Others, however, advocate the procedure in the absence of placenta previa or CPD.[39, 44] External version should be attempted carefully using real-time ultrasonography to follow the procedure and monitor the fetal heart. The anesthesia and operating teams should be available in the event of fetal distress, which occurs in 10% of cases. If external version is impractical, unsuccessful, or unavailable, and spontaneous rupture of the membranes or labor occurs with an abnormal lie (excluding certain breech presentations), cesarean section is the treatment of choice.[43, 45, 46] Fetal and maternal complications are unacceptably high for bipolar internal podalic version and breech extraction of the fetus in a transverse/oblique lie or an unstable presentation, and thus version and extraction have been abandoned[41] in modern obstetrics. (For recommendations on delivery of twins and breeches, see Chapters 19 and 20.) Other rare fetal presentations including brow, face, compound, and persistent occiput posterior presenta-

tions may cause dystocia. The old-fashioned internal manipulations such as difficult forceps rotations or cephalic fluxion have little to no role in modern obstetrics.

When the mentum is anterior or transverse, a trial of labor may be attempted, but the threat of dystocia remains high because of late engagement and the possibility of a large fetus or a contracted pelvis. Vaginal birth of a term live-born, third-trimester infant in a persistent mentum posterior position is impossible.

Brow presentations may undergo a trial of labor, because approximately ⅔ convert to either a vertex or face presentation as long as the head is not yet fixed at the inlet. Abdominal delivery is recommended for the persistent brow presentation, because the largest presenting diameter (occipito-mental) is 13 cm in the term fetus, and few pelves are large enough.

A compound presentation occurs when an extremity is prolapsed along with the presenting breech or vertex and is secondary to incomplete occlusion of the pelvic inlet by the presenting part. This is most commonly found when the fetus is smaller and/or premature. Rarely is a compound presentation an indication for abdominal delivery. The decision to perform a cesarean birth should be based on other coexisting complications, including cord prolapse.

The occiput posterior position is rarely an indication for cesarean section, because 90% of fetuses in this position will spontaneously rotate to the anterior. Most persistent cases will deliver vaginally spontaneously, with the aid of forceps, or with the vacuum extractor and a generous episiotomy. Manual rotation is often successful. Forceps rotation should be done only by the most experienced surgeon and with good indication after adequate clinical assessment of fetomaternal dimensions. Abdominal delivery is indicated in the face of "true" arrest of labor or fetal distress when vaginal delivery is not imminent.

Preterm delivery occurs in 9% of all live births and is responsible for 75% of neonatal deaths, excluding those from congenital malformations. Despite medical and social advances in the past 35 years, the rate of preterm birth has remained constant. Delivery of low birth weight (LBW, <2500 g) and very low birth weight (VLBW, <1500 g) infants has been controversial for the past 10 years as the survival rates for LBW and VLBW babies have improved. The main objective is as atraumatic a delivery as possible. Much debate has occurred over the delivery of a nonvertex preterm baby with management based on estimated fetal weight. This subject is addressed in Chapter 19.

Studies associating intracranial hemorrhage with the presence or absence of labor have been conflicting.[47–49] The recent data indicate no benefit of a cesarean section for delivery of the VLBW preterm infant presenting as a vertex.[50–52] However, there are clinical circumstances, such as maternal medical conditions, that require preterm delivery in the face of an unfavorable cervix, in which case cesarean section may be beneficial and less traumatic than a long and potentially morbid induction of labor. Current literature does not indicate clear evidence that either approach is beneficial to mother and/or neonate.

In a preterm delivery, the goal is to provide the neonatologist with an infant who is in the best possible condition. However, perinatal morbidity and mortality should be minimized with careful management in which risks and benefits are weighed.

On the other side of the coin is the macrosomic infant, who poses a different set of complications. It is well known that incidences of shoulder dystocia, birth injuries, perinatal death, and low Apgar scores are increased in macrosomic infants.[53] Macrosomia is detected clinically and confirmed by ultrasonic estimated fetal weight, and by comparing circumferences of fetal chest and head.[54, 55] Macrosomia has been defined by some as a weight of 4000 g or greater and by others as 4500 g or greater.[56–60, 96]

The most common associated complication with vaginal delivery of a macrosomic infant is shoulder dystocia. In one series, shoulder dystocia occurred in 3% of infants who weighed between 4100 and 4500 g and 8.2% of those who weighed more than 4500 g.[59] Another series reported a 47% injury rate secondary to shoulder dystocia in infants who weighed more than 4000 g and underwent midpelvic deliveries.[56] Figure 24–5 outlines a proposed management of the macrosomic fetus. Assessment of fetal weight and maternal pelvis is imperative.

If the estimated fetal weight is 4000 to 4500 g by ultrasonography and the patient has a clinically adequate pelvis, labor may be allowed. If labor is protracted or the second stage is prolonged, a cesarean section would avoid the possible trauma of a difficult vaginal delivery. Because of the greater morbidity associated with infants who weigh more than 4500 g, elective cesarean section is warranted.

The progress of labor may not predict shoulder dystocia. Therefore anesthesia personnel should be in the room for delivery of a baby estimated to weigh in excess of 4000 g and plans should be made to manage a potential shoulder dystocia.

If fetal anomalies are present, the indications for cesarean section depend on whether (a) the anomaly will cause dystocia, (b) fetal risks will be further increased by vaginal delivery, or (c) planned early delivery is necessary to prevent further deterioration of the particular fetal condition. The most commonly encountered defects diagnosed antenatally are neural tube defects, hydrocephalus, and abdominal wall defects. The etiology and prognosis of fetal hydrocephalus are varied. For the intrapartum management of a hydrocephalic fetus, three areas must be considered: (a) the isolated anomaly, (b) severe associated abnormalities that are incompatible with postnatal life, and (c) other associated abnormalities.

Infants with isolated hydrocephalus, even in extreme cases, such as substantial thinning of the cortical mantle, may have normal and sometimes superior intellectual function.[61–65] However, as a group, these infants have a greater incidence of mental retardation and death at an earlier age than does the general population.[61–64] Associated abnormalities may also go undetected, and the fetus may be incorrectly diagnosed to have isolated hydrocephalus.[66, 67] Keeping the fetus's best interests in mind, a cesarean section is indicated in hydrocephaly, in which the head is enlarged, as opposed to the alternative, cephalocentesis, which would be necessary for a vaginal delivery. Even under ultrasonic guidance in the most experienced hands, cephalocentesis results in a high perinatal mortality, fetal heart rate decelerations, and intracranial bleeding; it cannot be construed as promoting the best interests of the fetus.[67]

When hydrocephalus is associated with severe abnormalities incompatible with life, including bilateral renal agenesis, trisomy 18, and holoprosencephaly, there may be justification for cephalocentesis to enable vaginal delivery and avoid potential maternal morbidity resulting from an operative delivery.

For hydrocephaly associated with other abnormalities, including spina bifida, a cesarean section is recommended. These conditions have varying prognoses that cannot be adequately evaluated antenatally; therefore, the infant should have the least traumatic delivery method. Data are inadequate regarding the optimal mode of delivery for fetuses with spina bifida alone. Vaginal delivery could cause trauma to the defect and expose neural tissue to bacteria in the birth canal.[68–71] It has thus been suggested that the preferable mode of delivery is cesarean section.[68]

The method of delivery remains controversial

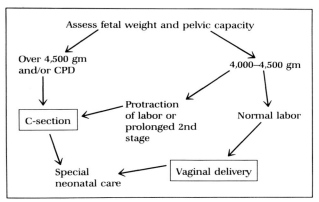

Figure 24–5. Proposed management of macrosomia. (Modified from Oskowitz SP. In Friedman, E (Ed), Obstetrical Decision Making. Trenton, N.J.: B.C. Decker, Inc., 1982.)

for fetuses having abdominal wall defects such as gastroschisis and oomphalocele. In several studies,[72-75] no improvement in outcome was shown for either defect as an isolated finding when cesarean section was performed in lieu of vaginal delivery.

Intrapartum events are responsible for nearly 20% of stillbirths, 20 to 40% of cases of cerebral palsy, and 10% of cases of severe mental retardation.[76] To avoid these complications and because of the threat of malpractice litigation, obstetricians have often resorted to cesarean deliveries for fetal distress, accounting for a 10 to 15% increase in the rate of cesarean section.[77, 78] Better education of physicians and nurses in the proper interpretation of fetal heart rate tracings would theoretically help reduce the rate of abdominal delivery for fetal distress. Use of fetal scalp blood sampling when tracings are equivocal to determine fetal acid/base status substantially reduces the need for cesarean deliveries for presumed fetal distress.[79]

Temporizing measures, i.e., positional changes, discontinuation of oxytocin, hydration, oxygen by face mask, tocolytics, and amnioinfusion, may be considered in certain clinical settings if delivery is expected within a reasonable period of time.[80] The obstetrician's major concern is to avoid brain damage to the fetus. It has been estimated that, in more than half the cases, the insult occurs in the antepartum period, and no correlation has been observed between intrapartum events and subsequent development of mental retardation and epilepsy.[81] The events leading to fetal brain damage are still not well defined, and until they are, cesarean deliveries will be performed for fetal distress, especially now that the atmosphere of malpractice litigation has increased the practice of defensive medicine.

The two most common maternal conditions in which cesarean section is indicated for fetal reasons are active genital herpes simplex virus (HSV) and idiopathic thrombocytopenia purpura (ITP). The exact incidence of genital HSV infections in pregnancy is unknown, but viral shedding occurs in approximately 0.1 to 0.4% of all deliveries.[82] The frequency of neonatal infection is actually much lower, occurring in approximately 0.01 to 0.04% of neonates, 90% of whose infection can be traced to a maternal source[83] (an ascending infection associated with ruptured membranes or colonization during birth). Approximately 50% of mothers who deliver vaginally with a primary genital HSV infection will give birth to an infected infant.[84, 85] Of those infected, 60% die in the neonatal period.[86] With recurrent infection at the time of delivery, fewer than 4% of mothers will have infected infants.[85]

For several reasons, the policy of obtaining weekly HSV cultures with vaginal delivery only if cultures were negative before labor or ruptured membranes had little impact on the overall incidence of neonatal HSV infection. There is no correlation between antepartum HSV infection and viral shedding at the time of delivery.[87] Mothers of infected infants usually have no history of infection and/or lesions at the time of delivery[88] and would not have met the criteria for weekly culturing. The current American College of Obstetricians and Gynecologists' recommendations[89] for pregnant women with a history of HSV infection include obtaining cultures of active lesions to confirm the diagnosis, allowing vaginal delivery in the absence of lesions, and performing cesarean deliveries in active labor with or without ruptured membranes in the presence of active lesions. Cesarean delivery does not always prevent neonatal infection. In fact, 12% of reported neonatal infections occurred in infants delivered by cesarean section with intact membranes.[88] Time elapsed from rupture of membranes does not seem to contribute to risk of neonatal infection. Uninfected neonates have been delivered after prolonged membrane rupture, and infected ones have been delivered within 2 hours of membrane rupture.[90]

The management of ITP during pregnancy and delivery remains controversial. There is no correlation between maternal and fetal platelet counts.[91, 92] Two maternal characteristics identified by one study indicate a low risk of severe (<50,000 platelets) neonatal thrombocytopenia: (a) absence of a history of ITP before pregnancy and (b) absence of circulating platelet antibodies in women with a previous history of ITP.[91] Earlier case reports documented intracranial hemorrhage in infants of mothers with ITP after delivery, leading many obstetricians to recommend delivery by cesarean section in the hope of lowering infant morbidity and mortality.[93, 94] Fetal scalp blood platelet counts have been proposed to avoid a cesarean birth for euthrombocytic fetuses.[95] Occasionally, insufficient samples or contamination with amniotic fluid may result in erroneously low counts and subsequently a wrong decision—cesarean section. Retrospectively,[92] the perinatal risk and the severity of the thrombocytopenia at delivery are far lower than had previously been anticipated. Therefore interventions associated with maternal or fetal morbidity, including cordocentesis, fetal scalp sampling, and delivery by cesarean section, cannot be justified for every pregnant patient with ITP.

SUMMARY

The cesarean section, once performed only to spare the life of an infant of a dying mother, has evolved into a procedure when indicated, to reduce maternal as well as neonatal morbidity. The indications for its use have been relaxed in the past two decades, as demonstrated by the dramatic rise in the rate of cesarean deliveries. In recent years, active management of labor and VBACs have resulted in a leveling off of the cesarean rate.

References

1. Young JH: The History of Caesarean Sections. London: H. K. Lewis, 1944.
2. Pickrell K: An inquiry into the history of cesarean section. Bull Soc Med Hist 4:414, 1935.
3. Rousset F: Traite Noveau de L'Hysterotomotokie au L'enfantément Cesarien. Paris, Denys de Val, 1581.
4. Fasbender H: Geschichte der Geburtshufe. Jena 979, 1906.
5. Naqui NH: James Barlow (1767–1839): Operator of the first successful caesarean section in England. Br J Obstet Gynaecol 92:468, 1985.
6. Sanger M: Der Kaiserschnitt bei Uterusfibromen nebst Verleichenden Methodik der Sectio Caesarea und der Porro Operation. Leipzig, Germany. Englemann, 1882.
7. Harris RP: The operation of gastro-hysterotomy (true cesarean section). Viewed in light of American experience and success; with the history and results of sewing up the uterine wound; and a full tabular record of the cesarean operations performed in the United States, many of them not hitherto reported. Am J Med Sci 75:313, 1878.
8. Harris RP: Special statistics of the cesarean operation in the United States, showing the success and failure in each state. Am J Obstet 14:341, 1881.
9. Williams JW: Obstetrics: A Textbook for the Use of Students and Practitioners, 6th Edition. New York: D. Appleton & Co., 1930.
10. Placek PH, Taffel SM: One-sixth of 1980 births by cesarean section. Public Health Rep 97:183, 1982.
11. National Center for Health Statistics: National Hospital Discharge Survey. Hyattsville, MD, August 28, 1990.
12. American College of Obstetricians and Gynecologists. New guidelines to reduce repeat cesareans. Statement presented by Dr. Luella Klein at news Conference on Vaginal Birth After Cesarean Section. Washington, DC, January 25, 1985.
13. Notzon FC: International differences in the use of obstetric interventions. JAMA 263:3286, 1990.
14. National Maternity Hospital, Dublin: Clinical Report for the Year 1988. Dublin: National Maternity Hospital, 1988.
15. Hibbard LT: Changing trends in cesarean section. Am J Obstet Gynecol 125:798, 1976.
16. Jones OH: Cesarean section in present day obstetrics. Am J Obstet Gynecol 126:521, 1976.
17. Minkoff HL, Schwarz RH: The rising cesarean section rate: Can it be safely reversed? Obstet Gynecol 56:135, 1980.
18. O'Driscoll K, Foley M: Correlation of decrease in perinatal mortality and increase in cesarean section rates. Obstet Gynecol 61:1, 1983.
19. National Institutes of Health consensus development statement on cesarean childbirth. Obstet Gynecol 57:537, 1981.
20. O'Driscoll K, Jackson RJ, Gallagher JT: Prevention of prolonged labour. Br Med J 2:477, 1969.
21. O'Driscoll K, Stronge JM, Minogue M: Active management of labour. Br Med J 3:135, 1973.
22. O'Driscoll K, Foley M, MacDonald D: Active management of labor as an alternative to cesarean section for dystocia. Obstet Gynecol 63:485, 1984.
23. Leveno KJ, Cunningham FG, Pritchard JA: Cesarean section: An answer to the House of Horne. Am J Obstet Gynecol 153:8383, 1985.
24. Hacker NF, Berek JS, Lagasse LD, et al.: Carcinoma of the cervix associated with pregnancy. Obstet Gynecol 59:735, 1982.
25. Minielly R, Yuzpe AA, Drake CG: Subarachnoid hemorrhage secondary to ruptured cerebral aneurysm in pregnancy. Obstet Gynecol 53:64, 1979.
26. Robinson L, Hall CJ, Sedzimer CB: Arterio-venous malformations, aneurysm and pregnancy. J Neurosurg 41:63, 1974.
27. AbuHamad AZ, Beydoun SN, Yasin S, O'Sullivan MJ: Determining factors for vaginal delivery in severe pre-eclamptic nulliparas at ≤34 weeks gestation (Abstract 528). Presented at the annual meeting of the Society of Perinatal Obstetricians, San Francisco, 1991.
28. Friedman EA: Labor. Clinical Evaluation and Management, 2nd Edition. New York: Appleton-Century-Crofts, 1982.
29. Peisner DB, Rosen MG: Transition from latent to active labor. Obstet Gynecol 68:448, 1986.
30. Cardozo LD, Gibb DMF, Studd JWW, et al.: Predictive value of cervimetric labour patterns in primigravida. Br J Obstet Gynaecol 89:33, 1982.
31. Koontz WL, Bishop EH: Management of the latent phase of labor. Clin Obstet Gynecol 25:111, 1982.
32. Caldeyro-Barcia R, Poseiro JJ: Oxytocin and contractility of the pregnant human uterus. Ann NY Acad Sci 75:813, 1959.
33. Hauth JC, Hankins GDV, Gilstrap LC, et al.: Uterine contraction pressures with oxytocin induction/augmentation. Obstet Gynecol 68:305, 1986.
34. Iams JD, Reiss R: When should labor be interrupted by cesarean delivery? Clin Obstet Gynecol 28:745, 1985.
35. Varner MW, Cruikshank DP, Lavke DW: X-ray pelvimetry in clinical obstetrics. Obstet Gynecol 56:296, 1980.
36. Katz VL, Datters DJ, Droegemueller W: Perimortem cesarean delivery. Obstet Gynecol 68:571, 1986.
37. Cruikshank DP, White CA: Obstetric malpresentations—twenty years' experience. Am J Obstet Gynecol 116:1097, 1973.
38. Edwards RL, Nicholson HO: The management of the unstable lie in late pregnancy. J Obstet Gynaecol Br Commonw 76:713, 1969.
39. Flowers CE: Shoulder presentation. Am J Obstet Gyencol 96:145, 1966.
40. Johnson CE: Abnormal fetal presentations. Lancet 84:317, 1964.
41. MacGregor WG: Aetiology and treatment of the oblique transverse and unstable lie of the faetus with particular reference to antenatal care. J Obstet Gynaecol Br Commonw 71:237, 1964.
42. Johnson CE: Transverse presentation of fetus. JAMA 187:642, 1964.
43. Cockburn KG, Drake RF: Transverse and oblique lie of the foetus. Aust NZ J Obstet Gynaecol 8:211, 1968.
44. Sandhur SK: Transverse lie. J Indian Med Assoc 68:205, 1977.
45. Yates MJ: Transverse foetal lie in labour. J Obstet Gynaecol Br Commonw 71:245, 1964.
46. Pelosi MA, Apuzzio J, Friechione D, et al.: The intra-abdominal version technique for delivery of transverse lie by low segment cesarean section. Am J Obstet Gynecol 136:1009, 1979.
47. Bejar R, Curbelo V, Coen R, et al.: Large intraventricular hemorrhage (IVH) and labor in infants >1000 g (Abstract). Pediatr Res 15:649, 1981.
48. Kosmetatos N, Dinton C, Williams M, et al.: Intracranial hemorrhage in the premature. Its predictive features and outcome. Am J Dis Child 134:855, 1980.
49. Tejani N, Rebold B, Tuck S, et al.: Obstetric factors in the causation of early periventricular-intraventricular hemorrhage. Obstet Gynecol 64:510, 1984.
50. Barrett J, Boehm F, Fisher D: Neonatal survival of the tiny infant: The challenge. Presented at the annual meeting of the Society of Perinatal Obstetricians, San Antonio, 1985.
51. Main D, Main E, Maurer M: Cesarean section versus vaginal delivery for the breech fetus weighing less than 1500 g. Am J Obstet Gynecol 146:580, 1983.
52. Olshan A, Shy K, Tuthy D, et al.: Cesarean birth and neonatal mortality in very low birth weight infants. Obstet Gynecol 64:267, 1984.

53. Spellacy WN: Macrosomia: Maternal characteristics of infant complications. Obstet Gynecol 66:158, 1985.
54. Hopwood HG: Shoulder dystocia—Fifteen years' experience in a community hospital. Am J Obstet Gynecol 144:162, 1982.
55. Seigworth GR: Shoulder dystocia—review of 5 years' experience. Obstet Gynecol 28:764, 1966.
56. Benedetti TJ, Gabbe AG: Shoulder dystocia—a complication of fetal macrosomia and prolonged second stage of labor with midpelvic delivery. Obstet Gynecol 52:526, 1978.
57. Boyd ME, Usher RH, McLean FH: Fetal macrosomia—prediction, risks, and proposed management. Obstet Gynecol 61:715, 1983.
58. Modanlou HD, Dorchester WL, Thorosian A, et al.: Macrosomia—maternal, fetal, and neonatal implications. Obstet Gynecol 55:420, 1980.
59. Golditch IM, Kirkman K: The large fetus—management and outcome. Obstet Gynecol 52:26, 1978.
60. Modanlou HD, Komatsu G, Dorchester W, et al.: Large for gestational age neonates: Anthropometric reasons for shoulder dystocia. Obstet Gynecol 60:417, 1982.
61. Lorber J: The results of early treatment of extreme hydrocephalus. Dev Med Child Neurol [Suppl] 16:21, 1981.
62. McCullough DC, Balzer-Martin LA: Current prognosis in overt neonatal hydrocephalus. J Neurosurg 57:378, 1982.
63. Chervenak FA, Duncan C, Ment LR: The outcome of fetal ventriculomegaly. Lancet 2:179, 1982.
64. Shurtleff DB, Floz EL, Loeser JD: Hydrocephalus: A definition of its progression and relationship to intellectual function, diagnosis, and complications. Am J Dis Child 125:688, 1973.
65. Kavnar EM, Case WS, Volpe JJ: Development and marked reconstitution of cerebral mantle after postnatal treatment of intrauterine hydrocephalus. Neurol 34:840, 1984.
66. Chervenak FA, Berkowitz RL, Romero R, et al.: The diagnosis of fetal hydrocephalus. Am J Obstet Gynecol 147:703, 1983.
67. Chervenak FA, Berkowitz RL, Tortora M, Hobbins JC: The management of fetal hydrocephalus. Am J Obstet Gynecol 151:933, 1985.
68. Chervenak FA, Duncan C, Ment J, et al.: Perinatal management of meningomyelocele. Obstet Gynecol 63:376, 1984.
69. Ralis ZA: Traumatizing effect of breech delivery on infants with spina bifida. J Pediatr 87:613, 1975.
70. Ralis Z, Ralis HM: Morphology of peripheral nerves in children with spina bifida. Dev Med Child Neurol [Suppl] 27:109, 1972.
71. Stark G, Drummond M: Spina bifida as an obstetric problem. Dev Med Child Neurol [Suppl] 22:157, 1970.
72. Sipes SL, Weiner CP, Sipes DR, et al.: Gastroschisis and omphalocele: Does either antenatal diagnosis or route of delivery make a difference in perinatal outcome? Obstet Gynecol 76:195, 1990.
73. Kirk EP, Wah RH: Obstetric management of the fetus with omphalocele or gastroschisis: A review and report of one hundred twelve cases. Am J Obstet Gynecol 146:512, 1983.
74. Carpenter MW, Curie MR, Dibbins AW, Haddow JE: Perinatal management of ventral wall defects. Obstet Gynecol 54:646, 1984.
75. Sermer M, Benzie RJ, Pitson T, et al.: Prenatal diagnosis and management of congenital defects of the anterior abdominal wall. Am J Obstet Gynecol 156:308, 1987.
76. Antenatal Diagnosis: Report of the Consensus Development Conference Sponsored by the National Institute of Child Health and Human Development (No. 79-1983). Washington, DC: U.S. Government Printing Office, 1979.
77. National Institutes of Health Consensus Development Task Force statement on cesarean childbirth. Am J Obstet Gynecol 139:902, 1981.
78. National Institutes of Health consensus development statement on cesarean childbirth: The Cesarean Birth Task Force. Obstet Gynecol 57:537, 1981.
79. Zolar RW, Quilligan EJ: The influence of scalp sampling on the cesarean section rate for fetal distress. Am J Obstet Gynecol 135:239, 1989.
80. Nageotte MP: Cesarean section for fetal distress. Clin Obstet Gynecol 28:770, 1985.
81. U.S. Department of Health and Human Services: Prenatal and Perinatal Factors Associated with Brain Injury (Publication (PHS) 85-1149). Bethesda, MD: Public Health Service, National Institutes of Health, 1985.
82. Brown ZA, Pontier LA, Benedetti J, et al.: Genital herpes in pregnancy: Risk factors associated with recurrences and asymptomatic viral shedding. Am J Obstet Gynecol 153:24, 1985.
83. American Academy of Pediatrics, Committee on Fetus and Newborn, Committee on Infectious Diseases: Perinatal herpes simplex virus infections. Pediatrics 66:147, 1980.
84. Stagno S, Whittley RJ: Herpes virus infections of pregnancy. Part II: Herpes simplex virus and varicella zoster virus infections. N Engl J Med 313:1327, 1985.
85. Brown ZA, Vontver LA, Benedetti J, et al.: Effects on infants of a first episode of genital herpes during pregnancy. N Engl J Med 317:1246, 1987.
86. Visintine AM, Nahmias AJ, Josey WE: Genital herpes. Perinatal Care 2(9):32, 1978.
87. Arvin AM, Hensleigh PA, Prober CG, et al.: Failure of antepartum maternal cultures to predict the infant's risk of exposure to herpes simplex virus at delivery. N Engl J Med 315:796, 1986.
88. Stone KM, Brooks CA, Guinan ME, et al.: Neonatal herpes—results of one year's surveillance (Abstract 515). In Abstracts of the 25th Interscience Conference on Antimicrobial Agents and Chemotherapy. Washington, DC: American Society for Microbiology, 1985.
89. Perinatal Herpes Simplex Virus Infections (Technical Bulletin 122). American College of Obstetricians and Gynecologists, Washington, D.C. 1988.
90. Grossman JH III: Herpes simplex virus (HSV) infections. Clin Obstet Gynecol 25:555, 1982.
91. Samuels P, Bussel JB, Braitman LE, et al.: Estimation of the risk of thrombocytopenia in the offspring of pregnant women with presumed immune thrombocytopenia purpura. N Engl J Med 323:229, 1990.
92. Burrows RF, Helton JG: Low fetal risks in pregnancies associated with idiopathic thrombocytopenia purpura. Am J Obstet Gynecol 163:1147, 1990.
93. Murray JM, Harris RE: The management of the pregnant patient with idiopathic thrombocytopenic purpura. Am J Obstet Gynecol 126:449, 1976.
94. Kitzmiller JL, Autoimmune disorders: Maternal, fetal, and neonatal risks. Clin Obstet Gynecol 21:385, 1978.
95. Patriario M, Sze-Ya Y: Immunological thrombocytopenia in pregnancy. Obstet Gynecol Surv 41:661, 1986.
96. Gross TL, Sakal RJ, Williams T, et al.: Shoulder dystocia: A fetal–physician risk. Obstet Gynecol Surv 42:692, 1987.

25

Operative Techniques for Cesarean Section

Alfred Abuhamad
Mary J. O'Sullivan

Before the end of the 19th century, the cesarean section was performed as a last resort to save the life of the mother or child. When natural birth was obstructed, little could be done for the laboring woman, because cesarean section was the most fatal of surgical operations. The major cause of death was peritoneal inflammation, resulting from the escape of lochia into the peritoneal cavity. Physicians were reluctant to close the uterus, fearing the sutures would cut through the contracting myometrium and cause bleeding and infection. In 1882, Sanger,[1] a German physician, described his procedure of closure of the uterine incision by inverting the peritoneal edges over a muscular layer, and thereby provided the basis for the modern cesarean section. This technique, later modified by several physicians, allowed more liberal use of the cesarean section to resolve some obstetric problems.

PATIENT PREPARATION

Patients scheduled for elective cesarean section should be kept fasting for at least 8 hours. It is important that at least type-specific blood is available and a recent hemoglobin level noted in the chart. A nonparticulate oral antacid (e.g., sodium citrate) administered within 30 minutes of the start of anesthesia will decrease potential morbidity associated with a rarely occurring aspiration. A large-bore (e.g., 16 gauge) intravenous line should be available with an infusion of crystalloid solution started. Although a Foley bladder catheter is commonly placed on the operating table, the procedure may be done without this because the bladder can be emptied abdominally using a syringe and needle. An empty bladder improves the exposure and decreases the risk of bladder trauma.

The tradition of an abdominoperineal shave has been criticized. Shaving has been associated with a tenfold higher rate of wound infection than when hair is removed by a depilatory[2] or hair clippers.[3] Commercially available surgical clippers remove all types of hair, including pubic hair, without causing skin trauma. The infection rate is lowest when shaving is done immediately before the skin preparation at operation. The operative field is usually scrubbed with an antiseptic agent for 2 to 10 minutes. The current three most widely used antiseptic agents are hexachlorophene, povidone-iodine, and chlorhexidine.[4, 5] Sterile draping is placed over the prepped area, leaving only the operative field accessible (Fig. 25–1). Although careful preparation of the patient is necessary to reduce the risk of wound infection, the surgeon should not forget the fetus and the need to know the presentation, position, and heart rate.

MATERNAL POSITION

The adverse effects of inferior vena cava and aortic compression by the pregnant uterus near term have been recognized for many years.[6, 7] "Supine hypotensive syndrome" or "aortocaval compression syndrome" describes the decreased

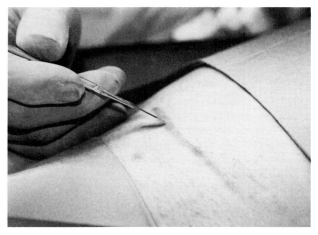

Figure 25–1. The abdomen prepared and draped for the skin incision for repeat cesarean delivery. Attempt to incise perpendicular to the plane of the skin.

venous return to the heart from the lower extremities and pelvis that causes a fall in cardiac output, hypotension, and decreased organ perfusion. If a cesarean section is performed under regional anesthesia, peripheral vasodilatation of the lower extremities further decreases venous return.

Lateral displacement of the uterus, either by tilting the patient with a wedge[8] or lateral table tilt[9] or by operating with the mother in the left lateral recumbent position,[10] allows normal venous return and improved fetal oxygenation.[9–13] Whereas marked improvement in newborn oxygenation occurs with tilt position under regional anesthesia, the benefits from this position are less evident under general anesthesia. Surgical access to the uterus is superior with a right rather than a left lateral tilt. However, studies on lower-limb arterial pressures and blood flow indicate that a tilt to the left is more effective in preventing both uterine compression of the inferior vena cava and partial obstruction of the abdominal aorta.[14–16] In 60 mothers with normal placental function, significant maternal hypotension occurred more frequently with right tilt.[17] The clinical and biochemical status of the fetus was generally more favorable with a left lateral tilt, as was the maternal-to-fetal blood gas gradient. The benefits of the left lateral position are more significant for the infant at risk than for the healthy fetus. The advantages gained by avoiding aortocaval compression easily offset any increased technical difficulties faced by the surgeon.

ABDOMINAL INCISIONS

The choice of an abdominal incision for cesarean section is usually determined by the surgeon's training and level of comfort. Unfortunately, incisions are infrequently individualized. Before making the incision, the surgeon should consider several factors: simplicity of the procedure, exposure and accessibility to the uterus, previous abdominal surgery, option for enlarging the incision, wound healing, and ultimate cosmetic results. Because most patients undergoing cesarean section are young, cosmetic results become important. Laparotomy incisions currently used by obstetricians for cesarean sections are shown in Figure 25–2.

In general, abdominal incisions can be divided into vertical and transverse. In a comparison of these incisions, the strain on the suture line of the vertical incision was 30 times greater than that on the suture line of the transverse incision.[18] As demonstrated by Sloan,[18] the force required to bring the edges of the fascia together in longitudinal incisions increased in proportion to the square of the length of the incision. In 2175 cesarean sections, there was an eightfold increase in wound dehiscence in vertical incisions (2.94%) compared with transverse incisions (0.37%) of the

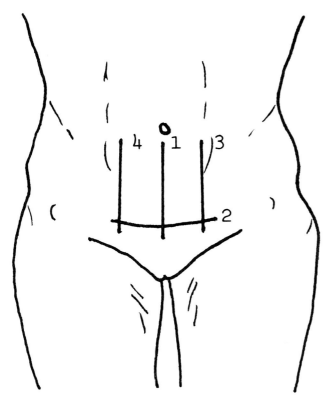

Figure 25–2. Laparotomy incisions used for cesarean delivery. 1—Midline vertical; 2—transverse; 3—left paramedian; 4—right paramedian.

abdominal wall.[19] Post-operatively, transverse incisions are usually accompanied by less discomfort and fewer respiratory infections due to respiratory splinting. From the patient's viewpoint the cosmetics of a transverse incision are favored, because the scar is in the lower abdomen or hidden by pubic hair.

Transverse incisions, however, have some disadvantages. Timones and colleagues[20] found the time from transverse incision to delivery significantly increased over that of a midline incision. It took 4 minutes or less in 56% of cesarean sections using the vertical incision versus 28% using the Pfannenstiel incision. The time difference was even greater if the cesarean section was performed through a secondary incision. Comparing two types of transverse incisions, Ayers and Morely[21] noted that ease of delivery correlated negatively with incision size. Defining difficult delivery as "forceful maternal abdominal pressure required to overcome relative dystocia of the abdominal wall incision,"[21] they found that 75% of cesarean sections with an incision less than 13 cm long fulfilled that criterion. When incision size was 15 cm or longer, the incidence of difficult delivery was significantly reduced. Transverse incisions involve division of multiple layers of fascia and sometimes muscle, with formation of potential spaces that increase the risk of hematoma formation.

The best choice of abdominal incision in the

massively obese patient is not yet clear. Most studies[22–26] in which this issue was addressed contained small series of patients. The advantage of the transverse incision is that the thickness of adipose tissue above the pubis is minimal and abdominal closure is more secure. Some oppose this incision because of an increased risk of infection because the area is so moist. Our experience, however, does not support this. The area can usually be kept dry with dressing changes or a towel. Disadvantages of the transverse approach include a longer operating time, greater blood loss, and less exposure. The cephalic retraction of the panniculus, sometimes needed in a transverse approach, may adversely affect maternal respiratory and cardiovascular function. Because of the panniculus, the anatomical location of the umbilicus is changed. Therefore a midline incision may have to be above the umbilicus, especially for a classic cesarean section. If the patient is morbidly obese and a midline incision is chosen, long retractors and instruments may be necessary for exposure.

Vertical Midline Incision

The abdomen is opened precisely in the midline, identified by the linea nigra. The skin is incised down to the fascia from just above the symphysis pubis to just below the umbilicus, although the exact length will depend on the size of the fetus and the contour of the maternal abdomen. The underlying fascia is usually incised near the umbilicus. Hemostasis is secured by thermocoagulation or ligation of open branches of the superficial epigastric vessels. The fascial incision is extended to the margins of the skin incision inferiorly and superiorly with scissors. A branch of the external pudendal artery is often encountered in the caudal end of the fascial incision; clamping and ligating it help prevent hematoma formation.

Transversalis fascia and preperitoneal fat are incised to the underlying peritoneum. In obese patients with a thick preperitoneal fat pad, identifying the urachus will help identify the peritoneum. The peritoneum should be grasped with nontoothed tissue forceps or hemostats; elevated at its upper third; and visually and palpably inspected to ensure exclusion of bowel, bladder, or omentum. The peritoneum is then carefully incised with either the knife or scissors and the incision extended cephalad, then caudad toward the dome of the bladder. When the abdomen is entered through a previous scar, the peritoneum is incised near the umbilicus to avoid injury to an adherent bladder. The surgeon should be even more careful about possible adhesions of bowel or omentum to the anterior abdominal wall.

Paramedian Incision

The skin and subcutaneous fatty tissues are incised in a vertical direction about 2 cm from the lateral edge of the rectus muscle (5 to 6 cm from the midline). The incision is carried through the muscle aponeurosis until the muscle edge can be identified. The rectus muscle is then displaced toward the midline. The posterior sheath of the rectus and the peritoneum are incised along with the transversalis fascia by a vertical incision about 2 cm from the lateral reflection of the sheath. Blood vessels encountered are grasped, divided, and ligated.

In a study comparing midline and paramedian incisions, Guillon and co-workers[27] found little difference between incisions in terms of wound infection, dehiscence, and respiratory complications. Increased bleeding and operating time and the possibility of damage to the rectus muscle are arguments against the paramedian incision. Possible remaining indications in obstetrics for this approach include the extraperitoneal cesarean birth and cases of suspected appendicitis.

Transverse Incisions

PFANNENSTIEL INCISION

In the Pfannenstiel incision,[28] the skin is incised horizontally, two finger breadths above the symphysis pubis. Subcutaneous fat and superficial fascia are similarly incised transversely down to the aponeurosis (Fig. 25–3). Care must be taken to expose and ligate the superficial epigastric vessels. The fascia is then incised in the midline with a scalpel and extended laterally with scissors. The

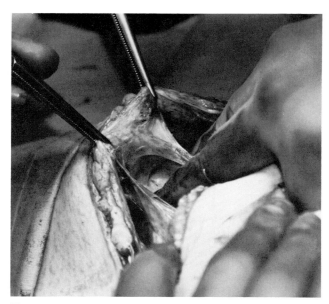

Figure 25–4. Low abdominal transverse incision: dissecting the subfascial planes on each side of the midline raphe toward the symphysis pubis.

fascia is then freed cranially from the underlying rectus abdominal muscles using blunt dissection. The heavier linea alba fibers have to be cut sharply with scissors. The same steps are repeated caudally (Fig. 25–4). Hemostasis is particularly important to avoid a post-operative subfascial hematoma. The rectus muscle is then separated in the midline and the peritoneum opened as described for the vertical midline incision (Figs. 25–5 and 25–6).

JOEL-COHEN MODIFICATION

In this method,[29] the tissues of the anterior abdominal wall are bluntly separated. After the transverse skin incision is made, the subcutaneous

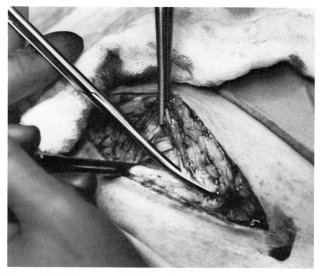

Figure 25–3. Transverse incision of the skin and fascia. (Courtesy Warren C. Plauché, M.D. and Karen Lanier, M.D.; photographed by Rita Letellier.)

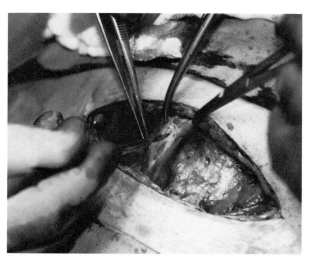

Figure 25–5. To enter the peritoneal cavity, pick up the peritoneal fold between two hemostats. Be sure no bowel is adherent. Incise the fold carefully with a scalpel.

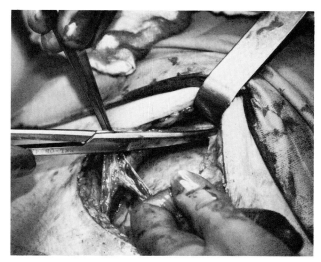

Figure 25–6. Low abdominal transverse incision: open the peritoneal cavity vertically, under direct vision to protect the underlying structures.

fat, superficial fascia, and deep fascia are divided by a scalpel centrally to about 2 to 3 cm on each side of the midline. Using both index fingers inserted in the deep fascial space created by the knife, the surgeon bluntly divides the fascia and subcutaneous tissue transversely. Thereafter, the rectus muscles are retracted laterally, with the surgeon taking care to avoid trauma to the inferior epigastric vessels. The peritoneum is entered, either transversely or cephalocaudally with scissors or bluntly with fingers. Using this approach, the blood vessels are pushed aside and not transected. Consequently, bleeding is very slight. With practice, the surgeon can enter the abdomen very rapidly. Difficulty can be encountered, however, where a great deal of exposure is needed, i.e., with obesity and/or abdominal wall scarring.

TRANSVERSE-MUSCLE-CUTTING INCISION

The limitation of operative exposure encountered with the Pfannenstiel incision can be improved by using the transverse-muscle-cutting incision advocated by Maylard.[30] By transecting the rectus muscles, the surgeon obtains excellent exposure for any type of pelvic procedure. The incision requires identification and ligation of the inferior epigastric vessels to avoid hematoma formation in the lateral margins of the incision. The major disadvantages are the increased time required to cut the muscles and the potential injury to the ilioinguinal and iliohypogastric nerves. For these reasons, the transverse-muscle-cutting incision is not popular among obstetricians.

CHERNEY INCISION

In 1941, Cherney[31] described dividing the fibrous, tendinous recti close to their insertion into the pubis, thus affording excellent pelvic exposure. This should be considered the procedure of choice when a transverse incision is desired but is inadequate to deliver the infant safely and expediently.

UTERINE INCISIONS

After the abdomen is opened, the uterus should be palpated to determine the precise location of the uterine vessels. This is easily done by feeling for the round ligament located anteriorly near the upper portion of each side of the uterus. The uterus will frequently be dextrorotated, which places the left round ligament closer to the midline. Rotation of the uterus 180 degrees may rarely occur and will be diagnosed before delivery if uterine artery palpation is routinely performed.

It is crucial to assess the adequacy of the operating space to permit an easy delivery before making the uterine incision to avoid interruption of uteroplacental blood flow.[32] It is our observation that difficulty in placement of the bladder retractor, after development of a bladder flap, is often associated with an obstructed abdominal delivery. Moistened laparotomy packs may be placed in each lateral colonic gutter to help absorb blood and amniotic fluid and prevent meconium granuloma formation.[33] This involves stretching of the peritoneum, which may produce nausea and vomiting in patients who are under regional anesthesia.

The peritoneal reflection between the bladder and uterus should be identified, regardless of the type of uterine incision. The loose visceral peritoneum is picked up with forceps about 1 cm below the uterine attachment and incised in the midline (Fig. 25–7). It is separated from the underlying uterus laterally with the closed scissors and divided to the lateral margins of the uterus, toward the round ligaments. The surgeon's finger bluntly separates the lower flap and posterior bladder wall

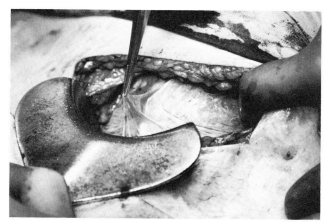

Figure 25–7. Retract the lower wound edge downward with a Balfour retractor. Pick up the fold of loose peritoneum overlying the lower uterine segment and incise transversely the width of the lower segment.

from the lower uterine segment by applying pressure to the uterus rather than to the bladder. Development of an adequate bladder flap is important because it increases exposure, facilitates repair, and decreases the risk of bladder damage.

The surgeon feels for the lie and the presentation of the fetus because these will affect the type of uterine incision. By preoperatively knowing the various options available, the operator can anticipate potential problems at delivery and handle them safely and wisely. Finally, a pair of forceps (preferably Kjelland or Elliott forceps) or the vacuum extractor should be available to aid in the delivery of the floating head if the need arises.

The uterine incision may be in the upper or lower segment of the uterus. The lower segment progressively increases in width and length as pregnancy advances, and its thickness decreases. Further thinning occurs during labor as the upper segment actively contracts and gets progressively thicker. The lower uterine segment can be recognized by its location posterior to the bladder.

The uterus may be entered vertically or transversely (see Fig. 25–8). The low transverse or Kerr incision[34] (Figs. 25–9 and 25–10) is most popular and is used in more than 90% of all cesarean births. The incision offers many advantages. It is easy to perform, the incised area is less vascular, and it is easier to repair. Adhesion formation to the uterine incision is markedly reduced because the operative site is completely covered by the bladder flap. The greatest advantage of the low transverse incision is that it has a low probability of dehiscence and rupture in a subsequent pregnancy, allowing a trial of labor. In a review of the literature, Keeping and co-workers[35] found uterine rupture rates of 2 to 4.7% after previous classic incisions and 0.5 to 1.0% after low-segment operations. Similar results were found on review of a total of 20,427 deliveries reported in the literature.[36]

Disadvantages of the low transverse incision include the risk of lateral extension into the uterine vessels, which results in increased blood loss. Limitation of the incision by the width of the lower segment depends on development of the segment itself.

Other options available to the surgeon include the low vertical or Kronig incision[37] and the classic uterine fundal incision. The low vertical incision is preferred over the low transverse incision when an underdeveloped lower segment is encountered. Adequate space can be obtained by extending the vertical incision superiorly into the upper segment. Its disadvantages include the need for greater separation of the bladder from the lower uterine segment, the risk of extension caudally into the

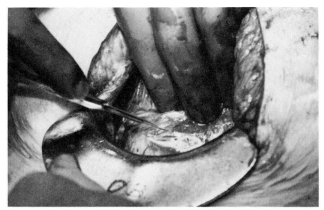

Figure 25–9. Begin the transverse uterine incision with short, shallow transverse strokes of the scalpel blade.

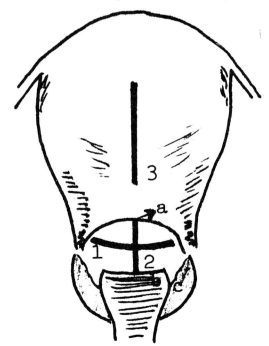

Figure 25–8. Uterine incisions. 1—Low transverse (Kerr); 2—low vertical (Kronig); 3—classic; a—visceral peritoneal reflection; b—bladder retractor; c—bladder.

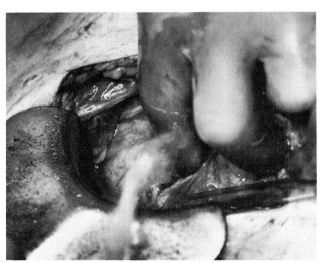

Figure 25–10. Stop the incision when the amniotic membranes are seen or when amniotic fluid escapes, as shown above.

Table 25–1. USUAL INDICATIONS FOR VERTICAL
UTERINE INCISION

Underdeveloped, narrow lower segment
Lower segment pathology (fibroids, adherent bladder, or large
  varicosities)
Anterior placenta previa
Transverse lie (back down or oligohydramnios)
Fetal anomalies (e.g., hydrocephaly)
Carcinoma of the cervix
Rapid delivery required

bladder and/or vagina, and the need for repeat cesarean section in subsequent pregnancies, especially if the upper segment is entered.

The classical cesarean section is a vertical incision in the upper uterine segment or fundus. Its primary advantage is that it allows rapid delivery when circumstances dictate such a need. Disadvantages include increased blood loss, difficulty of repair, increased risk of rupture in future pregnancies, and adhesion formation between the incision and abdominal organs or the anterior abdominal wall.

The choice of uterine incisions is largely dictated by the conditions at the time of surgery. One does not want to avoid a traumatic vaginal delivery only to have a difficult cesarean birth. The uterine incision depends on the fetal and placental position and the anatomy encountered on opening the abdomen. Table 25–1 lists various conditions in which a vertical uterine incision should be considered.

Controversies still exist regarding the choice of uterine incision in the abdominal delivery of the preterm fetus and the breech. The low vertical and classical incisions have been advocated by some for the very premature fetus.[35, 38] Westgren and Paul,[39] however, found no differences between incision types in the incidence of maternal/fetal complications in preterm infants. In this series, all incisions were believed adequate, and upper segment entrapment was believed to be responsible for the trauma incurred. The comparative safety of the low transverse versus the low vertical uterine incision for cesarean delivery of the breech infant was evaluated by Schutterman and Grimes[40] in 1983. Reviewing 416 cesarean deliveries, the authors found that standardized perinatal mortality rates, the incidence of low Apgar scores, extension of the uterine incision, the incidence of blood transfusion, and maternal fever were not significantly different between the two incisions. However, only 6.3% of the patients in the low transverse group and 8.7% of those in the low vertical group were less than 29 weeks pregnant.

Surgical Techniques

The transverse uterine incision is initiated by incising the uterine musculature at least two fin-

ger breadths above the remaining bladder attachment for a distance of about 2 to 3 cm. Continuous suctioning of the field is important to avoid injury to the baby, which commonly occurs in posterior cephalic and breech presentations, especially with prolonged rupture of the membranes and a lower segment well applied to the infant. Using Allis clamps to elevate the edges of the uterine incision or entering the endometrial layer with a hemostat or the handle of the knife will help avoid injury. Once the amniotic cavity is entered, two fingers are inserted to elevate the muscle from the fetal parts. Bandage scissors are used to cut the remaining lower segment in an upward concave arc under direct vision, taking care to avoid the uterine vessels (Fig. 25–11). Some surgeons enlarge the uterine incision by spreading the muscle laterally using both index fingers. Javanovic[41] reported a lack of control using this technique, causing laceration of the uterine vessels and the possibility of a downward curve that would result in a smaller transverse incision. Our experience supports that of Javanovic.

A vertical uterine incision is approached similarly. A small midline vertical incision is made in the lower segment into the amniotic cavity and extended upward and downward with bandage scissors until adequate space for delivery of the baby is obtained. In a term pregnancy, a 10- to 12-cm uterine incision is ideal. Because the lower segment is seldom sufficiently developed to provide adequate space for delivery, the incision frequently involves the body of the uterus.

Delivery of the Infant and Placenta

Before the delivery, the surgeon clinically confirms the lie and presentation of the fetus, the

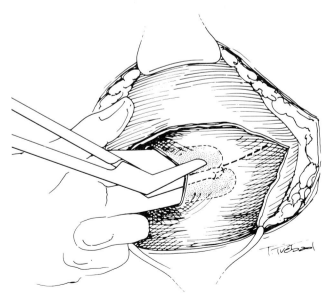

Figure 25–11. Following entry of the amniotic cavity, extend the uterine incision with bandage scissors. Insert fingers as shown to protect against fetal injury. (From Phelan JP, Clark SL: Cesarean Delivery, New York: Elsevier Science Publishers, 1988, p. 209.)

station of the presenting part, and the location of the placenta. This information affects the choice of uterine incision and the delivery approach. A third assistant should be available in the delivery room to help dislodge a deep presenting part if the need arises.

The interval between the uterine incision and delivery of the infant has a direct bearing on neonatal outcome. An interval of more than 3 minutes has been associated with a significantly higher incidence of low Apgar scores and acidotic infants.[42] In mothers under regional anesthesia, infants delivered after prolonged intervals had significantly lower cord pH values and increased umbilical arterial norepinephrine concentrations.[32]

After an adequate uterine incision, the surgeon's hand is introduced into the space between the anterior uterine wall and the presenting part of the fetus (Fig. 25–12). When the presentation is cephalic, flexion of the head during elevation will offer a smaller diameter coming through the uterine incision (Fig. 25–13). Forceps may be required to assist difficult extractions (Fig. 25–14).

When the head has been delivered, the nasal and oral passages are suctioned with a bulb syringe. If meconium is present, a wall suction on a low setting is used. With the help of an assistant, fundal pressure is applied and the body is delivered. In order to facilitate drainage of lung fluid, the shoulders may be delivered, leaving the body in the cavity. Uterine compression on the chest wall simulates compression of the chest and forces out fluid. Whether this maneuver decreases the incidence of wet lung is unknown, but when practiced it is surprising how much fluid is extruded. At this time, oxytocin is added to the infusion to help stimulate uterine contractions. After delivery of the body, the umbilical cord is doubly clamped and cut, and the baby is handed carefully to the resuscitation team. Blood is obtained from the

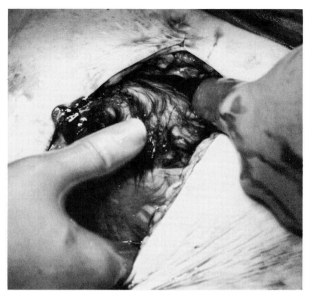

Figure 25–13. Extracting the vertex at cesarean delivery. Work the fingers down below the presenting part. Elevate the vertex into the incision without exerting leverage against the lower portion of the uterine incision.

placental end of the cord for possible laboratory analysis. If uterine bleeding is not excessive, spontaneous separation of the placenta can be allowed and removal completed by gentle cord traction. Manual removal of the placenta is another option, especially in the presence of heavy bleeding. After delivery of the placenta, the uterine cavity is inspected and remnants of membranes and placental fragments are removed digitally.

Wound Closure

For closure, the uterus may be left in situ or delivered onto the maternal abdominal wall; the

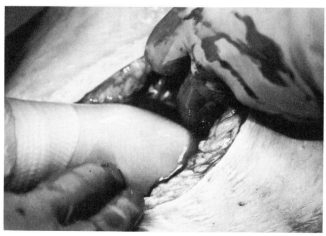

Figure 25–12. Extracting the vertex at cesarean delivery with the surgeon standing to the right, the right hand is inserted between the head and the lower uterine segment.

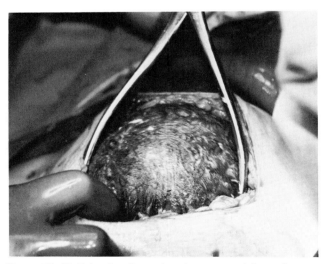

Figure 25–14. Extracting the vertex at cesarean delivery: forceps application. The forceps blades enclose the parietal bones with the tips of the forceps over the baby's cheeks. Gently elevate the head into the incision.

latter makes it easier to suture the incision (Fig. 25–15). Hershey and Quilligan[43] reported on 386 consecutive cesarean sections in which uteri were randomly exteriorized or left in situ for closure. Both groups showed similar results with respect to overall morbidity. A subgroup exhibiting increased blood loss included significantly more patients in the noneventrated group. Emesis occurred in 3.4% of patients in the eventrated group and was directly related to fundal traction under regional anesthesia.

A number of different suturing procedures have been tried over the years for uterine closure, using one or two layers of continuous or interrupted suture. A single-layer closure has been shown to give an excellent anatomic result and is at least as strong as, if not stronger than, a multilayered closure.[44–48] Lal and Tsomo,[49] using hysterography at 3 months post partum, demonstrated that single-layer interrupted suture uterine closure had substantially more normal hysterograms than the conventional two-layer closure using continuous sutures. Nonetheless, most physicians close the uterus in two layers using continuous running sutures with the second layer covering the first.

It is important to begin the closure with the initial stitch just beyond the angle of the incision. The stitches should be securely placed approximately 1 cm from the edge of the incision, ensuring that the edges can be inverted without a need to employ pressure on the suture line to the point of tearing tissue (Fig. 25–16). Although most surgeons prefer to use chromic catgut, polyglycolic acid (Dexon), polyglactin (Vicryl), and polydioxanone (PDS) are gaining wide support. We could not find any randomized studies in which efficacies of different suture materials on the uterine incision were compared. The choice is frequently motivated by emotion rather than scientific thought.

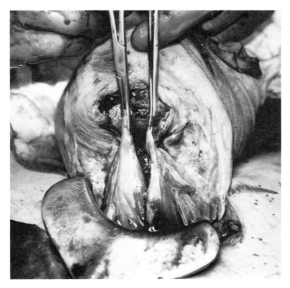

Figure 25–15. Exteriorizing the uterus to obtain additional room for repair of the vertical cesarean incision.

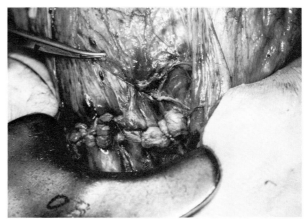

Figure 25–16. The transverse cesarean incision extends very close to the large vessels at the lateral margin of the uterus. Carefully close the lateral angles of the incision to ensure complete hemostasis.

Investigators[50] have suggested that incorporation of the decidua with the myometrium during closure of the uterine incision be avoided. One concern is that a suture including the decidua would increase abdominal wall scar endometriosis. However, there is no scientific proof for this theory. Besides, this complication is rare, reported to occur in about 0.03% of cesarean sections.[51] Surgical endometriosis in the uterine wound is another concern.

Repair of a low vertical uterine incision is similar to the repair of a low transverse incision (Fig. 25–17A). A three-layer closure is frequently needed for the classic scar. We usually run a continuous first layer and interrupt the second. We take care not to extend the sutures beyond the incision margins to avoid the large venous sinuses in the body of the uterus. The final layer is inverted with an absorbable suture with minimal tissue reaction to reduce the potential for adhesion formation (Fig. 25–17B).

After the uterine incision has been closed, the vesicouterine serosa may be reapproximated with a fine suture. The ovaries and fallopian tubes are inspected for evidence of pathology. The paracolic gutters and cul-de-sac may be cleaned with a wet sponge. Closing the parietal peritoneum as a separate layer appears to play no significant role in healing of the laparotomy wound.[52] We do not routinely close the peritoneum. If closure is chosen, a fine suture with low tissue reactivity is recommended.

The fascia is usually closed with a running synthetic absorbable suture. Wide bites should be taken at a minimum distance of 1 cm. If there is a significant risk of wound dehiscence (see Table 25–2), a permanent, continuous, monofilament suture in a mass closure technique appears to be superior to other conventional methods of closure.[53–56] In cases in which adequate hemostasis is not established, subfascial and subcutaneous suc-

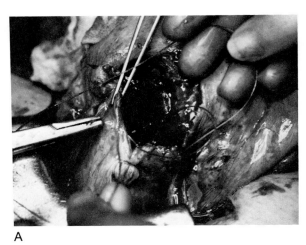

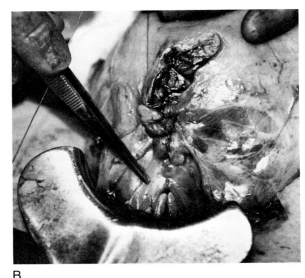

A   B

Figure 25–17. *A,* The lower portion of this vertical uterine incision is closed with a single layer of suture. Suture placement excludes the endometrial layer, inverting it into the endometrial cavity. *B,* The thick upper portion of many vertical uterine incisions requires closure in two or three layers.

tion drains should be used. The skin edges are reapproximated either with running subcuticular fine synthetic suture or with staples. The staples are removed 72 hours later and replaced with Steri-Strips. Nonabsorbant subcuticular suture (nylon) can be removed at the same time or several weeks later.

EXTRAPERITONEAL CESAREAN SECTION

The extraperitoneal approach to the uterine cavity was originally described by Physick[57] in 1824. Popularized in the preantibiotic era, the operation was an attempt to avoid the high mortality rate caused by peritoneal infection. By avoiding contamination of the peritoneal cavity by infected amniotic fluid, peritonitis, pelvic abscess formation and adhesions were dramatically reduced. In the United States, this operation reached its peak in the 1940s. However, with the availability and widespread use of antibiotics, a few saw a true need for the operation.

Proponents of the extraperitoneal approach cite many benefits to the operation. Perkins[58] reported 93 cases of extraperitoneal cesarean section, comparing findings with those of normal and high-risk control groups. The mean time from induction of anesthesia to delivery, mean duration of surgery,

Table 25–2. RISKS FOR WOUND DEHISCENCE

Obesity
History of hernia or wound dehiscence
Contaminated wounds
Previous abdominal surgery
Poor nutritional status

and mean decrease in post-operative hematocrit level were similar among the groups. One-minute Apgar scores were significantly lower in the extraperitoneal group than in either control group, probably related to the anatomic restrictions at the operative site, as explained later. Although 67% of the patients who underwent extraperitoneal cesarean section were febrile before surgery, the incidence of prolonged hospitalization and febrile morbidity did not differ among the groups. In Perkins' series, there were two inadvertent bladder injuries (2.2%).

In a trial[59] conducted at a large referral center in Africa, 239 intraperitoneal cesarean sections were compared with 173 extraperitoneal operations using Crichton's[60] modification. Benefits resulting from the latter approach included a fivefold reduction in the occurrence of pelvic abscess. Although all patients were treated with antibiotics, this patient population consisted of women with such gross infection that they hardly compared with a patient population in the United States.

Hanson[61] reported data from 346 personally conducted extraperitoneal procedures and concluded that the operation is a viable alternative to the transperitoneal cesarean section. This enthusiasm, however, was not shared by many. Wallace and co-workers[62] in a prospective randomized fashion, compared the extraperitoneal cesarean section with the transperitoneal approach. Although there was a trend toward enhanced post-operative recovery in the extraperitoneal group, this technique offered no significant advantage in the prevention of post-cesarean endomyometritis.

In a retrospective analysis of 186 primary cesarean sections, Haesslein and Goodlin[63] found that of those who would have benefited most from an extraperitoneal approach, for technical reasons, none were candidates. Of the cases of unsuspected pelvic pathology, 57% would have been missed if an indicated extraperitoneal cesarean section had been performed. Contraindications to extraperitoneal cesarean section include a low-lying anterior placenta previa, a previous cesarean section, an estimated fetal weight of greater than 4000 g, a need for abdominal exploration, fetal distress, transverse lie, and lack of experience of a qualified surgeon.[64]

Surgical Techniques

Epidural anesthesia is usually preferred because of the increased time that may be required from incision to delivery. The abdominal wall is incised through either a left paramedian or a low transverse incision. In the Latzko[65] method, a dye solution (300 to 400 mL) is infused into the bladder to help identify its limits. The midline transversalis fascia overlying the distended bladder is opened at approximately the midpoint between the symphysis and the dome of the bladder, either transversely or vertically. Care should be taken not to extend the vertical incision above the peritoneal reflection at the bladder dome. By blunt paravesical dissection, the fatty tissue and bladder are retracted laterally and inferiorly off the overlying peritoneum to the patient's right. It is advisable to continually inspect the uterine surface while carrying out the blunt dissection, to avoid

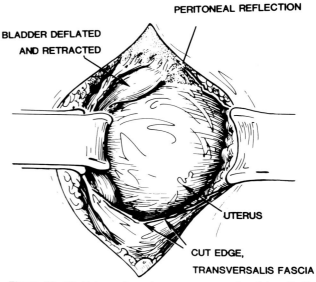

Figure 25–19. Extraperitoneal cesarean operation (step 2). The bladder is deflated and retracted to the right following dissection of the vesicouterine fascia, thus exposing the uterine surface. (From Phelan JP, Clark SL: Cesarean Delivery, New York: Elsevier Science Publishers, 1988, p. 196.)

injury to the uterine vessels and ureter. Because the uterus is most commonly dextrorotated, there is more room on the left, which is why everything is retracted to the right (Fig. 25–18). A layer of fascia (the endopelvic fascia) separates the lower uterine segment from the bladder. This must be entered sharply, and is retained on the posterior bladder wall as the bladder with its fascia is now separated from the uterus and vesicouterine peritoneal fold. The bladder is emptied and retracted inferiorly by the standard bladder retractor (Fig. 25–19). A transverse lower uterine segment incision is then made in the standard manner approximately 2 to 3 cm below the peritoneal reflection. A pair of forceps or the vacuum extractor should be kept on the operating table to assist delivery of the baby if difficulties are encountered because of the decreased space compared with the 10- to 12-cm lower segment incision of a transperitoneal cesarean section.

After delivery of the placenta, the uterus is closed in the usual way, either one or two layers. Bladder integrity should be checked by reinflation. Injury is most likely to occur in the dome and should be repaired in two layers using 3-0 chromic catgut. Retrovesical and subfascial drains are placed and brought out through separate stab wounds. The abdominal wall is then closed in the usual manner.

The peritoneal exclusion technique, originally described by Frank[66] in 1907 and later modified, involves opening the peritoneal cavity in the standard manner through either a midline or transverse incision, although the latter is much easier, because the peritoneum can be opened transversely. The bladder flap is developed as in the

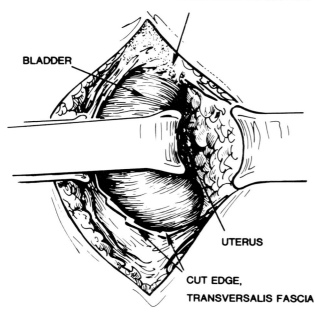

Figure 25–18. Extraperitoneal cesarean operation (step 1). The bladder is exposed in this vertical skin incision and retracted to the patient's right following incision of the fascia. The uterus can be seen behind the paravesical fat. (From Phelan JP, Clark SL: Cesarean Delivery, New York: Elsevier Science Publishers, 1988, p. 195.)

low-segment transverse cesarean. The cephalad portion of the peritoneum is teased off the uterus to its reflection. This cephalad visceral peritoneum is then sutured to the cephalad parietal peritoneum with chromic catgut. In a similar manner, the caudad parietal portion is sutured to the lower bladder-flap peritoneum. Although not watertight, this technique theoretically decreases peritoneal contamination and has the advantage of allowing intra-abdominal exploration before the lower uterine segment is opened, unlike the extraperitoneal procedure. Disadvantages include the time it takes to develop the flaps and suture back the peritoneum, and the compromised space for delivery of the infant.

References

1. Sanger J: Der Kaiserschnitt bei Uterusfibromen nebst-Vergleichender Methodik der Sectio Caesarea und der Porro Operation. Leipzig: W. Engelmann, 1882.
2. Seropian R, Reynold BM: Wound infections after preoperative depilatory versus razor preparation. Am J Surg 121:251, 1971.
3. Alexander JW, Aerni S, Pletner JP: Development of a safe and effective one-minute preoperative skin preparation. Arch Surg 120:1357, 1985.
4. Joress SM: A study of disinfection of the skin: A comparison of povidone-iodine with other agents used for surgical scrubs. Am Surg 155:296, 1962.
5. Lowbury EJL, Lilly HA: Use of 4% chlorhexidine detergent solution (Hibiscrub) and other methods of skin disinfection. Br Med J 1:510, 1973.
6. McRoberts WA Jr: Postural shock in pregnancy. Am J Obstet Gynecol 62:627, 1951.
7. Howard BK, Goodson JH, Mengert WF: Supine hypotensive syndrome in late pregnancy. Obstet Gynecol 1:371, 1953.
8. Crawford JS, Burton M, Davies P: Time and lateral tilt at cesarean section. Br J Anaesth 44:477, 1972.
9. Downing JW, Coleman AJ, Mahomedy MC, et al.: Lateral table tilt for cesarean section. Anaesthesia 29:696, 1974.
10. Waldron KW, Wood C: Cesarean section in the lateral position. Obstet Gynecol 37:706, 1971.
11. Ansari I, Wallace G, Clemetson CAB, et al.: Tilt caesarean section. J Obstet Gynaecol Br Commonw 77:713, 1970.
12. Kerr MG, Scott DB, Samuel E: Studies of the inferior vena cava in late pregnancy. Br Med J 1:532, 1964.
13. Goodlin RC: Importance of lateral position during labor. Obstet Gynecol 37:698, 1971.
14. Downing JW, Bees LT: The influence of lateral tilt on limb blood flow in advanced pregnancy. S Afr Med J 50:728, 1976.
15. Drummond GB, Scott SEM, Lees MM, Scott DB: Effects of posture on limb blood flow in late pregnancy. Br Med J 4:587, 1974.
16. Eckstein KL, Marx GF: Aorto-caval compression and uterine displacement. Anesthesiology 40:92, 1974.
17. Baley RJR, Downing JW, Brock-Utne JG, Cuerden C: Right versus left lateral tilt for cesarean section. Br J Anaesth 49:1009, 1977.
18. Sloan GA: A new upper abdominal incision. Surg Gynecol Obstet 45:678, 1927.
19. Mowat J, Bonnar J: Abdominal wound dehiscence after cesarean section. Br Med J 2:256, 1971.
20. Timonen S, Castren O, Kivalo I: Cesarean section: Low transverse (Pfannenstiel) or low midline incision. Ann Chir Gynaecol Fenn 59:173, 1970.
21. Ayers JWT, Morley GW: Surgical incision for cesarean section. Obstet Gynecol 70:706, 1987.
22. Hodgkinson R, Husain FJ: Caesarean section associated with gross obesity. Br J Anaesth 52:919, 1980.
23. Sicuranza BJ, Tisdall LH: Cesarean section in the massively obese. J Reprod Med 14:10, 1975.
24. Ahern JK, Goodlin RC: Cesarean section in the massively obese. Obstet Gynecol 51:509, 1978.
25. Morrow CP, Hernandez WL, Townsend DE, Disaia PJ: Pelvic celiotomy in the obese patient. Obstet Gynecol 127:335, 1977.
26. Vanghan RW, Bauer S, Wise L: Volume and pH of gastric juices in obese patients. Anesthesiology 43:686, 1975.
27. Guillon PJ, Hall TJ, Donaldson DR, et al.: Vertical abdominal incisions—a choice? Br J Surg 67:359, 1980.
28. Pfannenstiel HJ: Uber die Vortheile des suprasymphysaren Fascienguerschnitt fur die gynaekologischen Koeliotomien. Samml Klin Vortr Gynaekol (Leipzig) Nr 268, 97:1735, 1900.
29. Cohen SJ: Abdominal and Vaginal Hysterectomy. London: Heinemann, 1972.
30. Maylard AE: Direction of abdominal incisions. Br Med J 2:895, 1907.
31. Cherney LS: A modified transverse incision for low abdominal operations. Surg Gynecol Obstet 72:92, 1941.
32. Bader AM, Datla S, Arthur R, et al.: Maternal and fetal catecholamines and uterine incision-to-delivery interval during elective cesarean. Obstet Gynecol 75:600, 1990.
33. Freedman SI, Ang EP, Herz MG, et al.: Meconium granulomas in post-cesarean section patients. Obstet Gynecol 59:383, 1982.
34. Kerr JMM: The technic of cesarean section with special reference to the lower uterine segment incision. Am J Obstet Gynecol 12:729, 1926.
35. Keeping JD, Morrison J, Chang AMZ: Classical caesarean section in preterm deliveries. Aust NZ J Obstet Gynaecol 20:103, 1980.
36. O'Sullivan MJ, Fumia F, Holsinger K, McLeod ACW: Vaginal delivery after cesarean section. Clin Perinatol 8:131, 1981.
37. Kronig B: Transperitonealer Cervikaler Kaiser-Schnitt. In Doderlein A, Kronig B (eds.): Operative Gynakologie. 1912, p. 879.
38. Faranoff AA, Merkatz JR: Modern obstetrical management of the low birth weight infant. Clin Perinatol 4:215, 1977.
39. Westgren M, Paul RH: Delivery of the low birth weight infant by cesarean section. Clin Obstet Gynecol 28:752, 1985.
40. Schutterman EB, Grimes DA: Comparative safety of the low transverse versus the low vertical uterine incision for cesarean delivery of breech infants. Obstet Gynecol 61:593, 1983.
41. Javanovic R: Incisions of the pregnant uterus and delivery of low birth weight infants. Am J Obstet Gynecol 152:971, 1985.
42. Datta S, Ostheimer GW, Weiss JB, et al.: Neonatal effect of prolonged anesthetic induction for cesarean section. Obstet Gynecol 58:331, 1981.
43. Hershey D, Quilligan E: Extraabdominal uterine exteriorization at cesarean section. Obstet Gynecol 52:189, 1978.
44. Greenhill JP, Bloome B: Histologic study of uterine scars after cervical cesarean section. JAMA 92:21, 1929.
45. Potter M, Johnston DC: Uterine closure in cesarean section. Am J Obstet Gynecol 67:760, 1954.
46. Backer K: Hysterography of cesarean section scar. Surg Gynecol Obstet 100:690, 1955.
47. Poidevin L: Histopathology of cesarean section wounds. J Obstet Gynaecol Br Emp 68:1025, 1961.
48. Wojdeski J, Grynsztajn A: Scar formation in the uterus after cesarean section. Am J Obstet Gynecol 107:322, 1970.
49. Lal K, Tsomo P: Comparative study of single layer and conventional closure of uterine incision in cesarean section. Int J Gynecol Obstet 27:349, 1988.
50. Sortor RF, Brines OA: Endometriosis involving cesarean section abdominal scar. Report of a case. Obstet Gynecol 10:425, 1957.

51. Chatterjee SK: Scar endometriosis: A clinicopathologic study of 17 cases. Obstet Gynecol 56:81, 1980.
52. Ellis H, Heddle R: Does the peritoneum need to be closed at laparotomy? Br J Surg 64:733, 1977.
53. Fagniez PL, Hay JM, Lacaine F, Thomsen C: Abdominal midline incision closure: A multicentric randomized prospective trial of 3,135 patients, comparing continuous vs interrupted polyglycolic acid sutures. Arch Surg 120:1351, 1985.
54. Knight CD, Griffen FD: Abdominal wound closure with a continuous monofilament polypropylene suture. Experience with 1000 consecutive cases. Arch Surg 118:1305, 1983.
55. Archie JP, Feldtman RW: Primary abdominal wound closure with permanent, continuous running monofilament sutures. Surg Obstet Gynecol 153:721, 1981.
56. Richards PC, Balch CM, Aldrete JS: Abdominal wound closure: A randomized prospective study of 571 patients comparing continuous vs. interrupted suture techniques. Ann Surg 197:238, 1982.
57. Physick P: Extraperitoneal cesarean section. In Dewees WP (ed.): A Compendious System of Midwifery. Philadelphia: H. C. Carey I. Lea, 1824, p. 580.
58. Perkins RP: The merits of extraperitoneal cesarean section: A continuing experience. J Reprod Med 19:154, 1977.
59. Mokgokoug ET, Crichton D: Extraperitoneal lower segment caesaren section for infected cases. A reappraisal. S Afr Med J 48:788, 1974.
60. Crichton D: A single technique of extraperitoneal lower segment cesarean section. S Afr Med J 47:2011, 1973.
61. Hanson HB: Current use of the extraperitoneal cesarean section: A decade of experience. Am J Obstet Gynecol 149:31, 1984.
62. Wallace RL, Eglinton GS, Yonekura ML, Wallace TM: Extraperitoneal cesarean section: A surgical form of infection prophylaxis? Am J Obstet Gynecol 148:172, 1984.
63. Haesslein HC, Goodlin RC: Extraperitoneal cesarean section revisited. Obstet Gynecol 55:181, 1980.
64. Perkins RP: Role of extraperitoneal cesarean section. Clin Obstet Gynecol 23:585, 1980.
65. Latzko W: Uber den extraperitonealen Kaiserschmtl. Zentralbl Gynaekol 33:275, 1909.
66. Frank F: Extraperitonealen Kaiserschmtl. Arch F Gynak 81:46, 1907.

26

Problems Encountered During Cesarean Delivery

Salih Y. Yasin
David L. Walton
Mary J. O'Sullivan

■ INTRAOPERATIVE COMPLICATIONS OF CESAREAN SECTION
■ BOWEL INJURY
■ BLADDER INJURY
■ URETERAL INJURY

■ EXTENSION OF UTERINE INCISION
■ UTERINE DEFECTS
■ FETAL EXTRACTION
■ FETAL INJURIES

The mortality rate for cesarean section during the 90-year period ending in 1789 in Paris was 100%.[1] In the past 50 years significant advances have been made, resulting in a marked decrease in both the morbidity and the mortality of cesarean delivery. Of 121,217 cesarean sections performed in Massachusetts between 1976 and 1984, there were 27 maternal deaths, for a mortality rate of 22.3 per 100,000 cesarean births.[2] A prospective Swedish study in 1984 reported an intraoperative cesarean complication rate of 11.6%, with elective sections having a lower complication rate than emergency operations (4.2% vs. 18.9%).[3] Minor

complications included blood transfusion, injury to the infant, minor lacerations of the isthmic portion of the uterus, and difficulty in delivering the infant. Major complications included bladder, cervical, or vaginal injury and laceration through the broad ligament with or without involvement of the uterine arteries.

Complications of operative entry can be categorized according to anatomic location as abdominal wall incision, intraperitoneal entry (adhesions and bowel injury), and bladder and uterine extensions. In the following sections we discuss the management of each location.

BOWEL INJURY

Although rare, bowel injury or entry into the abdomen during cesarean delivery may lead to serious morbidity. The risk of trauma increases with previous intra-abdominal surgery, pelvic inflammatory disease, or other conditions that result in adhesion formation.[1]

Significant morbidity may be decreased when injuries are recognized early and properly managed. Management depends on the type of injury, part of intestine affected, severity of adhesions, and extension of the injury into the lumen. Because the bowel is rarely prepared preoperatively, as it is in oncologic surgery, injuries involving the lumen may lead to intra-abdominal fecal spillage with resultant peritonitis and/or abscess formation.

Blunt dissection of thick adhesions may result in serosal tears and lacerations because the tensile strength of some of these adhesions is more than that of the bowel wall. Sharp dissection with a scapel or scissors may result in injuries involving bowel lumen. Bowel may also be injured with clamps (e.g., Kelly clamp or hemostats[4]) or during abdominal closure with a needle or suture. All the aforementioned injuries may involve the visceral peritoneum, muscularis, and lumen.

Other factors that may increase the risk of surgical complications include a need to enlarge the incision to maximize exposure for an atraumatic delivery, blind attempts to control excess blood loss, and the need to deliver the fetus quickly.

The mainstay of management of bowel injury is prevention—by careful entry into the abdominal cavity. Knowledge of the patient's previous medical, obstetric, and anesthetic complications and a review of previous surgical records are helpful in anticipating the potential extent and nature of adhesions.[1] Also of importance is fetal status, i.e., whether the section is primary or repeat and the size, lie, and position of fetus. Adequate exposure, accurate knowledge of the surgical anatomy, and avoidance of blind manipulation with surgical instruments are essential. A combination of "gentle" blunt dissection of filmy adhesions and careful sharp dissection of thick adhesions is the safest approach. A stapling gun for transection of adhesions and hemostasis may be of value where extensive adhesions are expected but is of no value when the uterus is densely adherent to the anterior abdominal wall. In the event of trauma, depending on hospital practice and the experience of the surgeon, a general surgery intraoperative consultation to assist in management of these injuries may be wise. This approach optimizes patient care.

Once bowel injury is suspected, it is important to assess the extent of the injury and the layers involved. If the lumen has been entered, to avoid spillage into the peritoneal cavity, the operator may wrap the involved section in moist laparotomy pads and isolate the proximal and distant portions of the affected bowel by gastrointestinal clamps. Inspection for lacerations of the mesenteric vascular supply is imperative to decrease blood loss, prevent hematoma formation, and decrease the likelihood of ischemic bowel injury. Once the injury is identified, inspected, and isolated, the operator may proceed with the cesarean section, because the empty contracted uterus makes any necessary further exploration easier and provides better exposure for repair.

Tears in the small bowel serosa are weak points with a danger of later perforation. If they are superficial and few in number, they can be left without repair or oversewn with 3–0 or 4–0 absorbable or nonabsorbable suture. When serosal tears are numerous, excessive suture placement may further complicate the course. In the absence of bleeding they could be left alone; otherwise an end-to-end anastomosis might be considered.

If the muscularis is involved, repair can be accomplished using a single layer of interrupted nonabsorbable suture, such as 4–0 silk, at right angles to longitudinal direction of the bowel. Likewise, a two-layer technique may be used, approximating the muscularis with simple interrupted absorbable material, such as 3–0 or 4–0 chromic catgut, and approximating the serosal layer with nonabsorbable, 4–0 silk. When the lumen has been entered accidentally, repair is accomplished in two layers as just described, at right angles to the longitudinal axis of the bowel to prevent stenosis. When multiple lacerations involving the lumen or transection of the small bowel has occurred, optimal results are attained with resection and re-anastomosis (Figs. 26–1A through C).

Trauma to the colon is also rare at cesarean section. A small laceration with no fecal spill could be safely oversewn as in small bowel injury. In the presence of multiple lacerations or a significant spill, a diverting colostomy is the safer route.

Either of two methods may be used for resection and anastomosis: (a) the classical suture technique or (b) automated surgical stapling[5] (Fig. 26–2). The mesentery is usually opened in a V-shaped fashion starting at the edge of intact bowel. After resection of the involved traumatized segment of bowel, an end-to-end anastomosis is performed in layers, using interrupted absorbable suture in the inner layer and nonabsorbable in the outer layer (Figs. 26–1D and E). It is important to avoid inclusion of mesenteric vessels in the anastomosed bowel segment, because this may cause hematoma formation with possible disruption of the anastomosis. After the anastomosis by either technique, defects or holes in mesentery are repaired to prevent internal bowel herniation.

Post-operative care of patients with bowel injury depends on the severity of the trauma and whether a resection was done. The general principles of

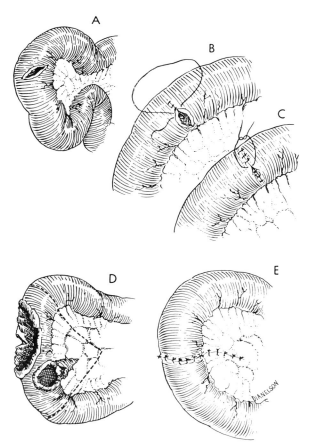

Figure 26–1. Small bowel injuries. A—simple laceration; B,C—two-layer closure. D,E—extensive injury with end to end reanastomosis. (From Greenlee HB: Surgery of the Small and Large Intestine, plate 58. Chicago: Year Book Medical Publishers, 1973.)

management include bowel rest until spontaneous intestinal activity resumes; hyperalimentation if the recovery period is expected to be prolonged; surveillance for potential infection, ileus, and obstruction; and, finally, timely management of such complications should they occur.

BLADDER INJURY

In a retrospective chart review of 7527 cesarean sections, Eisenkopp and co-workers[6] reported an incidence of .31% for bladder injury and .09% for ureteral injury. There were 23 accidental as well as 29 intentional cystotomies. Most (.6%) cystotomies occurred at repeat section; however, .19% occurred during primary sections. The most common cause was difficulty encountered during dissection of the bladder off the lower uterine segment. Bladder trauma during the uterine incision was the next most common cause, followed by extension of the uterine incision into the bladder.

It is generally recommended that the bladder flap be separated from the lower uterine segment before uterine entry.[7, 8] This provides better visualization of the lower uterine segment and drops

the ureters out of the field. Before incising the myometrium, the surgeon should be aware of the location of the dome of the bladder relative to the uterus in order to avoid entering the bladder on the way into the uterus. Overaggressive blunt bladder dissection may increase the risk of bladder injury. It is essential to recognize and properly repair such injuries. A red, vascular appearance of the muscularis, urine draining through the dome, or visualization of the Foley bulb are all telltale signs of bladder wall laceration. Hematuria may be indicative of bladder wall trauma but is not specific for cystotomy.

If there is suspicion of a bladder perforation, sterile milk (infant's formula), methylene blue, or indigo carmine injected into the urethral catheter with observed leakage into the abdomen confirms lack of integrity of the lower urinary tract. Sterile milk has the advantage of not staining, but the dyes are more readily available in the operating room. If a defect is identified, repair should be immediate for three reasons: (a) to prevent contin-

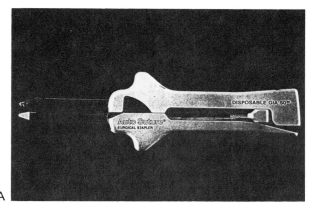

A

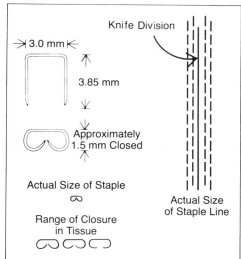

B

Figure 26–2. A, B, Automated stapler with schematic representation of the stapling and cutting mechanism. (From Sevin BU, Penalver MA: Reconstruction of bowel continuity with automated stapling instruments. In Knapstein PG, Friedburg V, Sevin BU (eds.): Reconstructive Surgery in Gynecology. New York: Thieme Medical Publishers, 1990.)

ual leakage of urine into the operative field, (b) because later the defect may become difficult to identify, and (c) to prevent enlargement of the defect during the ensuing operation.

Cystotomy is best repaired in two layers. We prefer to isolate the limits of the incision with Allis clamps, being certain the trigone and the ureteral orifices are clear and injury free. The submucosa and intermediate muscularis layer are reapproximated with continuous, nonlocking suture, either 3–0 chromic catgut or delayed absorbable suture, avoiding suture in the mucosa. The overlying muscularis and serosa are then sewn with the same suture. The integrity of the repair should be confirmed by distending the bladder gently, as previously described. Bladder drainage either suprapubicly or via a Foley catheter should be maintained for at least 5 days. There is evidence that 1 day may be sufficient if injury is away from the trigone. If injury to the bladder wall is only superficial, a single-layer closure with 2–0 or 3–0 absorbable suture will suffice. Bladder drainage is not required. Cystotomy recognized and properly repaired does not increase cesarean section morbidity.[6]

URETERAL INJURY

Although uncommon, ureteral injuries can occur as a result of extension of the uterine incision or secondary to hemostatic ligatures in the base of the broad ligament.

If there is suspicion of ureteral compromise, a cystotomy allowing direct visualization of the ureteral orifices for efflux of dye after intravenous administration of indigo carmine will establish a diagnosis. Eisenkopp and colleagues[6] have stressed the importance of symmetric appearance of dye in ruling out partial obstruction. Dye may also be injected directly into the ureter using a 22-gauge needle above the suspected obstruction. Resistance to injection or nonappearance of dye at the ureteral orifice will confirm obstruction. If dye appears in the operative field in the region of the ureter, then ureteral trauma (laceration or transection) is likely. If a ligature has caused ureteral occlusion, it should be released and the tissue inspected for viability. If the ureter appears normal, the area adjacent to the site should be drained to prevent formation of a urinoma. Suction drainage is preferred over a Penrose drain. Any questions of viability may require a stent or resection of the devitalized segment, depending on the size of the insult. An obstruction diagnosed post-operatively may be treated by passing a ureteral catheter through the bladder, or even doing so by radiologic guidance through the renal pelvis. Ureteral fistulas may be managed similarly, with a real possibility of nonsurgical repair. For all ureteral injuries, a urologist should be consulted and participate in the decision making and repair.

If the ureter is transected, the repair may involve a ureteroureterostomy or ureteroneocystotomy, depending on the site of transection. When the transection occurs within 8 cm of the bladder, it is best to perform a ureteroneocystotomy: The distal ureter is ligated, the proximal ureter is spatulated distally, and 3–0 or 4–0 absorbable sutures are placed at the site of spatulation. After the bladder is incised, the sutures are passed through the incision, sutured to the bladder wall, and tied with the knots outside the bladder mucosa. The periureteral tissue as it passes through the bladder muscularis is sutured at that site. An alternative technique is to tunnel the ureter for 3 cm within the bladder wall before bringing it out in the lumen of the bladder, with the intention of preventing ureteral reflux. Ureteral transection above the pelvic junction is best repaired with an end-to-end anastomosis or transureteroureterostomy. When ureteroureterostomy is performed, stents should be placed. Tension on the ureter should be relieved by tacking the distal and proximal ends to the psoas muscle. Retroperitoneal suction drains should be placed. Interested readers are referred to reference texts[9, 10] for further information on these procedures.

EXTENSIONS OF UTERINE INCISIONS

Nielsen and Hokegard[3] reported minor extensions of the uterine incision in 85 and major extensions of the uterine incision in 23 of 1319 patients. A minor extension was defined as small lacerations into the lower part of the uterus, whereas major extensions included tears into the cervix or vagina laterally from the uterine arteries, with bleeding and lacerations either involving most of the corpus uteri or extending around posteriorly beyond the broad ligament.

Transverse Incision

The type of uterine incision determines the direction of an extension. Transverse incisions tend to extend into the uterine vessels, whereas vertical incisions extend into the cervix, vagina, or bladder. The transverse incision is best effected by incising the myometrium until the amnionic sac is encountered. The incision is then extended under direct guidance using bandage scissors with two fingers inserted into the uterine cavity, ideally before rupture of the membranes. Intact membranes allow for optimal visualization, without obscuring the field by amnionic fluid, and permit easier manipulation of a fetus that may be entrapped in the fundus secondary to contraction of the physiologic contraction ring. The incision is extended upward in a curvilinear fashion, avoiding the lateral uterine vessels. Although some prefer the finger-spreading technique, the circular configuration of the muscles of the lower uterine segment will cause a downward slope to this incision, resulting in a smaller incision prone to extend into the uterine vessels.

Usually recognized after delivery, extension into the uterine vessels can result in profuse hemorrrhage and resultant shock in a short time. Uterine artery ligation can be accomplished by elevating the puerperal uterus, passing a large atraumatic needle containing an absorbable suture through the myometrium and out into the avascular area of the broad ligament, both above and below the uterine incision from anterior to posterior. Ligation of the ovarian-uterine anastomosis, which provides collateral supply, can be done just below the attachment of the uteroovarian ligament and accomplishes the same as ligation of the uterine vessels above the uterine incision (Fig. 26–3). This will result in both distal and proximal control.[11] Collateral flow is adequate for proper healing, and the vessels eventually recanalize if they have not been completely transected. If uterine artery ligation fails to control bleeding, pressure should be applied to the bleeding site and ligation of the ipsilateral hypogastric artery undertaken. The retroperitoneal space is entered posteriorly, lateral to the common iliac artery and medial to the infundibulopelvic ligament, or anteriorly between the round and infundibulopelvic ligaments. The common iliac artery is identified at the site where the ureter passes over it. The ureter is retracted medially and the vessel traced to the bifurcation of the internal (hypogastric) and external iliac ar-

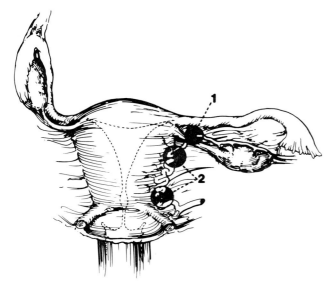

Figure 26–3. Sites for ligation of uterine (2) and utero-ovarian (1) vessels. (From Cruikshank SH: Management of postpartum and pelvic hemorrhage. Obstet Gynecol 29:218, 1986.)

tery. The external iliac is the lateral structure. Below the bifurcation, the hypogastric artery is stripped of areolar tissue for 2 cm; much of the dissection of the retroperitoneal space when it is entered anteriorly can be done with the tonsil tip sucker. A right-angle clamp is inserted generally from lateral to medial, taking care not to disrupt the accompanying vein. Two sutures of No. 0 silk are pulled through, and the artery is doubly ligated. When possible, the suture should be placed distal to the bifurcation of the superior gluteal artery; however, placing the ligature proximal to this point rarely causes loss of blood supply to the buttocks. If hemostasis is not obtained, contralateral utero-ovarian and hypogastric artery ligation is performed. Clark and co-workers[12] reported that hypogastric artery ligation was effective only 42% of the time. In cases of ineffective artery ligation, there was a 20% incidence of intraoperative cardiac arrest, whereas no patient undergoing emergency hysterectomy without hypogastric ligation suffered such an event. In their opinion, complications were most often attributable to delay in instituting definite therapy (i.e., hysterectomy). Therefore, if hemostasis is still not obtained after hypogastric ligation, then coagulopathies must be treated immediately and cesarean hysterectomy undertaken without delay.

Vertical Incision

The advantages and disadvantages of a vertical incision are the same as those of a transverse incision; i.e., the incision can extend or be extended, unintentionally or intentionally, quite easily. As with the transverse incision, the vertical incision is best extended under direct vision with bandage scissors. Uncontrolled tearing can result in deep cervical and vaginal tears that may be irreparable and necessitate hysterectomy. The dome of the bladder is also at greater risk with a low vertical incision.

Proper exposure is essential to identify the extent of the defect and to accomplish repair. The bladder should be isolated from the operating field and the laceration repaired with continuous, absorbable suture in two running layers. The surgeon must be aware of the course of the ureters, by identifying and tracing their course near the operative field. As previously described, dyes may be used to determine functional integrity as necessary.

UTERINE DEFECTS

If a uterine dehiscence is discovered at cesarean section, repair is easily effected by excising the fibrotic edges and closing the myometrium in two layers. Animal studies[13] have demonstrated that after repair of a uterine incision it is more likely for tearing to occur in the muscle region instead of in the scarred area. Therefore, unless the patient's wound-healing capability is demonstrably impaired, only the location of the defect and its size should determine future mode of delivery.

FETAL EXTRACTION

The most common uterine incision in modern obstetrics is the low-segment, transverse incision. Because of its retroperitoneal location, it prevents intra-abdominal infection. Moreover, blood loss is decreased and healing improved compared with a classic incision. These factors also affect the postoperative course in terms of anemia, infection, ileus, adhesions, ambulation, and long-term prognosis for future vaginal delivery. However, although they should be limited, vertical (classic) incisions may be necessary to prevent fetal injury or for technical reasons, such as absent or inadequate development of the lower uterine segment or inadequate exposure of the lower segment as a result of myomas, marked vascularity or adhesions from previous surgery (e.g., uterus adherent to the anterior abdominal wall), or fetal malpresentation. Vertical incisions are frowned on because of the short-term risks of bleeding, infection, ileus, adhesions, and intestinal obstruction, as well as the long-term risks of intestinal obstruction due to adhesions and poor healing quality of the active muscular segment, leading to potential rupture in a subsequent pregnancy. If the vertical incision is limited to a sufficiently well-developed low segment, then healing is the same as the transverse incision.

Vertex Presentation

The most common indication for cesarean section in a vertex presentation is cephalopelvic disproportion after arrest of the active phase of labor. Therefore the lower segment should be sufficiently well developed to allow a transverse incision. If a vertical incision must be done for technical reasons (e.g., a myoma on one side), whether the incision will be confined to the lower segment will depend on its development. In a term pregnancy with a normal head, approximately 10 to 12 cm of uterine incision is needed.

Planning delivery of the head will depend on its position and its location in relation to the pelvis. Introducing the fingers or hand into the uterus to deliver the head may cause stretching of the incision. Therefore, serious considerations in the transverse incision are its shape and location. If the cervix is fully dilated and retracted, the surgeon may inadvertently perform a transverse vaginal incision (a laparoelytrotomy). Originally de-

scribed to avoid a uterine incision,[14] the procedure was recently redescribed by Goodlin and co-workers[15] (Fig. 26–4). By definition, this is not a cesarean section because the infant is not delivered through a uterine incision. Under the circumstances described, the head is well down in the pelvis, with the biparietal diameter below the inlet, following development of the bladder flap; the distended vagina is visible over the vertex, free of major vessels; and a transverse incision is made. After delivery, the vagina is irrigated with an antibiotic solution and closed in two layers of running, locked, absorbable suture. We have described four unplanned laparoelytrotomies recognized when, after delivery, the cervix was visualized above the incision. All patients did well. However, we have seen at least one such unplanned procedure with massive hemorrhage from laceration of the lateral vaginal vessels, necessitating hysterectomy to control hemorrhage.

In the operating room, before the cesarean section is performed, a pelvic examination should be done to be certain vaginal delivery is not imminent and to check the cervix. If it is fully dilated and retracted, the bladder will be high on the lower segment, and minimal development will be necessary to enter the lower segment transversely. When the presenting part is deep in the pelvis, the operator's attempt to lift the head from above using a hand markedly increases the chances for an extension. Should an extension occur despite a curvilinear incision, it will usually occur inferiorly in the medial section of the wound. On the other hand, an incision extended transversely by fingers

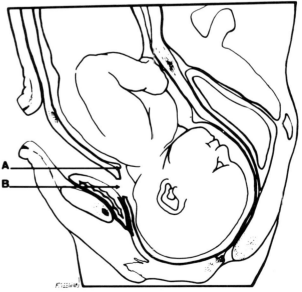

Figure 26–4. Laparoelytrotomy with the fetal head in the vagina. A—fully dilated, retracted cervix; B—vaginal incision with bladder retracted anteriorly. (From Goodlin RC, Scott JC, Woods RE: Laparoelytrotomy or abdominal delivery without uterine incision. Am J Obstet Gynecol 144:990, 1982.)

is likely to extend into the broad ligament and inferiorly.

There are several alternate maneuvers for delivery of the head to avoid such extensions. One is for an assistant to retract the shoulder superiorly, which will aid in lifting the head, while the surgeon insinuates a hand between the head and the lower segment. An alternative is to disengage the head before starting the operative procedure. Probably the most successful maneuver, with the least associated complications, is for an assistant to cup and lift the head into the lower segment transvaginally while the surgeon then delivers it. This can be accomplished either with the patient in the usual position and as the surgeon is opening the lower segment the head is elevated, or with the patient placed in the Whitmore position, which is similar to that used for laparoscopy (i.e., a modified lithotomy with thighs moderately abducted and flexed 135 degrees). The advantage of the latter technique is that the thighs and perineum are properly prepared and draped. An assistant stands in front of the patient, displacing the head, while the surgeon provides steady fundally directed pressure on the shoulder. As the head enters the lower segment, the surgeon then lifts it outward[16] (Figs. 26–5A and B).

Several methods have been described to deliver the head from the uterine cavity. When most uterine incisions were vertical, the head was rotated so the face was in the wound, and forceps were applied such that the pelvic curve of the blades was toward the symphysis pubis.[17, 18] The chin was then lifted out over the cephalic end of the incision and the head was delivered by flexion (Figs. 26–6A and C). A single blade of any forceps, including the posterior blade of Barton forceps, has also been used to act as a shoehorn-type vector to lift out the head (Fig. 26–7). Murless[19] described a special extractor to be inserted into the uterus "folded" and then extended after the curved blade had been positioned (Figs. 26–8A and B). In transverse incisions, the face may be manually rotated posteriorly and the head elevated by the hand between the head and lower uterine segment, so that the head delivers by extension.[20] Today, most surgeons rotate the head to a transverse position and lift it out manually by lateral flexion of the neck. Forceps may also be applied, ideally the Elliott or Kjelland forceps, each of which has minimal pelvic curve (Fig. 26–9). The cephalic application should be correct, with the apex of the blades pointing toward the chin and the head delivered by lateral flexion. Another useful method is fundal pressure by an assistant while the surgeon depresses the edges of the incision around the fetal head (Fig. 26–10).

When the head is high in the uterus, fundal pressure will generally bring it down. The vacuum extractor can be used to assist with descent and extraction. Before the cup is placed over the posterior fontanelle, the occiput is identified by palpating the anterior fontanelle and chin.[21]

Forceps may also be applied to the high head in the transverse position or by rotating the face posteriorly and applying the blades with the pelvic curve away from the symphysis (Fig. 26–9). The head is brought down in the occipitoanterior posi-

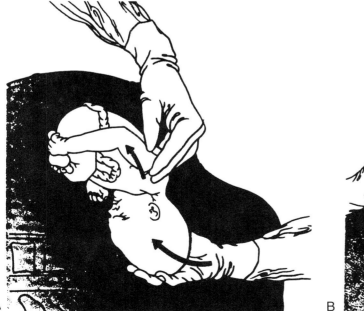
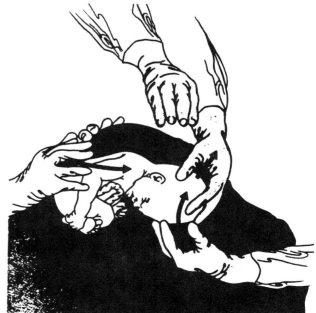

Figure 26–5. *A,* Disengaging the impacted head. The head is lifted into the lower uterine segment, and the shoulder is raised toward the fundus to assist elevation. *B,* The surgeon grasps the intrauterine head, elevating it through the uterine incision, while the assistant exerts fundal pressure. (From Landesman R, Graber EA: Abdominovaginal delivery: Modification of the cesarean section operation to facilitate delivery of the impacted head. Am J Obstet Gynecol 148:707, 1984.)

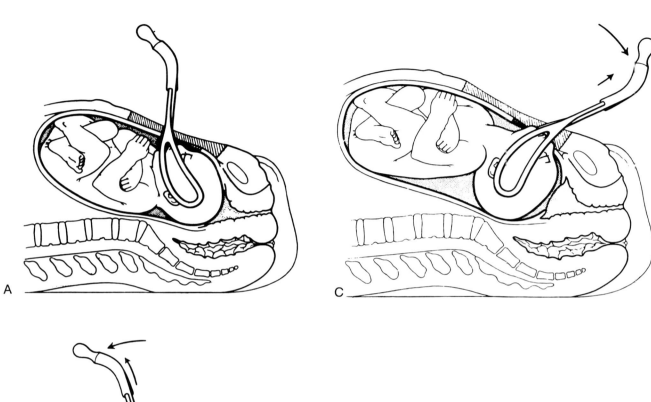

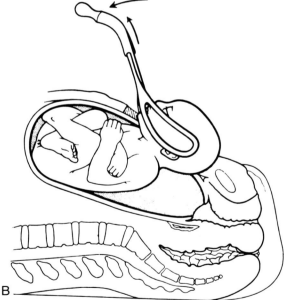

Figure 26–6. *A,* Delivery through a vertical uterine incision using Hale forceps. The blades are applied with a cephalic curve toward the symphysis pubis. *B,* Head extended to lft the chin up over the upper aspect of the uterine incision. *C,* Head delivered by flexion and outward extraction. (From Zuspan F, Quilligan E: Douglas-Stromme Operative Obstetrics, 5th Edition. Norwalk, Connect cut: Appleton & Lange, 1988, p. 442.)

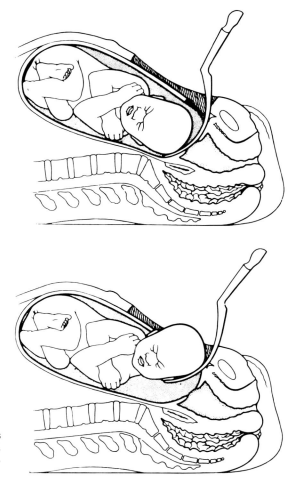

Figure 26–7. The forceps acting as a vector (shoehorn)—using the symphysis pubis as the fulcrum to deliver the head by lateral flexion. (From Zuspan F, Quilligan E: Douglas-Stromme Operative Obstetrics, 5th Edition. Norwalk, Connecticut: Appleton & Lange, 1988, p. 451.)

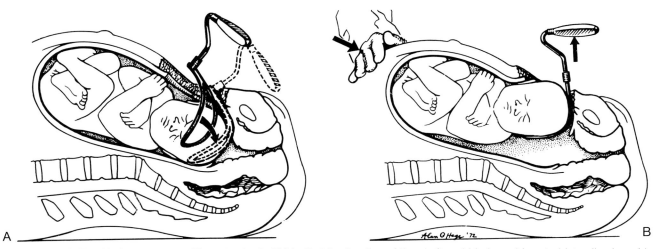

A   B

Figure 26–8. A, The Murless extractor. The extractor is "folded" at the junction of the shaft and blade and inserted laterally alongside the fetal forehead and rotated toward the pelvis, to lie along the inner lateral aspect of the head. B, The shaft is then straightened and the sliding sleeve is locked. The head is lifted up and delivered by lateral flexion. (From Zuspan F, Quilligan E: Douglas-Stromme Operative Obstetrics, 5th Edition. Norwalk, Connecticut: Appleton & Lange, 1988, p. 448.)

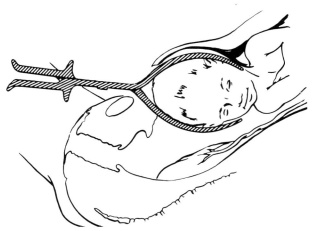

Figure 26–9. Kielland forceps for delivery either by lateral flexion or by rotation to the occiput anterior position and delivery by extension. (From Warenski J: A technique to facilitate delivery of the high floating head at cesarean section. Am J Obstet Gynecol 139:625, 1981.)

tion and delivered by extension or in the occipitotransverse position and delivered by lateral flexion.

When the head is deflexed, as in a brow or mentum presentation, an attempt should be made to flex the head before delivery through the uterine incision. This is done by placing the intrauterine hand behind the occiput, flexing the head, rotating it to the transverse position, and lifting it out by lateral flexion.

Although the transverse incision is preferred in the vertex presentation, there are circumstances in which a vertical incision may be a better choice. These include a contraction ring, abnormalities of the fetal head, locked twins, and abnormalities of the lower uterine segment. It is likely, however, that to obtain enough room, the upper active portion of the uterus will have to be entered, unless the cervix is fully dilated. A contraction ring, rarely seen in modern obstetrics in developed countries, occurs in multiparas with obstructed labor and impending rupture of the lower segment. If the contraction ring remains unrelieved by amyl nitrate, intravenous nitroglycerine, or deep general anesthesia, it may need to be transected for the fetus to be delivered. For the unusually enlarged head, e.g., hydrocephaly, macrocephaly, or bicephaly, the vertical incision is essential, because destructive procedures are generally not accepted. In these cases, the incision will invariably extend into the contractile portion of the uterus. It is the rare patient who comes to cesarean delivery with an unrecognized abnormally enlarged head. If this occurs and a transverse incision has already been made, the options are to convert it to a "J" or hockey-stick incision; a trap-door incision (i.e., extending superiorly in both sides); or, the worst choice because of its poor healing qualities, an inverted T incision. All three of these incisions will involve the contractile portion of the

uterus. Any suspicion of an abnormality of the head should be followed up by a sonogram or, if a sonogram is not available, at least a flat plate of the abdomen to help plan the uterine incision. A bicephalic fetus may be delivered through a low-segment, transverse incision because only one head is delivered at a time.

Malpresentations

The two major malpresentations that result in cesarean birth are the breech presentation and the transverse lie.

Breech Presentation. Most third-trimester breech deliveries can be conducted through a low transverse incision, if it is cut in a curvilinear fashion, making full use of the space. In contrast to the vertical incision extended into the active portion of the uterus, the low transverse incision does not decrease in size during surgery, at least not to the same degree as the vertical incision, because there are considerably less contractile fibers in the lower uterus compared with the corpus. Therefore, on entering the abdomen, the surgeon must carefully assess development of the lower uterine segment, the space available, and the presence of space-occupying fetal anomalies; these factors enter into the decision on the type of uterine incision.

When the low vertical incision was compared with the low transverse incision for breech deliveries, no difference in short-term outcome, mater-

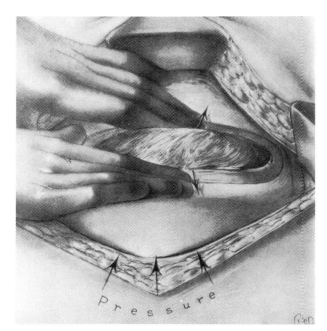

Figure 26–10. Delivery of the head at cesarean section by retracting the uterine incision around the head with concomitant fundal pressure by an assistant. (From Eastman NH, Hellman LM: Williams' Obstetrics, 12th Edition. New York: Appleton-Century-Crofts, 1981, p. 1189.)

nal or fetal, was noted with the type of incision chosen in 416 abdominal breech deliveries over 4½ years.[22] On the one hand is the aim of an atraumatic fetal delivery; on the other is maternal morbidity, both short term (blood loss, infection, ileus, and obstruction) and long term (risk of uterine rupture). The actual conduct of the breech delivery should be the same as in the vaginal route (see Chapter 19), and complications should be managed similarly. The head can become entrapped during abdominal delivery when the uterus contracts down around the fetal neck. The uterine incision must be extended to release the head. The transverse incision could be curved upward into the active segment, or a vertical incision could be enlarged superiorly. With a hyperextended head, the incision of choice may be vertical, unless there is a large low segment, because there is no opportunity to flex the head until the time of cephalic delivery, at which point the uterus is contracted down, leaving little space. Nonetheless, the Mauriceau-Smellie-Viet maneuver is used to deliver the vertex, with the head in the transverse (which in our opinion is easier) or the occiputoanterior position.

In a footling breech presentation, when one or both feet have descended into the pelvis, care must be taken not to fracture the long bones during delivery. The breech infant should be dislodged upward and into the incision with the back either anterior or oblique. Extraction of the buttocks and dorsiflexion of the spine will facilitate fetal hip flexion. The most easily accessible extremity is then further flexed toward the fetal abdomen until the knee comes up into the uterus and can be flexed by rotating the femur gently laterally on the fetal abdomen with the operator's index finger parallel to the femur. The other fingers then encircle the lower leg, grasp the foot, and extract it. If both extremities are prolapsed, a similar procedure is carried out on the opposite side.

Transverse Lie

Planning the surgery is vital to decrease maternal and/or fetal risks. The aim is to deliver the live fetus atraumatically at minimal risk to the mother. Therefore, the degree of development of the lower segment, although important, may not be the deciding factor. Ideally, sonographic determination of the position of the fetus and location of the feet and placenta are vital in deciding the surgical approach.

Once the abdomen is opened and before the uterine incision is made (except in cases of fetal distress or prolapsed cord), an intra-abdominal extrauterine version should be attempted, preferably to a vertex presentation. Although in the presence of decreased amniotic fluid it probably

will not succeed, if it does, then a transverse incision is more likely.

In the back-down transverse lie with ruptured membranes despite a well-developed lower segment, a transverse incision may result in prolapse of the shoulder through the incision, compromising delivery. In this case, or where there is an anterior placenta, a low vertical incision may be a better choice. With the back up, membranes intact, and the lower segment developed, a transverse incision is ideal, assuming the placenta is not in the way. As many as 25% of abnormal presentations are associated with a trapped head in a transverse incision.[23, 24] Therefore, the surgeon should be prepared to extend the incision superiorly should entrapment occur. Where the lower segment is either not developed or poorly developed, then a midline vertical uterine incision should be made, regardless of the location of the back. In the presence of an intrauterine fetal death, maternal benefits should take priority, and if at all possible a transverse incision should be done.

Once the uterus is entered, the infant is most commonly delivered by podalic version and extraction. Knowing the exact location of the lower extremities facilitates management of delivery. With the back up, the lower extremities are more easily accessible; however, arms and legs can be confused, because they are often together. If membranes are ruptured and the uterus is molded around the baby, space will be minimum. Administration of terbutaline, .25 mg subcutaneously, just before starting the operation may aid uterine relaxation. General anesthesia providing uterine relaxation may be necessary.

The surgeon, who is usually standing on the right if right handed (left if left handed), should insert the operating hand into the uterus to the buttocks, follow the thighs to the legs, grasp both feet if possible, and extract them gently while the assistant helps by pushing the head toward the fundus. If the head is on the same side as the surgeon, it can be raised by the surgeon's free hand.

For the back-down transverse lie, the procedure is similar except the feet are generally in the fundus. In this case, it is more important to grasp both feet or at least the posterior (lower) leg first to keep the back up. When the anterior leg and foot are delivered first, the body rotates so the abdomen is up. This can be prevented by gentle rotation of the hip as it is delivered, with the operator's hand first placed on the buttock, then reaching up to grasp the other leg. After extraction of the feet, the delivery proceeds as a total breech extraction using all the maneuvers and gentleness previously described (Chapter 19). After delivery of the placenta, an oxytocic such as an ergotrate or 15-methyl prostaglandin $F_2\alpha$ may be necessary to prevent atony if uterine relaxation was part of the procedure or, in the case of placenta previa, if atony of the lower segment is more likely to result in extensive hemorrhage because of the large space occupied by the placenta and the inability of the lower segment to contract as well as the fundus in closing off the sinusoids.

Preterm/Immature Malpresentation

It is not our purpose to discuss the pros and cons of the method of preterm delivery, i.e., vaginal versus abdominal, an issue that has been dealt with elsewhere (Chapters 19 and 20). Our interest is in the uterine incision when cesarean delivery has already been decided. The main reason for cesarean delivery of the premature/immature fetus, at least in breech presentations, is to decrease fetal trauma. Thus, choice of incision for fetal benefit must be weighed against maternal risks. In an era when the transverse cesarean section was well entrenched in obstetrics because of its benefits, and the classical incision was rarely used, along came the call for cesarean delivery of the very low birth weight infant (4500 g).[25-28] As a result, many obstetricians who have delivered fetuses as early as 25 to 26 weeks have routinely done classical sections. Although the method of delivery is currently in debate, we encourage careful deliberation and selection of the low-segment transverse incision wherever there is any possibility it will be sufficient.

In a comparison of the long-term outcomes in pregnancies after classical versus low-segment transverse incisions for preterm delivery, the former were associated with a higher repeat cesarean section rate, although both had a greater than 80% repeat section rate.[29] In repeat surgeries, 12.8% of scars from classical sections were abnormal, whereas no abnormalities were noted in the transverse-section scars.[29] In this study, 76% of the classical sections, as opposed to 32% of the low-segment procedures, were performed for breech presentation or transverse lie. Seven (13.5%) patients required an extension of the transverse incision. In the remaining 45 patients with breech presentation or transverse lie, a classical incision was avoided.

Two other studies have shown no differences in short-term outcome for mother or infant in premature/immature deliveries, regardless of the uterine incision.[22, 30] During the year of 1989 in our institution, of the 102 cesarean births of 29 weeks' gestation or earlier, 23.5% were classical and 4.9% low vertical. The majority—71.5%—were low transverse. Between 30 and 33 weeks' gestation, at which time there is better development of the lower segment, 89.8% were low transverse and 2.7% low vertical, whereas 9.5% of the total were classical. Although in terms of percentage of the total the majority of classical procedures were performed for the very low birth weight infant, there were almost an equal number of classical procedures in pregnancies at 34 weeks' gestation or later as there were at 29 weeks or earlier (26 vs. 24) (Table 26–1).

The placenta has a 40% chance of occupying the anterior uterine wall. Knowing exactly where the placenta is by sonography before the cesarean certainly helps in planning. Therefore, when performing a classical section, in order to minimize potential blood loss from the immature/premature infant, the placenta should be avoided if possible or separated rather than cut. The cord of the infant should be clamped as soon as it can be identified, even before delivery, to decrease fetal blood loss, or delivery should be performed as rapidly but safely as possible. Blood can be collected via a syringe irrigated with 1:10,000 units of heparin from the umbilical cord and immediately transfused to the infant if the child appears shocked and pale.

Druzin[31] described a splint procedure for the delivery of the very low birth weight infant (Fig. 26–11). With a vertical incision, the hand is inserted into the cavity to cup the fetal head, and the fetal trunk rests against the forearm, with the buttocks resting near the antecubital fossa. The transverse lie is then converted to a longitudinal lie, and the infant is delivered totally splinted or splinted up to the umbilicus, then extracted.

FETAL INJURIES

Most fetal injuries occur during labor and delivery. Many of those that occur as a result of cesarean delivery also occur during vaginal delivery. Because of changes in obstetric management during labor and delivery, the incidence of injuries resulting in perinatal mortalities has de-

Table 26–1. TYPES OF CESAREAN SECTIONS VERSUS GESTATIONAL AGE AT JACKSON MEMORIAL HOSPITAL, JANUARY–DECEMBER 1989

Type	Gestational Age in Weeks			Total No. of Cesarean Sections	% of Total No.
	≤29	30–33	≥34		
Low vertical	4.9%	2.7%	.7%	27	1.0
Low transverse	71.6%	87.8%	98.3%	2697	96.7
Classical	23.5%	9.5%	1.0	64	2.3
Total no. of cesarean sections	102	148	2538	2788	—
% of total no.	3.7	5.3	91.0	—	100.0

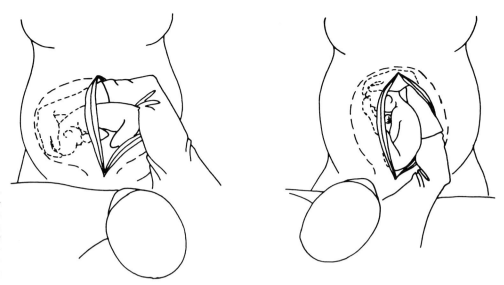

Figure 26–11. The splint procedure for delivery of the very low birth weight infant. (From Druzin ML: Atraumatic delivery in cases of malpresentation of the very low birth weight infant at cesarean section: The splint technique. Am J Obstet Gynecol 154:941, 1986.)

creased,[32, 33] and new injuries have occurred, e.g., scalp abcesses. The overall incidence varies from 2 to 7%, and most injuries are mild and self-limiting over time,[34, 35] although others require early diagnosis and proper management to prevent or decrease long-term sequelae.

By far, the most common injuries are soft-tissue injuries, including bruising/ecchymosis, which is more common in the very premature than in the term infant because of the delicacy of the subcutaneous blood vessels in these infants. Contributory factors are a small uterine or abdominal incision, which may increase the risk of trauma; haste during delivery, which is dependent on the indication for surgical intervention; and the amount of manipulation necessary for delivery. The premature/immature infant in breech presentation or transverse lie may have ecchymosis about the ankles where they are grasped during extraction. This seems to be more common where membranes have been ruptured, amniotic fluid is decreased, and the patient is in labor, all of which make delivery more difficult than when the amniotic fluid volume is sufficient. Forceps are rarely used for delivery, but when they are, there is also a risk of facial bruising or abrasions. However, this is minimal because the duration of blade application is usually very short. Of course, the vacuum extractor if used, will result in a caput or aggravate one already present and, rarely, will lead to a cephalohematoma, which could also occur with forceps.

Rarer still, but specifically related to cesarean section, are fetal skin lacerations, usually superficial, sustained during entry into the uterine cavity. Such lacerations are far more likely with oligohydramnios and a thinner uterine musculature than is expected, and depend on the experience of the primary surgeon. Prevention includes (a) being aware of the amniotic fluid volume and location of the presenting part; (b) ensuring adequate visualization by suctioning and/or pressure on either side of the uterine incision to decrease bleeding into the operative field; (c) gently elevating the incision site away from the fetus using Allis clamps; and (d) cutting through some of the uterine muscle and then using the opposite end of the handle to separate the last fibers when the nearness of the decidua is sensed. On cutting through muscle, fetal skin can look surprisingly the same and pouch through into the incision. Lacerations are more common when the breech or vertex infant fills the lower uterine segment. Parents, pediatricians, and nurses are greatly upset by these usually very small lacerations, especially if they occur on the cheeks, and rightly so. However, most require only steri Steri-Strips and have unrecognizable scars several months later. Rarely does the laceration need to be sutured; if it does, suturing should be done using plastic surgical technique.

The next group of injuries are skeletal and almost invariably occur in relation to breech extraction or version and extraction. Even though they rarely occur in abdominal deliveries, the same injuries that occur vaginally may occur with cesarean delivery. Humerus fractures are more likely with nuchal arms and occur during displacement maneuvers, illustrating the importance of the operator's splinting the long bones with his or her fingers, using gentleness, and avoiding haste during displacement. Clavicular fractures can also occur with raised or nuchal arms. In our institution during the last 12 years, only two femur fractures are known to have occurred in abdominal deliveries. Both were term infants, in labor with ruptured membranes. One was a classical cesarean section in a 500-lb woman with a transverse lie; the other was a low-segment, transverse cesarean in a 350-lb woman with a foot prolapsed to the introitus through an incompletely dilated cervix. Both were difficult deliveries; however, both babies did well treated in the standard fashion with traction and spica casts. To our knowledge, there has been only one humeral and no clavicular fractures in more than 20,000 abdominal deliveries.

Most injuries of long bones occur during extraction. The fractures may be green-stick, complete, or through either the diaphysis or epiphyseal plate. If there is any suspicion an injury has occurred, communicating this to the pediatrician and following up on the findings and management is wise. The family expects the surgeon to know what is happening, and all physicians should be speaking the same language regarding the injury and its prognosis. Most of these fractures heal quickly, leaving no residual effect.

Brachial plexus palsy may occur as a result of lateral extension of the neck during an extraction of the head made difficult because of entrapment by an insufficient incision, a contraction ring, or raised arms. Prognosis will depend upon extent of the nerve injury and whether avulsion of the nerve roots occurred.[36]

Although cesarean delivery has had a significant impact on decreasing the risk of spinal cord trauma in breech infants with a hyperextended head,[37-40] the problem may still occur in abdominal deliveries, especially where the incision has been inadequate.[41] Injuries to the facial bones or subluxation of the temporomandibular joint are possible with the Mauriceau-Smellie-Viet maneuver during breech delivery. Trauma to the floor of the mouth or pharynx with development of a pseudodiverticulum has also occurred.

Intra-abdominal trauma to the liver and spleen especially, and occasionally the kidney or adrenals, may occur particularly when the surgeon's hands are inappropriately compressing abdominal viscera during delivery. The first manifestations are a shocked, hypotensive infant with a distended abdomen. Despite early diagnosis and management, the mortality rate from a ruptured liver or spleen is high.[42, 43]

In summary, any injury that occurs in a vaginal delivery is possible in an abdominal delivery. Only by (a) planning the surgical procedure individually, keeping in mind gestational age, indication for surgery, and fetal status; (b) carefully assessing the uterus; and (c) performing a controlled, gentle, nonrushed delivery, not panicking at unexpected complications but simply reassessing the situation, can injuries be avoided and the best surgical procedure planned for mother and infant.

References

1. Rogers RE: Complications at cesarean section. Obstet Gynecol Clin North Am 15:673, 1988.
2. Sachs BP, Yeh J, Acker D, et al.: Cesarean section-related mortality in Massachusetts, 1954–1985. Obstet Gynecol 71:385, 1988.
3. Nielsen TF, Hokegard KH: Cesarean section and intra-operative complications. Acta Obstet Gynecol Scand 63:103, 1984.
4. Hawkins J, Hudson CN: Treatment of wounds of the intestine; Management of intestinal fistulae, colostomy. In Shaw's Textbook of Operative Gynecology, 5th Edition. New York: Churchill-Livingston, 1983, p. 369.
5. Sevin BU, Penalver MS: Reconstruction of bowel continuity with automated stapling instruments. In Knapstien PG, Friedburg V, Sevin BU (eds.): Reconstructive Surgery in Gynecology. New York: Thieme Medical Publishers, 1990, p. 255.
6. Eisenkop SM, Richman R, Platt LD, et al.: Urinary tract injury during cesarean section. Obstet Gynecol 60:591, 1982.
7. Field CS: Surgical techniques for cesarean section. Obstet Gynecol Clin North Am 15:657, 1988.
8. Cunningham FG, MacDonald PC, Gant NF: Williams Obstetrics, 18th Edition. Norwalk, CT: Appleton-Century-Crofts, 1989, p. 448.
9. Mattingly RF, Thompson JD: Telinde's Operative Gynecology, 6th Edition. Philadelphia: J.B. Lippincott, 1985, p. 325.
10. Newton M, Newton ER: Complications of Gynecologic and Obstetric Management. Philadelphia: W.B. Saunders, 1988.
11. O'Leary JL, O'Leary JA: Uterine artery ligation for control of postcesarean section hemorrhage. Obstet Gynecol 43:849, 1974.
12. Clark SL, Phelan JP, Yeh SY: Hypogastric artery ligation for obstetric hemorrhage. Obstet Gynecol 66:353, 1985.
13. Dunnihoo DR, Otterson WN, Mailhes JB: An evaluation of uterine scar integrity after cesarean section in rabbits. Obstet Gynecol 73:390, 1989.
14. Garrigues HJ: On gastro-elytrotomy. NY Med J 28:449, 1878.
15. Goodlin RC, Scott JC, Woods RE, et al.: Laparoelytrotomy or abdominal delivery without uterine incision. Am J Obstet Gynecol 144:990, 1982.
16. Landesman R, Graber EA: Abdominovaginal delivery: Modification of the cesarean section operation to facilitate delivery of the impacted head. Am J Obstet Gynecol 148:707, 1984.
17. Moir JC, Myerscough PR: Munro-Kerr's Textbook of Obstetrics. Baltimore: Williams & Wilkins, 1971.
18. Greenhill JP: In Obstetrics. 11th Edition. Philadelphia: W.B. Saunders, 1955, p. 986.
19. Murless BC: Lower segment cesarean section: A new head extractor. Br Med J 1:1234, 1945.
20. Eastman NJ, Hellman LM: Williams Obstetrics, 12th Edition. New York: Appleton-Century-Crofts, 1961, p. 1185.
21. Boehm F: Vacuum extraction during cesarean section. South Med J 78(12):1502, 1985.
22. Schutterman E, Grome D: Comparative safety of the low transverse versus low vertical uterine incision for cesarean delivery of breech infants. Obstet Gynecol 61:593, 1983.
23. Cockburn KG, Drake RF: Transverse and oblique lie of the fetus. Aust NZ J Obstet Gynaecol 8:211, 1968.
24. Pelosi MS, Apuzzio J, Fricchione D, et al.: The intra-abdomen version technique for delivery of transverse lie by low segment cesarean section. Am J Obstet Gynecol 136:1009, 1979.
25. Stewart A, Reynolds EOR: Improved prognosis for infants of very low birth weight. Pediatrics 54:724, 1974.
26. Lubchenko LO, Bard H, Goodman AL, et al.: Neonatal intensive care and long term prognosis. Dev Med Child Neurol 16:421, 1974.
27. Davies PA, Tizard JPM: Very low birthweight and subsequent neurologic defects (with special reference to spastic dysplegia). Dev Med Child Neurol 17:3, 1975.
28. Keiping JD, Morrison J, Chang AM: Two classical caesarean sections in pre-term deliveries. Aust NZ J Obstet Gynaecol 20:103, 1980.
29. Halperin ME, Movie DC, Hannah WJ: Classical versus low segment transverse incision for preterm caesarean section:

Maternal complications and outcome of subsequent pregnancies. Br J Obstet Gynaecol 95:990, 1988.

30. Druzin ML, Hutson JM, San Roman G: Uterine incision and maternal morbidity after cesarean section for delivery of the very low birthweight fetus. Surg Gynecol Obstet 169:131, 1989.

31. Druzin ML: Autraumatic delivery in cases of malpresentation of the very low birth weight fetus at cesarean section: The splint technique. Am J Obstet Gynecol 154:941, 1986.

32. Arey JB, Dent J: Causes of fetal and neonatal death with special reference to pulmonary and inflammatory lesions: J Pediatr 42:205, 1953.

33. Valdes-Dapena MA, Arey JB: The causes of neonatal mortality: An analysis of 501 autopsies in newborn infants. J Pediatr 77:366, 1970.

34. Rubin A: Birth injuries: Incidence, mechanisms and end results. Obstet Gynecol 23:218, 1964.

35. Mangurten H: Birth injuries. In Fanaroff AA, Martin RJ (eds.): Behrman's Neonatal-Perinatal Medicine: Diseases of the Fetus and Infant, 4th Edition. St. Louis, Mosby: 1987, pp. 317–342.

36. Greenwald AG, Schute PC, Shiveley JL: Brachial plexus birth palsy: A ten year report on the incidence and prognosis. J Pediatr Orthop 4:689, 1984.

37. Abrams J: Cervical cord injuries secondary to hyperextension of the head in breech presentations. Obstet Gynecol 41:369, 1973.

38. Ballas S, Toaff R: Hyperextension of the fetal head in breech presentations: Radiologic evaluation and significance. Br J Obstet Gynaecol 83:201, 1976.

39. Hellstran B, Sallmander U: Prevention of spinal cord injury in hyperextension of the fetal head. JAMA 204:1041, 1968.

40. Towkin A: Latent spinal cord and brain stem injury in newborn infant. Dev Med Child Neurol 11:54, 1969.

41. Slagan WB, Liang K, Piligian J, et al.: Thoracic spinal cord (T3-T4) transection in a breech-presenting cesarean section delivered preterm infant. Am J Perinatol 4:233, 1987.

42. Eraklis AJ: Abdominal injury related to trauma at birth. Pediatrics 39:421, 1967.

43. Matsuyama S, Suzuki N, Nagamuchi Y: Rupture of the spleen in the newborn: Treatment without splenectomy. J Pediatr Surg 11:115, 1976.

VII

Peripartal Operations

27

Peripartal Hysterectomy

Warren C. Plauché

- INTRODUCTION
- HISTORICAL PERSPECTIVES
- INDICATIONS
- OPERATIVE TECHNIQUE

- POSTOPERATIVE CARE
- COMPLICATIONS, MORBIDITY, AND MORTALITY
- SUMMARY

Peripartal hysterectomy implies removal of the uterus at or near the time of obstetric delivery. The term peripartal hysterectomy includes both cesarean hysterectomy and postpartum hysterectomy. These operations were developed to address some of the most distressing problems facing the obstetrician.

Peripartal hysterectomy began as a technique to make emergency cesarean delivery safer. It evolved into a method of last resort to control life-threatening obstetric hemorrhage and infection. The operation became much safer with advances in surgical technique, anesthesia, blood transfusion, and antibiotics. Indications gradually expanded to include nonemergency problems and even elective removal of the uterus at the time of delivery.

Pharmacologic and surgical advances gave obstetricians new and more effective methods for addressing peripartal bleeding and infection problems. These improved methods reduced the need for emergency peripartal hysterectomy. The operation all but disappeared from the repertory of routine obstetric training in some obstetric departments.

Under emergency conditions, such as massive uterine rupture, peripartal hysterectomy is among the most complex operations confronting the obstetric surgeon. Rapid, accurate technique is necessary to control the severe blood loss that threatens the life of the patient. Anatomic relationships are often distorted by uterine tears and pelvic hematomas. There may be injuries to other abdominal organs. All obstetricians can be prepared to perform peripartal hysterectomy with proper training opportunities. The time for this training is during preplanned cases that are not obstetric emergencies.

HISTORICAL PERSPECTIVES

The development of peripartal hysterectomy can be divided into four historical eras: early explorations, the Porro era, the expansionist era, and the present.

Early Explorations

Joseph Cavallini of Italy in 1768 conceived the idea that the uterus could be safely removed at the time of obstetric delivery. The obstetric practices of the time must be appreciated to understand the importance of Cavallini's idea.

Before the end of the nineteenth century, mothers with fetopelvic disproportion labored to exhaustion. Most of their babies died. Obstetricians, when they were available to these unfortunate mothers, used fetal destructive operations to extract the dead infants. Maternal suffering and injuries were severe. Hemorrhage, exhaustion, and dehydration often brought the parturient what was described as "a merciful death."

Operative abdominal delivery was uniformly fatal in all the centuries before the nineteenth. Bleeding, peritonitis, and septicemia were untreatable complications of cesarean delivery. There were no antibiotics or blood transfusions or fluid and electrolyte replacement. Surgical antisepsis was not widely practiced. Surgeons did not even recognize the need to close the uterine incision.

The incidence of obstructed labor was high in the eighteenth and early nineteenth centuries. Nutritional principles were not established. Pelvic deformities caused by rickets were common. Women with pelvic contraction did not have effective contraception or safe abortion techniques to protect them from the dangers of pregnancy. When these women became pregnant, their lives were at great risk.

Cavallini, a Florentine scientist, published in 1768 the results of animal experiments that tested his theory that "the uterus is not at all necessary for life."[1] He proposed that the uterus could be removed with impunity in animals, even pregnant ones. He wrote that further studies were necessary to know if the uterus could be removed from humans.

Professors Michaelis of Marburg and Blundell of London performed further surgical research on pregnant animals in the early 1800s.[2] Both of these influential obstetric teachers felt that the cesarean operation would be less dangerous if the uterus were removed as part of the delivery procedure.

Fogliata of Pisa, Rein of St. Petersburg, and Porro of Pavia experimented with hysterectomy in pregnant rabbits and dogs in the 1860s and early 1870s.[3] These experiments supported the development of cesarean hysterectomy in human subjects.

Gynecologic hysterectomy was not accepted as a legitimate operation until late in the nineteenth century. Extirpation of the uterus was condemned in a London surgical review in 1825 as "a cruel, bloody, and ill-judged operation."[3]

The first documented cesarean hysterectomy on a living human patient was performed in the United States in July of 1868 by Horatio Robinson Storer of Boston.[1] Storer studied obstetrics with James Young Simpson of Edinburgh after graduating from Harvard Medical School. He was America's first declared specialist in the diseases of women.

Storer was an aggressive innovator. He was one of the first to wear rubber gloves in the operating room. He performed the fourth hysterectomy ever in the United States. These and other audacities resulted in his dismissal from the Harvard medical faculty in 1866.

Two years later, Storer consulted on a case involving an obstetric patient in labor with a large uterine tumor obstructing the pelvis below the fetal head. Fetal destructive procedures to relieve the woman were not possible although the baby was dead. Storer executed what he believed to be the only feasible choice and removed the macerated fetus by cesarean incision under chloroform anesthesia.

Storer's assistant, G. H. Bixby, recorded that life-threatening hemorrhage led to a decision to remove the uterus with its fibrocystic tumor the size of a baby's head.[4] Storer obtained hemostasis with metal ligatures that encircled the cervix and the pedicle of the tumor. A chain-crushing device slowly constricted the mass. The uterus and the pelvic mass were removed, and the cervical stump was cauterized within the pelvis with a hot iron. The abdominal wound was then closed with a mass closure of silver wire sutures. The patient recovered from the anesthetic but died on the third postoperative day.

The Porro Era

Eduardo Porro of Pavia, Italy, reported the first successful cesarean hysterectomy in 1876, 8 years after Storer's operation.[5] Porro held the Chair of Obstetrics at the University of Pavia at that time. He later directed the prestigious School of Obstetrics in Milan.

Porro had previously performed a cesarean delivery on a young woman with a rachitic pelvis. No woman of Pavia had ever survived a cesarean delivery. Porro's patient was no exception. He began his animal experiments determined to improve the safety of cesarean delivery. Porro planned and rehearsed removal of the uterus after cesarean delivery. It is a dramatic coincidence of history that his first patient bore the surname of Cavallini.

Julia Cavallini was a dwarf with rickets whose first pregnancy was complicated by a markedly distorted pelvis. Porro estimated the diagonal conjugate diameter of her pelvic inlet to be 7 cm. Porro wrote "It was obvious that absolute disproportion existed and that cesarean section was mandatory."[5]

Julia Cavallini was carefully observed during the last weeks of her pregnancy. The decision was made to attempt abdominal delivery after membranes had been ruptured for 6 hours, and strong labor pains persuaded the patient to accept the operation.

The latest surgical techniques were followed. The amphitheater was heated to a precise 18°C. The operators washed their hands with dilute carbolic acid. Chloroform anesthesia was induced. A 12-cm vertical midline infraumbilical incision was performed. A vertical incision in the uterus allowed the 3300-g female infant to be delivered by version and extraction.

Attempts at manual and suture control of bleeding after removal of the placenta were unsuccessful. Porro stated, "It was providential that we had made all the preparations necessary for hysterectomy; otherwise the patient would surely have died."[5]

An assistant elevated the uterus out of the abdominal wound. Porro slipped the wire noose of a Cintrat constrictor over the uterus, both fallopian tubes, and the ovaries. The loop was tightened about the neck of the uterus to obtain hemostasis. The uterus and adnexa were then sliced away. The cul-de-sac was drained through the vagina, and additional drains were placed in the abdominal wound.

The cervical stump was treated with perchloride of iron. Both the cervical stump and the Cintrat constrictor were exteriorized onto the abdominal wall. The abdominal wound was closed around them with silver wire sutures. The entire operation was completed in 26 minutes.

The Cintrat constrictor was left on the cervical stump under dressings for 4 days. The wound sutures were removed on the seventh postoperative day. The ischemic pedicle sloughed 7 days later. The patient was pronounced cured on the fortieth day. She and the Porro operation entered the pages of obstetric history.

Porro's operation was widely publicized. It was performed with little success by several famous obstetricians in the 2 years succeeding the presentation paper. Inzana of Parma, Hegar of Freiburg, and Previtali of Bergamo each lost their first patients.[1, 2] Physicians in the Vienna Lying-In Hospital, where no patient had survived a cesarean delivery in 100 years, were eager to try the new operation despite reported failures. Obstetricians in Belgium and Switzerland also adopted Porro's procedure.

Müller of Berne was the first to modify the Porro operation.[3] Müller elevated the uterus from the peritoneal cavity before opening it in a case of severe chorioamnionitis. Prevention of gross contamination of the peritoneal cavity allowed the mother to survive. Müller also suggested the use of an elastic tube tourniquet, such as those used in limb amputations, to constrict the uterus. Müller placed his tourniquet through a large incision in the abdomen prior to elevating the uterus. Asphyxia of the child was described by Richardson as "usual in a Müller operation."[6]

The frequency of cesarean hysterectomy in the late nineteenth century is recorded in the 1880 review of the world literature by Robert P. Harris.[7] He was able to collect only 50 cases from seven countries. The maternal mortality rate at that time was 58%, and the fetal survival rate was 86%.

Isaac Taylor of New York performed the first Porro operation in the United States in 1880.[1] His patient unfortunately died of pulmonary embolism more than 3 weeks after an apparently successful operation.

Richardson reported the first Porro operation with maternal survival in the United States in 1881.[6] Richardson offered an important further modification of the Porro-Müller procedure. After amputating the uterus, he cauterized the cervix with carbolic acid, replaced it, and completely closed the abdominal wound.

Spencer Wells of Great Britain executed the first cesarean total hysterectomy in 1881 in a pregnant patient with carcinoma of the cervix.[3]

Clement Godson of Great Britain studied 134 cesarean hysterectomy cases in 1884.[8] The most common indication for operation was still a contracted pelvis caused by rickets (66%). The maternal mortality rate in this group was 45%. Death was most commonly due to peritonitis (27%), shock (12%), and septicemia (6%).

Godson offered an important modification of the cesarean operation.[8] He suggested a transverse incision at the junction of the lower and middle thirds of the uterus. Godson felt that tearing the uterine muscle was accomplished more rapidly and with less blood loss than was cutting the muscle.

Technical innovations increased rapidly toward the close of the nineteenth century. Lawson Tait of Great Britain published modifications of the Porro procedure that became widely adopted.[9] For several decades, the procedure was called the Tait-Porro operation. The new century held bright prospects for Porro's operation.

The Expansionist Era

Two events occurred in the year 1900 that hold the key to a lasting division of opinion about the proper use of cesarean hysterectomy. Reed codified the indications for cesarean hysterectomy in 1900.[10] He recognized only those circumstances that were life-threatening to the mother.

Duncan and Targett of Great Britain in that same year recorded the first cesarean hysterectomy performed for sterilization.[11] Conservative surgeons clung to Reed's "emergency only" indication list. Aggressive surgeons extended the indications to incorporate gynecologic disorders and sterilization.

Lash and Cummings in the United States included maternal diseases and sterilization among the cases in their 1935 study.[12] Wilson reported in 1937 that 8.7% of patients having cesarean delivery in Rochester had concomitant hysterectomy.[1] Myomata uteri and sterilization were among the indications listed by this group. Morbidity and mortality figures steadily improved during the 1930s and 1940s.

M. Edward Davis of Chicago stated in 1951 that cesarean hysterectomy was justified ". . . in women nearing the end of their reproductive period, in whom the uterus no longer serves a useful function. . . ."[13] Davis reported a 19% incidence of hysterectomy among a series of 736 cesarean deliveries. Davis' recommendation that cesarean hysterectomy was a "logical development in obstetrics" proved very influential.[13]

John Weed's study from New Orleans a few years later added to the enthusiasm of the time for hysterectomy at the time of obstetric delivery.[14] Weed followed the gynecologic fate of 400 of his cesarean patients. Over 20% of these women later required hysterectomy for gynecologic disorders. The mean time between cesarean delivery and hysterectomy was 6.3 years. This paper was widely quoted by authors who argued for elective cesarean hysterectomy.

Those on the other side of the controversy argued that peripartal hysterectomy should be reserved for life-threatening emergencies. Brenner and colleagues, in 1970, wrote that complications outweighed the benefits in peripartal hysterectomy performed for sterilization.[15] The Brenner group and others held that tubal ligation after cesarean or vaginal delivery was the safer procedure. This argument continued in the obstetric literature for 3 decades.

The New Orleans experience with cesarean hysterectomy began at Charity Hospital in 1938.[16] Two large groups of cases reported by Barclay[17] and Mickal and colleagues[18] supported the use of planned peripartal hysterectomy in certain gynecologic disorders. These groups performed many hysterectomies after multiple previous cesarean deliveries. The religious order that directed Charity Hospital forbade operations purely for sterilization. The "defective or dangerous cesarean scar" became a common indication for obstetric hysterectomy.

The New Orleans groups realized an unanticipated benefit from their liberal cesarean hysterectomy policy. Cesarean hysterectomy was performed frequently by upper-level residents. Residents attained a level of mastery that allowed them to operate skillfully and rapidly with few serious complications.

Obstetricians with such training accepted cesarean hysterectomy as part of routine obstetric practice. In the 1960s and the 1970s, a number of studies detailed the experiences of both public and private hospitals in the New Orleans region.[17–22]

The Current Era

The literature of the 1970s and the 1980s continued the controversy over elective cesarean hysterectomy. University services published studies heavily weighted with critical emergency cases.[23–25] Conservative obstetricians expressed alarm at the blood loss, transfusion rates, and complications detailed in these reports. It is clear that much of the morbidity resulted from the conditions treated, not the operation chosen. However, these reports exerted a restraining influence on cesarean hysterectomy on some obstetric services.

Collections of elective cesarean hysterectomy cases from private services recorded few complications. Blood loss was limited, and transfusion rates were low.[20, 21, 32] These reports counterbalance the impression of excessive morbidity.

The use of peripartal hysterectomy in the United States varies by region. Some obstetric services use it regularly to solve coexisting obstetric delivery problems and gynecologic disorders. Some of these services include sterilization among their indications. Other services employ peripartal hysterectomy only in dire emergencies. These regional variations reflect legitimate differences of professional opinion and training experience.

INDICATIONS

What is the place of peripartal hysterectomy in current obstetric practice? Advances in obstetric health care have changed the management of many of the conditions that formerly required peripartal hysterectomy.

Severe malformations of pelvic architecture are rare in modern obstetric practice. A pelvis distorted by rickets or poliomyelitis is seldom encountered. Minor interruptions of the progress of labor are now managed aggressively. Cesarean delivery usually occurs long before prolonged labor causes uterine rupture, tissue necrosis, or severe infection.

Forty-eight percent of the early Charity Hospital cases were done for Couvelaire uterus.[26] This intramyometrial hemorrhage associated with abruptio placentae often causes transient uterine atony. This form of atony usually responds, in the absence of coagulopathy, to diligent use of oxytocin and prostaglandins. Hysterectomy is only occasionally indicated.

Postpartal hemorrhage as a result of uterine atony from other causes was the indication for 7.5% of early Charity Hospital cases.[26] The mech-

Table 27–1. PERIPARTAL HYSTERECTOMY INDICATIONS: CHARITY HOSPITAL OF NEW ORLEANS,
LOUISIANA STATE UNIVERSITY OBSTETRIC SERVICE, 1975 to 1983 (n = 110)

Emergency	No.	Indicated Nonemergency	No.	Elective	No.
Placental Disorders					
Accreta-fundal	3	Fibroids	13	Multiple	
Previa accreta	2	CIN*	10	Repeat CS†	30
Previa + postpartum	4	Defective CS scar	8	Primary CS + sterilization	
hemorrhage	2	Chorioamnionitis + sepsis	6	Grandmultiparity	7
Abruptio + postpartum				Fetal distress	10
hemorrhage					
Uterine Rupture					
Previous CS	3				
Spontaneous	4				
Postpartum Hemorrhage					
Atony at CS	5				
Uterine artery laceration at CS	3				
TOTALS	26		37		47

*CIN—Cervical intraepithelial neoplasia.
†CS—Cesarean section.

anisms that control bleeding after obstetric delivery are now better understood. Conservative management of uterine atony is successful in a high percentage of cases. Prostaglandins, administered by the intramuscular or intramyometrial routes, control many previously resistant cases of atony. Coagulopathies are more rapidly identified and more effectively managed with replacement blood products. Unresponsive cases of uterine atony may still require hysterectomy as a life-saving measure.

Rupture of the pregnant uterus and uterine scar dehiscences are increasingly managed by suture repair, without removal of the uterus. Catastrophic rupture of the uterus remains an important current indication for peripartal hysterectomy. Chapter 13 discusses the subject of uterine rupture in detail.

Uterine infections often respond to modern antibiotic therapy. Premature rupture of membranes and fetal demise are aggressively managed. Obstetricians rarely see advanced cases of chorioamnionitis and sepsis that threaten the life of the patient. Neglected cases can develop multiple abcesses or recalcitrant uterine atony that require hysterectomy for cure.

Many elective cesarean hysterectomies are performed after the last of a number of cesarean deliveries. Vaginal birth after cesarean delivery may reduce the number of cases done for this indication.

Classification of Current Indications

Indications for peripartal hysterectomy are divided into emergency cases, indicated nonemergencies, and elective cases.[27] A review of the Louisiana State University Obstetrical Service at Charity Hospital of New Orleans (LSU series) from 1975 to 1983 revealed that 24% of peripartal hysterectomies were emergencies. Thirty-three percent were indicated nonemergencies, and 43% were elective cases.[27] Table 27–1 outlines these indications.

Emergency indications are the least controversial. The majority of emergency peripartal hysterectomies are performed to manage problems of obstetric hemorrhage resulting from placental problems, resistant uterine atony, or uterine rupture.

Placenta accreta, particularly placenta previa accreta, is increasing with the rising number of cesarean scars.

Spontaneous uterine ruptures and rupture of previous cesarean scars each caused half of the uterine ruptures in the LSU series. Laceration of the uterine vessels at the time of cesarean delivery with pelvic hematoma formation necessitated hysterectomy in several cases.

The second indication category is labeled "indicated nonemergencies." Cases in this category have been labeled "planned" or "anticipated" cesarean hysterectomies by other authors.[28, 29] The operations are performed for gynecologic disorders in patients requiring cesarean delivery.

Leiomyomata uteri and cervical intraepithelial neoplasia are the most prevalent reasons for indicated nonemergency operations. The philosophy guiding these cases is to perform cesarean delivery and indicated hysterectomy during a single hospitalization and anesthetic exposure.

McNulty,[28] in 1984, reviewed the 10-year experience of 80 planned cesarean hysterectomies from eight southern California private hospitals. The most prevalent diagnoses in this series were leiomyomata uteri or previous myomectomies (25%) and thinned scars or multiple previous cesarean operations (28%). Previous gynecologic conditions, such as menorrhagia, dysmenorrhea, endometriosis, and adhesions accounted for 20% of indications. Five percent of patients were operated on for pelvic malignancies. This mix of indications closely resembles the 1986 report by Sturdee and Rushton[29] of a 5-year experience from Birmingham Maternity Hospital in England.

Other reports contain a larger percentage of patients with pelvic malignancies. Park and Duff[3] stated that most of the experience with cesarean hysterectomy at Walter Reed Army Medical Center was with radical operations performed on pregnant patients with invasive cervical cancer.

Hysterectomy at delivery is occasionally performed for other malignancies. An example is hysterectomy with bilateral salpingo-oophorectomies to control advanced breast cancer metastases. Ovarian cancer diagnosed during pregnancy or encountered at the time of cesarean delivery accounts for a small number of peripartal hysterectomy cases.

Defective previous cesarean scars were the reason for indicated nonemergency cesarean hysterectomy in approximately 20% of cases reviewed. The surgeons in these cases feared the possibility that a broad, translucent, thin uterine scar would rupture with future pregnancy. The experience with such scars at the time of trial of labor after cesarean indicates that the risk ascribed to these scars may have been overestimated in the past.

Dehiscence of an infected uterine cesarean incision may result in broad attachment of the uterus to the anterior abdominal wall, bowel, and omentum. This special type of scar defect is difficult to securely repair at the time of the next cesarean delivery. Many surgeons choose cesarean hysterectomy for these rare cases.

Chorioamnionitis, in its ordinary guises, is not an indication for either cesarean delivery or hysterectomy. Most patients respond to intensive antibiotic therapy appropriate to the organism causing the infection. Chorioamnionitis with sepsis was the indication for six peripartal hysterectomies in the LSU series. These cases were examples of prolonged rupture of membranes or prolonged labors referred with advanced infections. Uteri removed for advanced myometritis displayed many micro- and macroabcesses. There was often coexistent uterine atony with hemorrhage.

Elective cases constitute the most controversial indication category. McNulty reported multiparity and "desired hysterectomy" as the indication for 15% of his California series.[28] Hysterectomy after multiple cesarean deliveries, with normal scars, was the indication for another 15% of McNulty's cases and 27% of the cases in the LSU series. Hysterectomy was performed electively at the time of first cesarean delivery in a very few cases. Our service does not encourage primary abdominal delivery to create opportunities for surgical sterilization.

Summary of Current Indications

Peripartal hysterectomy remains important as a life-saving procedure in cases of severe obstetric hemorrhage. Patients who have both an indication for abdominal delivery and an indication for hysterectomy are well served by a single peripartal procedure. Elective cases remain controversial, particularly when the only reason for the surgery is sterilization.

OPERATIVE TECHNIQUE

Precautions

Performance of hysterectomy in pregnant patients is different from gynecologic hysterectomy in several ways. The blood vessels supplying the uterus are greatly enlarged. Collateral vessels, which might be unnoticeable in the nonpregnant patient, are numerous and prominent.

The pregnant uterus is much more bulky and difficult to manipulate than the nonpregnant uterus. Tissues are friable and edematous. Pedicles are thick and shrink in size as edema subsides. The ureter is dilated and sluggish.

Tissue planes dissect easily in most pregnant patients. Dense adhesions may replace the loose adventitial plane between the bladder and the lower uterine segment in patients who have had previous cesarean deliveries. Operative injuries to the bladder and the ureter are more common than in gynecologic hysterectomy and are difficult to detect.

The physiologic changes of pregnancy call for alterations in standard hysterectomy technique (Table 27–2). Hemostasis must be meticulous. Dilated vessels and multiple collaterals are unforgiving of the careless operator. The surgeon must often apply extra clamps to avoid "back-bleeding" blood loss from collateral circulation.

Thick, edematous pedicles must be ligated with transfixing sutures to prevent blood vessels from slipping from hemostatic control. Hematomas can result from transfixing sutures passing directly through blood vessels. Avoid these by first placing a ligature that encompasses the entire pedicle. Place the transfixing ligature distal to this suture.

Keep pedicles small. Clamp tissues only in the most efficient distal third of clamps where they will be held securely. Pedicle clamps should be supported, not manipulated, during passage of sutures. Tugging on clamps risks stripping pedicles away from adjacent tissues. This opens venous bleeders that are difficult to safely clamp and suture.

Know the location of the ureter at all phases of the operation. Never hesitate to dissect the course of the ureter if there is any question of its safety.

Table 27-2. OPERATIVE STEPS FOR PERIPARTAL HYSTERECTOMY: DELAYED LIGATION TECHNIQUES

1. Open abdominal wall
2. Assess pelvis and abdomen
3. Complete delivery of baby and placenta
4. Close uterine incision with clamps or suture
5. Double clamp and cut right round ligament
6. Open avascular window in right broad ligament
7. Triple clamp and divide right adnexal pedicle
8. Skeletonize right uterine vessels
9. Double clamp right uterine vessels
10. Double clamp and cut left round ligament
11. Open avascular window in left broad ligament
12. Triple clamp and divide left adnexal pedicle
13. Skeletonize left uterine vessels
14. Double clamp left uterine vessels
15. Double suture left uterine vessel pedicle (transfix)
16. Clamp, divide, and suture upper left cardinal ligament
17. Suture left round ligament (transfix)
18. Double suture left adnexal pedicle (transfix)
19. Double suture right adnexal pedicle (transfix)
20. Suture right round ligament (transfix)
21. Double suture right uterine vessels (transfix)
22. Clamp, divide, and suture upper right cardinal ligament (amputate uterus if necessary for exposure)
23. Dissect bladder flap downward
24. Clamp, divide, and suture lower cardinal ligaments on both sides
25. Clamp, divide, and suture uterosacral ligaments
26. Identify location of upper vagina
27. Open vagina posteriorly
28. Excise cervix
29. Place vaginal angle support sutures, including cardinal and uterosacral pedicles
30. Suture vaginal cuff
31. Reperitonealize
32. Clean up and perform sponge and instrument count
33. Close abdominal wall

Take special care dissecting the band of adhesions between the bladder and the lower portion of the uterus. Use meticulous sharp dissection. Detect small or hidden perforations of the bladder wall by filling the bladder with a colored solution during the operation. Repair any defects promptly.

Avoid bacteria-laden lochia spills when developing the vaginal cuff. Hemostatic technique at the vaginal cuff must be meticulous to avoid late bleeding and hematoma formation.

Operative Technique Using a Tourniquet

Rapid control of the blood supply to the uterus is essential in all peripartal hysterectomy techniques. Some surgeons utilize a tourniquet about the lower uterine segment, as did Porro and his successors.

Complete the cesarean delivery as usual. Place the tourniquet in the following manner. Elevate the uterus into the wound. Transilluminate the broad ligaments to identify avascular windows. Thrust Kelly clamps through these windows at the level of the lowest part of the uterine incision. Pass a rubber catheter, drain, or similar flexible

length of material through the openings in the broad ligament. Pull the tourniquet tight and secure it with a clamp at the back of the uterus. Proceed with hysterectomy by your chosen technique.

Leon Guillard taught this technique for many years at one of the affiliates of the LSU obstetric service. He believed that blood loss was reduced by the tourniquet technique. The technique certainly helps control blood loss from the uterine vessels. Collateral circulation from the ovarian vessels is not controlled by the tourniquet. The delayed ligation technique described next offers quick control of all uterine blood supply.

Delayed Ligation Technique

The principle that distinguishes the delayed ligation technique from other techniques for peripartal hysterectomy is the rapidity of control of all vascular supply to the uterus. This is accomplished by clamping each individual vascular pedicle and quickly proceeding to the next pedicle. Suture ligation is delayed until all major uterine vascular bundles are clamped.

Three sets of clamps are placed in preplanned order on each side of the dissection (Fig. 27-1). These clamps control the round ligament, the utero-ovarian vessels, and the uterine vessels. This controls all blood supply to the uterus except for the cervical branches of the vaginal arteries.

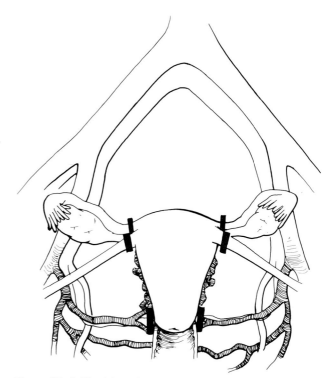

Figure 27-1. Black bars indicate the three sites on each side of the uterus where clamps must be placed to control the blood supply to the postpartum uterus.

Dyer and colleagues[19] described the delayed ligation technique in 1953 in a study from the Tulane Obstetric Service of Charity Hospital of New Orleans. The operation is described in this chapter as though performed for catastrophic spontaneous rupture of the pregnant uterus. The method discussed developed over a period of years to make the operation safe, to address common intraoperative problems, and to prevent postoperative problems.

Preoperative evaluation carefully defines the level of blood loss, the stability of the patient, and her coagulation status. The blood bank readies blood replacement products. Anesthesia consultants choose the appropriate general anesthetic. Discuss the situation with the patient and her family. Obtain informed consents. Assemble a team consisting of an experienced nurse circulator, scrub technician, and assistant surgeon. When time permits, review the details of procedure with the team to ensure maximum efficiency.

Choose the instruments and sutures to be used before the operation begins. A single type of suture for the entire operation facilitates the job of the technical team. Procedural delays should be as short as possible in emergency cases.

Blood transfusion begins before surgery in most unstable patients. Prompt operative hemostasis is required, however, for continuing intra-abdominal bleeding.

Administer prophylactic antibiotics before or during surgery to patients who have been in labor. These antibiotics are not continued after surgery unless overt infection is encountered.

Peripartal hysterectomy can be performed through either vertical or transverse abdominal wall incisions. This author prefers a vertical paramedian infraumbilical incision. This incision can be performed very rapidly. It offers extensive exposure for exploration of the abdomen and can be easily extended, if necessary.

Visually inspect and palpate the abdominal and pelvic contents. Remove blood in the peritoneal cavity by suction and sponging to facilitate exposure. Consider using the cell-saver blood-filtering apparatus when the volume of hemoperitoneum is over 500 mL. This device filters blood clots from intraperitoneal blood and prepares it for retransfusion. A portion of the patient's blood loss can be replaced with her own blood.

Determine the extent of hematoma formation in the broad ligament or elsewhere. Note any anatomic distortion or organ displacement.

The large pregnant uterus restricts the general examination of the abdomen at this stage. Bleeding from the uterus takes first surgical priority. Abdominal exploration, if not completed at this time, must not be forgotten. At some time during the procedure, examine the bladder, ureters, colon, small bowel, and adnexal structures for injury. Check the pelvic side walls and presacral space for

hematomas, neural injuries, or vascular injuries. Explore the liver, kidneys, spleen, and upper abdomen for lacerations or hematomas.

The first step in peripartal hysterectomy is the cesarean delivery, unless the baby has been expelled into the peritoneal cavity through a rupture of the uterine wall. Perform the cesarean delivery in standard fashion with one exception. Extend the incision of the bladder flap peritoneum overlying the lower uterine segment laterally to the round ligaments. The incision meets each round ligament 2 to 4 cm from its insertion on the uterus (Fig. 27–2).

Peripartal hysterectomy can be accomplished with either vertical or transverse uterine incisions for the cesarean delivery. The author prefers a vertical incision in the uterine wall for planned peripartal hysterectomy. One need not worry about scar rupture with future pregnancy. There is less risk that a vertical incision will extend into the uterine vessels when the baby is delivered. The edges of the vertical wound are quickly and easily clamped for hemostasis. Use of the assistant's finger in the apex of the vertical uterine incision is a good traction device in later operative steps. Complete the cesarean delivery as usual, including delivery of the placenta.

The hysterectomy phase of the operation begins immediately after the cesarean delivery. The anterior leaf of the broad ligament was partly dissected with the bladder flap incision. Complete this dissection by dividing the round ligaments.

Doubly clamp the right round ligament with straight Ochsner (Kocher) clamps placed 2 and 3 cm from the lateral wall of the uterus (Fig. 27–3). Be careful to control Sampson's artery. This artery courses parallel to the round ligament in most patients. The vessel is inconsequential in gynecologic hysterectomy but is much larger in pregnant patients. Steady blood loss occurs if the vessels are not secured during peripartal hysterectomy. Divide the round ligament between the clamps. The distal pedicle and clamp drop from the field to be sutured later.

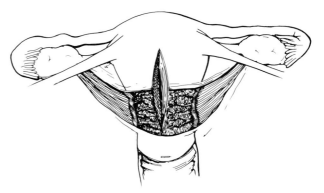

Figure 27–2. Peripartal hysterectomy procedure. The visceral peritoneum of the bladder flap is incised out to each round ligament. A vertical cesarean incision is shown in the postpartum uterus.

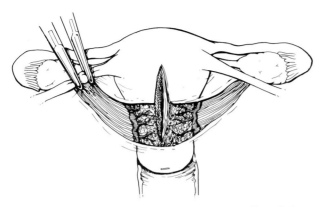

Figure 27–3. Peripartal hysterectomy procedure. Two Ochsner clamps are placed on the right round ligament near its origin at the uterine cornu. The tips of the clamps are within the opening in the anterior broad ligament.

Thrust a curved Kelly clamp through an avascular window in the posterior leaf of the broad ligament (Fig. 27–4). Open the instrument to enlarge the opening. Reposition the proximal Ochsner clamp on the right round ligament to encompass the uterine insertion of the round ligament, the utero-ovarian ligament, and the fallopian tube (Fig. 27–5).

Place two additional Kelly or Ochsner clamps across the utero-ovarian pedicle and the fallopian tube 1 cm lateral to the first clamp. Place the tips of these clamps within the opening in the broad ligament to ensure that all vessels are controlled. Sever the pedicle between the proximal and two distal clamps (see Fig. 27–5). Allow this pedicle with its two clamps to drop from the field, to be sutured later.

Next, address the right uterine vascular bundle.

The assistant retracts the uterus sharply upward. A finger placed in the apex of the vertical cesarean incision facilitates this maneuver. A tumor tenaculum on the upper fundus can serve the same purpose. Adnexal tissues near the uterine cornu, used for traction in gynecologic hysterectomy, are very friable and not suitable for vigorous traction.

Dissect the peritoneum of the posterior broad ligament to skeletonize the right uterine vessels (Fig. 27–6). Carefully strip away loose connective tissues from around the uterine vessels.

Doubly clamp the isolated uterine vascular bundle with two curved Heaney clamps (Fig. 27–7). The proper location is opposite the inferior extent of the cesarean incision in most cases. Clamp higher on the uterine wall if there is a question of anatomic proximity of the ureter or distortion of anatomic relationships by a broad ligament hematoma. Do not sever the right uterine vascular pedicle at this time.

The blood supply to the right side of the uterus is now completely controlled. Attention quickly turns to the left side of the dissection.

Clamp and cut the round ligament and adnexal pedicles on the left, as was done on the right side. Skeletonize and clamp the left uterine vessels.

All major blood vessels supplying the uterus are now controlled. The dissection to this point can be done by an experienced team faster than it can be described. The team prepares to suture all previously clamped pedicles in reverse order. A self-retaining retractor can be placed in the abdominal incision at this stage if exposure is inadequate.

The next steps replace all clamps previously set aside with sutures. The left uterine vascular pedicle receives attention first. The assistant must

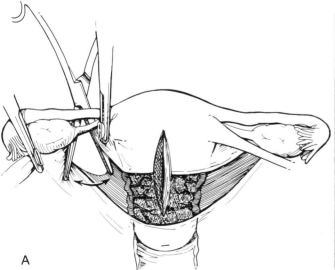

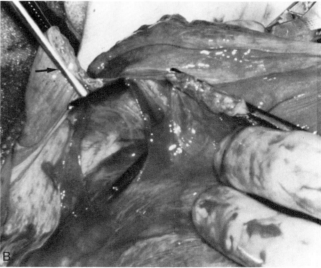

Figure 27–4. *A,* Peripartal hysterectomy procedure. A Kelly clamp is thrust through an avascular portion of the posterior broad ligament to create a site for clamping the adnexal structures. *B,* Upper left, clamped and severed right round ligament. Center, a Kelly clamp makes a window in an avascular portion of the right broad ligament. (Photographed by Lester V. Bergman; courtesy LTI Medica and the UpJohn Company. Copyright 1988 by Learning Technology Incorporated.)

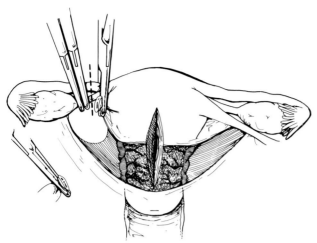

Figure 27–5. Peripartal hysterectomy procedure. The proximal round ligament clamp is moved to include the fallopian tube, the utero-ovarian ligament, and the round ligament. Two Ochsner clamps are placed lateral to this clamp across the adnexal structures. The tips of these clamps lie in the developed broad ligament opening. The round ligament distal clamp and the two adnexal distal clamps are allowed to drop from the surgical field.

support the clamps placed on this vascular bundle, not use them for traction. Any pull on these clamps strips the pedicle from the uterine wall and opens small vessels. Place a Heaney or Ochsner clamp on the ascending branches of the uterine vessels above the dissection to control collateral bleeding.

Incision to develop the uterine vascular pedicle begins with a small scalpel and continues with Mayo scissors to a point beyond the tip of the first clamp but not past the second (Fig. 27–8). A small amount of tissue is left distal to the clamp to

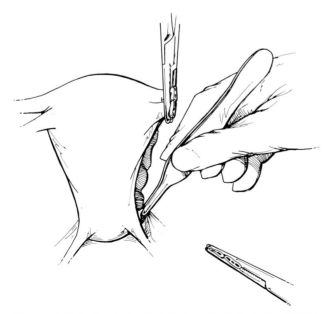

Figure 27–6. Peripartal hysterectomy procedure. Loose connective tissue is stripped away from the uterine vascular bundle on the right. Lower right, clamped and severed adnexal pedicle.

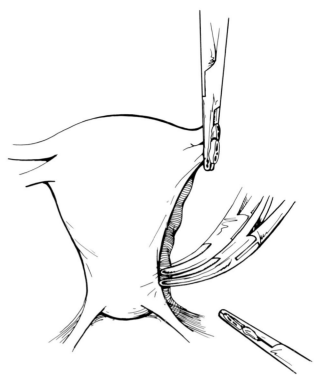

Figure 27–7. Peripartal hysterectomy procedure. Two Heaney clamps are placed on the uterine vascular bundle at a level just below the lowest extent of the cesarean incision or approximately at the internal cervical os. Clamping the right uterine vascular bundle.

prevent the escape of the uterine vessels from the clamp.

Pass the swaged needle of a 0 chromic or 00 polyglycolic-polyglactin suture at the tip of the distal (back) clamp. This clamp is removed as the first throw of a surgeon's knot is drawn tight. A second suture passes at the tip of the remaining clamp, around the back of the clamp, and through the center of the pedicle (Heaney stitch) (Fig. 27–9). This suture is tied back of the clamp as the clamp is withdrawn.

Clamp a 1-cm portion of the uppermost cardinal ligament with a straight Ochsner (Kocher) clamp. This tissue supports the uterine vascular pedicle. Incise the pedicle with a scalpel and secure it with a single suture. Tie this suture around the uterine vascular pedicle to prevent the stripping open of small veins near the vascular bundle during later manipulations.

Next, replace the clamp on the left round ligament with a single transfixing suture (Fig. 27–10).

The left adnexal pedicle receives two sutures. The assistant carefully elevates the adnexal clamps. Replace the proximal (back) clamp with a single circumferential tie. Pass a second suture through the center of the pedicle between the circumferential tie and the distal remaining clamp. Pass the suture around both sides of the

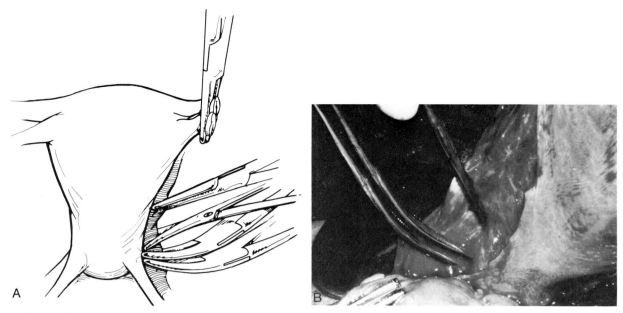

Figure 27–8. *A,* Peripartal hysterectomy procedure. An Ochsner clamp is placed above the uterine vascular clamps to prevent retrograde bleeding. The uterine vascular pedicle is incised with Metzenbaum scissors. *B,* Clamping the left uterine vascular bundle. (Photographed by Lester V. Bergman; courtesy LTI Medica and the UpJohn Company. Copyright 1988 by Learning Technology Incorporated.)

clamp and tighten it as the assistant removes the clamp (Fig. 27–11). Transfixing this suture in the tissue prevents escape of the vessels if reduction of edema loosens the free tie.

Next, suture the right adnexal pedicle as was done on the left. The right round ligament then receives a single transfixing suture. Suture the right uterine vascular pedicle as was done on the left, including the first cardinal ligament bite.

All vessels to the uterus have now been tied. It is possible to amputate the uterus above the ligatures. The posterior cervix often bleeds at the time of such amputation. Considerable blood supply remains from ascending cervical branches of the vaginal arteries.

The team may now take a breather. Explore the bowel and upper abdomen at this stage of the operation if this was not done previously. Pack the bowel out of the pelvis and place a self-retaining retractor. This author prefers an O'Conner-O'Sullivan retractor for thin patients and a large Balfour retractor for obese patients.

We recommend total hysterectomy for all but the most unstable cases. It is particularly embarrassing to complete a subtotal hysterectomy for rupture of the uterus only to find that the patient is still bleeding from undetected extension of the rupture into the cervix.

Patients frequently do not see physicians for regular pelvic examination or Papanicolaou

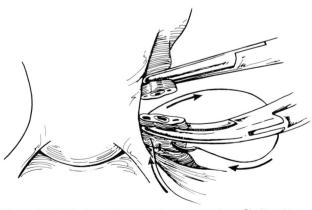

Figure 27–9. Peripartal hysterectomy procedure. Similar clamping and development of the pedicle are done on both sides. The vascular pedicles are then tied in reverse order. This drawing shows replacement of the clamps on the right uterine vessels with a circumferential first suture and a second transfixing (Heaney) suture.

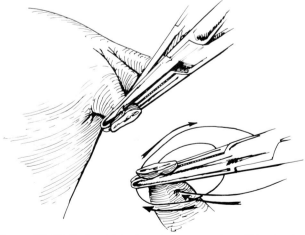

Figure 27–10. Peripartal hysterectomy procedure. This drawing illustrates the securing of the round ligament pedicle with a transfixing suture.

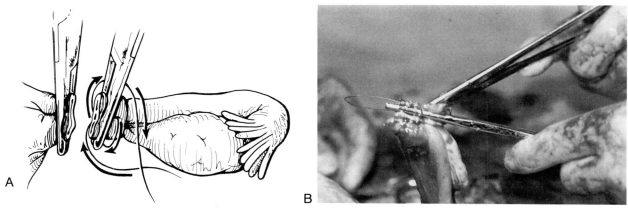

Figure 27–11. *A,* Peripartal hysterectomy procedure. Securing the adnexal pedicle first with a circumferential tie at the site of the distal clamp. The distal clamp is replaced with a transfixing suture, as illustrated. *B,* Placing the transfixing second suture on the right adnexal pedicle. (Photographed by Rita Letellier.)

smears after hysterectomy. Carcinoma may develop to advanced stages in a retained cervical stump before it is recognized. Removal of the cervix prevents these tragedies. However, it does take time and increases the risk of damage to the bladder and ureter.

The dissection to this point requires only the amount of bladder reflection necessary for the cesarean delivery. Cervical dissection demands further mobilization of the bladder.

Elevate the peritoneum of the bladder flap and begin careful detachment of the posterior bladder wall from the upper cervix. A plane of wispy, edematous connective tissue normally permits easy separation. An inch or more of dense adhesions obscures this plane of dissection when the patient has previous cesarean scars. Careful dissection of this zone is necessary to avoid injury to the bladder.

Lateral dissection around the bladder pillars produces troublesome bleeding in an area where clamping and suturing are dangerous. Concentrate dissection near the midline with sharp scissor dissection with the blades turned toward the cervix. Small, blunt dissectors made of rolled pledgets of umbilical tape in the jaws of a Kelly clamp can help. Large pushing motions with sponge sticks are dangerous. The moistened, gloved finger is a good dissection tool once the principal adhesions are traversed.

Bladder dissection need not advance more than 1 cm beyond the level of current cardinal ligament dissection. Exercise care with the bladder retractors. Swinging these retractors from side to side can slice open the friable posterior bladder wall.

The cardinal ligaments are successively clamped exactly against the side of the cervix. One or two bites are taken on the right side, then one or two on the left side to maintain a symmetric dissection (Fig. 27–12). An Ochsner clamp incorporates 1.5 to 2.0 cm of cardinal ligament and slides off the body of the cervix in the clamping motion. Incise

the pedicle with a scalpel to the tip of the clamp. Pass a suture exactly beneath the tip. Tighten the knot down the back of the clamp, including only cardinal ligament tissue as the clamp is removed.

Take each cardinal ligament bite medial to the previous bite. As successive pedicles fall laterally, the ureter falls away from the dissection, out of danger. It is often possible to palpate the ureter in the cardinal ligament tunnel under normal conditions. The ureter may be difficult to palpate if edema, inflammation, or a hematoma distorts the broad ligament.

The uterosacral ligaments insert into the posterior aspect of the upper cervix. These ligaments may be stretched and attenuated or thick and edematous. The surgeon must decide whether or not to incorporate the uterosacral ligament into a low cardinal ligament bite (Fig. 27–13). Clamp and suture the ligament separately if it is large or under tension. Continue the cardinal ligament dissection until the upper vagina is approached.

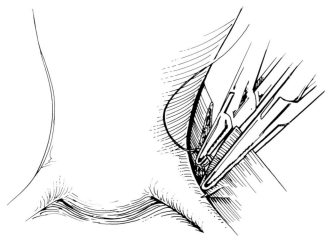

Figure 27–12. Peripartal hysterectomy procedure. The upper right cardinal ligament is clamped with an Ochsner clamp, severed and replaced with a suture ligature placed carefully just at the tip of the clamp.

Next, prepare to excise the cervix. It is often difficult to be certain where the cervix ends and the vagina begins. Feel for the cervix by grasping the upper vagina between the thumb and forefinger and milking upward. When the patient has been in labor and the cervix is effaced and dilated, identification may not be possible by this maneuver. Double glove, open the uterine incision, and palpate the lowest extent of the cervix from within the cervical canal for guidance. This procedure introduces an element of bacterial contamination to the operative site.

Place a fresh laparotomy sponge in the cul-de-sac before opening the vagina. Assistants should prepare to remove any lochia spill by suction.

Incise the vagina transversely with Mayo scissors on its posterior aspect, just below the cervix (Fig. 27–14). Introduce one blade of the scissors into the vaginal opening. Incise the upper vagina circumferentially at its attachment to the cervix under direct vision.

This dissection ensures that the entire cervix is removed and the vaginal length is preserved. The bladder is protected from injury by direct visualization during dissection. An extra length of upper vagina is easily dissected when necessary for cases of intraepithelial neoplasia.

Assistants grasp the edge of the upper vagina as it is opened with Allis clamps at 3, 6, 12, and 9 o'clock (Fig. 27–15). These clamps are kept on gentle upward tension to reduce lochia spill from the upper vagina. Vaginal tissues are fragile, par-

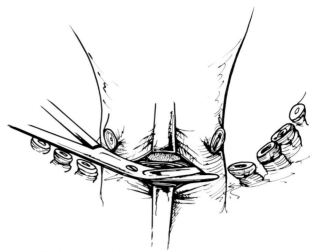

Figure 27–14. Peripartal hysterectomy procedure. After ensuring that the cardinal ligament dissection is below the level of the cervix, the vagina is opened on its posterior aspect.

ticularly if the patient has been in labor. They tear easily with traction. Check the excised uterus to be sure the cervix is completely removed. Hand the freed uterine specimen off the field.

The vaginal cuff can be managed with an open or closed technique. The open technique is favored when fluids are expected to collect in the pelvis. I prefer the closed technique when there is good hemostasis, no infection, and no injury to bowel or bladder.

Place a running locked suture for the closed vaginal cuff technique. Start the suture at one corner of the vaginal cuff. The first bite includes anterior vaginal epithelium, cardinal ligament pedicle, uterosacral pedicle, and posterior vaginal epithelium (Fig. 27–16).

Each pass of the needle catches both anterior and posterior vaginal epithelium. The epithelium has a tendency to slip downward away from the dissection. Postoperative bleeding occurs from vessels in the subepithelial layer if the vaginal epithelium is not secured.

The open cuff technique oversews the anterior and posterior vaginal edges separately with running locked sutures.

The vaginal cuff must be adequately supported whether it is left open or closed. The cardinal ligaments and the uterosacral ligaments are the principal supports of the vaginal apex. Reattach these ligaments to the lateral corners of the vaginal cuff to prevent cuff prolapse (see Fig. 27–16). Plicate the anterior and posterior endopelvic fascia over the closed cuff if additional support of the vagina is needed. The round ligaments are elongated by pregnancy. They contribute little to vaginal support.

Provide for surgical drainage if fluids will collect at the operative site. Drains are required in cases of incomplete hemostasis, extensive pelvic infection, or peritonitis. Drains are also placed at the

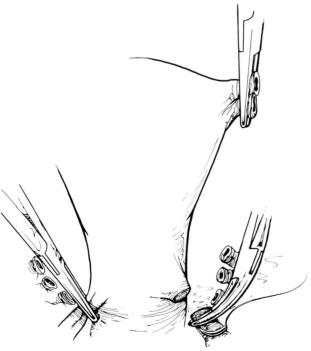

Figure 27–13. Peripartal hysterectomy procedure. The uterosacral ligament may be clamped separately if large and secured with a single suture ligature *(right)*. It may be included with the lowest cardinal ligament pedicle if small *(left)*.

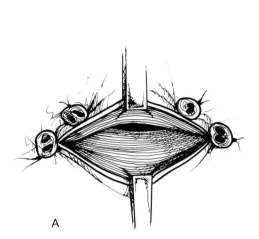
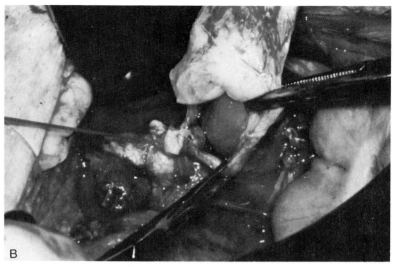

Figure 27–15. *A,* Peripartal hysterectomy procedure. The specimen is excised. The anterior and posterior vagina are grasped with Allis clamps. *B,* Incision of the vaginal cuff. The cervix is visible between the vaginal epithelial clamps in the center of the photograph. A traction suture is on the left cardinal ligament. An Allis clamp supports the posterior vagina. (Photographed by Lester V. Bergman; courtesy LTI Medica and UpJohn Company. Copyright 1988 by Learning Technology Incorporated.)

repair sites of injuries to the urinary tract or large bowel. Simple drains that exit through the vagina offer dependent gravity drainage of cul-de-sac fluids. We currently prefer suction drainage that exits through a separate stab wound in the anterior abdominal wall for most pelvic drainage.

Test the integrity of the bladder by filling it with sterile milk or dye solution. Milk should be available in presterilized bottles from the nursery. The milk is drawn into a bulb syringe and introduced through the urethral catheter. It has the advantage of high visibility and it does not stain tissues.

Dye solutions are made by introducing an ampule of indigo carmine or methylene blue into a collapsible liter bag of normal saline. Dyes stain tissues and may obscure later testing of the site of bladder repair.

The circulator introduces the chosen test solution into the bladder by connecting the intravenous tubing to the transurethral catheter with an adapter. The preparation steps can all be done before the operation begins.

Simply lifting the bag fills the bladder with dye solution. Three or four hundred milliliters sufficiently distend the bladder. Inspect all surfaces of the bladder for dye leaks. If the bladder is intact, the circulator lowers the bag to drain the dye. Repair any defects in the bladder wall with the two-layer technique, as described in Chapter 23.

Practices are changing regarding reperitonealization of the pelvis after hysterectomy. Many surgeons believe that peritoneal closure is an unnecessary step that increases the chances of adhesion formation. The author prefers a neat peritoneal closure with all pedicles placed outside the peritoneal cavity.

Irrigate and cleanse the pelvis. Remove all sponges and instruments. Complete the sponge and instrument count. Close the abdominal wall as described in Chapter 3 on wounds.

Figure 27–17*A–D* illustrates additional steps in the parametrial and pelvic node dissections required for cesarean radical hysterectomy.

POSTOPERATIVE CARE

The care of the patient after peripartal hysterectomy is similar to care of the patient after cesarean delivery. The patient may breast-feed or a system of lactation suppression may be instituted. Avoid lactation suppression drugs that increase the risk of phlebothrombosis and thromboembolism, such as those that employ high doses of steroid hormones.

Institute prompt leg exercises and early ambulation of the patient. We have not routinely em-

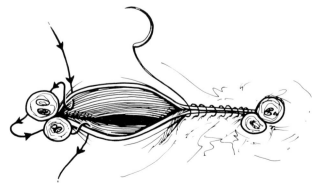

Figure 27–16. Peripartal hysterectomy procedure. The left side of the drawing shows a transfixing suture that includes the anterior vagina, cardinal ligament pedicle, uterosacral ligament pedicle, and posterior vagina. The right side illustrates a continuous suture closing the upper vagina.

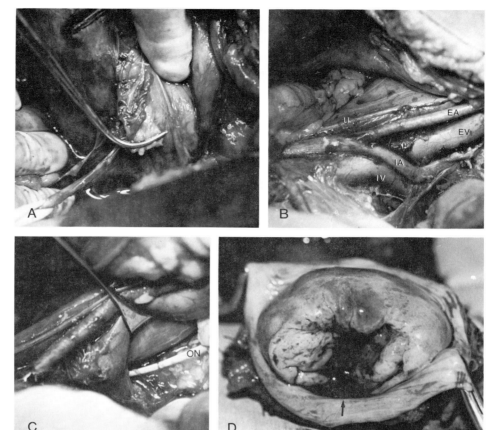

Figure 27–17. Cesarean radical hysterectomy. *A,* Dissection of the right parametrium. The curved clamp encloses the uterine vascular bundle. *B,* Dissection of the external, internal, and common iliac lymph nodes on the left pelvic side wall exposes from above, downward the ureter (U), the external iliac artery (EA), the external iliac vein (EV), the internal iliac artery (IA), and the internal iliac vein (IV). *C,* Further pelvic node dissection exposes the obturator nerve (ON) in the obturator fossa. *D,* The excised surgical specimen shows a stage IB epidermoid carcinoma involving the posterior lip of the cervix. Note the generous vaginal cuff margin around the cervix. (Courtesy Ruth Higdon, M.D.; photographed by Rita L. Letellier.)

ployed anticoagulation to avoid thrombosis, since many of these patients have coexisting severe blood loss or coagulopathies. Antiembolism fitted stockings are of some value. Periodic pneumatic compression of the calves has been recommended. Early and frequent ambulation is the most cost-effective means to prevent phlebothrombosis.

Observe the patient closely for excessive vaginal bleeding or signs of internal bleeding. Check serial hematocrit levels at 6, 12, and 24 hours. A significant fall in the hematocrit level in a stable patient or after transfusion demands complete re-evaluation. Evaluation includes physical examination of the abdomen, wound site, vaginal cuff, and pelvis. Radiologic and sonographic imaging techniques help localize collections of blood.

Blood loss may not be external. It may escape the most careful examination and imaging. The patient who becomes hemodynamically unstable after adequate transfusion must be re-explored for hidden bleeding.

Remove drains in the pelvis or subcutaneous spaces in 24 to 48 hours or as soon as drainage is minimal. Remove urinary catheters as soon as possible. The incidence of urinary infection is directly related to the time the transurethral catheter remains in the bladder.

Postoperative fever in patients after peripartal hysterectomy necessitates careful evaluation. Vaginal cuff cellulitis, pelvic cellulitis, and wound and urinary tract infections are the common causes of postoperative fever. Early fever should not be attributed to pulmonary atelectasis or breast engorgement without careful evaluation. Virulent organisms, such as β-hemolytic streptococci, can cause a febrile response as early as 12 to 24 hours after colonization of the operative site.

Work-up of the patient with fever includes cultures of the vaginal cuff and wound drainage sites. Add blood cultures if septic fever spikes are noted. Institute antibiotic regimens in therapeutic doses that will cover the common aerobic and anaerobic gram-positive and gram-negative organisms. Alter the antibiotics depending on culture reports and the patient's course. Give antibiotic regimens at least a 48-hour trial before altering the mix of drugs.

Continue intravenous fluid support for at least 24 hours. The diet progresses from clear liquids to soft foods to solid foods beginning on the first postoperative day. The patient without postoperative complications is usually walking on her own and eating solid food by the third day after surgery.

COMPLICATIONS, MORBIDITY, AND MORTALITY

Peripartal hysterectomy carries a perceived burden of operative risk that influences its use. The principal points of concern are operative mortality, blood loss, injury to the urinary tract, and postoperative bleeding or infection.

Mortality Rates

The mortality risk for all hysterectomies was examined by Wingo and colleagues from the Centers for Disease Control in 1985.[31] This group processed data collected by the Commission on Professional and Hospital Activities during 1979 and 1980. They found 477 deaths among 317,389 women having abdominal hysterectomies. The overall mortality rate was 12 per 10,000 procedures. Their estimated mortality risk for nonradical abdominal hysterectomy in patients who were not pregnant was 6 per 10,000 procedures.

A large percentage of the deaths (61%) in the Wingo study occurred in hysterectomies for cancer or hysterectomies performed for pregnancy complications. There were 5435 hysterectomies in pregnant patients. The standardized mortality rate for this group was 29.2 per 10,000 procedures.[31] These data appear to indicate a five times greater overall risk of dying from hysterectomy performed during pregnancy.

Wingo and colleagues made no effort to correct for mortality related to the disease for which the surgery was performed. They did not separate peripartal hysterectomy cases to arrive at a procedure-specific mortality rate. Elective cases were not separately examined. It is important to try to separate deaths related to the operative procedure from those related to the disease treated. Attributing causes of death in retrospective case reviews is necessarily subjective. When we attempted this analysis, less than half of peripartal hysterectomy deaths appeared directly related to the operation.

Three of the seven patients who died after peripartal hysterectomy in the LSU series were moribund on admission (see Table 27–5). Their deaths resulted from prior hemorrhage or sepsis. A fourth patient died of advanced pelvic malignancy. Three deaths were related to complications of the operative procedure. Two of these patients died of unrecognized postoperative bleeding. One died of the complications of overwhelming postoperative infection.

Maternal mortality in the cumulative series of cesarean hysterectomies collected by Park and Duff[3] was 28 of 3913 cases (71 per 10,000). Barclay's early Tulane Service-Charity Hospital series reported a 130 per 10,000 mortality rate.[17] The current LSU Service-Charity Hospital series records 7 deaths in 1008 cases for a mortality rate of 69 per 10,000 procedures.

Studies from university services in public hospitals contain a disproportionate share of emergency cases. The acuity of illness is high. The general condition of the patients is often unfavorable. Arrival or referral late in the course of an obstetric catastrophe is common. Many of the members of operating teams at such hospitals are in training.

Obstetric surgeons in private practice describe a patient mix with many more elective cases. They report much lower mortality rates. No maternal deaths were recorded in 543 peripartal hysterectomies reported by three private groups in the New Orleans region[20, 21, 32] (Table 27–3).

Park and Duff[3] found 11 collections of cesarean hysterectomies, many preplanned or elective, with no maternal deaths. They concluded, "when corrected for mortality associated with underlying obstetric catastrophe, the mortality rate of the procedure (cesarean hysterectomy) is not significantly higher than that of cesarean section or abdominal hysterectomy alone."[3]

Morbidity Risks

Postoperative morbidity is influenced by the patient population, environmental conditions, and circumstances surrounding the operation. Table 27–3 exhibits a comparison between reports from private practices and public hospitals. The private groups record 19% shorter operating times, 50% fewer patients given blood transfusions, and 42% fewer intraoperative complications. Private series record one-third the general incidence of febrile morbidity and total morbidity.

Table 27–3 represents a time sample that is not strictly applicable to present-day practices. Transfusion indications and frequency have changed from the decades of 1950 to 1970, as represented by these studies. Blood transfusion is quite rare with current elective cesarean hysterectomies performed in the private sector.

Intraoperative Complications

The most frequent complications during the performance of peripartal hysterectomy are bleeding and injury to the urinary tract (Table 27–4).

Table 27–3. MORBIDITY AND MORTALITY OF CESAREAN HYSTERECTOMY: COMPARISON OF PRIVATE AND TRAINING CENTER CASES

	Private Series* (n = 543)	Training Center Series† (n = 1335)
Average operating time	93 min	114 min
Patients given blood transfusions	32%	63%
Operative complications	11.3%	19.2%
Postoperative febrile morbidity	13.4%	40.5%
Total morbidity	20.5%	52.5%
Maternal mortality	0	1.2/1000

*Ward and Smith,[20] Schneider and Tyrone,[21] Plauché, Gruich, and Bourgeois.[32]

†Mickal and Begneaud,[17] Barclay,[13] Dyer and colleagues.[19]

Bleeding problems can occur at any time during the procedure. Many of the most serious bleeding problems relate to events that occurred before surgery. Traumatic uterine rupture and placental abruption are examples of such events.

The most common cause of excessive blood loss from surgical technique is loss of control of a uterine vascular pedicle. This usually occurs during manipulation of clamps or during suture ligation. Blood may be lost into the operating field or an expanding broad ligament hematoma may develop.

Bleeding can also occur from the adnexal pedicles. An ovarian vessel may be torn during manipulation of the adnexal pedicle. A suture may pierce a blood vessel that is not controlled by a more proximal tie. Reduction of edema may loosen adnexal ties. The ovarian vessels are on tension and easily retract out of a single clamp or suture. The result in all cases is an expanding adnexal hematoma that must be dissected. Unilateral salpingo-oophorectomy is often necessary to control the problem. Double clamping and suturing of the adnexal pedicle using a distal transfixing suture prevents most of these problems.

Ten percent of Barclay's early cases from Charity Hospital, reported in 1969, required unilateral salpingo-oophorectomy for control of adnexal bleeding.[17] Adnexal hematoma required resection in 6% of the more recent series from Charity Hospital reported in 1983 by Plauché and colleagues.[24]

There are many dilated collateral vessels in the pelvis of the pregnant woman. Each must be controlled to prevent steady blood loss throughout the operation. Blood lost from uncontrolled collateral circulation is commonly seen as "back bleeding" from severed pedicles. Control of excessive blood loss during peripartal hysterectomy depends on meticulous hemostatic surgical technique and careful management of all vascular pedicles.

Table 27–4. OPERATIVE AND POSTOPERATIVE COMPLICATIONS OF CESAREAN HYSTERECTOMY REVIEW: 1951 TO 1984 (n = 5185)

Problem	Incidence per 1000 Cases
Postoperative hemorrhage requiring packing, suture, or reoperation	33
Urinary tract injury	39
Inadvertent cystotomy	28
Ureteral injury	4.4
Fistulas	5.7
Vesicovaginal	4.6
Ureterovaginal	0.9
Wound complications	171
Abdominal wound (abscess or dehiscence)	50
Vaginal cuff (abscess or hematoma)	121
Thromboembolism	5.2
Intestinal obstruction	3.3
Febrile morbidity	350
Maternal mortality	7
Procedure-related deaths	3
Disease-related deaths	4

Urinary tract structures are subject to injury at several points during peripartal hysterectomy. Unrecognized injuries become serious postoperative problems. Recognized and repaired injuries usually heal well and do not lengthen hospital stays or cause lasting disability.

Inadvertent injury to the bladder most often occurs when the bladder is dissected from the lower uterine segment in patients who have previous cesarean scars. Plauché and colleagues[24] reported a 3% incidence of inadvertent operative cystotomy among 100 cesarean hysterectomies. Careful sharp dissection technique avoids many unintended cystotomies. The cystotomy is not a tragedy, provided it is recognized and properly repaired. Filling the bladder with dye near the end of the procedure helps detect unrecognized defects in the bladder wall. The technique for repair of the bladder is described in detail in Chapter 23.

The bladder may also be injured by inclusion in a clamp or a tight suture. These injuries occur when the vaginal cuff is clamped or sutured. Cross-clamping the upper vagina before excising the uterus increases the risk of inadvertent bladder injury. There is danger of inclusion within the clamp of the lateral bladder wall where it is tented by the bladder pillars. The injured bladder wall may undergo necrosis, particularly if there is a vaginal cuff infection after surgery.

Ureteral injury most often occurs when the anatomic relationships of the ureter are distorted by hematomas or pelvic tumors. Visualization, palpation, and dissection of the ureter avoid most injuries.

Guard against high ureteral injury by visualizing the ureter before clamping adnexal pedicles. Prevent injury to the ureter at the level of the cervix by placing clamps exactly against the wall of the uterus and cervix, always inside the previous pedicle. When hematomas distort the course of the ureter, one cannot be sure of its location. Its course should be traced or dissected to ensure its safety. Dissection in the cardinal ligament region in pregnant patients may provoke brisk bleeding. Bring all care and experience to this dissection. Chapter 23 describes the management of the injured ureter.

Some authors express concern about incomplete removal of the cervix at the time of peripartal hysterectomy. This is of particular importance if the operation is employed to manage cervical premalignant or malignant disease. Plauché and colleagues[24] found three instances of incomplete removal of the cervix among 100 cesarean hysterectomies. Excision of the cervix under direct vision as described in this chapter ensures its complete removal (see Figs. 27–14B and 27–17D).

Postoperative Complications

Table 27–5 outlines the most frequent postoperative complications encountered on the LSU Charity Hospital service.

Postoperative bleeding is most often from an escaped adnexal or uterine vessel. Adnexal bleeding can be difficult to detect. Blood that collects in retroperitoneal flank spaces makes diagnosis difficult and often delayed. Instability of vital signs is often the first and only sign of this hidden bleeding. Magnetic resonance imaging and computed tomography help detect collections of blood in retroperitoneal spaces.

Bleeding from uterine vessels may be external or remain hidden. Blood may collect within the broad ligament or in the large presacral space. After surgery, the region above the vaginal cuff is heavily colonized with vaginal bacteria. A cuff hematoma often becomes infected. Evaluation reveals a febrile patient with a mass above the vaginal cuff. It is often possible to drain such hematomas through the vaginal cuff. Symptoms and signs rapidly resolve after adequate drainage. However, it is risky to attempt vaginal drainage when the mass does not point near the midline of the cuff.

Reoperation is necessary for enlarging hematomas that are not accessible to vaginal drainage. Imaging procedures help follow the expansion of hematomas. The patient who shows instability of vital signs after peripartal hysterectomy must be evaluated for hidden bleeding. The patient receives blood transfusion as necessary. Reoperation is indicated if instability of vital signs or falling hematocrit levels return after transfusion. The physician should resist the natural reluctance to reoperate, since delay may result in irreversible shock.

Laparotomy for bleeding after peripartal hysterectomy was required in 1.6% of the entire LSU series of over 1000 cases.[16] Park and Duff reported an incidence of reoperation for bleeding of 0.97%.[3]

Infections are among the most common complications after peripartal hysterectomy. Febrile morbidity is reported in 8 to 48% of cases. Groups of cases from public hospitals report febrile morbidity of 30% or more. Private groups report incidences near 10%.

Table 27–5. POSTOPERATIVE COMPLICATIONS: CESAREAN HYSTERECTOMY, LSU SERVICE-CHARITY HOSPITAL OF NEW ORLEANS (n = 1008)

Complication	Percent
Urinary tract infections	17.0
Vaginal cuff hematoma or infection	12.8
Wound infection or separation	5.3
Pulmonary complications	4.1
Laparotomy for postoperative bleeding	1.6
Fistula formation	1.0
Vesicovaginal	(0.8%)
Ureterovaginal	(0.2%)
Intestinal obstruction	0.3
Thromboembolism	0.2
Febrile morbidity	30.0
Maternal mortality (7 cases)	0.69
Procedure-related (3)	
Disease-related (4)	

The LSU series indicated an incidence of vaginal cuff hematoma or infection of 12.8%.[16] Park and Duff reported an 8.7% incidence of pelvic or cuff cellulitis.[3] Antibiotic therapy is effective treatment for most cases of vaginal cuff cellulitis. Vaginal cuff abscesses or pelvic abscesses occur in 5.2% of cases.[3] Abscesses necessitate operative drainage in addition to intensive antibiotic treatment.

Urinary tract infections relate directly to the length of time indwelling catheters remain in place. Seventeen percent of the LSU Charity Hospital series and 9.8% of the collected cases of Park and Duff developed urinary infections.[3, 16] The incidence at Charity Hospital among recent cases decreased to 6%.[24] This improvement most likely is because of an increase in prophylactic antibiotic use and a policy of early removal of catheters.

Wound infections and or dehiscence occurred in 5.3% of the LSU-Charity Hospital cases and 4.8% of Park and Duff's collected cases.[3, 16] Meticulous hemostasis, avoidance of bacterial contamination of the operative site, and prophylactic antibiotics for patients who have been in labor reduce the incidence of wound infections.

SUMMARY

Peripartal hysterectomy was proposed 2 centuries ago to solve the problems of unremitting obstetric bleeding and infection. It still fulfills these functions. Generations of innovative surgeons modified and refined the operation to increase its safety and utility.

Heroic obstetric manipulations are no longer part of obstetric practice. Few difficult birth extractions that result in injury to maternal organs are performed by modern obstetricians. We no longer see prolonged, impacted labors. New drugs combat infection and obstetric bleeding. These changes reduce the need for emergency peripartal hysterectomy.

Advances in surgery and anesthesia allowed expansion of the indications for peripartal hysterectomy beyond emergencies. The operation is presently performed for coincident gynecologic disease and occasionally for elective sterilization. These indications, particularly the latter, remain controversial.

The arguments over peripartal hysterectomy lie not in its utility or results but in its difficulty and complications. The operation can be exceptionally challenging when performed under conditions of life-threatening emergency. Morbidity and mortality risks under these conditions exceed, by perhaps a factor of five, those of cesarean section or gynecologic hysterectomy. Only one half of the excess morbidity and mortality can be assigned directly to complications of the operative procedure.

Complications are dramatically reduced when the operation is performed as a preplanned procedure. Morbidity and mortality risks under these conditions are only marginally greater than those of cesarean section with tubal ligation or gynecologic hysterectomy.

The controversy over peripartal hysterectomy for sterilization stems from different training philosophies and different perceptions of the magnitude of risk. The existence of this controversy places the obstetric surgeon at increased medicolegal risk should a complication occur.

Some of the most important obstetric emergencies necessitate hysterectomy to save the mother's life. It is very difficult to learn the techniques that make the operation quick and safe under emergency conditions. We encourage the teaching of the basic concepts and techniques of peripartal hysterectomy to all obstetric residents under nonemergency conditions. Peripartal hysterectomy should be in the repertory of all consultant obstetricians.

References

1. Durfee RB: Evolution of cesarean hysterectomy. Clin Obstet Gynecol 12:575, 1969.
2. Young JH: Caesarean section. The history and development of the operation from earliest times. London: H.K. Lewis & Co. Ltd., 1944, pp. 93–105.
3. Park RC, Duff WP: Role of cesarean hysterectomy in modern obstetric practice. Clin Obstet Gynecol 23:601, 1980.
4. Bixby GH: Extirpation of the puerperal uterus by abdominal section. J Gynaec Soc Boston 1:223, 1869.
5. Porro E: Dell'amputazione utero-ovarica come complemento di taglio cesareo. Ann univ med e chir 237:289, 1876.
6. Richardson E: Caesarean section with removal of uterus and ovaries after the Porro-Müller method. Am J Med Sci 81:36, 1878.
7. Harris RP: Results of the first fifty cases of caesarean ovaro-hysterectomy: 1869–1880. Am J Med Sci 80:129, 1880.
8. Godson C: Porro's operation. Br Med J 1:142, 1884.
9. Tait L: Address on the surgical aspect of impacted labour. Br Med J 1:657, 1890.
10. Reed CAL: Caesarean hysterectomy indications. Am J Obstet 42:71, 1900.
11. Duncan W, Targett JH: Porro-caesarean hysterectomy with retro-peritoneal treatment of the stump in a case of fibroids obstructing labour; with remarks upon the relative advantages of the modern Porro operation over the Sanger caesarean in most other cases requiring abdominal section. Trans Obstet Soc Lond 42:244, 1900.
12. Lash AF, Cummings WC: Report on the outcome of caesarean hysterectomy. Am J Obstet Gynecol 30:199, 1935.
13. Davis ME: Complete cesarean hysterectomy—logical advance in modern obstetric surgery. Am J Obstet Gynecol 62:838, 1951.
14. Weed JC: The fate of the postcesarean uterus. Obstet Gynecol 14:780, 1959.
15. Brenner P, Sall S, Sonnenblick B: Evaluation of cesarean section hysterectomy as a sterilization procedure. Am J Obstet Gynecol 108:335, 1978.
16. Plauché WC: Cesarean hysterectomy. In Schiarra J (ed.): Gynecology and Obstetrics, Vol. 2, Ch. 84, 1986, p. 1.
17. Barclay DL: Cesarean hysterectomy: Thirty years experience. Obstet Gynecol 35:120, 1970.
18. Mickal A, Begneaud WP, Hawes TP: Pitfalls and complications of cesarean section hysterectomy. Clin Obstet Gynecol 12:660, 1969.
19. Dyer I, Nix GF, Weed JC, et al.: Total hysterectomy at cesarean section and the immediate puerperal period. Am J Obstet Gynecol 65:517, 1953.
20. Ward SV, Smith H: Cesarean hysterectomy: Combined section and sterilization. Obstet Gynecol 26:858, 1965.
21. Schneider GT, Tyrone CH: Cesarean total hysterectomy: Experience with 160 cases. South Med J 59:927, 1968.
22. Barclay DL, Hawks BL, Frueh DM, et al.: Elective cesarean hysterectomy: A five-year comparison with cesarean section. Am J Obstet Gynecol 124:900, 1976.
23. Clark SL, Yeh ZY, Phelan JP, et al.: Emergency hysterectomy for obstetric hemorrhage. Obstet Gynecol 64:376, 1985.
24. Plauché WC, Wycheck JS, Iannessa M, et al.: Cesarean hysterectomy on the LSU Service of Charity Hospital, 1975–1981. South Med J 76:1261, 1983.
25. Chestnut DH, Eden RD, Gall SA, et al.: Peripartum hysterectomy: A review of cesarean and postpartum hysterectomy. Obstet Gynecol 65:792, 1984.
26. Bowman EA, Barclay DL, White LC: Cesarean hysterectomy: An analysis of 1,000 consecutive operations. Bull Tulane Med Faculty 23:75, 1964.
27. Plauché WC: Cesarean hysterectomy: Indications, technique and complications. Clin Obstet Gynecol 29:318, 1986.
28. McNulty JV: Elective cesarean hysterectomy—revisited. Am J Obstet Gynecol 149:29, 1984.
29. Sturdee DW, Rushton DI: Caesarean and post-partum hysterectomy 1968–1983. Br J Obstet Gynecol 93:270, 1986.
30. Hay DL, van Fraunhofer JA, Masterson BJ: Hemostasis in blood vessels after ligation. Am J Obstet Gynecol 160:737, 1989.
31. Wings PA, Huezo CM, Rubin GL, et al.: The mortality risk associated with hysterectomy. Am J Obstet Gynecol 152:803, 1985.
32. Plauché WC, Gruich FG, Bourgeois MO: Hysterectomy at the time of cesarean section: Analysis of 108 cases. Obstet Gynecol 58:459, 1981.

Puerperal Tubal Sterilization

Haywood L. Brown
Joseph G. Pastorek II

Surgical sterilization is the most frequently used method of contraception in the United States. Tubal ligation in the puerperium following vaginal or cesarean delivery has long been a primary method of operative sterilization. There has been a significant upward trend in tubal sterilization over the last 2 decades. Bopp and Hall[1] demonstrated a decrease in the tubal ligation to delivery ratio from 1 to 421 in 1959 to 1 to 5.1 between 1967 and 1968 at their institution. A review by Edwards and Hadakson in 1973[2] showed a drop in the ratio of sterilization to delivery from 1 to 17.4 between 1958 and 1967 to 1 to 4.3 in 1970 to 1971.

Prior to the 1970s, major indications for sterilization included high parity, medical and obstetric complications, and socioeconomic considerations. Until 1969, even the American College of Obstetricians and Gynecologists observed the rule that required a woman to have the magic number of 120 in her history (multiplying age times parity) before she could be eligible for sterilization. For example, a woman 30 years of age would have to have had four living children or a woman aged 40 would have to have had three children before sterilization could be considered. In addition, the request often had to be signed by the patient, her husband, and two physicians, and then counter-signed by the chief of service. Although present restrictions imposed by the federal government often discourage voluntary sterilization among financially underprivileged women, these restrictions are far fewer than they were years ago.

In the United States, tubal sterilization is for the most part now available on patient demand. In contrast to the years prior to the 1970s, women who now request sterilization are of lower parity, younger age, and from all socioeconomic strata. Even though federally subsidized women must sign sterilization consent 30 days before surgery, a woman of at least 21 years of age can obtain sterilization regardless of parity or marital status.

In comparison to interval sterilization procedures, tubal sterilization following delivery in the early puerperium is convenient, simple, and cost-effective. Early puerperal sterilization also has the advantage of a single hospitalization and utilization of the same anesthetic as was used for delivery, unless there are maternal or infant complications that suggest that the procedure be deferred. Because interval sterilization remains a viable alternative, puerperal sterilization is considered inappropriate if fetal health is uncertain or maternal condition is less than optimal.

HISTORY OF TUBAL LIGATION

Samuel Lungren of Toledo, Ohio, is credited with performing the first tubal interruption for sterilization in the United States over 100 years ago.[3] He ligated the oviducts with a strong silk ligature about 1 inch from their uterine attachment following the woman's second cesarean delivery. Prior to this time, female sterilization methods included surgical removal of both ovaries, fimbrial or ovarian sequestration in peritoneal pouches, removal of both tubes and ovaries leaving the uterus, radiotherapy to the pelvic viscera, cauterization of the endometrium with hot vapors, and removal of the uterus with or without the cervix.

Tubal sterilization at the time of cesarean delivery became even more popular in the United States after 1881. Some of the described methods for tubal interruption included single and double silk ligatures, ligatures of kangaroo tendon, excision of a segment of tube between ligatures, excision of the entire tube, burial of a cut portion of tube in peritoneal folds, crushing of the tubes, crushing and tying the tubes, and cauterization of the tubes with chemicals or heat.[4] These historical methods of interfering with tubal continuity pioneered the modern techniques for tubal sterilization in use at present.

Needless to say, surgical sterilization, particularly by tubal interruption, has never been without opponents. There were and still are the obvious religious objections to purposeful sterilization. In addition, the 1944 review by Young lists arguments by many prominent gynecologists as to the morality of sterilization in otherwise healthy women, as opposed to those women of the "depraved pauper class, patients illegitimately pregnant, women likely to become a burden to the state, mental incompetents, and social derelicts."[4]

PREOPERATIVE ASSESSMENT

The patient interested in sterilization should have thorough counseling in the antenatal period. If practical, the counseling session should include the woman's partner. During this session, alternatives to permanent female sterilization, including male sterilization and other available female contraceptive methods, should be discussed. The technique being considered should be reviewed in detail along with the timing of the procedure, side effects, complications, potential for failure and reversibility, and sexual and menstrual ramifications. Operative sterilization permits should be signed and witnessed within the appropriate time span.

Prior to surgery, the preoperative history should be reviewed and physical examination should be performed to determine if there are any contraindications to elective surgery. The status of the newborn should also be re-evaluated, and the infant should be confirmed to be healthy.

Preoperative laboratory tests should include hematocrit and hemoglobin levels and urinalysis. The patient's predelivery laboratory tests usually are adequate unless excessive blood loss or other complications have occurred during the delivery. If the sterilization operation is being performed after vaginal delivery, the patient's bladder should be emptied immediately prior to the operation to minimize the risk of bladder injury during surgery.

TIMING POSTPARTUM STERILIZATION

Tubal sterilization may be performed after closure of the uterine incision and bladder peritoneum during cesarean delivery or following completion of a vaginal delivery.

Up to several days after vaginal delivery, tubal sterilization is technically simple because the uterine fundus is at the level of the umbilicus, making the oviducts readily accessible through a small periumbilical abdominal incision.

If there are no maternal contraindications and if the condition of the infant is good, puerperal sterilization can be performed immediately after vaginal delivery. Sterilization at this time permits the use of the same anesthetic for both delivery and tubal interruption, especially if conduction anesthesia has been used during labor and delivery. If immediate tubal sterilization is not possible, the procedure can be performed within the first 24 to 48 hours or even up to 72 hours post partum. Often the epidural catheter can be left in place overnight, thereby eliminating the need for a new anesthetic. The major advantage of postponing sterilization for at least 24 hours is that this time delay allows a longer period for assessment of the newborn infant's condition. In addition, after 12 to 24 hours, the risk of postpartum hemorrhage in the multiparous woman requesting sterilization has significantly decreased.

In the late 1940s, Hellman[5] and Whitacre and colleagues[6] suggested that a longer vaginal delivery to sterilization time interval is correlated with an increased risk of histologic salpingitis from ascending bacterial invasion of the fallopian tubes and increased maternal morbidity. This theory was strongly supported by Overstreet, who believed that puerperal sterilization should be limited to within a 48-hour period after delivery if significant maternal morbidity was to be avoided.[7] Subsequent studies failed to demonstrate a relationship between histologic salpingitis, clinical complications, and maternal morbidity, even when the delivery to sterilization interval extended to 5 days post partum.[2, 8–11] Therefore, it seems that postoperative morbidity is the same, regardless of the delivery to tubal surgery time interval.

TUBAL STERILIZATION TECHNIQUES

Incision

Puerperal sterilization after vaginal delivery may be easily performed through a 1- to 5-cm periumbilical semilunar incision. This type of incision is cosmetic and usually disappears completely into the umbilicus after healing. If the procedure is delayed for several days or if the patient undergoing tubal ligation has a significantly involuted uterus, as might be found after delivery of a preterm infant, then a small, vertical midline abdominal incision at the level of the fundus may be more appropriate. A small vertical incision under these circumstances facilitates easier delivery of the oviduct through the abdominal incision for ligation.

In the periumbilical approach, once the skin incision is made, the blunt end of a scissors is used to expose the underlying fascial sheath, which can then be grasped with hemostats. The fascia is opened transversely, exposing the peritoneum, which can then be entered gently.

The uterine fundus is visible through the umbilical incision, and with manipulation and retraction, the tubes can be visualized and grasped with a Babcock clamp. The tubes are exposed until the fimbriated end is identified. Appropriate identification is imperative because a major cause of tubal ligation failure is mistakenly ligating the round ligament, falsely identified as the tube.

After tubal ligation has been performed, the abdominal incision can be closed. We prefer separate peritoneal and fascial closures. The peritoneum is closed with a 2–0 delayed absorbable polyglycolate suture in a purse-string fashion and the skin with a 3–0 or 4–0 polyglycolate absorbable suture in a subcuticular manner.

The Pomeroy Technique

The Pomeroy technique for tubal sterilization is the most simple and commonly performed puerperal sterilization procedure (Fig. 28–1). The Pom-

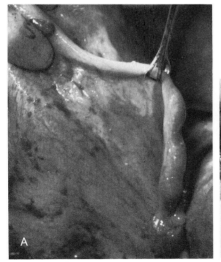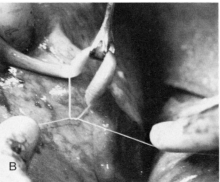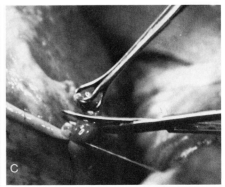

Figure 28–1. *A,* Pomeroy tubal ligation. Grasping the midportion of the tube with a Babcock clamp. *B,* A single ligature of 00 plain catgut ties off a loop of fallopian tube. *C,* A segment of the ligated tube is excised with Metzenbaum scissors.

eroy method was first published after Pomeroy's death by Bishop and Nelms in 1930.[12] The original operation consisted of a loop of tube being ligated in the middle with a double strand of 1–0 chromic catgut, followed by resection of the top of the ligated loop. The rationale for this tubal ligation technique is based on prompt absorption of the suture ligature, with subsequent separation of the cut ends of the tube, which then become sealed over by spontaneous reperitonealization and fibrosis. There should be a natural gap of 2 or 3 cm between the severed proximal and distal segments.

The principal method of failure of the Pomeroy method is by recanalization in a tube that did not complete its cycle of spontaneous separation and fibrosis. Bishop and Nelms felt it necessary to avoid crushing the tube—a principal component of the Madlener tubal technique. They believed that crushing the tube and using permanent suture prohibited spontaneous separation and contributed to a higher failure rate.

In keeping with this theory for tubal failure, we, as others, prefer to use a 00 plain catgut suture for the Pomeroy technique and to cut each limb of the tubal knuckle separately to avoid crushing the sides together. Cautery of the cut ends of the tube is unnecessary and in fact causes more reactive tubal exudate; this may lead to adherence of the cut ends of the tubes prior to ligature absorption, thereby predisposing to failure.

Obviously, many modifications of the Pomeroy technique have been described. The most common involves ligating the proximal end of each tube with a nonabsorbable suture. This modification probably is not harmful as long as the permanent suture is placed several centimeters proximal to the resected loop. The Pomeroy technique, properly performed, has a failure rate of 1 in 300 to 500, or 2 to 4 per 1000.[13–15]

Garb, in 1957,[16] and Overstreet, in 1964,[7] reported failure rates as high as 1 in 50 when the Pomeroy method of tubal ligation was used at the time of cesarean delivery. These studies prompted many clinicians to avoid the Pomeroy technique

during cesarean section. Such high failure rates at cesarean delivery were not explainable, and subsequently, several authors reported contrary data.[8, 17, 18] However, a recent report by deVilliers quoted a 1.35% failure rate with the Pomeroy technique during cesarean section.[19]

We believe that when the Pomeroy technique is performed in the manner we have described, whether at cesarean section or after vaginal delivery, the failure rate should be no greater than 1 in 300 to 500 patients.

The Parkland Technique

The midsegmental resection, or Parkland technique, for tubal ligation was designed to avoid the intimate approximation of the cut ends of the tube that occurs with the Pomeroy technique, thereby eliminating the risk of secondary adherence and subsequent recanalization of the cut ends of the tube (Fig. 28–2).[20]

After the tube is identified down to its fimbriated end, an avascular area is identified in the mesosalpinx directly under the tube. This avascular site is perforated with a hemostat, and the jaw of the hemostat is opened to spread the mesosalpinx, thereby freeing approximately 2.5 cm of oviduct. If an avascular site is not readily identifiable, the Bovie tip can be used to cauterize small vessels in the mesosalpinx before perforating it with the hemostat. This modification eliminates bleeding, which can occur when small vessels in the area inadvertently disrupted.

The freed tube is then ligated proximally and distally with 0 or 00 plain or chromic suture, and a 1 to 2-cm segment of tube between the two ligatures is removed and sent for pathologic confirmation. The finished Parkland technique represents the designed aim of the Pomeroy method after dissolution of the sutures in that the tubal ends can heal and reperitonealize without initially being in proximity.

Failure rate with this method is approximately

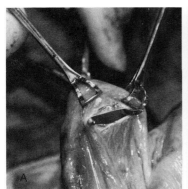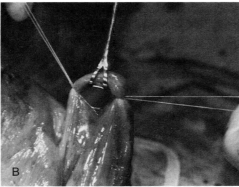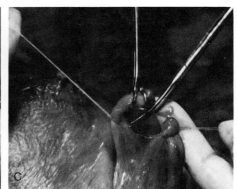

Figure 28–2. *A,* Parkland tubal ligation. The midportion of the tube is elevated with Babcock clamps. A hemostat is thrust through an avascular portion of the mesosalpinx. *B,* Two 00 chromic catgut sutures ligate each end of a 2-cm segment of fallopian tube. *C,* A segment of tube approximately 1 cm long is excised between the occluding sutures.

0.25% (1 in 400) if the technique is strictly followed.[20]

The Uchida Technique

In the mid 1940s, Hajime Uchida developed what he termed a simple and effective method for tubal sterilization that could be carried out rapidly during the early puerperium or as an interval procedure (Fig. 28–3). At the 1961 World Congress of Obstetrics and Gynecology, Uchida reported his experience of 5000 tubal sterilizations with no failures.[21] He subsequently reported on his personal experience with over 20,000 tubal sterilizations over 28 years without a known failure.[22] During the puerperium and especially at the time of cesarean delivery, Uchida modified the sterilization procedure by including fimbriectomy. This fimbriectomy involved a single ligation and excision of that portion of the mesosalpinx that lies below the distal tubal segment. Uchida believed that this important modification further added to the minimal repeat pregnancy rate following sterilization.

The Uchida procedure can be performed either through the usual periumbilical incision after vaginal delivery or at the time of cesarean section.

After mobilization of the tube, the tubal serosa is raised from the muscularis by subserosal injection of a dilute (1:100,000) saline solution of phenylephrine or epinephrine, or of plain saline. We prefer using a plain saline injection subserosally in the area where the incision is to be made. After saline injection, a linear incision is made in the ballooning serosa on the antimesosalpingeal aspect of the tube with a sharp knife. The tubal serosal peritoneum is grasped on both sides of the incision with hemostats, and a third hemostat is used to bluntly dissect and reflect the serosa and the surrounding areolar tissue from the tubal muscularis. With the tubal muscularis exposed, a relatively long (up to 5 cm) segment of tubal muscularis is ligated proximally and distally with 2–0 plain catgut suture and resected. The raw serosal edges are then reapproximated, burying the proximal cut tubal end within the leaves of the broad ligament and exteriorizing the distal end from the broad ligament. We do not perform fimbriectomies in conjunction with the Uchida sterilization.

The Uchida procedure has a very high success rate, which approaches 100% in published series. Explanation for the failures encountered with this operation are attributable to surgical errors in deviations from the original technique.[23]

Because such a long segment of tubal muscularis

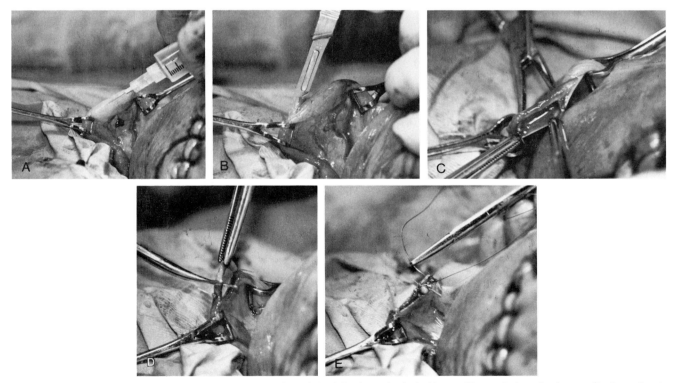

Figure 28–3. *A,* Uchida tubal sterilization. The midportion of the fallopian tube is held up with two Babcock clamps. Sterile saline is injected beneath the serosa of the tube to form a large wheal. *B,* A small scalpel incises the anamesenteric serosal covering of the tube, exposing the tubal muscularis layer for 3 to 5 cm. *C,* Two hemostats grasp the serosal peritoneum while a third dissects the fallopian tube free of surrounding areolar tissue. *D,* The denuded fallopian tube is ligated at two sites at least 2 cm apart with 00 plain catgut. A 1-cm segment of fallopian tube is excised with Metzenbaum scissors. *E,* Uchida tubal sterilization. The procedure is completed by closing the peritoneal incision with 000 Vicryl suture, burying only the proximal ligated end of the tube within the leaves of the mesentery.

is removed in the Uchida operation, the potential for reversal if the need arises seems poor. However, we know of no data on attempts at reversal of the Uchida operation to support such a conclusion.

As with the midsegmental resection, the most bothersome problem encountered in performing the operation is bleeding when the mesosalpinx is stripped off the tube. This makes the Uchida procedure more time-consuming and difficult than standard Pomeroy and midsegment resection methods. In addition, there are occasional problems in initiating a wheal when injecting saline, thereby making it difficult to dissect the serosa free of the muscularis. The problem is most notably encountered in women with post-inflammatory changes, as is often the case with patients who have had multiple cesarean operations. Attempts at dissection of the serosa from the muscularis in these cases often lead to troublesome bleeding, resulting in frustration and abandonment of the procedure in favor of Pomeroy or midsegment resection.

Nonetheless, the Uchida technique is an excellent procedure for women with medical or obstetric indications that absolutely contraindicate further pregnancy.

The Irving Method

Frederick Irving of Boston published his method for tubal sterilization in 1924 (Fig. 28–4).[24] The procedure was designed specifically to be used in conjunction with cesarean delivery. Irving developed this procedure primarily because of his dissatisfaction with available methods for tubal ligation with cesarean section. The Irving method requires a larger operating field and generous exposure of the uterus and oviducts, thus making them easily accessible. This procedure is not appropriate for the routine postpartum vaginal delivery patient.

The Irving tubal method involves separation of the tube near its midportion. The isolated segment is dissected from the underlying mesosalpinx so that the proximal segment is free. It is important to identify a segment of tube where the mesosalpinx is fairly avascular so that bleeding from small vessels is avoided. Coagulation of small vessels within the mesosalpinx with the Bovie tip will aid in making the dissection less bloody. The segment of tube is tied proximally and distally with 2–0 delayed absorbable polyglycolate suture, and the ligature on the proximal segment is left long. A small segment is removed for pathologic confirmation. The proximal segment is buried in a small tunnel in the myometrium on the anterior surface of the uterus. The tunnel is formed by making a small 0.5-cm incision through the serosa into the muscle of the uterus just above the insertion of the round ligament. With the use of a hemostat placed through this incision, a space of 1.0 to 1.5 cm in length is created for the proximal tubal segment to be pushed into. The long ligature on

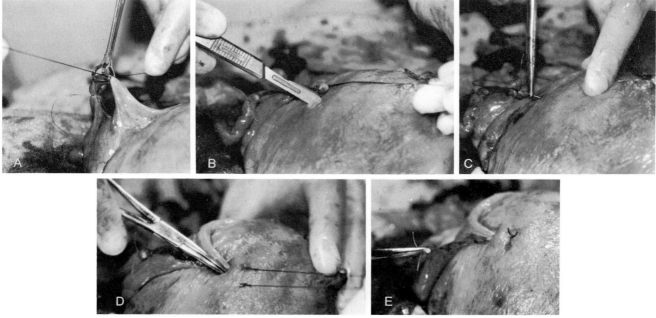

Figure 28–4. *A,* Irving tubal sterilization. The tube is first isolated, doubly ligated, and then divided, as in the Parkland technique. The proximal suture is held for later use. *B,* A 1- to 1.5-cm incision is made in the cornual portion of the uterus at a point accessible to the proximal end of the tube. *C,* Each end of the suture on the proximal end of the tube is threaded on a large half-circle needle. The needle passes into the myometrial incision and out onto the surface of the uterus. *D,* A hemostat pushes the proximal end of the tube into the myometrial incision while the holding suture draws the end of the tube into the depths of the myometrial incision. *E,* The suture is tied. The proximal end of tube is buried within the myometrium. The distal ligated tube retracts away from the uterus.

the proximal segment is threaded on a half-curved needle and carried through the tunnel until it emerges at its base, thereby guiding the proximal tubal end into the tunnel. The suture is tied, leaving the proximal end of the tube anchored inside of the tunnel. An additional option is to bury the distal end of the tube between the leaves of the broad ligament, as originally described by Irving.[24] However, we do not consider this addition any great advantage and have not adopted this practice.

The advantage of burial of the tubal end is that it prevents recanalization and failures. Irving had performed over 800 such procedures by 1950 without any failures.[25] The Irving procedure is undoubtedly the most reliable puerperal tubal sterilization method. Up until a report by Lopez-Zeno and colleagues in 1990,[26] only two other failures had been reported in over 1300 Irving procedures,[27, 28] thus bringing the total number of failures reported with this method to three.

Major disadvantages of the Irving tubal ligation procedure are that it can only be employed at cesarean section, has poor potential for reversal, and is extremely time-consuming. Also, it is often complicated by significant bleeding from the mesosalpinx and myometrium tunnel site. Bleeding from the tunnel site is often difficult to control. Several minutes of firm pressure or suturing with a single figure-of-eight stitch across the incision line usually controls the bleeding. Nonetheless, in cases in which repeat pregnancy is absolutely contraindicated, the Irving method is an excellent choice.

The Madlener Technique, the Kroener Fimbriectomy, the Oxford Technique, and the Simple Ligation Method

These tubal ligation techniques have all been popular in the past as methods of tubal sterilization; however, most have fallen into disfavor because of an unacceptably high failure rate.

The Madlener technique is one of the oldest methods of tubal ligation. The technique consists of crushing across a knuckle of tube near its midportion and ligating it with a nonabsorbable suture, such as silk.[29] The procedure is similar to the Pomeroy method, except that no portion of the tube is resected. This procedure has a high failure rate, apparently caused by the tendency of the nonabsorbable suture to cut through the tube, thereby facilitating fistula formation or recanalization of the tube.[18, 30, 31] Early experience with the Madlener technique at other institutions indicated a failure rate of about 7%.[20] For this reason, permanent or nonabsorbable suture placed about the tube in a circumferential fashion should always be avoided.

Kroener popularized the fimbriectomy method of tubal ligation; the main advantages were ease of performance and lack of interference with ovarian or tubal blood supply.[32] The procedure consisted of excision of the distal portion of each tube and ligation of the cut end with a nonabsorbable suture, such as silk. Although Kroener and others demonstrated excellent results with this method, failure rates as high as 3% have been reported.[33] The failures were believed to result from the presence of residual fimbrial tissue, fimbria ovarica, and tuboperitoneal fistulas.[34–36] The major disadvantage of this method of tubal ligation is its poor chance of reversal if the need arises.

The Oxford method was popularized by Williams.[37] The procedure is very similar to the midsegmental resection. After ligating the tube proximally and distally, a small segment of the tubal isthmus is removed and the cut ends are separated by tying the proximal and distal tubal ends on opposite sides of the round ligament.[37] This procedure has been primarily used in England and has never been popular in the United States. It is more complex than the commonly employed Pomeroy and midsegment resection methods and necessitates a larger abdominal incision. However, after reversal of the Oxford technique, an excellent pregnancy rate has been reported.[37]

Mehta described the single-stitch tubal ligation technique, which involved ligating the tube in its midisthmic portion with a 1-mm ligature of Barbour linen.[38] The advantage of this procedure was that if reversal was desired, reanastomosis would be more easily accomplished. However, this procedure was found to have a significantly high failure rate and at present has no place in modern medicine as a tubal ligation method.

Clips and Rings

Various types of clips and rings have been employed in the puerperium.[29] These mechanisms for tubal sterilization had a promised advantage of minimal tubal damage, higher successful reversal rates, and easier and more rapid application.

Hulka has the most extensive experience with clip application in the puerperium.[39, 40] The Hulka spring-loaded clip consists of two plastic-toothed jaws hinged by a metal pin and closed with a stainless steel spring. The clip involves only 3 to 4 mm of tube and has the advantage of excellent reversal potential. However, when used in the puerperium, the Hulka clip has a post-tubal failure rate of approximately 10%, in comparison with a corrected pregnancy rate of 0.2 to 0.6% when performed as an interval sterilization procedure.[39–41] The Haskins tantulum clip had a similarly high failure rate of 11%,[42] as did the Wheeless two-clip technique[43] when these methods were used in the puerperium. The Bleier plastic snap-shut clip, at least the American variety, also has an unacceptably high failure rate of 8.2 to 10.2% when employed in the puerperium.[44]

The Falope ring, developed by Yoon in 1973,[45] is made of non–tissue-reactive silicone rubber. The Falope ring has been as effective as other methods when employed as an interval sterilization procedure. The Falope ring has also been successfully placed in the puerperium, although postpartum tubal edema would seem to prohibit appropriate application. Failure rates for puerperal ring placement of 1.3% are significantly less than failure rates for clip methods employed post partum.[46]

COMPLICATIONS

Morbidity attributable to tubal surgery is low. The most commonly reported complications following puerperal tubal ligation include bleeding or hematoma formation at the site of ligation and postoperative infection at the site. However, death secondary to broad-ligament hematoma after cesarean delivery with tubal ligation has been reported.[9]

The most frequently discussed complication following tubal ligation is the "post-tubal ligation syndrome." The constellation of symptoms attributable to the syndrome include pelvic discomfort, ovarian cystic changes, and menorrhagia. Post-tubal ligation syndrome is said to occur in 5 to 51% of women after sterilization.[47] It has been suggested that such symptoms occur as a result of disruption of the utero-ovarian blood supply, with resultant disturbances of ovulatory function after ligation of the tubes.[48, 49] Whether tubal ligation induces any of these changes remains controversial. Kasonde and Bonnar[50] noted that women who presented with menorrhagia after sterilization usually had a history of the problem before sterilization or had been using oral contraceptives prior to operative sterilization, which likely had an effect on menstrual flow. DeStefano and co-workers[51] reported on menstrual changes 2 years after tubal sterilization surgery in 2456 women and found no increase in the prevalence of adverse menstrual function except for menstrual pain among women who underwent unipolar electrocoagulation procedures. In fact, for all menstrual variables, more than 50% of women with adverse menstrual function preoperatively had an improvement by 2 years after tubal sterilization. In a follow-up study by DeStefano and co-workers in 1985, which compared the menstrual characteristics of women who had tubal sterilizations and women whose partners had undergone vasectomy, the tubal ligation group did not have a statistically significant increase in menstrual cramps and adverse menstrual bleeding.[52] However, in follow-up intervals longer than 2 years, the tubal sterilization group had significantly increased risk of menstrual disturbance. This risk of abnormal menstrual function for all menstrual variables was dependent on presterilization menstrual status and seldom developed unless it was present before sterilization.

Donnez and co-workers,[53] in an evaluation of luteal function after sterilization, found that women who had undergone tubal sterilization by electrocoagulation had a significantly lower mean midluteal progesterone level than did a group of unsterilized women and those who had been sterilized using Hulka-Clemens clips. They concluded that clip sterilization may offer the protection of preservation of utero-ovarian artery blood flow and maintenance of luteal function in comparison to electrocoagulation sterilization. Other investigators have failed to show disturbances in luteal phase function after tubal sterilization.[54] Although these findings of altered ovarian endocrine function after clip sterilization may be accurate, they have little bearing on the puerperal patient, in whom clips and electrocoagulation are rarely used for sterilization.

Obviously, patients who have pelvic pain and menstrual disturbances before sterilization should be advised that these symptoms may continue after tubal ligation. In these women, it may be important to disrupt the vasculature within the mesosalpinx as little as possible. Puerperal sterilization techniques, such as the midsegmental resection and the Pomeroy method, should not compromise the blood supply to the ovary, at least when performed in the conventional manner.

The most significant concern of the clinician is the patient's later regret of sterilization and her desire for restoration of reproductive function. Studies of women undergoing sterilization reversal indicate that younger women who are unhappily married, as well as those who feel forced by financial circumstances into having sterilization performed, are most likely to be unhappy with their decisions.[55–57] In young women with low parity in particular, it may be necessary for the clinician to provide more extensive presterilization counseling and often defer to interval sterilization at a later date if this problem is to be minimized.

SUMMARY

Puerperal tubal ligation is a safe and effective approach to female sterilization that is associated with minimal maternal morbidity and mortality. However, it is critical for the clinician to remember that puerperal sterilization is an elective procedure. If there is any question about the condition of the mother or the infant, it is more appropriate to defer puerperal tubal ligation and perform an interval procedure at a later date. The physician can choose among the quick and simple Pomeroy technique or midsegmental resection technique, which has slightly higher but acceptable failure rates or the Uchida method or the Irving method which is appropriate when chance of failure is unacceptable. The Uchida and Irving methods are especially appropriate if performed in conjunction with cesarean delivery.

Most important, strict presterilization counseling and a careful explanation of the risks, complications, and failure rates of each procedure are imperative for all patients undergoing tubal sterilization.

References

1. Bopp JR, Hall DG: Indications for surgical sterilization. Obstet Gynecol 35:760, 1970.
2. Edwards LE, Hakanson EY: Changing status of tubal sterilization: An evaluation of fourteen years' experience. Am J Obstet Gynecol 115:347, 1973.
3. Lungren SS: A case of cesarean section twice successfully performed on the same patient. Am J Obstet 14:78, 1881.
4. Young JH: The history of cesarean section. London: HK Lewis, 1944, pp. 235–244.
5. Hellman LM: Morphology of the human fallopian tube in the early puerperium. Am J Obstet Gynecol 57:154, 1949.
6. Whitacre FE, Loeb W, Loeb L: The time for postpartum sterilization: Report of 150 cases. Bacteriologic studies on the postpartum uterus. Am J Obstet Gynecol 52:1041, 1946.
7. Overstreet EW: Techniques of sterilization. Clin Obstet Gynecol 7:109, 1964.
8. Mabray CR, Malinak R, Flowers CE: Tubal sterilization: Morbidity on a charity hospital service. Obstet Gynecol 36:204, 1970.
9. White CA: Tubal sterilization. A 15 year survey. Am J Obstet Gynecol 95:31, 1966.
10. Mustafa MA, Pinkerton JHM: Bacteriology of fallopian tube in relation to puerperal sterilization. J Obstet Gynecol Br Commonw 77:171, 1970.
11. Laros RK Jr, Zatuchni GI, Andros GJ: Puerperal tubal ligation: Morbidity, histology, and bacteriology. Obstet Gynecol 41:397, 1973.
12. Bishop E, Nelms WF: A simple method of tubal sterilization. NY State J Med 30:214, 1930.
13. Haynes DM, Wolfe WM: Tubal sterilization in an indigent population: Report of 14 years experience. Am J Obstet Gynecol 106:1044, 1970.
14. Little WA: Current aspects of sterilization: The selection and application of various surgical methods of sterilization. Am J Obstet Gynecol 123:12, 1975.
15. Poulson AM: Analysis of female sterilization techniques. Obstet Gynecol 42:131, 1973.
16. Garb AE: A review of tubal sterilization failures. Obstet Gynecol Survey 12:291, 1957.
17. Husband ME Jr, Pritchard JA, Pritchard SA: Failure of tubal sterilization accompanying cesarean section. Am J Obstet Gynecol 107:966, 1974.
18. Wortman J: Tubal sterilization: Review of methods population reports, series C, No 7, Washington, DC: George Washington University Center, 1976.
19. deVilliers VP, Morkel DJ: Postpartum sterilization by the Irving technique: A report of 200 cases at Paarl Hospital, CP. S Afr Med J 71:253, 1987.
20. Cunningham FG, MacDonald PC, Gant NF: William's Obstetrics, 18th Edition. Norwalk, Connecticut: Appleton-Century-Crofts, 1989, pp. 936–937.
21. Uchida H: Uchida's abdominal sterilization technique. Proceedings of the 3rd World Congress of Obstetrics and Gynecology, Vol. 1. Vienna, 1961, p. 26.
22. Uchida H: Uchida tubal sterilization. Am J Obstet Gynecol 121:153, 1975.
23. Stock RJ: Tubal patency following Uchida tubal ligation. Obstet Gynecol 56:521, 1980.
24. Irving FC: A new method of insuring sterility following cesarean section. Am J Obstet Gynecol 8:335, 1924.
25. Irving FC: Tubal sterilization. Am J Obstet Gynecol 60:1101, 1950.
26. Lopez-Zeno JA, Muallem NS, Anderson JB: The Irving sterilization technique: A report of a failure. Int J Fertil 35(1):23, 1990.
27. Hornstein S, Kay SA: Abdominal pregnancy following Irving tubal ligation: Report of a case. Obstet Gynecol 13:337, 1959.
28. Wittich AC: Failure of Irving tubal sterilization. Obstet Gynecol 57:505, 1981.
29. Green LR, Laros RK: Postpartum sterilization. Clin Obstet Gynecol 23:647, 1980.
30. Dippel AL: Tubal sterilization by the Madlener method: A critical analysis of failures. Surg Gynecol Obstet 71:94, 1970.
31. World Health Organization. Female sterilization: Guidelines for the development of services. Geneva: World Health Organization, Publication 26, 1976.
32. Kroener WJ: Surgical sterilization by fimbriectomy. Am J Obstet Gynecol 104:247, 1969.
33. Taylor ES: Editorial comments. Obstet Gynecol Surv 27:168, 1972.
34. Metz KGP: Failure following fimbriectomy. Fertil Steril 28:66, 1977.
35. Metz DGP: Failure following fimbriectomy: A further report. Fertil Steril 30:269, 1978.
36. Soderstrom RM: Sterilization failures and their causes. Am J Obstet Gynecol 152:395, 1985.
37. Williams EA: Aspects of fallopian tube surgery. In Stallworthy J, Bourne G (eds.): Recent Advances in Obstetrics and Gynaecology, Number 12, Edinburgh: Churchill Livingstone, 1977.
38. Mehta V, Bhatia DL, Pai DN: Evaluation of single-stitch tubal ligation in postpartum women. Obstet Gynecol 51:567, 1978.
39. Hulka JF, Omran KF, Phillips JM Jr, et al.: Sterilization by spring clips: A report of 1000 cases with a 6 month followup. Fertil Steril 26:1122, 1975.
40. Hulka JF, Ulberg LC: Reversibility of clip sterilization. Fertil Steril 26:1132, 1976.
41. Kumarasany T, Hulka JF, Mercer JP, et al.: Spring clip tubal occlusion: A report of the first 400 cases. Fertil Steril 26:1116, 1975.
42. Haskins AL: Oviductal sterilization with tantalum clips. Am J Obstet Gynecol 114:370, 1972.
43. Wheeless CR: Laparoscopically applied hemoclips for tubal sterilization. Obstet Gynecol 44:752, 1974.
44. Adelman R: High failure rate of the plastic tubal (Bleier) clip. Obstet Gynecol 64:721, 1984.
45. Yoon IB, King TN, Parmley TH: A two year experience with Falope ring sterilization procedure. Am J Obstet Gynecol 127:109, 1977.
46. Sotrel G, Edelin K, Lowe EW: Puerperal sterilization with silastic band technique. Surg Forum 28:514, 1977.
47. Rioux JE: Late complications of female sterilization: A review of the literature and a proposal for further research. J Reprod Med 19:329, 1977.
48. Radwanska E, Berger GS, Hammond J: Luteal deficiency among women with normal menstrual cycles requesting reversal of tubal sterilization. Obstet Gynecol 54:189, 1979.
49. Radwanska E, Headley SK, Dmowski P: Evaluation of ovarian function after tubal sterilization. J Reprod Med 27:376, 1982.
50. Kasonde JM, Bonnar J: Effect of sterilization on menstrual blood loss. Br J Obstet Gynaecol 83:572, 1976.
51. DeStefano F, Greenspan JR, Dicker RC, et al.: Complications of interval laparoscopic tubal sterilization. Obstet Gynecol 61:153, 1983.

52. DeStefano F, Perlman JA, Peterson HB, Diamond EL: Long term risk of menstrual disturbances after tubal sterilization. Am J Obstet Gynecol 152:835, 1985.

53. Donnez J, Wauters M, Thomas K: Luteal function after tubal sterilization. Obstet Gynecol 57:65, 1981.

54. Ladehoff P, Lindholm P, Quist K, Sorenson T: Gonadotrophin and estrogens before and after laparoscopic sterilization. Acta Obstet Gynecol Scand (suppl) 93:77, 1980.

55. Divers WA: Characteristics of women requesting reversal of sterilization. Fertil Steril 41:233, 1984.

56. Gomel V: Profile of women requesting reversal of sterilization. Fertil Steril 30:39, 1978.

57. Leader A, Galan N, George R, et al.: A comparison of definable traits in women requesting reversal of sterilization and women satisfied with sterilization. Am J Obstet Gynecol 145:198, 1983.

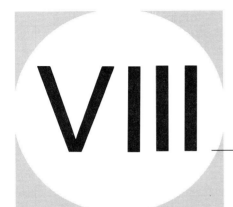

VIII

Fetal Surgery

Fetal Invasive Procedures

Jane Chueh
Mitchell S. Golbus

Over the last decade, significant advances have been made in the diagnosis of birth defects in utero. One reason for this has been the growth of molecular genetics, which has been successful in characterizing single-gene defects. Another reason has been the improvement in sonographic techniques, which has accelerated visual diagnosis of anomalies and aided in the precise localization of fetal tissues that need to be sampled. As a result of this ability to diagnose heritable conditions early in pregnancy, the obstetrician and the patient are now faced with new and increasingly sophisticated options for fetal therapy. This chapter discusses the choices for invasive fetal diagnosis available today, describes widely practiced closed fetal procedures, such as fetal intrauterine intravascular transfusion, and introduces some experimental techniques, such as open fetal surgery.

AMNIOCENTESIS

The standard method of genetic investigation of the at-risk fetus is amniocentesis. Advanced maternal age is the most common indication for prenatal diagnosis. Most clinicians recommend prenatal testing when the patient will be 35 years old at the time of delivery because at this age the chance of a chromosomally abnormal fetus exceeds the often-quoted 0.5% complication risk of amniocentesis. Approximately 2.5% of fetuses assessed for maternal age are aneuploid; the risks of this condition being present range from 0.9% for maternal age 35 to 36 years to 7.8% for maternal age 43 to 44 years.[1] Other risk factors for fetal aneuploidy include a previous child with aneuploidy. If the parents have normal karyotypes, there may be a 1 to 2% recurrence risk. If one of the parents is a balanced translocation carrier, there is an increased risk, approximately 10% if the carrier is the mother and 2 to 3% if the carrier is the father.[2] If the parental translocation is discovered because of a previously affected child, this risk is increased. Many metabolic disorders can be detected prenatally through enzyme assays on cultured amniotic fluid cells or amniotic fluid. For example, Tay-Sachs disease may be detected through the absence of hexosaminidase A in amniotic fluid or in cultured amniotic fluid cells.

Abnormal values of maternal serum α-fetoprotein (AFP) often require amniocentesis as part of the diagnostic assessment. This protein is found in very low concentrations (1 to 2 ng/mL), except in fetuses, pregnant women, and patients with certain tumors, such as hepatomas and germ-cell malignancies. The fetal yolk sac and liver produce AFP in large amounts. Alpha-fetoprotein normally enters the amniotic fluid through fetal urination and appears in the maternal circulation through direct transfer across fetal membranes. The association between open neural tube defects in the fetuses and elevated levels of amniotic fluid AFP detected by Brock and Sutcliffe[3] in 1972 can be explained by diffusion of AFP across exposed capillaries. Other anomalies that lack normal skin integrity, such as ventral wall defects, sacrococcygeal teratomas, cystic hygromas, and fetal demise all result in elevated serum and amniotic fluid AFP levels. Placental abnormalities, such as abruption, may also be associated with elevated serum AFP, presumably because of altered permeability across fetal-maternal membranes.

The procedure for maternal serum AFP (msAFP) screening involves measuring the level of this protein in pregnant women who are between 15 and 20 menstrual weeks. The cutoff value chosen for further evaluation depends on the prevalence of neural tube defects in the population tested and the desired sensitivity and specificity. We use the value 2.5 times the multiple of median as the upper limit of normal and a sliding scale related to maternal age for the lower limit of normal. For msAFP levels above the cutoff value at a gestational age less than 18 weeks, repeat sampling is recommended because 45% to 50% of women with an initial elevated msAFP value have a normal value on repeat testing. In the event of an elevated second value, or in those gestations beyond 18 weeks, a basic ultrasonographic examination is performed to rule out twins, fetal demise, anencephaly, incorrect gestational age, or a gross anomaly. If no abnormalities are found, amniotic fluid is obtained by amniocentesis to assess AFP and acetylcholinesterase. If these are abnormal, a targeted ultrasonographic examination is performed to search for anomalies. If both amniocentesis and ultrasonographic results are normal, the pregnancy falls into the subgroup at risk for nonspecific "poor obstetric outcomes." Serial antepartum testing and sonographic assessment for fetal growth are recommended.

Low levels of msAFP have been associated with the Down syndrome. Risk tables based on maternal age and serum AFP have been constructed. Most centers now offer amniocentesis to women less than 35 years of age when low msAFP indicates an increased risk for a chromosomally abnormal fetus. Using low msAFP in conjunction with maternal age, one can detect one quarter to one third of fetuses with the Down syndrome. If amniocentesis were limited to women over 35 years of age, only 20% of infants with the Down syndrome would be diagnosed.[4]

Abnormally low levels of msAFP necessitate basic sonography to rule out incorrect gestational dating. If the sonogram confirms the gestational age, amniocentesis is recommended for karyotyping. If the sonogram redates the pregnancy so that the msAFP was obtained before 15 weeks, the patient should have repeat testing at the appropriate time because she has not been effectively screened.

Complications of amniocentesis include infection, rupture of membranes, and spontaneous abortion. The risk of complications after amniocentesis varies from institution to institution, but the commonly quoted figure is 0.5%.[1] Perhaps the most significant risk of amniocentesis is finding a positive result, and appropriate counseling before the procedure is very important.

Amniocentesis involves basic sterile technique with concurrent sonographic guidance. After counseling and consent to the procedure, a basic sonogram establishes gestational age and searches for gross fetal anomalies. Placentation, amount of amniotic fluid, number and presentation of fetuses, and maternal pelvic structures are visualized and recorded. Standard amniocentesis performed between 15 and 21 menstrual weeks allows sufficient time for the result to influence management prior to 24 weeks. The largest pocket of fluid away from fetal parts is identified. The mother's abdominal area is prepared in a sterile fashion. One percent lidocaine without epinephrine may be injected subcutaneously and intradermally over the area of anticipated needle entry, although some clinicians prefer to use no anesthetic. A 22-gauge needle is inserted into the amniotic cavity under direct sonographic guidance, and 24 mL of fluid is removed (Fig. 29–1).

Women who present too late for chorionic villus sampling (CVS) and too early for standard amniocentesis may be offered early amniocentesis as an option. Indications for early amniocentesis are basically the same as those for standard amniocentesis, but testing is performed between 12 and 15 menstrual weeks. Studies to determine efficacy and complications are currently ongoing. Luthy and colleagues performed 495 early amniocenteses and found a higher incidence of gross rupture of membranes, unsuccessful taps, and culture failures in such procedures.[5] Follow-up data on 298 of 541 early amniocenteses performed by Crandall and colleagues showed a miscarriage rate within 2 weeks of the procedure of 1.7%, compared with 0.4% in their experience with standard amniocentesis.[6] They found no significant difference in growth between cells obtained early and those obtained at the traditional time. One potential disadvantage of early amniocentesis is the inability to assess AFP this early in gestation. At the present time, data about AFP in early pregnancy are being collected, but the correlation with normal and abnormal pregnancies is not yet established. Acetylcholinesterase appears to be normally present in amniotic fluid at this gestational age.[7] The technique for early amniocentesis is essentially the same as standard amniocentesis, although a smaller amount of fluid is taken based on the gestational age at which the procedure is performed.

CHORIONIC VILLUS SAMPLING

The indications for CVS are very similar to those for amniocentesis. The majority of procedures are performed for advanced maternal age, but the detection of inborn errors of metabolism and DNA analysis are also possible.[8] However, a neural tube defect risk cannot be evaluated by CVS.

The technique of CVS evolved from sampling through a hysteroscope[9] to blind aspiration for early sexing of the fetus[10] to the sonographically guided transcervical and transabdominal approaches performed today. Although metal-tipped cannulas, brushes, and rigid forceps have been used, the most popular technique involves transcervical aspiration through a flexible catheter between 9 and 12 menstrual weeks. The loss rate increases outside this time window. Prior to 9 weeks, there are more spontaneous abortions, and after 12 weeks, increased manipulation and tissue disruption occur in sampling a placenta that is more organized and located higher in the pelvis.

Contraindications are uncommon. Populations at high risk for herpes or gonococcal infections should be tested prior to sampling. Marked anteversion or retroversion of the uterus usually can be corrected by manipulation of the cervix with a tenaculum or by bladder distension. Sampling of twin pregnancies is controversial because failure to sample both gestations occurs in 3 to 4% of cases.

The major complication of CVS is pregnancy loss. For transcervical CVS, the National Institute of Child Health and Human Development (NICHD) collaborative study found a pregnancy loss rate 0.8% higher than that seen in patients undergoing amniocentesis.[11] A randomized, collaborative study from Canada reported a 0.6% difference in pregnancy loss between patients sampled by CVS and those undergoing amniocentesis.[12] The increased loss rates were not statistically significant in either study. Other complications include immediate rupture of membranes (0.1%), oligohydramnios, chorioamnionitis (isolated cases), and the potential for fetal-maternal hemorrhage to cause Rh isoimmunization.

Chorionic villus sampling has the potential to cause fetal-maternal hemorrhage, which theoretically might sensitize Rh-negative mothers. Knott and co-workers studied serum AFP levels in 11 pregnant women undergoing CVS and found that

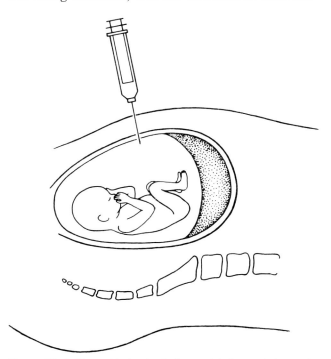

Figure 29–1. The gold standard of prenatal diagnosis is amniocentesis, which is performed between the 15th and 20th weeks of gestation. The technique is performed to obtain amniocytes for karyotyping and biochemical analysis and is also useful for the diagnostic work-up of an elevated or depressed maternal serum α-fetoprotein.

72% had more than 50% of the original value of AFP within 2 to 3 hours of CVS.[15] The level then stabilized and gradually returned to normal. By 16 to 18 weeks, the AFP level was in the normal range. The magnitude of this increase did not predict the likelihood of spontaneous abortion. Even the pregnancies with the most substantial rises in AFP progressed normally to delivery. However, because the rise in AFP reflects placental bed disruption leading to fetal-maternal hemorrhage, the administration of rhesus immune globulin (RhIg) prophylaxis may be advisable in nonsensitized Rh-negative mothers following CVS.

Chromosome mosaicism and maternal cell contamination of chorionic villi are two difficulties of CVS interpretation. Data from the first 5484 chorionic villus samples at our institution showed 46 cases of autosomal mosaicism, only three of which were confirmed by subsequent amniocentesis (unpublished data). The NICHD collaborative study found such pseudomosaicism in 0.8% of 2278 CVS samples.[11] The phenomenon was most commonly observed in direct chromosome preparations, suggesting post-zygotic nondisjunction limited to the placenta as the predominant underlying mechanism. For this reason, long-term CVS culture should be employed. However, this will not eliminate all cases of pseudomosaicism, and midtrimester amniocentesis should be offered to CVS patients when mosaicism is encountered.

Maternal cell contamination occurs in 4 to 27% of long-term CVS cultures.[13, 14] Careful washing and dissection of villus tissue, the use of pronase in preparing villi for CVS cultures,[13] and the use of both short-term ("direct") preparations and long-term cultures reduce the risk of maternal cell contamination.[14]

Transabdominal CVS arose as an alternative approach to placentas that were difficult to sample transcervically. Some conditions that may obviate a safe and successful transcervical approach include vaginismus, vaginitis, inaccessible cervical canal, extreme flexion of the uterus, multiple pregnancy, previous failure of transcervical sampling, and gestational age greater than 12 weeks. Brambati and colleagues evaluated the efficacy and risks in 1159 transabdominal CVS procedures in the first trimester and the early second trimester.[16] An adequate amount of chorionic tissue was obtained by two needle insertions in 99.7% of cases. A second needle insertion was required in only 3.5% of cases. The only early complication was local peritoneal reaction, which occurred in 0.3% of cases and had no adverse effect on maternal or fetal outcome. The pregnancy loss rate up to 28 weeks was 2.4%, and the rate of late obstetric complications or perinatal morbidity and mortality compared favorably with the rates in the general population. Smaller tissue samples are obtained with the transabdominal approach, but this difference does not influence the rate of culture success.

Other theoretic advantages include a lower risk of maternal and fetal infection and the wider range of gestational ages over which the procedure can be performed.

Fetal karyotyping in the second and third trimesters is usually achieved through amniocentesis. However, for amniocentesis, 2 to 3 weeks are required to obtain culture results, and this may be unacceptable when rapid karyotyping is needed for proper pregnancy management. The alternative method of cordocentesis has excellent safety and success rates in experienced hands. Obtaining blood samples from umbilical cord vessels can be a difficult procedure for inexperienced operators or when amniotic fluid volumes are abnormal. In such cases, transabdominal CVS can be useful in the second and third trimesters.

Even though the mitotic index in cytotrophoblast cells decreases, successful karyotypes through CVS have been performed even late in the third trimester.[17] Holzgreve and colleagues performed 224 chorionic villus samplings during late second and third trimesters with successful karyotyping in all but three cases.[18] Of these, 171 were performed for abnormal sonographic findings and 20% had aneuploidy. Oligohydramnios was present in 43% of the cases, which would have made fetal blood sampling difficult. Pijpers and colleagues performed 127 late chorionic villus samplings and were successful in karyotyping all but four cases.[19]

Following late transabdominal CVS, Holzgreve and colleagues noted a pregnancy loss of 2.03% if the sonogram was normal and 14.29% if the sonogram was abnormal.[20] Given the 20% rate of chromosomal abnormalities in fetuses with abnormal sonograms, late CVS appears to benefit these high-risk pregnancies. In pregnancies with sonographically normal fetuses, the benefit of late CVS can be evaluated only with further knowledge of its risks.

CHORIONIC VILLUS SAMPLING TECHNIQUES

For transcervical CVS, the patient is placed in the dorsal lithotomy position with a full bladder. The bladder aids in sonographic visualization of the gestational sac and its surrounding tissue. A flexible sterile 16-gauge catheter with a wire guide is used to sample the villi (Fig. 29–2). A technician conducts an abdominal sonogram while the operator performs the sampling. The catheter is bent appropriately to accommodate the position of the uterus and the location of the villi. The catheter is visualized by sonography on its entry into the cervix and guided to the villus tissue. The wire guide is removed, and while the catheter is held steady, a 20-mL syringe is attached to the end of the catheter to aspirate the tissue. Negative suc-

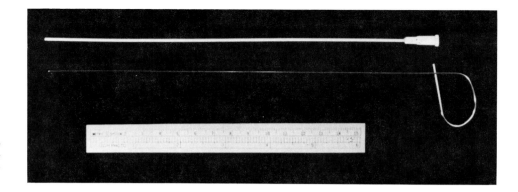

Figure 29–2. The flexible sterile 16-gauge catheter with wire guide used for transcervical chorionic villus sampling.

tion of 10 to 15 mL is maintained on the syringe while the catheter is slowly withdrawn (Fig. 29–3).

For transabdominal CVS, most investigators use a free-hand sonographically guided fine needle aspiration technique with a 20-gauge spinal needle. The abdomen is prepared and draped as for amniocentesis, and a sampling site is selected. The 20-gauge needle is inserted into the placenta under direct ultrasonographic guidance, and tissue is aspirated. The yield of tissue is increased by directing the needle in several directions and aspirating before exiting the needle from the uterus (Fig. 29–4).

One additional advantage of the transabdominal approach is patient acceptability. Monni and colleagues[21] asked 72 patients who were sampled both transcervically and transabdominally in separate pregnancies about their preferences. Of these, 71 patients preferred the transabdominal technique, describing it as being less embarrassing, more comfortable, rapid, and practical, while being less painful and associated with less bleeding in the days following the procedure. Considering that this technique can be performed after 9 to 12 menstrual weeks and that its risk is similar to that of the transcervical approach, transabdominal CVS should be considered a valuable adjunct to transcervical CVS.

CLOSED FETAL PROCEDURES

Percutaneous Umbilical Blood Sampling

The management of Rh-sensitized pregnancies demonstrates the evolution of an invasive technique as an aid in the treatment of a disease. In 1961, A. W. Liley described the spectrophotometric analysis of amniotic fluid as a means of assessing the severity of Rh-sensitization.[22] Elevated optical density of 450 μm values were indications for intrauterine transfusion or delivery, depending on gestational age. Until 1982, intrauterine transfusion was accomplished by depositing red cells into the fetal peritoneal cavity. However, success of this procedure depended on the absorption of blood through the fetal subdiaphragmatic lymphatic vessels. Absorption was erratic and inconsistent, particularly in severely hydropic fetuses.

Since 1982, numerous groups have reported successful intrauterine, intravascular transfusions of

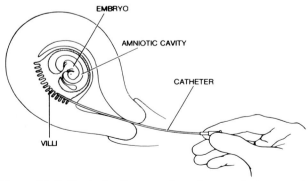

Figure 29–3. Chorionic villus sampling—transcervical approach: the 16-gauge catheter is inserted through the cervix and advanced to the villous tissue under direct sonographic guidance.

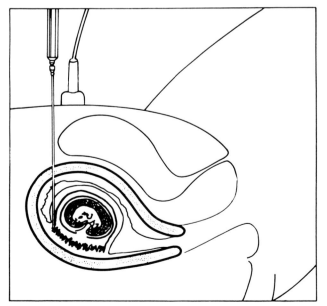

Figure 29–4. Chorionic villus sampling—transabdominal approach: the 20-gauge spinal needle is inserted abdominally, and the villous tissue is sampled under direct sonographic guidance.

severely erythroblastotic fetuses. A major advantage of the intravascular route is its beneficial effect on the hydropic fetus. Grannum and co-workers[23] reported 80% survival of transfused, hydropic fetuses, and 81% of these had complete reversal of hydrops. Barss and colleagues[24] reported 23 pregnancies receiving 45 intrauterine transfusions, with an overall survival rate of 85.7% and 83% among hydropic fetuses. Another advantage is access to the fetal intravascular compartment, with the ability to quantitate preprocedure and post-procedure hematocrit levels.

The technique of percutaneous umbilical blood sampling (PUBS) has been useful in other situations. Fischer and colleagues[25] reported treatment of chronic massive fetal-maternal hemorrhage managed by serial fetal intravascular transfusions. Percutaneous umbilical blood sampling has been used to evaluate fetal platelet counts in women with autoimmune thrombocytopenia purpura to determine the appropriate route of delivery.[26] It also can be used in selected cases to determine fetal status through cord gases[27] or to diagnose intrauterine starvation of the fetus through assessment of amino acid ratios.[28]

The reported incidence of serious side effects associated with PUBS has been extremely low. In general, significant complications occur in 1% of procedures.[29] The most common adverse effects are bleeding from the umbilical cord and bradycardia, both of which are usually transient. However, acute fetal distress can occur and can result in a severely compromised fetus or death. Benacerraf and colleagues[30] reported one case of fetal distress in 42 PUBS procedures which, because of prompt immediate delivery, resulted in survival. Sutro and colleagues[31] reported sonographic observation of an umbilical cord hematoma after PUBS, leading to fetal death. However, bleeding into the umbilical cord is usually limited by tension created by the Wharton jelly, and only rarely, if the cord surface is ruptured, does significant bleeding into the amniotic cavity occur.[32] Jauniaux and colleagues[32] reported a twin pregnancy at 21 weeks that resulted in a very large umbilical cord hematoma after PUBS, causing fetal death 6 days after the procedure. Wilkins and co-workers[33] reported a case of amnionitis and associated septic respiratory distress in the mother following PUBS. Pathologic examination of 50 umbilical cords by Jauniaux and colleagues collected between 1 hour and 20 weeks after PUBS showed macroscopic evidence of needle entry in 37 cases. By one week after PUBS, the vessel wall was partially reformed and there were no morphologic differences between needle entry into a vein or into an artery. They found no thromboses of the umbilical vessels. There was no relationship between transient fetal bradycardia or bleeding from the cord puncture site to the size of intrafunicular hemorrhage. Potentially serious injuries can occur during PUBS, but the more common small umbilical hematoma probably does not affect fetal umbilical circulation.

Percutaneous Umbilical Blood Sampling Technique

The sampling technique that allows direct access to the fetal circulation evolved from fetoscopy. Fetoscopy carried a relatively high risk of fetal complications, including fetal death (2 to 5%), amniotic fluid leakage (4 to 5%), and preterm labor (8 to 12%).[34, 35] In contrast, PUBS is performed under direct ultrasonic guidance with a 22-gauge spinal needle (Fig. 29–5). If an anterior placenta is present, access to the umbilical vessels is usually easier and entry is optimal at the cord root where it joins the placenta. When an anterior placenta is not present or when the cord insertion is not well visualized, insertion into a free loop of cord may be the only option.

When fetal movement complicates the visualization or needle entry, fetal neuromuscular blockade may be useful.[36] A variety of agents, including tubocurarine, vecuronium, atracurium, and pancuronium bromide, have been used, with good results. Vecuronium is primarily excreted by the liver and is not a good choice in Rh-affected fetuses. These agents are usually administered intravenously, but intramuscular injection can be performed in cases such as for skin biopsy, where intravascular access is unnecessary, or in situations in which paralysis is necessary before intra-

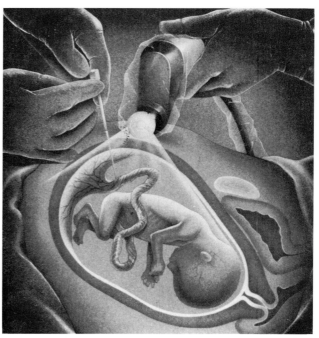

Figure 29–5. Percutaneous umbilical blood sampling. In addition to rapid fetal karyotyping, this technique is useful in a variety of clinical situations in which access to the fetal circulation is desired.

vascular access can be achieved. Disadvantages include requirement of a second amniotic puncture and risk of possible injury to structures in the fetal thigh. The use of a 25-gauge needle can theoretically reduce the incidence of complications.

Percutaneous umbilical blood sampling is gaining widespread acceptance for diagnostic and therapeutic fetal procedures. Although not a complex technique, it is difficult and potentially dangerous when performed by inexperienced operators. Like any technique, attainment of this skill follows a learning curve, with the rates of safety and success directly related to the operator's experience. Angel and colleagues[37] developed an instructional model for PUBS that allowed more individuals to be trained in this skill at no patient risk and little expense.

Selective Termination

In a singleton pregnancy with a birth defect, the option for termination is relatively straightforward. In multiple gestations, the decision is complicated by the presence of one or more other fetuses that are normal. Prior to 1978, the option was to abort the pregnancy and sacrifice a normal fetus or to continue the pregnancy and accept the burden of a child with a birth defect. In 1978, the report of a successful selective birth from a twin pregnancy discordant for the Hurler syndrome introduced a third option: to selectively terminate the affected fetus and continue the gestation of the normal fetus.[38]

A variety of techniques have been reported. The first case described cardiac puncture and aspiration of blood, resulting in death by exsanguination of the affected fetus.[38] Subsequent attempts using this method failed to reliably achieve fetal termination. Rodeck performed second trimester fetal terminations using air embolization through a fetoscope.[39] Intracardiac injections of calcium gluconate and potassium chloride have been used successfully.[40]

The development of CVS, along with the increase in multiple pregnancies from ovulation induction and in vitro fertilization, has allowed selective termination in the first trimester. The first selective terminations during the early months of pregnancy were performed by aspiration of the amniotic fluid sac, either transabdominally or transvaginally.[40] In 68 first- and second-trimester selective terminations of multiple gestations at the University of California at San Francisco, (UCSF), our most reliable results in dichorionic pregnancies were obtained by fetal intracardiac or intrathoracic injection of potassium chloride. In the first trimester, the needle is placed into the heart or in the pericardial region of the chest, whereas in the second trimester the needle is placed directly into a cardiac cavity. A sterile

potassium chloride solution (2 mEq/mL) is then injected rapidly in 2-mL increments until cardiac asystole is confirmed ultrasonographically. The total amount of potassium chloride required ranged from 4 to 14 mEq, with the dose being related to gestational age.

The two most prominent factors associated with poor outcome following selective termination are preterm labor and the presence of monochorionic placentation. A review of 22 reported pregnancies delivered after fetal viability showed a preterm birth rate of 50%.[40] Our preterm labor rate ranged from 20% for first-trimester selective terminations to 43% for second-trimester procedures. Further reductions in the rate of preterm labor and early delivery may be seen as techniques improve. Decreased intrauterine manipulation and a reduction in the procedure time required to perform the potassium chloride injections may be important.

The high failure rate of selective birth in monochorionic twins stresses the necessity to diagnose chorionic status to determine the method of choice of selective termination. Monochorionic pregnancies commonly share placental vessels that could lead to the death or possible compromise of the normal fetus after termination of the abnormal fetus. Thus, the only option for selective termination in monochorionic pregnancies appears to be to block the affected fetal circulation, either by removal of the entire fetus or by ligation of the umbilical cord. If identification and ligation of the umbilical cord could be performed with ease, this option might result in less uterine manipulation and thereby reduce the risk of preterm labor. At UCSF, we offer hysterotomy with removal of the abnormal twin for the motivated patient who understands the experimental nature of the procedure and agrees to the restrictions it puts on the remainder of that pregnancy and the effect it has on all subsequent gestations.

Fetal Liver Biopsy

Indications for fetal liver biopsy include fetuses at risk for ornithine transcarbamylase deficiency or carbamyl phosphate synthetase deficiency, in which DNA studies are noninformative, and von Gierke glycogen storage disease (type IA). Between June 1982 and May 1986, eight liver biopsies were performed at UCSF.[41] Satisfactory results were obtained in seven out of eight cases, and there were no spontaneous abortions or preterm deliveries. All dignoses were confirmed after delivery.

The technique involves direct sonographic guidance of a 16.5-gauge thin-walled needle directly below the right costal margin and into the fetal liver. The samples are centrifuged immediately to separate liver tissue from blood contamination. If frozen immediately, samples remain stable without losing inherent enzyme activity (Fig. 29–6).

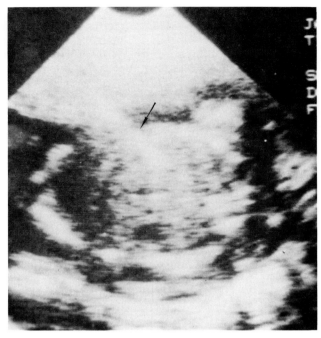

Figure 29–6. Fetal liver biopsy: the linear sonolucency entering the fetal liver from the left side of the picture is the 16.5-gauge thin-walled needle used to sample this fetal liver for a diagnosis of possible ornithine transcarbamylase deficiency.

Fetal Skin Biopsy

Conditions that can be diagnosed with fetal skin biopsy include ichthyosis, epidermolysis bullosa, and autosomal dominant ichthyosiform erythroderma. Of 15 skin sampling procedures performed at UCSF between January 1979 and December 1987, satisfactory samples were obtained in 14.[41] The results of one test performed for ichthyosiform erythroderma showed a normal skin biopsy, but a mildly affected infant was revealed at birth. All other cases had diagnoses confirmed after delivery or termination. Although one pregnancy resulted in spontaneous abortion with chorioamnionitis 2 days after the sampling, a meaningful complication rate cannot be derived because of the small number of cases. The world-wide experience suggests a 3 to 4% spontaneous abortion rate after fetal skin biopsy.

Fetal skin samples are obtained under sonographic guidance. A trochar is introduced into the uterus while the mother is under local anesthesia, and a biopsy forceps is passed through the cannula to obtain approximately 2 mm of skin. The samples are placed in appropriate fixative for electron and light microscopy (Figs. 29–7 and 29–8).

Catheter Placement

Catheters have been used in the past for shunting abnormal amounts of fluid from the cerebral

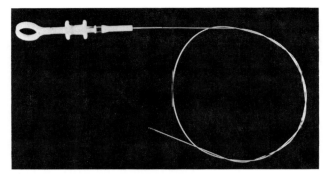

Figure 29–7. The flexible sterile biopsy forceps is passed through a trocar sleeve (not shown) to sample the fetal skin under direct sonographic guidance.

ventricular space or from an obstructed urinary bladder. Increasing evidence exists, however, that the shunting procedure is difficult and fraught with complications, such as blockage and dislodgement. At the present time, there is no clear benefit from intrauterine shunting for ventriculomegaly.[42] For bladder outlet obstruction, open fetal surgery is usually more definitive if the lesion is discovered in the early second trimester; however, catheters may be useful for the shorter periods of time necessary when the lesion is found late in the second trimester (Fig. 29–9).

OPEN FETAL SURGERY

A fetal anomaly can be managed in one of several ways. Those incompatible with life, such as trisomy 13 or trisomy 18, are best managed by pregnancy termination. Defects that do not interfere with the normal course of intrauterine development or labor and delivery are best managed after full-term delivery. These include mild structural defects (e.g., mild hydrocephalus, small neural tube defects, small sacrococcygeal teratoma, and unilateral hydronephrosis) and the majority of metabolic defects (e.g., phenylketonuria, maple syrup urine disease, homocystinuria, tyrosinemia, galactosemia, and hypothyroidism). A

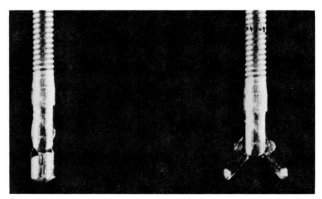

Figure 29–8. Close-up view of the biopsy forceps used for fetal skin sampling.

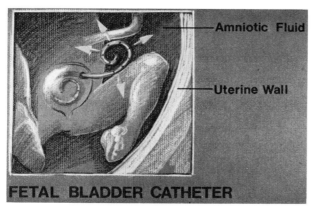

Figure 29–9. Fetal bladder catheter: a catheter can establish necessary communication between the obstructed fetal bladder and the amniotic fluid cavity to allow for a few weeks of continued fetal development. However, because these catheters inevitably become blocked or dislodged, open fetal surgery may be a better option if the goal is to achieve months of intrauterine growth and development.

third category may necessitate some form of prenatal intervention. Some cases, including progressive hydrocephalus, worsening hydronephrosis, fetal hydrops, and intrauterine growth retardation, may require preterm delivery for early correction of a defect. Cases such as Rh-sensitization, fetal cardiac arrhythmias, and fetal coenzyme deficiencies respond to medical treatment in utero with the appropriate drug, vitamin, or transfusion.

Finally, a minority of cases are suitable for in utero open surgery. These include very selected cases of bilateral obstructive uropathy, congenital diaphragmatic hernia, cystic adenomatoid hyperplasia, "stuck twins," and monozygotic twins with discordant anomalies. The indications for each of these are discussed briefly below.

INDICATIONS

Obstructive Uropathy

The consequences of unrelieved obstruction of the fetal urinary system range from unilateral hydronephrosis to bilateral megaureters, megacystis, and oligohydramnios. When complete obstruction occurs, oligohydramnios, pulmonary hypoplasia, and Potter facies result. Persistent ureteral reflux under pressure can lead to renal dysplasia.

Because prognosis and therefore management depend heavily on the pattern of anomalies found in each case, a skillful and thorough sonographic examination is essential. Important distinctions that must be made include (1) partial versus complete obstruction, (2) unilateral versus bilateral obstruction, (3) degree of oligohydramnios, and (4) degree of renal dysplasia. Fetuses with unilateral obstruction without oligohydramnios usually do well and deliver near term and can be eliminated

as candidates for intervention. Cases of bilateral obstruction and oligohydramnios are uniformly fatal and, therefore, the mother may be appropriately offered intrauterine surgery if there is not already evidence of renal damage.

The assessment of renal dysplasia is difficult but can be made with a combination of sonography and laboratory information. In a review of cases by Mahoney and colleagues,[43] the presence of cortical cysts on sonogram for predicting renal dysplasia had a specificity of 100% but a sensitivity of only 44%. Increased echogenicity had a slightly better sensitivity (57%) but less specificity (89%). The degree of hydronephrosis was the least predictive. Furthermore, the absence of all three elements did not rule out renal dysplasia. The use of fetal urine electrolytes in conjunction with ultrasonography offers a better estimate of prognosis. Hypotonic urine (Na < 100 mEq/L, Cl <90 mEq/L, Osm <210 mOsm/L) with normal-appearing kidneys on ultrasonography has been correlated with good renal function.[44] Another good prognostic sign is lack of longstanding obstruction.

Cases appropriate for intrauterine surgical intervention are those pregnancies that would be fatal to the fetus if allowed to progress naturally. These include fetuses with bilateral hydronephrosis, oligohydramnios, normal urine electrolytes, and normal karyotype. Of these, the best outcomes appear to occur with male fetuses that have suffered a relatively short duration of oligohydramnios.

Congenital Diaphragmatic Hernia

The defect in congenital diaphragmatic hernia (CDH) results from a failure of the pleuroperitoneal canal to close by 10 weeks, at the time the intestines return to the abdomen. As a result, abdominal contents herniate into the thoracic cavity, compressing the ipsilateral (and often the contralateral) lung, thus retarding pulmonary development. The natural history of congenital diaphragmatic hernia is dismal. In a retrospective review of in utero diagnosed cases from North America, Adzick and colleagues[45] found that only 20% of fetuses with CDH diagnosed in utero survived, despite optimal perinatal care including maternal transport, planned delivery, and aggressive resuscitation. Of the nonsurvivors, 16% had associated lethal anomalies and 5% were aneuploid. The outcome was not affected by gestational age at diagnosis, early delivery, or mode of delivery. All fetuses with bilateral lesions died.

Prenatal diagnosis of CDH is made by ultrasonography, usually on a patient referred for size greater than dates or incidentally on routine, screening sonogram. Sonography is diagnostic if herniated abdominal organs are seen in the chest but other signs, such as polyhydramnios, shift of the mediastinum, or absence of a normally positioned stomach bubble, should prompt a more careful examination. Amniography using contrast medium to visualize the anatomy of the fetal gastrointestinal tract may be useful in subtle cases. Because 16 to 40% of fetuses have associated nonchromosomal anomalies, a careful assessment of fetal anatomy should be performed.[46–49] Fetal karyoptyping is also important because chromosomal abnormalities have been reported to occur in 5 to 21% of fetuses with CDH.[46–49] Right-sided hernias with large amounts of liver present in the chest cavity are inoperable because of technical difficulties.

At the present time, intrauterine repair is controversial. Large lesions that herniate early in gestation are usually fatal without intervention, and animal studies suggest that intrauterine correction would allow normal growth and development of the lung. Although still in an experimental phase, it would appear that the best cases for intrauterine surgical intervention are those chromosomally normal fetuses devoid of other anomalies, with large left-sided hernias compressing both lungs and without liver herniation into the chest.

Twins

Two subsets of twin pregnancies may benefit from intrauterine surgery. The first is the diamniotic, monochorionic, monozygotic twin pregnancy with discordant anomalies. Over 90% of such twin pregnancies with this type of placentation share circulation, thereby making selective termination of one twin hazardous to the wellbeing of the other. Because of shared circulation, the technique of aborting the anomalous fetus by injecting intracardiac potassium chloride also places the other fetus at risk. Such cases can be managed only by opening the uterus and directly removing the anomalous twin. Sonography aids in identification of the anomalous fetus, and the incision is made in the uterus such that entry into the normal fetal sac or near the placenta is avoided. The abnormal fetus is delivered, followed by clamping, cutting, and tying off the cord, leaving its placenta behind.

The phenomenon of "stuck twin" was first described by Mahoney and colleagues[50] in 1985. The pregnancy is characterized by discordant growth of the fetuses, the smaller one existing in a sac devoid of fluid with membranes collapsed around it, making it appear "stuck" against the uterine wall. In contrast, the larger twin exists in a hydramniotic sac. Although the exact pathophysiology of the entity is not understood, numerous series have documented the poor natural history of the "stuck twin" pregnancy. Without intervention, 84% of 48 affected twin pregnancies died.[51] Most of these adverse outcomes are related to

preterm labor and delivery, with the resulting complications of extreme prematurity, or to sudden intrauterine demise. Almost all of the described "stuck twin" pregnancies are monochorionic, diamniotic pregnancies, and therefore selective termination of the stuck twin using intracardiac potassium chloride is not an option. These patients are first offered a treatment that consists of serial amniocentesis to remove generous amounts of fluid from the hydramniotic sac. Petty and co-workers have reported reaccumulation of fluid in the oligohydramniotic sac in "stuck twin" pregnancies treated in this manner, resulting in improved survival of both twins.[51] At UCSF we have had two "successes" and a number of "failures" with this technique. If patients refuse this option or if the treatment is not successful because of the poor natural history of the pregnancy, selective delivery of the "stuck twin" is offered for pregnancies in which gestation is less than 24 weeks at the time of diagnosis. Removal of the growth-retarded "stuck twin" has been associated with normal development of the remaining twin, resulting in the salvage of one fetus rather than the loss of both fetuses (unpublished data from UCSF).

Cystic Adenomatoid Malformation

Congenital cystic adenomatoid malformation of the lung is a distinct pathologic entity within the general group of congenital cystic diseases of the lung. Although the exact nature of the disease is not known, the most widely accepted theory is that it represents a hamartoma. The resulting tumor has characteristic microscopic features, including an "adenomatoid" increase of terminal respiratory structures in the lungs, with formation of cysts lined by either respiratory or cuboidal epithelium, a polypoid growth of mucosa with increased elastic tissue in the walls, absence of cartilage, and no inflammation.[52] A subclassification of congenital cystic adenomatoid malformation was suggested by Van Dijk and Wagenvoort, who divided this entity into a cystic type, an intermediate type, and a solid type.[52] Prognosis depends on the amount of lung affected and the degree of tumor compression of normal lung tissue, which results in pulmonary hypoplasia. Obstruction of venous return by the expanding pulmonary mass can also lead to fetal hydrops. Theoretically, surgical resection of the mass should allow proper expansion and development of the remaining normal lung tissue. However, Saltzman and colleagues[53] have reported several cases of congenital cystic adenomatoid malformation that regressed spontaneously, resulting in survival. Fetuses that develop hydrops, however, do not survive. In utero surgical intervention should be limited to these hydropic fetuses that otherwise have no chance for survival. Unfortunately, once hydrops fetalis occurs, these fetuses are poor candidates for intrauterine surgery. Not only do hydropic fetuses have a poor survival rate but once the disease has progressed to this point, surgical correction of the defect by intrauterine surgery does not always reverse the disease. Finally, once a fetus develops hydropic changes, the mother may develop symptoms very similar to pre-eclampsia. This has been called the "mirror syndrome."[54] Because of increased placental mass, maternal hypertension, proteinuria, and edema develop. These changes may remain even after intrauterine surgery has corrected the fetal anomaly. Inevitably, delivery is required for maternal indications even after the fetal defect has been surgically corrected.

Techniques

The management protocol for open fetal surgery can be divided into several sections. Adequate *fetal evaluation and selection* are required. Evaluation for potentially correctable fetal anomalies is performed through the fetal treatment program and the prenatal diagnosis center at UCSF. Many of these patients are referred from great distances, and the initial evaluation is often performed in the referring institution with consultation with the UCSF group. Once a fetal case is determined to be appropriate for intervention (an isolated, potentially correctable lesion with no other chromosomal or anatomic defects), the family is offered further evaluation at UCSF. The family meets with the surgeons, who describe the procedure as well as the risks and complications, as mentioned previously. The responsible obstetricians also review with the family the procedure, the risks and complications, the difficulties in obstetric management of the pregnancy, and the subsequent delivery. Counselors independently discuss the social, emotional, and logistic problems that the family must face in allowing the fetus to undergo such surgery. If intervention is deemed medically appropriate according to the guidelines mentioned previously, the family is counseled by the members of the fetal treatment team on at least two separate occasions, with adequate time to reflect on the information and ask questions before arriving at a decision regarding fetal intervention.

Preoperative preparation includes admitting the patient to the hospital the night before planned surgery to receive a full medical and obstetric assessment. The patient is given one 50-mg indomethacin suppository the night before surgery and one just prior to the surgery for prophylaxis for preterm labor. Perioperative antibiotics are also given. The patient signs a consent for the experimental procedure as well as the standard surgical consent and speaks with the anesthesia group the night before the surgery.

Intraoperative management begins in the oper-ating room with preparation of the operative site in a sterile fashion. Intraoperative sterile sonography is performed to locate the fetus and determine its presentation. The uterine incision is made at an appropriate location on the uterus to provide adequate access to the fetal anomaly; therefore, its orientation varies depending on the patient. Special care is taken to avoid the placenta and other large venous lakes apparent in the uterus. The amniotic sac is entered by deepening the uterine incision, and approximately 500 mL of amniotic fluid is removed to facilitate surgery while not compromising the fetus or the cord during the procedure.

After the fetal surgery is completed, the original amniotic fluid or sterile isotonic saline is replaced, along with an antibiotic (500 mg of nafcillin). The uterus is then closed in two layers, the first being a through and through running suture (0 Prolene) that incorporates the amniotic membranes; the second is a running imbricating layer of 0 Prolene. Halothane general anesthesia, which passes through the placenta to the fetus, is used throughout the operation. A pulse oximeter is attached to a fetal limb to monitor fetal oxygen saturation, and electrocardiographic leads allow continuous monitoring of the fetal heart rate (Fig. 29–10).

Intensive *postoperative management* is crucial to success. A maternal epidural catheter is placed for morphine pain control, and the patient remains in an intensively monitored environment until she is fully recovered. Postoperative management is aimed at total suppression of uterine activity through a combination of tocolytic therapy and activity restriction. Indomethacin suppositories, 50 mg every 6 hours per rectum are begun postoperatively and used for a minimum of 48 hours or continued as necessary. Magnesium sulfate is started immediately postoperatively and continued for a minimum of 48 hours or until uterine con-

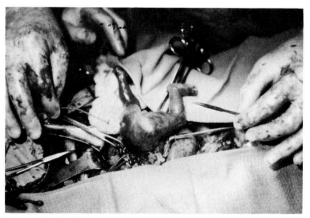

Figure 29–10. Open fetal surgery: this procedure exposes the mother and her extremely preterm fetus to numerous risks and potential complications. This experimental procedure should be performed only at experienced centers and limited to extremely motivated mothers and otherwise moribund fetuses that have isolated, potentially correctable lesions.

tractions are completely controlled. Serum levels of magnesium are monitored to achieve therapeutic levels (4 to 8 mg/dL). The patient is maintained at bed rest with a Foley catheter for at least 48 hours. The patient is allowed out of bed only when uterine contractions are completely controlled. She is usually restricted to bathroom privileges for the first 5 days. Intravenous fluids are continued until the patient is taking adequate fluids by mouth. Intravenous antibiotics are administered for 3 to 5 days. The patient is then weaned off intravenous tocolytic agents, and oral β-mimetic agents are begun. The patient is observed for a few days to make certain she is stable before discharge. Fetal evaluation consists of continuous fetal heart rate monitoring, with daily portable sonograms for biophysical profiles.

Outpatient management begins after the patient has fully recovered and when there is no evidence of uterine activity while she is on oral tocolytics. The patient is managed as an outpatient for a week to allow adjustment of tocolytic medication with increasing activity. After the patient returns home, the management of the remainder of the pregnancy is a joint effort between the physicians performing the surgery and the referring physician. In general, the patient remains on oral tocolytics and her activity is restricted until the time of delivery.

Delivery is by planned cesarean section, preferably prior to the onset of labor. The patient should not be allowed to undergo labor with her relatively recent hysterotomy incision; therefore, uncontrollable preterm labor necessitates timely cesarean section for maternal safety. If preterm labor does not force early delivery at the referring institution, the preferred management is to transfer the patient back to UCSF at 34 weeks' gestation. Fetal lung maturity is documented by serial amniocentesis. When mature levels are attained, an elective cesarean section is performed with a full neonatal team available for resuscitation and post-delivery management. An alternative management is planned cesarean section at the time of lung maturity at the referring institution. This should be considered only if it can be performed at a perinatal center with a full neonatal team that is prepared to work in close concert with the UCSF fetal treatment team in the management of the neonate. The cesarean section performed uses the same incision as the hysterotomy. The edges of the incision are freshened to eliminate any thinning of the scar and to minimize difficulties with subsequent pregnancies. All future pregnancies should be delivered by cesarean section.

COMPLICATIONS

The first major hurdle for the fetus is surviving the surgery itself. Being external to the uterine environment is stressful to the premature fetus; therefore, earlier gestations and longer surgeries fare worse.

If the fetus weathers the operation, a difficult recovery period remains. During this time, the major risks are preterm labor and premature rupture of membranes. Uterine contractions occur invariably but can be effectively checked with prolonged and aggressive tocolytic therapy. Rupture of membranes can lead to leakage of fluid through the vagina or, rarely, through the uterine incision into the peritoneal cavity. This latter event can cause the mother abdominal pain and necessitates reoperation for repair of the uterine incision. At our institution, we have begun using "fibrin glue" (manufactured from the father's blood), to strengthen the uterine closure. Since the start of its use, we have had no clinically significant amniotic fluid leaks.

CONCLUSIONS

With increased neonatal survival at early gestations, the "patient" to be treated becomes younger and younger. Fetal therapy is now a reality. It begins with early diagnosis, using invasive procedures such as transcervical and transabdominal CVS, early and standard amniocentesis, and blood and tissue sampling. Treatment spans the range from closed procedures, such as fetal intrauterine intravascular transfusion, catheter placement, and selective termination, to experimental open fetal surgery, which either removes the anomalous half of a twin pregnancy, leaving the normal twin intact, or corrects an otherwise fatal defect, allowing for further maturation in utero. More and more, the fetus is becoming the "patient." The obstetrician, to offer comprehensive, informed patient care, must be familiar with the options available for fetal diagnosis and the techniques being crafted in fetal therapy today.

References

1. Golbus MS, Loughman WD, Epstein CJ, et al.: Prenatal genetic diagnosis in 3000 amniocenteses. N Engl J Med 300:157, 1979.
2. Hamerton JL: Human cytogenetics, Vols. 1 and 2. New York: Academic Press, 1971.
3. Brock DHJ, Sutcliffe RG: Alphafetoprotein in the antenatal diagnosis of anencephaly and spina bifida. Lancet 2:197–199, 1972.
4. DiMaio MS, Baumgarten A, Greenstein RM, et al.: Screening for fetal Down's syndrome in pregnancy by measuring maternal serum alphafetoprotein levels. N Engl J Med 317:342–346, 1987.
5. Luthy D, Hickok D, Luthardt F, Resta R: Prospective evaluation of early amniocentesis for prenatal diagnosis: An alternative to chorionic villus sampling. Society of Perinatal Obstetricians 1986, abstract #68.
6. Crandall BF, Hanson FW, Tennant F, Perdue S: AFP levels

in amniotic fluid (AF) obtained between 11 and 15 weeks. Am J Hum Genet 43(3):0914 (abstract), 1988.

7. Burton BK, Nelson LH, Pettenati MJ: False-positive acetylcholinesterase with early amniocentesis. Obstet Gynecol 74:607, 1989.

8. Golbus MS, Appelman Z: Chorionic villus sampling. In: Eden RE, Boehm F eds.: Fetal assessment: physiological, clinical and medicolegal principles. East Norwalk, Connecticut: Appleton-Century-Crofts, 1988.

9. Hahnemann N, Mohr J: Genetic diagnosis in the embryo by means of biopsy from extraembryonic membranes. Bull Eur Soc Hum Genet 2:23–4, 1968.

10. Dept of ObGyn Tietung Hospital of Anshan Iron and Steel Company. Fetal sex prediction by sex chromatin of chorionic villi cells during early pregnancy. Chin Med J 1:117–126, 1975.

11. Rhoads GG, Jackson LG, Schlesselman SE: The safety and efficacy of chorionic villus sampling for early prenatal diagnosis of cytogenetic abnormalities. N Engl J Med 320:609–617, 1989.

12. Canadian collaborative CVS-Amniocentesis Clinical Trial Group. Multicentre randomised clinical trial of chorionic villus sampling and amniocentesis. Lancet 1(8628):1–6, 1989.

13. Hogge WA, Schonberg SA, Golbus MS: Prenatal diagnosis by chorionic villus sampling: Lessons of the first 600 cases. Prenat Diagn 5:393–400, 1985.

14. Cheung SW, Crane JP, Beaver HA, Burgess AC: Chromosome mosaicism and maternal cell contamination in chorionic villi. Prenat Diagn 7:535–542, 1987.

15. Knott PD, Chan B, Ward RHT, et al.: Changes in circulating alphafetoprotein and human chorionic gonadotrophin following chorionic villus sampling. Eur J Obstet Gynecol Reprod Biol 27:277–281, 1988.

16. Brambati B, Lanzani A, Oldrini A: Transabdominal chorionic villus sampling: Clinical experience of 1159 cases. Prenat Diagn 8:609–617, 1988.

17. Nicolaides KH, Southill PW, Rodeck CH, Warren RC: Why confine chorionic villus sampling to the first trimester? Lancet 1:543, 1986.

18. Holzgreve W, Miny P, Berlach B, et al.: Benefits of placental biopsies for rapid karyotyping in the second and third trimester (late CVS) in high risk pregnancies (in press).

19. Pijpers L, Jahoda MGJ, Wladimiroff JW, et al.: Transabdominal chorionic villus biopsy in second and third trimester pregnancies (in press).

20. Holzgreve W: Unpublished data.

21. Monni G, Giovanni O, Cao A: Patient's choice between transcervical and transabdominal chorionic villus sampling (letter). Lancet 1:1057, 1988.

22. Liley AW: Liquor amnii analysis in the management of pregnancy complicated by rhesus sensitization. Am J Obstet Gynecol 82:1359–1370, 1961.

23. Grannum PAT, Copel JA, Moya FR, et al.: The reversal of hydrops fetalis by intravascular intrauterine transfusion in severe isoimmune fetal anemia. Am J Obstet Gynecol 158:914–919, 1988.

24. Barss VA, Benacerraf BR, Grigoletto FD, et al.: Management of isoimmunized pregnancy by use of intravascular techniques. Am J Obstet Gynecol 159:932–937, 1988.

25. Fischer RL, Kuhlman K, Grover J, et al.: Chronic, massive fetomaternal hemorrhage treated with repeated fetal intravascular transfusions. Am J Obstet Gynecol 162:203–204, 1990.

26. Moise KJ, Carpenter RJ, Cotton DB, et al.: Percutaneous umbilical cord blood sampling in the evaluation of fetal platelet counts in pregnant patients with autoimmune thrombocytopenia purpura. Obstet Gynecol 72:346, 1988.

27. Pardi G, Buscaglia M, Ferraze E, et al.: Cord sampling for the evaluation of exygenation and acid-base balance in growth-retarded human fetuses. Am J Obstet Gynecol 157:1221–1228, 1989.

28. Econimides DL, Nicolaides KH, Gahl WA, et al.: Cordocentesis in the diagnosis of intrauterine starvation. Am J Obstet Gynecol 161:1004–1008, 1989.

29. Daffos F, Capella-Pavlovsky M, Forestier F: Fetal blood sampling during pregnancy with use of a needle guided by ultrasound: A study of 606 consecutive cases. Am J Obstet Gynecol 153:655–660, 1985.

30. Benacerraf BR, Barss VA, Saltzman DH, et al.: Acute fetal distress associated with percutaneous umbilical blood sampling. Am J Obstet Gynecol 156:1218–1220, 1987.

31. Sutro WH, Tuck SM, Lesevitz A, et al.: Prenatal observation of umbilical cord hematoma. AJR 142:801–802, 1984.

32. Jauniaux E, Donner C, Simon P, et al.: Pathologic aspects of the umbilical cord after percutaneous umbilical blood sampling. Obstet Gynecol 73:215, 1989.

33. Wilkins I, Mezrow G, Lynch L, et al.: Amnionitis and life-threatening respiratory distress after percutaneous umbilical blood sampling. Am J Obstet Gynecol 160:427–428, 1989.

34. Rodeck CH: Fetal blood sampling. In Caljaard H (ed.): The future of perinatal diagnosis. New York: Churchill Livingstone, 85–92, 1982.

35. March of Dimes Birth Defects Foundation. Special report: The status of fetoscopy and fetal tissue sampling. Prenat Diagn 4:79–84, 1984.

36. Moise KJ, Carpenter RJ, Deter RL, et al.: The use of fetal neuromuscular blockade during intrauterine procedures. Am J Obstet Gynecol 157:874–879, 1987.

37. Angel J, O'Brien WF, Mechelson J, et al.: Instructional model for percutaneous fetal umbilical blood sampling. Obstet Gynecol 73:669, 1989.

38. Aberg A, Miterian F, Cantz M, Geliler J: Cardiac puncture of fetus with Hurler's disease avoiding abortion of unaffected co-twin. Lancet 2:990–991, 1978.

39. Rodeck C, Mibashan R, Abramowitz J, Campbell S: Selective feticide of the affected twin by fetoscopic air embolization. Prenat Diag 2:189–194, 1982.

40. Golbus MS, Cunningham N, Goldberg JD, et al.: Selective termination of multiple gestations. Am J of Med Gen 31:339–348, 1988.

41. Golbus MS, et al.: Fetal tissue sampling: The San Francisco experience with 190 pregnancies. Western J Med 150:423–430, 1989.

42. Manning FA, Harrison MR, Rodeck C: Catheter shunts for fetal hydronephrosis. N Engl J Med 315:336–340, 1986.

43. Mahoney BS, Filly RA, Callen PW, et al.: Sonographic evaluation of fetal renal dysplasia. Radiology 152:143–146, 1984.

44. Golbus MS, Harrison MR, Filly RA, et al.: Prenatal diagnosis and treatment of fetal hydronephrosis. Semin Perinatol 7:102–105, 1983.

45. Adzick NS, Harrison MR, Glick PL, et al.: Diaphragmatic hernia in the fetus: Prenatal diagnosis and outcome in 94 cases. J Pediatr Surg 20(2):357, 1985.

46. Johnson DG, Deaner RM, Koop CE: Diaphragmatic hernia in infancy: Factors affecting the mortality rate. Surgery 62:1082, 1967.

47. Fitzgerald RJ: Congenital diaphragmatic hernia: A study of mortality factors. Ir J Med Sci 146:280, 1979.

48. Butler N, Claireaux AE: Congenital diaphragmatic hernia as a cause of perinatal mortality. Lancet 1:659, 1962.

49. Puri P, Gorman F: Lethal nonpulmonary anomalies associated with congenital diaphragmatic hernia: Implications for early intra-uterine surgery. J Pediatr Surg 19:29, 1984.

50. Mahoney BS, Filly RA, Callen PW: Amnionicity and chorionicity in twin pregnancies: Prediction using ultrasound. Radiology 155:205–209, 1985.

51. Petty CN, Mahoney BS, Luthy DA, et al.: The stuck twin phenomenon: Treatment with therapeutic amniocenteses. Society of Perinatal Obstetricians 1990, abstract #439.

52. Kwittken J and Teiner L: Congenital cystic adenomatoid malformation of the lung. Pediatrics 30:759, 1962.

53. Saltzman DH, Adzick NS, Benacerraf BR: Fetal cystic adenomatoid malformation of the lung: Apparent improvement in utero. Obstet Gynecol 71:1000–1003, 1988.

54. Nicolay KS, Gainey HL: Pseudotoxemic state associated with severe Rh isoimmunization. Am J Obstet Gynecol 89:42–45, 1964.

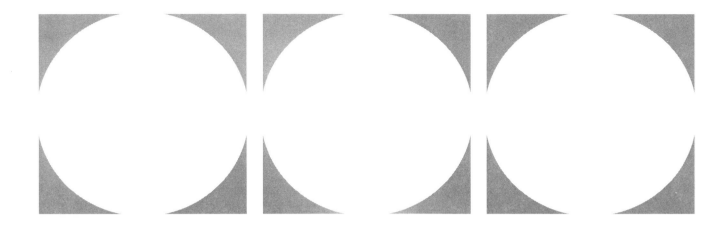

Index

Note: Page numbers in *italics* refer to illustrations; page numbers followed by t refer to tables.